Hsp90 Structure, Mechanism and Disease

Hsp90 Structure, Mechanism and Disease

Editor

Chrisostomos Prodromou

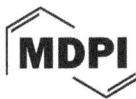 Basel • Beijing • Wuhan • Barcelona • Belgrade • Novi Sad • Cluj • Manchester

Editor
Chrisostomos Prodromou
Biochemistry and Biomedicine
University of Sussex
Brighton
United Kingdom

Editorial Office
MDPI
St. Alban-Anlage 66
4052 Basel, Switzerland

This is a reprint of articles from the Special Issue published online in the open access journal *Biomolecules* (ISSN 2218-273X) (available at: https://www.mdpi.com/journal/biomolecules/special_issues/Hsp90_Structure_Mechanism_Disease).

For citation purposes, cite each article independently as indicated on the article page online and as indicated below:

Lastname, A.A.; Lastname, B.B. Article Title. *Journal Name* **Year**, *Volume Number*, Page Range.

ISBN 978-3-0365-9714-0 (Hbk)
ISBN 978-3-0365-9715-7 (PDF)
doi.org/10.3390/books978-3-0365-9715-7

Cover image courtesy of Chrisostomos Prodromou

© 2023 by the authors. Articles in this book are Open Access and distributed under the Creative Commons Attribution (CC BY) license. The book as a whole is distributed by MDPI under the terms and conditions of the Creative Commons Attribution-NonCommercial-NoDerivs (CC BY-NC-ND) license.

Contents

About the Editor vii

Preface ix

Chrisostomos Prodromou
An Editorial on the Special Issue 'Hsp90 Structure, Mechanism and Disease'
Reprinted from: *Biomolecules* **2023**, *13*, 547, doi:10.3390/biom13030547 1

Chrisostomos Prodromou and Dennis M. Bjorklund
Advances towards Understanding the Mechanism of Action of the Hsp90 Complex
Reprinted from: *Biomolecules* **2022**, *12*, 600, doi:10.3390/biom12050600 5

Samarpan Maiti and Didier Picard
Cytosolic Hsp90 Isoform-Specific Functions and Clinical Significance
Reprinted from: *Biomolecules* **2022**, *12*, 1166, doi:10.3390/biom12091166 29

Daniel Jay, Yongzhang Luo and Wei Li
Extracellular Heat Shock Protein-90 (eHsp90): Everything You Need to Know
Reprinted from: *Biomolecules* **2022**, *12*, 911, doi:10.3390/biom12070911 51

Patricija van Oosten-Hawle
Organismal Roles of Hsp90
Reprinted from: *Biomolecules* **2023**, *13*, 251, doi:10.3390/biom13020251 71

Dennis M. Bjorklund, R. Marc L. Morgan, Jasmeen Oberoi, Katie L. I. M. Day, Panagiota A. Galliou and Chrisostomos Prodromou
Recognition of BRAF by CDC37 and Re-Evaluation of the Activation Mechanism for the Class 2 BRAF-L597R Mutant
Reprinted from: *Biomolecules* **2022**, *12*, 905, doi:10.3390/biom12070905 85

Sarah J. Backe, Rebecca A. Sager, Katherine A. Meluni, Mark R. Woodford, Dimitra Bourboulia and Mehdi Mollapour
Emerging Link between Tsc1 and FNIP Co-Chaperones of Hsp90 and Cancer
Reprinted from: *Biomolecules* **2022**, *12*, 928, doi:10.3390/biom12070928 111

Laura A. Wengert, Sarah J. Backe, Dimitra Bourboulia, Mehdi Mollapour and Mark R. Woodford
TRAP1 Chaperones the Metabolic Switch in Cancer
Reprinted from: *Biomolecules* **2022**, *11*, 274, doi:10.3390/coatings11030274 133

Abhinav Joshi, Takeshi Ito, Didier Picard and Len Neckers
The Mitochondrial HSP90 Paralog TRAP1: Structural Dynamics, Interactome, Role in Metabolic Regulation, and Inhibitors
Reprinted from: *Biomolecules* **2022**, *12*, 880, doi:10.3390/biom12070880 153

Anna G. Mankovich and Brian C. Freeman
Regulation of Protein Transport Pathways by the Cytosolic Hsp90s
Reprinted from: *Biomolecules* **2022**, *12*, 1077, doi:10.3390/biom12081077 167

Jeffrey Lynham and Walid A. Houry
The Role of Hsp90-R2TP in Macromolecular Complex Assembly and Stabilization
Reprinted from: *Biomolecules* **2022**, *12*, 1045, doi:10.3390/biom12081045 179

Peter William Piper, Julia Elizabeth Scott and Stefan Heber Millson
UCS Chaperone Folding of the Myosin Head: A Function That Evolved before Animals and Fungi Diverged from a Common Ancestor More than a Billion Years Ago
Reprinted from: *Biomolecules* **2022**, *12*, 1028, doi:10.3390/biom12081028 209

Siddhi Omkar, Tasaduq H. Wani, Bo Zheng, Megan M. Mitchem and Andrew W. Truman
The APE2 Exonuclease Is a Client of the Hsp70–Hsp90 Axis in Yeast and Mammalian Cells
Reprinted from: *Biomolecules* **2022**, *12*, 864, doi:10.3390/biom12070864 219

Kalliopi Ziaka and Jacqueline van der Spuy
The Role of Hsp90 in Retinal Proteostasis and Disease
Reprinted from: *Biomolecules* **2022**, *12*, 978, doi:10.3390/biom12070978 233

Huafeng Xu
Non-Equilibrium Protein Folding and Activation by ATP-Driven Chaperones
Reprinted from: *Biomolecules* **2022**, *12*, 832, doi:10.3390/biom12060832 253

Tanima Dutta, Harpreet Singh, Adrienne L Edkins and Gregory L Blatch
Hsp90 and Associated Co-Chaperones of the Malaria Parasite
Reprinted from: *Biomolecules* **2022**, *12*, 1018, doi:10.3390/biom12081018 277

About the Editor

Chrisostomos Prodromou

Chrisostomos Prodromou obtained a first-class honours degree in Applied Biology at Chelsea College, University of London, and a PhD in Yeast Molecular Genetics from Queen Mary College, University of London, in 1988. Following a brief spell at the University of Sheffield, he then moved to University College London in 1991, where he started working on the molecular chaperone Hsp90. Chris continued his work on Hsp90 at the Institute of Cancer Research, which he joined in 1999. In 2010, Chris accepted a senior research fellowship at the University of Sussex, and later became senior lecturer, where he continues his studies on Hsp90. Chris' research interests over the last 20 years have been directed towards the structure and mechanistic action of the Hsp90 chaperone complex. Chris' aims are to understand the molecular details by which Hsp90 and its cohort of co-chaperones bring about the maturation and activation of its client proteins. His structure of the N-terminal domain of Hsp90 in complex with ATP won him the award for the best postdoctoral paper within a decade to be published in the Department of Biochemistry and Molecular Biology at UCL. This work showed that Hsp90 was an active ATPase and changed the course of research within the field. At the Institute of Cancer Research, Chris was involved in developing the resorcinol class of Hsp90 inhibitors, as well as a number of inhibitors of Hsp90 based on the natural antibiotics radicicol and geldanamycin. He also solved the structure of the full-length Hsp90 protein, giving us our first insight into the closed, N-terminally dimerised, conformation of Hsp90. At the University of Sussex, Chris solved the first structure of an Hsp90 in complex with a C-terminally bound Hsp90 activator, LA1011, which shows excellent potential as a clinical candidate against Alzheimer's disease. Chris, together with a number of his colleagues, is a holder of the 2013 CRUK translational prize towards beating cancer.

Preface

The Hsp90 chaperone complex is responsible for the activation and maturation of a vast array of signaling proteins, which when disregulated often lead to disease. Recently, there has been a leap in our understanding of the molecular mechanisms involved in such regulation. The focus of this Special Issue is on the recent structural and biochemical advances of Hsp90 that provide insights into the mechanistic activation of Hsp90 client proteins. This special Issue brings together our current understanding of the role of the Hsp90 complex into a concise collection of articles that is aimed at researchers and scientists new to the field.

My sincere thanks go to all the authors that have contributed to this Special Issue, without whom this excellent collection of articles would not have been possible.

Chrisostomos Prodromou
Editor

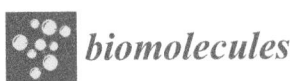

Editorial

An Editorial on the Special Issue 'Hsp90 Structure, Mechanism and Disease'

Chrisostomos Prodromou

School of Life Sciences, Biochemistry and Biomedicine, John Maynard Smith Building, University of Sussex, Falmer, Brighton BN1 9QG, UK; chris.prodromou@sussex.ac.uk

Hsp90 is known for its role in the activation of an eclectic set of regulatory and signal transduction proteins. As such, Hsp90 plays a central role in oncogenic processes [1,2]. Although the specific details of the chaperone cycle remained controversial for a significant amount of time, the development of small molecules to inhibit Hsp90 was intense, and recently, the inhibitor Pimitespib was approved against gastrointestinal stromal tumour [3]. It is now apparent that Hsp90's role reaches beyond what we first envisaged. The scope of this 'Special Issue' is to bring together this diverse information to better understand Hsp90 structure, mechanism and its role in disease. The articles not only highlight the most recent advances in our understanding, but present challenges that will need to be addressed by the scientific community. In total, six manuscripts were selected as 'Editor's Choice' articles.

The review by Bjorklund and Prodromou [4], an 'Editor's Choice' article, discuses recent advances in our understanding of the chaperone cycle and its regulation by co-chaperones by focusing on known structural complexes of Hsp90. Similarly, the mechanism of client protein activation by the Hsp90 complex is discussed, particularly for those of steroid hormone receptors and kinases. It appears that the Hsp90 complex is able to unfold client protein, allowing for their subsequent activation.

The article by Wengert et al. [5], also selected as an 'Editor's Choice' article, reviewed the impact of mitochondrial TRAP1 on the regulation of mitochondrial function. TRAP1 is often upregulated in transformed cells and contributes to the 'hallmarks of cancer'. It was reported that TRAP1 function is regulated by a number of post-translational modifications, which differentially impact on the function of TRAP1 in normal and cancer cells. Future progress towards understanding the post-translational or 'chaperone code' may inform therapeutic targeting of TRAP1 in cancer.

The review of Joshi et al. [6], another 'Editor's Choice' article, brings together work where there has been an increased appreciation of the importance of mitochondria in regulating diverse aspects of normal cell biology, cancer and neurodegenerative disease. Much remains to be learned about the regulation of mitochondrial function and the contributions provided by their proteostasis. Specifically, how TRAP1 modulates the balance between oxidative phosphorylation (OXPHOS) by the mitochondrial electron transport chain (ETC) to generate ATP and by the less efficient process of aerobic glycolysis in the cytoplasm is discussed. It appears that TRAP1 interacts with components of the ETC to modulate activity, while the loss of TRAP1 dramatically upregulates OXPHOS by association with ETC components and suppresses their activity, forcing cells to rely on glycolysis for energy. The functional significance of TRAP1 as a dimer or higher-order oligomers is also discussed. Ongoing studies will no doubt provide additional mechanistic insight into the role of TRAP1 as a component of the mitochondrial proteostasis network.

The article by Jay et al. [7] looks at the role of extracellular Hsp90 alpha (eHsp90α), which is emerging as a newly defined research topic. It appears that inducible cellular Hsp90α (eHsp90α) is a stress-responsive isoform primarily for extracellular tissue repair. Milestone findings of recent research are elegantly brought together, including how

Citation: Prodromou, C. An Editorial on the Special Issue 'Hsp90 Structure, Mechanism and Disease'. *Biomolecules* 2023, 13, 547. https://doi.org/10.3390/biom13030547

Received: 10 March 2023
Accepted: 16 March 2023
Published: 17 March 2023

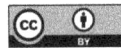

Copyright: © 2023 by the author. Licensee MDPI, Basel, Switzerland. This article is an open access article distributed under the terms and conditions of the Creative Commons Attribution (CC BY) license (https://creativecommons.org/licenses/by/4.0/).

eHsp90α is hijacked by tumours for their invasion and metastasis. It is anticipated that future therapeutic targeting of eHsp90α in wound healing and tumorigenesis could be safer and more effective than a pan inhibition of Hsp90 as a whole.

The 'Editor Choice' review by Backe et al. [8] looks at the large co-chaperones FNIP1, FNIP2 and Tsc1 that broaden the spectrum of Hsp90 regulators. These proteins have established roles in the regulation of tumour suppressor proteins FLCN and Tsc2. The authors discuss how their co-chaperone functions may explain their previously observed behaviour in cells and how they regulate numerous Hsp90 client proteins, including oncoproteins and tumour suppressors. Furthermore, these co-chaperones enhance Hsp90 binding to inhibitory drugs. These studies provide the groundwork for future investigations of these large co-chaperones in a pathological context as well as developing the next generation of cancer therapeutics.

The article by Ziaka and van der Spuy [9] extensively reviewed the critical role of Hsp90 in retinal proteostasis in health and disease. Current evidence highlights that the inhibition of Hsp90 as a therapeutic approach is a double-edged sword in the retina, with Hsp90 inhibition both inducing the neuroprotective upregulation of the heat shock response, but also leading to the degradation of key Hsp90 client proteins that can eventually lead to ocular toxicity. Based on the current understanding of the Hsp90 association with the retina-specific clients PDE6 and GRK1, critical components of the phototransduction cascade are reviewed. These insights will be of critical importance for the development of future next-generation molecules targeting Hsp90 proteostasis, either for the treatment of systemic or retina-specific disease.

The review by Dutta et al. [10] highlighted how the major cytosolic Hsp90 chaperone of the malaria parasite, *Plasmodium falciparum* (PfHsp90), and its associated co-chaperone complexes, display key structural and functional differences compared to the human Hsp90 system. While the core co-chaperones regulating client entry, ATPase activity and Hsp90 conformation are broadly conserved in *P. falciparum*, there are some major differences, such as the expression of two p23 isoforms, and the apparent absence of a canonical Cdc37. Overall, these differences in the co-chaperone network of PfHsp90 suggest that the elucidation of Hsp90–co-chaperone interactions can greatly extend our understanding of proteostasis and lead to the identification of novel inhibitors and drug candidates.

Piper et al. [11] bring together a review using a wealth of information on the folding of myosin heads which require a UCS (Unc45A and B, Cro1, She4) domain-containing co-chaperone for their efficient and expedient functional activation. The divergent role of Unc45 is discussed, where it appears that Hsp90α operates with Unc45B whereas Hsp90β utilises Unc45A. Given that these initial findings were first reported nearly 25 years ago, the important roles of UCS proteins are brought together, raising new questions to direct research activities.

In addition to assisting protein homeostasis, Hsp90 has been shown to be involved in the promotion and maintenance of proper protein complex assembly either alone or in association with other chaperones, such as the R2TP complex. The review by Lynham and Walid [12] looks at R2TP and its role in complex assembly. However, the molecular basis of function of Hsp90-R2TP in complex assembly has yet to be determined, and this review brings together the current understanding of the function of Hsp90-R2TP in the assembly, stabilization and activity of several client protein complexes.

The review by Mankovich and Freeman [13] shows that Hsp90 interacts with a broad array of client proteins, including a variety of factors involved in protein trafficking. Despite the numerous reports demonstrating a Hsp90 connection to protein transport, our understanding on how Hsp90 contributes to this complex process remains limited. Given the immense contributions that both Hsp90 and protein trafficking have to human health, a better comprehension on how these factors intersect is merited. The review brings together the latest research findings forming a platform to expediate research in this field of study.

The review by Maiti and Picard [14], an 'Editor's Choice' article, discusses the client and functional specificities of Hsp90α and Hsp90β isoforms and whether they have specific roles in cancer, neurodegeneration and aging. Beyond gaining a better fundamental understanding of why there are two distinct isoforms, recent progress in developing isoform-specific inhibitors raises the prospects of translating new knowledge into novel therapies, and evidence is presented where a pathological process is primarily supported by one particular isoform. In such cases, targeting the relevant isoform might be 'safer' since 'housekeeping' functions could still be provided by the other isoform. This view is supported by genetic evidence where yeast or mammalian cells are viable with a single isoform.

The review by van Oosten-Hawle [15] looks at the role of Hsp90 at an organismal level, where Hsp90 regulates the proteostasis cell-nonautonomously across tissues through its involvement in cross-tissue stress signaling responses. Recent advances in the field of organismal proteostasis and its regulation by Hsp90 at a tissue-specific and organismal level have major implications on how animals respond to environmental challenges and age-associated disease. Future aspects that need to be researched further will be to understand how the different tissue-specific roles of Hsp90 are integrated into an organism to regulate survival and behavioural cues with whole-organism benefits.

The 'Editor's Choice' article by Haufeng [16] discusses whether proteins always fold to a free-energy minimum or whether they can be maintained by energy-consuming processes in functional conformations with elevated free energies. The common view is that chaperones accelerate the kinetics of the folding process so that substrates reach their free-energy minimum. However, Xu challenges this view by presenting a theoretical model of non-equilibrium protein folding. It answers some long-standing questions in chaperone-assisted folding, including the necessity of ATP hydrolysis and how timing in the chaperone cycle affects the folding efficiency, and raises questions around protein structure predictions based on (free) energy minimization. Xu suggests new proteomic experiments to identify proteins that depend on ATP-dependent chaperones for the maintenance of their native structures and how to test such predictions.

The study by Omkar et al. [17] explored the importance of molecular chaperones for the activation of the Exonuclease APE2. Although APE2 has recently been demonstrated to be an important player in the DNA damage response and in a variety of human pathologies including cancer, there are currently no therapeutics that target APE2. The authors demonstrate that APE2 interacts with Hsp70 and Hsp90 in both budding yeast and mammalian cells. Furthermore, the inhibition of molecular chaperones using small molecule inhibitors promoted the rapid degradation of APE2. Taken together, this work suggests a novel way to manipulate APE2 function in cancer.

A second contribution by Bjorklund et al. [18] looks at the activation of the class 2 BRAF mutant L597R. The authors discuss how BRAF addiction for Hsp90 is broken upon dimerization of the kinase. A surprising finding was that although the L597R BRAF mutant was dimeric, it possessed no kinase activity. This has profound implications as this suggests that this class 2 mutant must therefore be dependent on RAS for its activation. Consequently, it appears that Hsp90's role, at least with BRAF, is not the direct activation, of the kinase, but to maintain an inactive kinase that may then be delivered to the membrane-bound RAS system for its activation. In the case for the L597R mutant, signaling could occur from a CRAF-L597R heterodimer. Clinically, this is important because it could determine the way such cancers are treated—by focusing on CRAF inhibition, rather than on the inactive L597R BRAF protein.

In conclusion, the 'Special Issue' brings together a series of review and research papers that concentrate on past and recent advances on Hsp90. It highlights its diverse role form the cytoplasm to the extracellular environment and even at the organismal level, and concentrates on the structure, mechanism and its pivotal position in disease. The articles bring together a diverse array of research findings into specific articles that will help drive research effectively towards making further progress in this fascinating research field that is Hsp90.

Acknowledgments: CP acknowledges Gregory L Blatch, Brian C. Freeman, Walid A. Houry, Stefan H. Millson, Len Neckers, Wei Li, Mehdi Mollapour, Didier Picard, Andrew W. Truman, Jacqueline van der Spuy, Patricija van Oosten-Hawle, Mark R. Woodford and Huafeng Xu for their individual contributions to this editorial.

Conflicts of Interest: The author declares no conflict of interest.

References

1. Whitesell, L.; Lindquist, S.L. HSP90 and the chaperoning of cancer. *Nat. Rev. Cancer* **2005**, *5*, 761–772. [CrossRef] [PubMed]
2. Pearl, L.H.; Prodromou, C.; Workman, P. The Hsp90 molecular chaperone: An open and shut case for treatment. *Biochem. J.* **2008**, *410*, 439–453. [CrossRef] [PubMed]
3. Kurokawa, Y.; Honma, Y.; Sawaki, A.; Naito, Y.; Iwagami, S.; Komatsu, Y.; Takahashi, T.; Nishida, T.; Doi, T. Pimitespib in patients with advanced gastrointestinal stromal tumor (CHAPTER-GIST-301): A randomized, double-blind, placebo-controlled phase III trial. *Ann. Oncol.* **2022**, *33*, 959–967. [CrossRef] [PubMed]
4. Prodromou, C.; Bjorklund, D.M. Advances towards Understanding the Mechanism of Action of the Hsp90 Complex. *Biomolecules* **2022**, *12*, 600. [CrossRef] [PubMed]
5. Wengert, L.A.; Backe, S.J.; Bourboulia, D.; Mollapour, M.; Woodford, M.R. TRAP1 Chaperones the Metabolic Switch in Cancer. *Biomolecules* **2022**, *12*, 786. [CrossRef] [PubMed]
6. Joshi, A.; Ito, T.; Picard, D.; Neckers, L. The Mitochondrial HSP90 Paralog TRAP1: Structural Dynamics, Interactome, Role in Metabolic Regulation, and Inhibitors. *Biomolecules* **2022**, *12*, 880. [CrossRef] [PubMed]
7. Jay, D.; Luo, Y.; Li, W. Extracellular Heat Shock Protein-90 (eHsp90): Everything You Need to Know. *Biomolecules* **2022**, *12*, 911. [CrossRef] [PubMed]
8. Backe, S.J.; Sager, R.A.; Meluni, K.A.; Woodford, M.R.; Bourboulia, D.; Mollapour, M. Emerging Link between Tsc1 and FNIP Co-Chaperones of Hsp90 and Cancer. *Biomolecules* **2022**, *12*, 928. [CrossRef] [PubMed]
9. Ziaka, K.; van der Spuy, J. The Role of Hsp90 in Retinal Proteostasis and Disease. *Biomolecules* **2022**, *12*, 978. [CrossRef] [PubMed]
10. Dutta, T.; Singh, H.; Edkins, A.L.; Blatch, G.L. Hsp90 and Associated Co-Chaperones of the Malaria Parasite. *Biomolecules* **2022**, *12*, 1018. [CrossRef] [PubMed]
11. Piper, P.W.; Scott, J.E.; Millson, S.H. UCS Chaperone Folding of the Myosin Head: A Function That Evolved before Animals and Fungi Diverged from a Common Ancestor More than a Billion Years Ago. *Biomolecules* **2022**, *12*, 1028. [CrossRef] [PubMed]
12. Lynham, J.; Houry, W.A. The Role of Hsp90-R2TP in Macromolecular Complex Assembly and Stabilization. *Biomolecules* **2022**, *12*, 1045. [CrossRef] [PubMed]
13. Mankovich, A.G.; Freeman, B.C. Regulation of Protein Transport Pathways by the Cytosolic Hsp90s. *Biomolecules* **2022**, *12*, 1077. [CrossRef] [PubMed]
14. Maiti, S.; Picard, D. Cytosolic Hsp90 Isoform-Specific Functions and Clinical Significance. *Biomolecules* **2022**, *12*, 1166. [CrossRef] [PubMed]
15. van Oosten-Hawle, P. Organismal Roles of Hsp90. *Biomolecules* **2023**, *13*, 251. [CrossRef] [PubMed]
16. Xu, H. Non-Equilibrium Protein Folding and Activation by ATP-Driven Chaperones. *Biomolecules* **2022**, *12*, 832. [CrossRef] [PubMed]
17. Omkar, S.; Wani, T.H.; Zheng, B.; Mitchem, M.M.; Truman, A.W. The APE2 Exonuclease Is a Client of the Hsp70-Hsp90 Axis in Yeast and Mammalian Cells. *Biomolecules* **2022**, *12*, 864. [CrossRef] [PubMed]
18. Bjorklund, D.M.; Morgan, R.M.L.; Oberoi, J.; Day, K.; Galliou, P.A.; Prodromou, C. Recognition of BRAF by CDC37 and Re-Evaluation of the Activation Mechanism for the Class 2 BRAF-L597R Mutant. *Biomolecules* **2022**, *12*, 905. [CrossRef] [PubMed]

Disclaimer/Publisher's Note: The statements, opinions and data contained in all publications are solely those of the individual author(s) and contributor(s) and not of MDPI and/or the editor(s). MDPI and/or the editor(s) disclaim responsibility for any injury to people or property resulting from any ideas, methods, instructions or products referred to in the content.

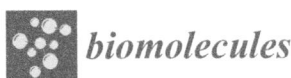

Review

Advances towards Understanding the Mechanism of Action of the Hsp90 Complex

Chrisostomos Prodromou * and Dennis M. Bjorklund

School of Life Sciences, Biochemistry and Biomedicine, John Maynard Smith Building, University of Sussex, Falmer, Brighton BN1 9QG, UK; dennis.bj90@gmail.com
* Correspondence: chris.prodromou@sussex.ac.uk

Abstract: Hsp90 (Heat Shock Protein 90) is an ATP (Adenosine triphosphate) molecular chaperone responsible for the activation and maturation of client proteins. The mechanism by which Hsp90 achieves such activation, involving structurally diverse client proteins, has remained enigmatic. However, recent advances using structural techniques, together with advances in biochemical studies, have not only defined the chaperone cycle but have shed light on its mechanism of action. Hsp90 hydrolysis of ATP by each protomer may not be simultaneous and may be dependent on the specific client protein and co-chaperone complex involved. Surprisingly, Hsp90 appears to remodel client proteins, acting as a means by which the structure of the client protein is modified to allow its subsequent refolding to an active state, in the case of kinases, or by making the client protein competent for hormone binding, as in the case of the GR (glucocorticoid receptor). This review looks at selected examples of client proteins, such as CDK4 (cyclin-dependent kinase 4) and GR, which are activated according to the so-called 'remodelling hypothesis' for their activation. A detailed description of these activation mechanisms is paramount to understanding how Hsp90-associated diseases develop.

Keywords: chaperone; co-chaperone; heat shock proteins; Hsp90; Aha1; immunophilins; p23; Cdc37; kinase; steroid hormone receptor; structure; mechanism; ATPase

1. Introduction

Heat shock protein 90 (Hsp90) is an ATP-dependant chaperone that is subject to regulation by a variety of co-chaperones [1,2]. Hsp90 consists of three domains, a C-terminal domain (CTD) that is inherently dimerised, a middle domain (MD) and an ATP-binding N-terminal domain (NTD) (Figure 1A). ATP binding and hydrolysis drive conformational changes that lead to the NTDs undergoing cycles of dimerisation and disassembly (recently reviewed [3–6]). During this cycle, the formation of a catalytically active unit leads to the hydrolysis of ATP. The chaperone cycle is thought to be the basis by which Hsp90 client proteins are regulated or matured into an active state, and it is thought that Hsp90 assists in the late stages of the folding of its client proteins [7,8]. The rate-limiting step of the cycle is the co-ordinated structural changes required to bring about the hydrolysis of ATP [9,10]. Client proteins include kinases, such as ErbB2, Cdk4 and Braf, as well as nuclear receptors, transcription factors and structural proteins, such as actin and tubulin. A full list of such protein clients can be found at https://www.picard.ch/downloads/Hsp90interactors.pdf (accessed on 16 April 2022).

The NTD is responsible for the binding of ATP and, together with the catalytic-loop arginine within the MD of Hsp90, they form a catalytically active unit able to hydrolyse ATP [5,11]. The NTD is the target of ATPase regulation by interaction with a series of co-chaperones, including p23 (Sba1 in yeast), Cdc37 and Aha1. The catalytic-loop arginine is essential for ATP hydrolysis and contacts the γ-phosphate of the N-terminally bound ATP [11]. Because of the essential nature of the catalytic-loop arginine, co-chaperones such as Cdc37, p23 and Aha1 may influence Hsp90's ATPase activity through interactions with the MD of Hsp90 [5,11–13]. In addition to these co-chaperones, many bind Hsp90 using a TPR domain that engages the conserved MEEVD motif of Hsp90 at its extreme C-terminus. Such co-chaperones include immunophilins such as FKBP51 (**FK506**-binding protein 51) and FKBP52, HOP (Sti1 in yeast), the phosphatase PP5, the E3 ligase CHIP, AIP and Tah1, amongst others. These co-chaperones may be either specific for a client protein or a class of client or may impart enzymatic activities that regulate Hsp90 for the activation or degradation of a client protein [3,4,14].

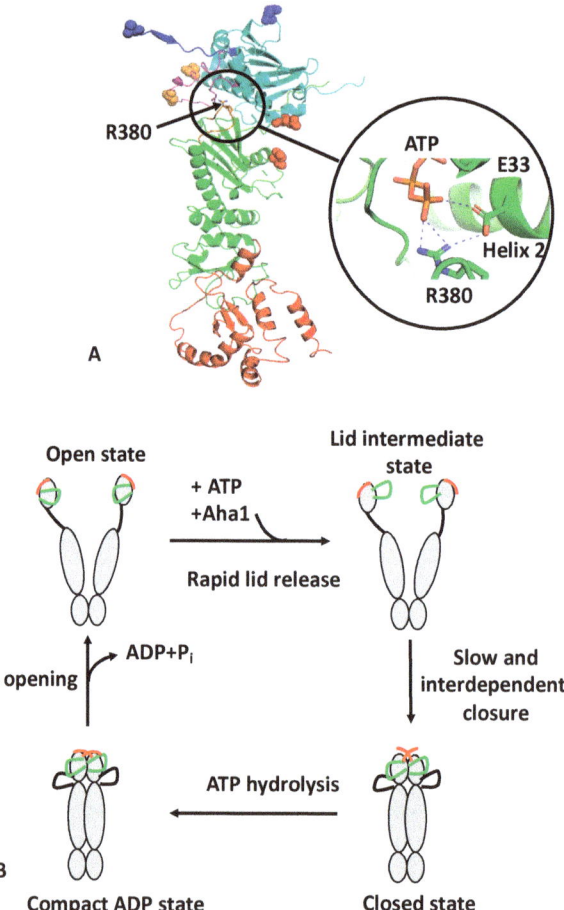

Figure 1. PyMol cartoon showing the structure and conformational switches of Hsp90 and its catalytic cycle. (**A**) Monomeric Hsp90 in the active, N-terminally dimerised closed conformation. Hsp90 consists of three domains: cyan, NTD; green, MD; and red, CTD. Four structural features are shown: blue, the structure involved in the N-terminal β-strand cross-subunit swapping; magenta, the lid-segment involved in lid closure; cyan and green, the NTD and MD domains involved in intra-subunit association; and magenta, the catalytic loop containing Arg 380 (shown as sticks). Attachment points for the fluorophore or Trp are shown as residues in sphere representation: blue, represents the N-terminal β-strand cross-subunit swapping switch pair (normally as a pair between both protomers); red, the NTD and MD intra-subunit association switch; and gold, the lid-closure switch. The close up shows the interaction of Arg 380 with the γ-phosphate of ATP and Glu 33. Dotted blue lines represent salt bridges.

(**B**) The catalytic cycle of Hsp90. The apo state of Hsp90 occupies a heterologous ensemble of open-conformers. The lid (green) and N-terminal β-strand (red) are highly mobile structural elements showing a sub-millisecond reconfiguration time. The binding of ATP to the NTD of Hsp90 leads to a rapid release of the lid segment to an intermediate conformational state, between the so-called open- and closed-lid states. The association of Aha1 can remodel the lid but also preassociates the N- and M-domains for accelerated closure. Cooperative action of conformational switches leads to full closure of the molecular clamp. This involves closure of the lid over the ATP-binding pocket, a cross-subunit swap of the β-strands, and association of the N- and M-domains, which collectively are slow and interdependent. The β-strand swapping is weakly coupled with the other motions. The cycle completes following the hydrolysis of ATP, which leads to a compact, ADP-bound conformation. The hydrolysis of ATP appears to be non-cooperative between the two protomers of Hsp90. Following ATP hydrolysis, Hsp90 then relaxes to an open state, with concomitant release of ADP and inorganic phosphate.

The structure and catalytic cycle of the Hsp90 chaperone has been extensively reviewed [2,3,14–16], and we direct readers to these. The current manuscript concentrates on advances in understanding the Hsp90 mechanism through recent structural and biochemical studies.

2. Concerted and Unconcerted Actions of the ATPase Cycle of Hsp90

The regulation of the ATPase cycle of Hsp90 was recently reviewed [3,4,14]. Formation of catalytically active Hsp90 involves the binding of ATP, which triggers a number of conformational changes. These include closure of the so-called N-terminal lid of each protomer, which traps the bound nucleotide and allows N-terminal dimerisation, an N-terminal β-strand exchange between the two protomers of the Hsp90 dimer, the association of the MD and NTD of each protomer and the release of the catalytic loop from the MD. The association of the N- and middle-domains (N/M-domains) is critically dependent on Arg 380 (yeast Hsp90) [9]. Mutation of Arg 380 to alanine abolishes lid closure, the β-strand swap, and N/M-domain association altogether [9]. Arg 380 interacts with the γ-phosphate of the bound ATP molecule [11] but additionally forms a salt bridge with the catalytic Glu 33 (yeast Hsp90) (Figure 1A). Arg 380, therefore acts as an important interaction site linking together ATP and the catalytic Glu 33 residue. Since Glu 33 is located on helix 2, which is directly involved in the interface between the N/M-domains, it would appear that Arg 380 acts as a sensor detecting the presence of bound ATP and the presence of Glu 33 in the ATP-bound conformation, which subsequently allows N/M association and provides stability to the N/M-domain interface.

Recently, structural changes at local sites within Hsp90 were probed using a reporter system based on fluorescence quenching by photo-induced electron transfer (PET) with nanosecond single-molecule fluorescence fluctuation analysis [9,17]. Unlike fluorescence resonance energy transfer (FRET), which occurs at 2–10 nm scales, PET quenching relies on van der Waals contacts at distances of ≤1 nm, which occur between the organic fluorophore and a tryptophan indole side-chain. The PET reporter system relies on the introduction of a Trp and Cys amino acid residue by site-directed mutagenesis, where the Cys residue acts as a point of fluorophore attachment, and Trp for fluorescence quenching. Three conformational switches were designed: lid-closure using two PET reporter systems (S51C-A110W and A110C-S51W), N/M-domain intra-subunit association (E192C-N298W) and N-terminal β-strand cross-subunit swapping (using a fluorophore on the N-terminus of one subunit (A2C) and Trp on the other (E162W)). The study showed that the ATPase activity of Hsp90 was correlated with the kinetics of the specific structural rearrangements that acted cooperatively on a sub-millisecond time scale. However, lid closure over the nucleotide-binding pocket was identified as a two-step mechanism (Figure 1B). The finding suggests that the lid of apo-Hsp90 is dynamic and populates an ensemble of conformers, which is then reconfigured rapidly, following ATP binding, to an intermediate state that most likely exposes the N-terminal dimerisation interface. Subsequently, the lid fully closes over the nucleotide-binding pocket, which occurs slowly and in a concerted manner with the N- and M-domain inter- and intra-subunit associations. The subunit swap of the N-terminal β-strands upon association of the N-domains, is facilitated by their highly mobile nature, as seen in apo-Hsp90. Consequently, the swapping of the terminal β-strands, the closure of the lid, and N- and M-domain associations are cooperatively coordinated to form the catalytically active Hsp90 conformation that can hydrolyse ATP. Ultimately, the hydrolysis of ATP opens the molecular clamp and reconstitutes the chaperone for its next catalytic cycle (Figure 1B).

The authors also showed that Aha1 substantially accelerated conformational changes. A ~40-fold acceleration in the mean rate constant of N/M-domain association was seen, which was in agreement with the enhanced ATPase activity. In contrast, a ~20-fold increase in the mean rate constant of lid closure and β-strand swapping was observed. Preorganization of the NTD and MD induced by Aha1 could perhaps explain the stronger acceleration of N/M-domain association compared to the other motions [18,19]. The effect of Aha1 was also investigated on the three conformational switches. As previously seen, Aha1 stimulates the ATPase activity of the Hsp90 F349A mutant (F349 is important for N/M association) to wild-type levels [18,19] and could accelerate all three of the local motions. The authors show that binding of Aha1 to apo-Hsp90 showed fluorescence quenching both for the wild-type and mutant F349A protein, suggesting that binding of Aha1 can influence the conformation of the lid. The most recent studies suggest that Aha1 may help "bypass" a slowly formed closed-lid intermediate of Hsp90 [18]. Although other work suggests that Aha1 initiates a partially closed lid conformation and acts late on the ATP-bound N-terminally-dimerised conformation [20]. However, PET-FCS provided evidence that Aha1 could mobilise the lid early in the apo-state of Hsp90 and this is also supported by NMR chemical shift perturbations that show weak and transient interactions of C-Aha1 with the NTD of Hsp90 [21]. The T101I lid mutation can also be re-activated by Aha1 [19], and consequently, it appears that lid mobilisation is an early mode of Aha1 action. Furthermore, it was shown that the mutations T101I and R380A (yeast), which disrupt Hsp90 ATPase activity, also abolish lid closure, β-strand swapping and N/M-domain association altogether, although the lid segment was still able to remodel rapidly. In contrast, the activating A107N mutation accelerated lid closure and N/M-domain association by ~5-fold, in agreement with previous studies [6,11]. Interestingly, the A107N effect on the β-strand swap was moderate.

The PET technique was further developed and combined with two-colour fluorescence microscopy. This allowed the simultaneous detection of two structural coordinates, one colour per coordinate, within a single protein molecule [9]. These experiments showed that the lid of the NTD and the N-terminal β-strand are highly mobile, with μs reconfiguration time constants [22]. These studies concluded that ATP binding rapidly remodels the lid, likely exposing the N-terminal dimerisation interface and priming inter-subunit dimerisation early in the cycle [22]. In conclusion, the recent data suggests a concerted mechanism involving a number of conformational switches that from the catalytically active state of Hsp90 (Figure 1B). However, mutations show that some decoupling of these switches is possible and this is evident with the effect of A107N on the rate of β-strand swapping, which was moderate in comparison to lid and N/M-domain association. Furthermore, Aha1 can accelerate N/M-domain association over that of lid-closure and the β-strand swapping of wild-type Hsp90. Consequently, Hsp90, through a cooperative mechanism, is highly efficient at establishing an active state but nonetheless can be modulated by co-chaperones and perhaps by client proteins themselves to meet the specific demands of client protein activation. Although the dimerisation of Hsp90 is cooperative, the hydrolysis of ATP by each monomer appears to be unaffected by the state of the adjacent protomer. Studies using a variety of Hsp90s show that despite having two ATP-binding sites, their ATPase activities follow simple, non-cooperative kinetics [23–26]. Consistent with such observations, the activity of the wild-type ATPase domain is unaffected by the adjacent protomer carrying a mutation that is either unable to bind or hydrolyse ATP [27,28]. An adaptation to the above model is seen with the TRAP1 (tumor necrosis factor receptor-associated protein 1) paralogue of Hsp90 [29]. In this model, ATP binding leads to an asymmetric dimer in which one protomer is buckled compared to the other, which remains in a similar conformation to the yeast Hsp90–Sba1-bound structure [11]. In this model the hydrolysis of ATP is sequential and deterministic, where the buckled protomer is better able to hydrolyse ATP. Subsequently, a flip in the MD and CTD asymmetry positions the opposite protomer in the buckled conformation, thus promoting hydrolysis of the second ATP and allowing TRAP1 to proceed through the cycle to its open state.

3. The Hsp90–Cdc37–CDK4 Complex

Cdc37 is an Hsp90 co-chaperone that delivers client kinases to Hsp90 and in doing so inhibits the ATPase activity of Hsp90 to allow client protein loading [30]. Structural work has shown how Cdc37 binds to the lid-segment of the NTDs of Hsp90 and prevents them from closing, which in turn prevents N-terminal dimerisation (PDB 1US7) [12] (Figure 2A). In addition, a key interaction between Arg 167 of Cdc37 and the catalytic residue Glu 33 (yeast) of Hsp90 inactivates the catalytic machinery of the chaperone [31]. The EM structure of Hsp90, in complex with Cdc37 and CDK4 at ~19 Å, was interpreted as showing the MD of Cdc37 sitting between the NTDs of Hsp90 and delivering CDK4, which engages with the NTD and MDs of Hsp90 [31] (Figure 2B). This structure may represent an early loading stage of the kinase complex. However, a higher resolution structure at 3.9 Å was presented using cryo-EM, which clearly represents a mature Hsp90–kinase complex (PDB 5FWM) [13]. In this structure, Hsp90 is in a closed conformation in which its NTDs are clearly dimerised (Figure 2C). Taking this higher resolution structure into account it is possible to interpret the lower resolution structure of this complex as being the same in terms of location of the individual domains. Nonetheless, it is clear that Cdc37 does engage with the lid-segment of the NTD of Hsp90 and that Cdc37 is able to inhibit Hsp90 ATPase activity. Thus, the spatial relationship of the proteins in an early-state complex and how the complex remodels to a later mature conformation remains to be confirmed.

In the higher-resolution structure or mature state, Cdc37 makes a number of interactions, including a very important interaction between a loop consisting of ^{20}HPNI^{23} in Cdc37 and the C-terminal lobe of CDK4 (Figure 2D). Although the resolution of the cryo-EM map of this complex is variable, from 3.5 to 6 Å, some potential interactions can be inferred, but nonetheless caution should be exercised in these predictions. The extreme NTD of Cdc37 (residues 1 to 18) sits between the interface of the NTD and MD of one of the Hsp90 protomers, and probably helps to stabilise the N/M-domain association of Hsp90 (Figure 2E). Potentially the side-chain hydroxyl group of Tyr 4 from Cdc37 may be able to form a hydrogen bond with the side-chain amine group of Gln 128 of the N-terminal domain of the adjacent Hsp90 protomer. The side-chain carboxyl group of Gln 128 also appears close enough to form a hydrogen bond with one of the amine side-chain groups of Arg 392 (Arg 380 in yeast Hsp90) from the catalytic loop, where the same amine group is also engaged with the γ-phosphate of the bound ATP. Additional contacts between the catalytic loop of Hsp90 and Cdc37 residues Tyr 4, Trp 7 and Asp 8 may help stabilise the catalytic loop in its active conformation. The side-chains of Asp 8 and His 9 may also interact with those of Lys 36 and Asp 188 of the NTD of Hsp90. The next segment of the NTD of Cdc37, residues 10 to 18, interacts with the long helix of the MD of Hsp90 (residues Gln 385 to Ala 408) and potentially a series of salt bridges involving side-chains occur from the following interactions: Asp 14 and Glu 16 of Cdc37 with Arg 405 of Hsp90, Asp 17 of Cdc37 and Lys 402 of Hsp90 and Glu 18 of Cdc37 with Lys 399 of Hsp90 (Figure 2E). As seen with Aha1, the interaction of Cdc37 with the MD long helix of Hsp90 likely aids the conformational change of the catalytic loop to its open active state [5,32]. In addition, the side-chain of Glu 11 of Cdc37 may form a salt bridge with the side-chain of Arg 39 and phospho-Ser 13 (pSer 13) may form a bridging interaction by forming salt bridges with both His 33 and Arg 36 side-chains from the N-terminal end of the coiled-coil region of Cdc37 and with Lys 406 of the MD long helix of Hsp90. These interactions are critical for helping to position the conserved HPNI motif of Cdc37 for interaction with the C-lobe of Cdk4 (Figure 2D,E). The HPNI interaction mimics the interaction of the αC–β4 loop from the N-terminal lobe of CDK4 (HPNV in Cdk4 or HVNI in BRAF) (Figure 2D) and complex formation with Cdc37 is likely aided by the propensity of kinases to unfold [33]. Exiting from the coiled-coil segment of Cdc37, a beta strand then interacts with the 1AC β-sheet of Hsp90 (2CG9 nomenclature) and places the MD and CTD of Cdc37 on the opposite side of the Hsp90 dimer (see PDB 5FWL), which may be centred above Trp 312 (yeast Hsp90, Trp 300 and Hsc90, Trp 296) and Phe 341 (yeast Hsp90, Phe 329 and Yeast Hsc90, Phe 325). Interestingly, Trp 300 was previously identified as a client binding site [32] (Figure 2C).

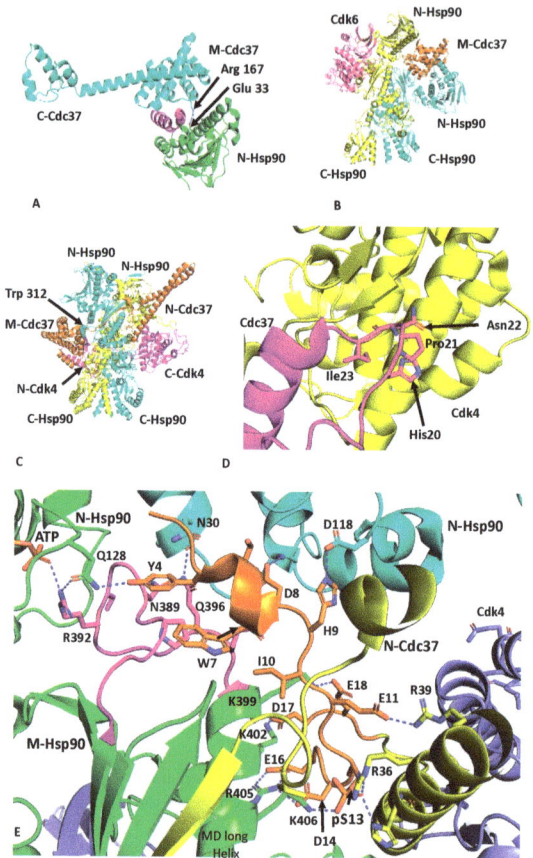

Figure 2. PyMol cartoons showing the interactions of Hsp90, Cdc37 and kinases. (**A**) The interaction of the MD and CTD of Cdc37 (cyan) with the NTD of Hsp90 (green). The Hsp90 lid is shown in magenta. Arg 167 of Cdc37 forms a salt bridge with Glu 33 of Hsp90. Residues are shown in stick format. (**B**) The negative stain EM structure of the Hsp90–Cdc37–Cdk4 complex, where Cdk6 was superimposed into the electron density of Cdk4 [31]. (**C**) The cryo-EM structure of the Hsp90–Cdc37–Cdk4 complex [13]. Note that the MD of Cdc37 is centered above Trp 312. (**D**) Interaction of the HPNI motif (sticks) of Cdc37 (magenta) with the C-terminal domain of Cdk4 (yellow). (**E**) Interaction of the NTD of Cdc37 (gold to yellow) with Hsp90 (green and cyan). Interactions are seen to occur with the catalytic loop (magenta) and the long helix of the MD and NTD of Hsp90. Phospho-Ser 13 (pS13) helps to stabilise the N-terminal loop of Cdc37 and forms important interactions with the base of the N-terminal end of the helix–turn–helix of the NTD of Cdc37. Some potential interactions are shown using dashed lines (blue). Blue, the CTD of Cdk4.

The cryo-EM structure also reveals that the β4 and β5 strands of the N-terminal lobe of CDK4 are pulled apart and the CDK4 polypeptide threads through the centre of the

Hsp90 dimer and positions the remaining N-terminal lobe on the adjacent Hsp90 protomer (Figure 2C). Interestingly, the structure from PDB 5FWL appears to show that the position of the remainder of the CDK4 N-terminal lobe is close to the long helix of the other MD of Hsp90. If this is the case, it appears that the NTD of Cdc37 may be able to influence the activation of one protomer of the Hsp90 dimer, while the client kinase may be aiding the other protomer and thus setting up hydrolysis of ATP by both Hsp90 protomers. Hydrolysis of ATP and dephosphorylation of pSer 13 by PP5 [34] may then destabilise the complex and release the kinase.

4. The Hsp90–Aha1 Complex

Aha1 remains the only potent activator of Hsp90 ATPase activity documented to date and is thought to be able to reduce the kinetic barrier presented by the rate-limiting conformational changes that Hsp90 has to undergo to produce a catalytically active unit [5,35]. Aha1 consists of an NTD separated from the CTD by a flexible ~60 amino acid linker. The structure of the NTD of Aha1 in complex with the MD of Hsp90 showed that Aha1 could modulate the catalytic loop of the MD of Hsp90 from an inactive to an active conformation, where Arg 380 (yeast Hsp90) could interact with the γ-phosphate of bound ATP [5]. The human NTD and the full-length structure of Aha1 were previously determined by NMR (PDB 7DMD and 7DME, respectively) [36].

Recent cryo-EM structures show that the activation of Hsp90 by Aha1 involves a multistep mechanism [8]. Binding of Aha1 to apo-Hsp90 leads to a partially closed Hsp90 dimer (EMD (Electron Microscopy Data Bank)-22238 and PDB 6XLB; 3.8 Å) (Figure 3A) that is bound by two molecules of Aha1. In this complex the NTD of Aha1 is engaged with a MD of Hsp90, as seen in the fragment crystal structure [35]. In contrast, each CTD of Aha1 is bound to the MDs of both Hsp90 protomers, and each contacts an amphipathic helix (residues Pro 324 to Asn 340) that was previously identified as a client–protein binding site [37]. The semi-closed conformation therefore represents a state in which the MDs are now closely associated and approach, but do not exactly match, the conformation seen in the yeast closed Hsp90–Sba1 structure [11]. To achieve this, a further 5° rotation of the Hsp90 MDs would be required. The binding of the CTDs of Aha1 appear to be incompatible with Hsp90 N/M-domain association, and the NTDs in the structure remained undefined. Binding of Aha1 to apo-Hsp90 therefore leads to the dissociation of the resting state for the N/M associated domains of Hsp90.

To achieve a fully closed state requires binding of nucleotide to Hsp90. With increasing concentrations of Aha1, in the presence of the non-hydrolysable nucleotide AMPPNP, a variety of Hsp90–Aha1 complexes were seen, with the equilibrium shifting from Hsp90 bound with one Aha1 molecule (with only the CTD being visible; HAc; EMD 22240 and PDB 6XLD; 3.66 Å) through to a Hsp90 complex with two Aha1 molecules bound, but with only the CTD visible (HAcc; EMD-22241 and PDB 6XLE; 2.74 Å) and finally to an Hsp90 complex in which two Aha1 molecules are bound, with two CTD and one NTD visible (HAncc; EMD-22242 and PDB 6XLF; 3.15 Å). In the HAncc structure, Hsp90 is now N-terminally dimerised and Aha1 binding has been restructured and forms a tighter bound complex. The NTD of Aha1 is found to be tilted by 30° relative to the state with apo-Hsp90, and consequently, the original interface with the MD of Hsp90, as seen in the fragment structure, is broken (Figure 3B) and new interactions are formed. Specifically, Aha1 residues 1 to 10 containing the conserved motif NxNNWHW are found bound across the dimer interface and appear to stabilise N-terminal dimerisation (Figure 3C). The two conserved Trp residues of the NxNNWHW motif also form stabilising interactions, where Trp 9 is engaged with the lid segment of one of the Hsp90 protomers and Trp 11 is engaged with the MD of the same Hsp90 protomer. Deletion of the N-terminal segment (residues 1 to 11) of Aha1 has previously been shown to reduce its ability to activate Hsp90 [38]. The interaction of the N-terminal segment of Aha1 is further supported by a small helix coil that binds over the N-terminal segment of Aha1 but also forms stabilising interactions with the lid segment of Hsp90, and Tyr 165 appears to be important in this interaction (Figure 3C).

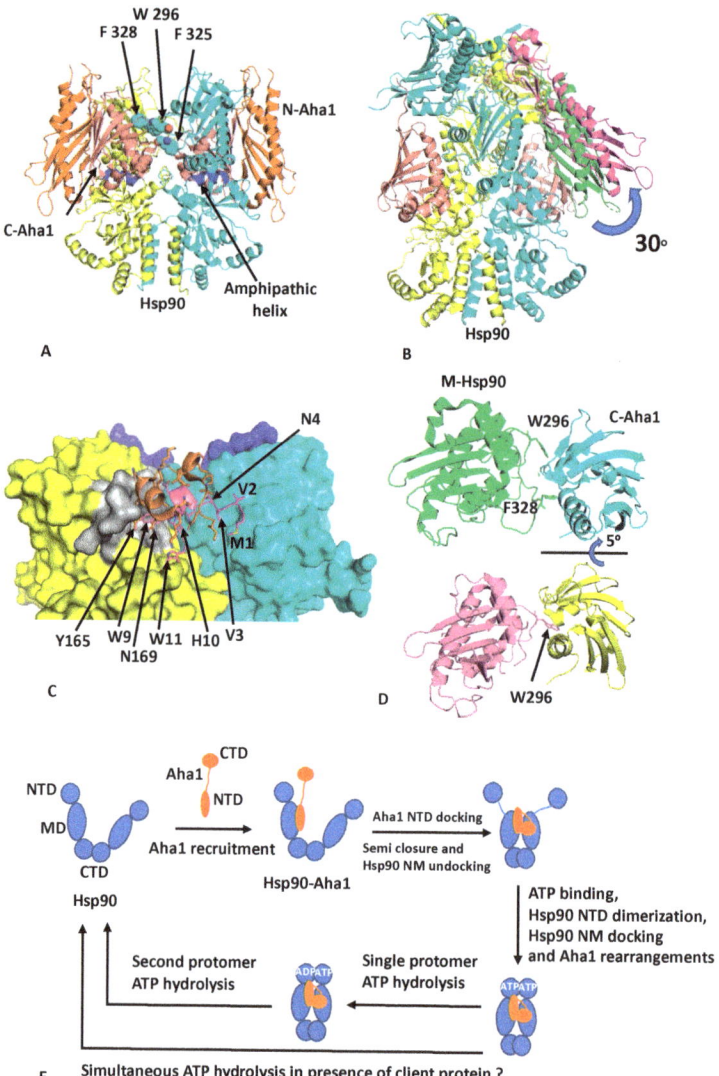

Figure 3. PyMol cartoons showing the Hsp90–Aha1 interactions. (**A**) apo-Hsp90 (yellow and cyan) in complex with two molecules of Aha1 (gold, N-Aha, and salmon, C-Aha1). Blue, amphipathic helix (**B**) AMPPNP-Hsp90 (yellow and cyan) in complex with two molecules of Aha1 (magenta and salmon), although only one N-terminal domain of Aha1 was observed in the complex. The rotation of the NTD of Aha1 from its apo-Hsp90 (green) to the AMPPNP-Hsp90 location (magenta) is shown. (**C**) Interaction of segments of Aha1 (magenta, residues 1–10 and gold, residues 154–170) with the NTDs of Hsp90 (yellow and cyan). Grey, surface lid segment of Hsp90. (**D**) Rotation of the CTD of Aha1 from its apo-Hsp90 (green and cyan) to the AMPPNP-Hsp90 location (salmon and yellow) results in changes of interaction from Phe 328 to Trp 296 of Aha1. (**E**) Chaperone cycles in response to Aha1 binding.

In addition to the changes that occur between the NTD of Aha1 and Hsp90, the interaction of the CTD of Aha1 also alters its interaction with Hsp90. The Aha1 residues Phe

264, Asn 267, Asn 268, Leu 287, Arg 327, Asn 331 and Tyr 335 no longer interact with the amphipathic loop (residues Pro 324 to Asn 340) but shift their interaction to a loop formed by residues Ser 297 to Leu 304 (Figure 3D). The shift in conformation from the apo-Hsp90 to the AMPPNP bound structure involves a 15° counter clockwise rotation as well as a deep pocket within the Aha CTD opening up to accommodate Trp 296 of Hsp90 (yeast Hsp90 Trp 300 and Human Hsp90b Trp 312), having switched from interacting with Phe 328 (yeast Hsp90 Phe 332 and human Hsp90β Phe 344). Trp 296 (yeast Hsp90 Trp300) is the same residue identified as a client–protein binding site [32], and also involved in interactions with CDK4 in the Hsp90–Cdc37–Cdk4 cryo-EM structure, discussed above. It would therefore appear that there is a series of aromatic amino acid residues (Yeast Hsp90 Trp 300, Phe 329 and 332; Yeast Hsc90 Trp 296, Phe 325 and 328 and human Hsp90β Trp 312, Phe 341 and 344;) that are involved in both client protein and co-chaperone binding (Figure 3A). Mutating yeast Trp 296 to either Ala or Gly has been shown to significantly reduce the ATPase activity of human Hsp90β, but the equivalent mutation in yeast Hsp90 (Trp 300A) did not affect its ATPase activity [8,32]. It therefore appears that interaction with these aromatic residues by co-chaperones and clients may act as a signal to regulate Hsp90 ATP hydrolysis by communicating the co-chaperone and client protein–bound state in the complex.

Another cryo-EM structure of Hsp90–Aha1 in complex with the slowly hydrolysable ATPγS (EMD-22243 and PDB 6XLG) contains a dimer of Hsp90 and two Aha1 molecules, where one NTD and two CTD are visible (HAnccg). This is equivalent to the AMPPNP structure discussed above, except that the Hsp90 protomer whose MD is bound by the NTD of Aha1 has hydrolysed the ATPγS to ADP and the other protomer still retains intact ATPγS. Collectively, these structures allowed the authors to propose a conformational cycle involving four steps towards hydrolysis of ATP by Hsp90 [8] (Figure 3E). Initially, Aha1 can be recruited to apo-Hsp90 by binding of its NTD to the MDs of Hsp90. This would produce a complex equivalent to the fragment structure determined by crystallography [35]. Next, the semi-closed Hsp90 state is formed by the binding of the CTDs of Aha1 to the MDs of Hsp90, which also displace the NTDs of Hsp90. However, the NTDs of Hsp90 are now primed for ATP binding and dimerisation as well as for Hsp90 N/M-domain association. ATP then binds and this signals a restructuring of the Hsp90–Aha1 complex to allow Hsp90 NTD dimerisation. Finally, Aha1 reorganises and helps stabilise the N-terminally dimerised state of Hsp90 and this in turn signals for ATP hydrolysis, which in the presence of a single molecule of Aha1 appears to occur sequentially for each protomer of Hsp90. The multistep activation of Hsp90 by Aha1 is consistent with the findings from an NMR study that found a two-step binding mechanism for Aha1 and that structural changes were induced near the ATP binding site of Hsp90, which conspire to activate Hsp90 [8]. Although, another model suggests that a single Aha1 molecule bound to Hsp90 can cause asymmetric activation of Hsp90 and thus fully activate it [21]. However, the Hsp90 'sequential ATP hydrolysis' model does not take into account the presence of client protein. Thus, the co-ordinated interaction of a client on one protomer of the Hsp90 dimer and a co-chaperone on the other might allow the simultaneous hydrolysis of ATP by both protomers of Hsp90. Clearly, further work to determine the exact timing of ATP hydrolysis by each protomer of an Hsp90—co-chaperone—client protein complex is therefore required.

5. The Hsp90–p23–FKBP51 and Hsp90–Sba1 Complex

Crystal structures of human FKBP51 (PDB 5OMP) and yeast Sba1 (PDB CG9) (p23 in humans) have been reported [11,39,40]. FKBP51 is an immunophilin and possesses peptidyl propyl isomerase (PPIase) activity, which catalyses the cis-trans isomerisation of proline and includes members such as FKBP52 and the cyclophilin Cyp40 [41]. FKBP 51 contains three distinct domains, a catalytically active N-terminal PPIase domain (FK1), an inactive PPIase MD (FK2) and a C-terminal tetratricopeptide (TPR) domain. FKBP51, FKBP52 and p23 have been reported as members of steroid hormone complexes [42,43], where they facilitate client protein activation and localisation [44–46]. FKBP52 was shown to potentiate the GR receptor activation when hormone levels where limiting, whereas

FKBP51 appears to block potentiation [45]. p23 is a CS domain–containing co-chaperone that appears to enter the Hsp90 activation cycle in its late stage and, as with FKBP51, favours the closed-nucleotide bound conformation of Hsp90 [11,39]. Sba1 in yeast appears to down regulate the ATPase activity of Hsp90 and stabilises the closed Hsp90 complex [11].

The role of p23 in Hsp90 complexes was previously determined in the context of steroid hormone activation, which has been elegantly reviewed previously [43,47,48]. The work described by these authors is relevant not only to this section but also to the subsequent sections that look at the loading and maturation complex for the glucocorticoid receptor (GR). Much of the work detailed by Pratt, WB, Toft, D, O and their co-authors showed that a Hsp90/Hsp70-based chaperone complex was responsible for regulating the steroid binding, trafficking and turnover of GR. An ATP-dependant activation cycle involving HOP, p23, Hsp40, FKBP51/52 and the Hsp90/Hsp70 complex is able to assemble ligand-binding domain (LBD) of the GR with Hsp90, in which the hydrophobic ligand-binding cleft is opened to allow access for steroid hormone binding. Much of this work has now been confirmed by the advances discussed below.

The crystal structure of Sba1 was determined in complex with Hsp90 (PDB CG9) [11] and is essentially similar to the cryo-EM structure of human p23 in complex with Hsp90 (PDB 7KRJ) [39,40]. Essentially, Sba1 is bound between the NTDs of N-terminally dimerised Hsp90 (Figure 4A) and contacts the closed lid-segment, the NTDs of both protomers and the MD of one Hsp90 protomer. Some critical interactions can be seen, which include a hydrogen bond between the side-chain of Asn 97 of p23 and the carbonyl main-chain of Leu 122 in the lid-segment of Hsp90, a salt bridge from the side-chains of Lys 95 of p23 and Glu 336 in the MD of Hsp90 and a hydrogen bond between the side-chains of Asn 104 of p23 and Asn 35 of Hsp90. Further interactions occur between the side-chain of Arg 71 of p23 and those from Ser 31 and Glu 22 of Hsp90 (Figure 4A). Collectively, the lid-segment, N-terminal dimerisation and N/M-domain association of Hsp90 are all stabilised. This is not too dissimilar to the action of Aha1, although for Sba1/p23 the ATPase activity is downregulated [35,49]. However, what is clear from these structures is that the binding of Aha1 and p23 to the same side of Hsp90 is incompatible (Figure 4A). A further set of interactions that is worthy of a mention is the interaction between the conserved yeast Sba1 residues Phe 121 (human Phe 103) and Trp 124 (human Trp 106), which sit in a hydrophobic pocket formed by Leu 315, Asp 373, Leu 376, Gln 385, Lys 387 and Val 391 of yeast Hsp90. These interactions may help stabilise the open conformation of the catalytic loop so that Arg 380 (yeast Hsp90) is able to interact with the γ-phosphate of bound ATP (Figure 4B). In fact, some analogies can be drawn between the Sba1 and Aha1 interactions with the MD long helix (residues Lys 399 to Ala 420) of yeast Hsp90 (Figure 4C). When comparing the interactions of the conserved Phe 121 (human Phe 103) and Trp 124 (human Trp 106) of Sba1 to those of Aha1, an analogous set of interactions occurs, where Aha1 residues bind into the same hydrophobic pocket(s) as those of Sba1. The interaction with Aha1 involves Ile 64, Leu 66 and Trp 11 (from the conserved NxNNWHW motif). Comparing the various structures of the human and yeast Hsp90–Aha1 complex, there is a gradual engagement of these residues as the closed conformation of Hsp90 is formed (Figure 4C). The least engaged situation is with the apo-Hsp90, in which two Aha1 molecules are bound (EMD-22238 and PDB 6XLB) and then closer engagement is seen in the yeast Aha1 fragment structure (PDB 1USU) and finally in the human AMPPNP bound structure (EMD-22242 and PDB 6XLF), where Aha1 has been tilted to fully engage with the NTD of Hsp90 (Figures 3B,C and 4C). The engagement of Sba1 and Aha1 with the MD long helix likely helps to stabilise the catalytic loop of the MD and N/M-domain association.

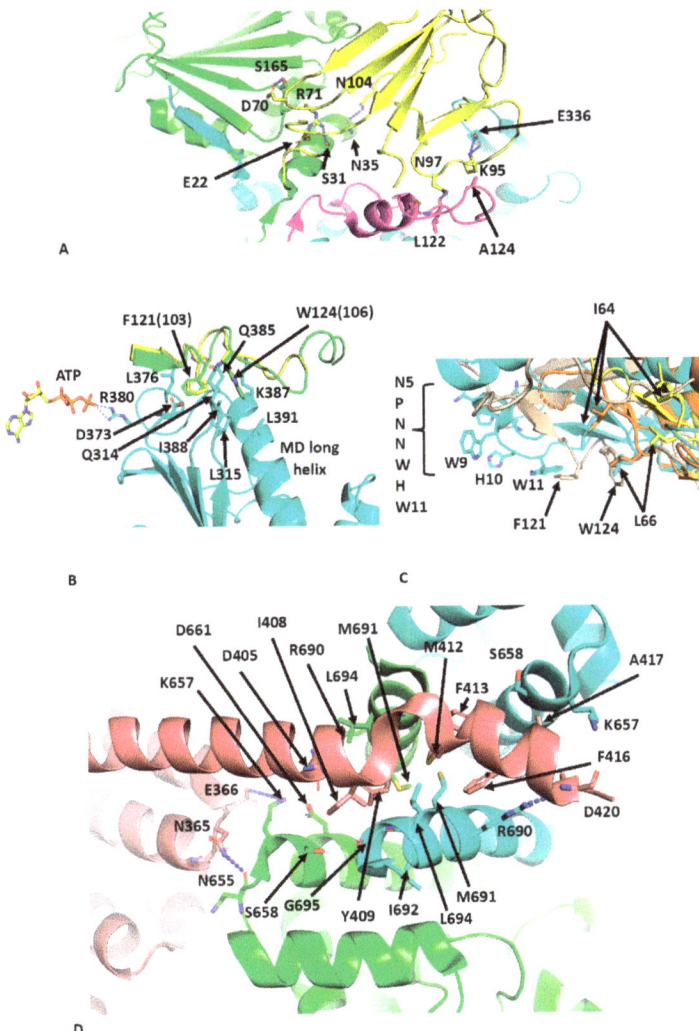

Figure 4. PyMol cartoons showing the Hsp90-p23 interactions. (**A**) Interaction of p23 (yellow) with the NTDs of both Hsp90 protomers (green and cyan) and the MDs of one Hsp90 protomer (magenta). (**B**) Interaction of the C-terminal unstructured segment of Sba1 (green) and p23 (yellow) with the long helix of the MD of Hsp90 (cyan). Numbers in brackets are for the human protein. (**C**) Comparison of the position of Phe 121 and W124 of Sba1 (wheat), which engage with the middle domain of Hsp90 (not shown) and the gradual engagement of specific Aha1 residues (yellow [apo-Hsp90-Aha1] to orange [Yeast Hsp90-Aha1] to cyan [Hsp90–AMPPNP–Aha1; fully tilted structure]) at similar positions with those from Sba1. Residues between Sba1 and Aha1 more or less overlap as the fully closed complex of the Hsp90–Aha1 complex is formed. Overlap of positions occur for Trp 11 and Leu 66 of Aha1, which mimic the position of Phe 121 and Trp124 of Sba1, respectively. (**D**) Interaction of the C-terminal helix 7 of FKBP51 (salmon) with the C-terminal hydrophobic pocket at the C-terminal dimer interface of Hsp90 (green and cyan). Interacting residues are shown in stick format and polar interactions as dotted blue lines.

There are many structures reporting the interaction of the conserved MEEVD motif of Hsp90 with TPR domain–containing proteins [50–53]. Recently, the cryo-EM structure of intact FKBP51 in complex with Hsp90 and p23 was reported (PDB 7L7I) [39]. The structure shows the expected TPR domain interaction with the MEEVD motif of Hsp90 but also an unexpected interaction with the C-terminal helix 7 extension of the TPR domain. The helix is kinked compared to the crystal structure of FKBP51 [54] and docks in a small hydrophobic cleft at the dimer interface at the C-terminal end of the CTD of Hsp90 (Figure 4D). Consequently, the stoichiometric binding of FKBP51, where helix 7 is also bound to dimeric Hsp90 is 1:1 [FKBP51: Hsp90 dimer]. FKBP51 helix residues Ile 408, Tyr 409, Met 412, Phe 413, Phe 416 and Ala 417 become unfolded and interact with Hsp90 residues that line the hydrophobic cleft (Leu 694, Lys 657, Ser 658, Asp 661, Arg 690, Met 691, Ile 692 and G695). Interestingly, Tyr 409, Met 412 and Phe 413 appear to be conserved among other immunophilin proteins. Additionally, the side-chain of Arg 690 from each Hsp90 protomer forms a salt bridge to the side-chains of Asp 405 and 420. Interactions are also seen between Hsp90 and residues on the H5–H6 loop of FKBP51, including the carboxyl main-chain of Asn 365 of FKBP51, which makes contact with the side-chain of Asn 655 in Hsp90 and possibly the side-chain of Asp 366 of FKBP51 with that of Lys 657 of Hsp90. Finally, some minor contacts are visible between the FK1 domain of FKBP51 and Hsp90 along the MD and adjacent to the substrate-binding loops. The affinity for the binding of FKBP51 was shown to be higher for the closed N-terminally dimerised state of Hsp90, and docking of the helix 7 extension with Hsp90 appears to be specific for the closed conformation of Hsp90 [39]. The catalytically active FK1 domain appears to be placed with its active site cleft facing the MD client–binding residues and modelling studies suggest that Pro 173 from CDK4 may be accessible to the active site of the FK1 domain [55]. Pro 173 is part of the highly conserved APE motif found at the base of the activation loop of kinases. Non-canonical APE motifs, such as AAE in ARAF, lead to a lower allosteric and catalytic activity as a result of a lower propensity to undergo homodimerisation, showing the importance of this motif in attaining an active state conformation [56]. The activation loop, including the APE motif, is very flexible [56,57] and the action of PPIase activity by immunophilins such as FKBP51 on the conserved proline residue may promote assembly of the activation segment into an active state. However, the mechanistic details that may link this to kinase dimerisation and activation, whether through allosteric activation and cis-autophosphorylation or by trans-phosphorylation [57–61], are yet to be established. However, it was also suggested that with particular clients, such as the glucocorticoid receptor (GR), that the FK1 domain may provide a scaffolding function and thus activation of GR is independent of the PPIase activity of the FK1 domain [39].

6. Hsp90–Hop–Hsp70–GR Loading Complex

Another client chaperone complex that was determined by cryo-EM is the loading complex for the glucocorticoid (GR) client with Hsp90, Hop and Hsp70 at 3.6 Å (PDB 7KW7) [62], which is thought to represent an early loading complex. The structure revealed some unexpected findings. Namely, two Hsp70 molecules were found in the complex, the first chaperoning the GR client and the second interacting with Hop, which itself was found to interact with all components within the complex. Within this structure, Hsp90 appears to adopt a semi-closed conformation, where the NTDs are oriented correctly but remain posed for dimerisation. The lid-segments of the NTDs remain open and are devoid of nucleotide, and the N-terminal β-strand, which can undergo strand exchange with the adjacent protomer, remains in place on its own NTD. The two Hsp70 molecules are bound by ADP and adopt an ADP-like conformation that is similar to that of the co-crystal structure (PDB 3AY9) [63]. Both Hsp70 molecules interact with Hsp90 in almost identical ways and there are two major interfaces between each Hsp70 molecule and its associated Hsp90 protomer. In the first heterodimeric interface a β-strand from the outer face of the MD β-sheet of Hsp90 inserts itself into the cleft between the subdomains IA and IIA of Hsp70 (Figure 5A). This cleft is only available in the ADP state of Hsp70. Side-chain interactions, within the first interface are seen between Lys 414, 418 and 419 of Hsp90 with the side-chains of Asp 213, 214 and 218 of Hsp70, respectively. In addition, the main-chain carbonyl of Asp 214 of Hsp70 makes a hydrogen bond with the side-chain Gln 334 of Hsp90, the main-chain amide of Gln 334 is hydrogen bonded to the carboxyl main-chain of Gly 215 of Hsp70 and the side-chain of Glu 332 of Hsp90 makes a set of interactions with the side-chains of Asn 174 and Thr 177 from Hsp70. Similarly, Arg 171 of Hsp70 makes side-chain interactions with Glu 336 and Asp 393 of Hsp90. In addition to these polar interactions there are several hydrophobic residues, Leu 334 and Val 411 from Hsp90 and Ile 216 and Phe 217 from Hsp70, which help to stabilise the interface. In the second interface between Hsp70 and Hsp90, Arg 60 and Tyr 61 of Hsp90 make side-chain interactions with Asp 160 from Hsp70 (Figure 5A). However, the presence of Hsp70 is incompatible with the closed N-terminally dimerised state of Hsp90, and transition to the closed state likely requires nucleotide exchange by an Hsp70 nucleotide exchange factor such as Bag1 in order to advance the complex.

Within the Hsp90–Hsp70–Hop–GR complex, only three domains of Hop were visible, TPR2A, TPR2B and the DP2 domain. These domains appear to be fully sufficient for full GR activation [64,65]. The TPR2A and TPR2B domains are bound by the conserved C-terminal -EEVD extensions of Hsp90 and Hsp70, respectively, and subdomain IIA of Hsp70 is found to be critical in positioning the relative positions of Hsp90 and HOP (Figure 5B). All three visible domains of HOP make contact with Hsp90 such that the Hsp90 protomers are fixed in their semi-closed conformation. Perhaps the most interesting interactions between HOP and Hsp90 are the interactions of the DP2 domain with two residues (Trp 606 and Met 614 in Hsp90a or Met 550 and Phe 554 in HTPG) previously identified in a set of conserved client-protein binding-site residues in HTPG (Glu 466, Trp 467, Asn 470, Met 546, Met 550, Leu 553 and Phe 554 and in human Hsp90α these are Glu 527, Tyr 528, Gln 531, Trp 606, Met 610, Ile 613 and Met 614, respectively) (Figure 5C) [66]. Collectively, a hydrophobic set of interactions involves Met 610, 614, 625 and 628, Ala 618 and Trp 606 from Hsp90 and Pro 502, Ala 503, Leu 506 and Ile 507 from DP2. In addition, a hydrogen bond is formed between the side-chains of Thr 624 of Hsp90 and Asp 501 from DP2 (Figure 5C).

Reminiscent in the way CDK4 is unfolded and passes through Hsp90 in the Hsp90–Cdc37–Cdk4 complex, the N-terminal segment of the GR domain threads through the lumen of Hsp90 (Figure 5D). While GR is poorly structured, some important interactions with Hsp90 can be inferred and include Trp 320 and Phe 349. In particular, Trp 320 (yeast Hsp82 Trp 300) was described as not only interacting with the GR (Figure 5D) but also with the DP2 domain of HOP and Aha1 as well as with the kinase client CDK4. Other potential interactions include the side-chain of Asp 626 of the GR with that of Thr 603 of Hsp90, the main-chain carbonyl of Lys 703 of the GR and the side-chain nitrogen of Lys 410 of Hsp90 and main-chain nitrogen of Lys 410 of the GR with the side-chain oxygen of Gln 405 of Hsp90 (Figure 5D). Residues from Ile 539 to Ser 550 of the GR pass through Hsp90 and connect to the GR ligand-binding domain (LBD) helix 1 that is cradled by a hydrophobic cleft in the DP2 domain of HOP (Figure 5E). The hydrophobic residues from the GR helix 1 include Leu 532, 533, 535 and 536, Val 538 and Ile 539 (conserved motif $L^{532}XXLL^{536}$) and residues forming the hydrophobic pocket of the DP2 domain include Met 499, Arg 505, Leu 508, Gln 512 and Leu 534 (Figure 5E). Finally, the upstream amino acid residues representing pre-helix-1 (residues Ala 523 to Thr 531) lead to Ser 519 through to Leu 525, which are bound within the substrate binding site of Hsp70 (Figure 5E). Overall, this complex holds the GR in an inactivated state, as is consistent with observations suggesting that Hsp70 inactivates hormone binding by the GR and that Hsp90 eventually restores its activity [67]. The loss of specific co-chaperones, such as Hsp70 and HOP, from the complex is therefore required for the maturation of the GR to the active state.

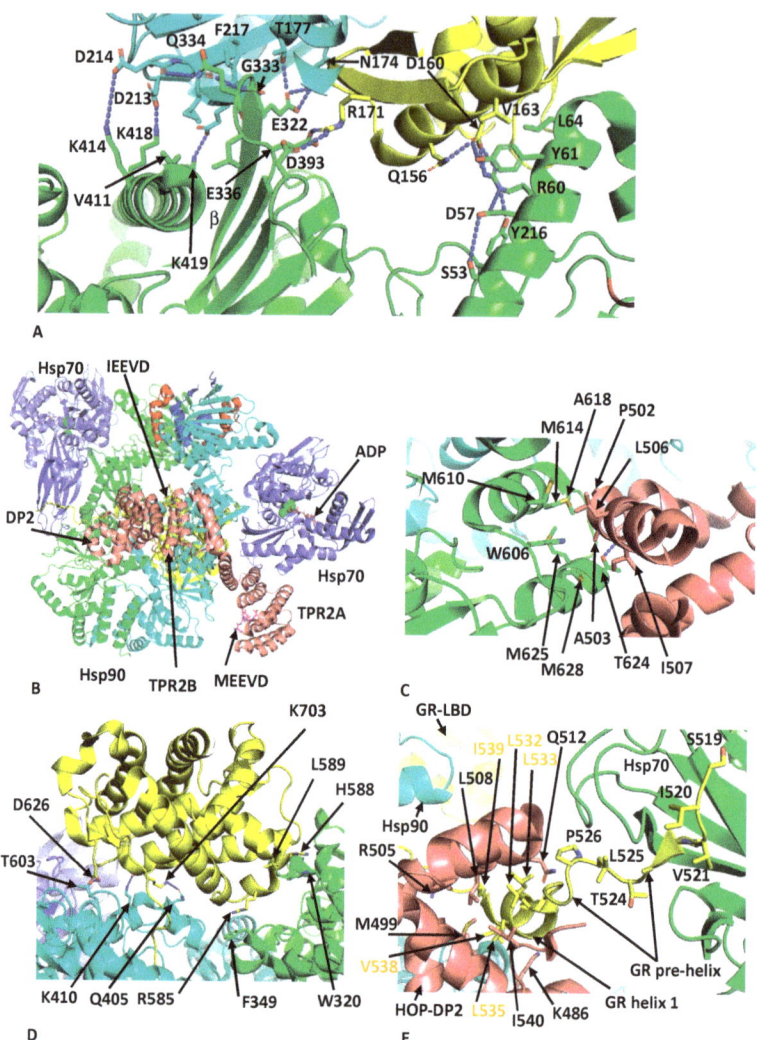

Figure 5. PyMol cartoons showing interactions within the Hsp90–Hsp70–HOP–GR loading complex. (**A**) Interface 1 and 2 of the Hsp90–Hsp70 interaction. A β-strand (β) from the outer face of the MD β-sheet of Hsp90 (green) inserts itself into the cleft between the subdomains IA and IIA of Hsp70 (cyan IIA and yellow, IA) in interface 1. This cleft is only available in the ADP state of Hsp70. Interface 2 is shown on the right-hand side of the panel. (**B**) The interaction of HOP and Hsp70 within the Hsp90–Hsp70–Hop-GR complex. Only three domains of Hop were visible, TPR2A, TPR2B and the DP2 domain, which appear to be fully sufficient for full GR activation. The binding of HOP is essential to maintaining the semi-closed conformation of Hsp90 and also for assembling the two bound Hsp70 molecules. Salmon, HOP; cyan and green, Hsp90 dimer; red, lid-segment of Hsp90; blue, N-terminal segments of Hsp90; and slate, Hsp70. (**C**) Interaction of the DP2 domain of HOP with the conserved client-protein binding-site residues of Hsp90. Green, Hsp90 dimer and salmon, HOP. (**D**) GR domain interactions with the Hsp90 complex. Yellow, GR; cyan and green, Hsp90 dimer; and slate, Hsp70. (**E**) Interaction of helix 1 and the pre-helix-1 segment of GR with DP2 and Hsp70, respectively. Yellow, GR; cyan, Hsp90; green, Hsp70 substrate-binding domain; and salmon, HOP DP2 domain.

7. Hsp90–p23–GR Maturation Complex

The cryo-EM structure of the Hsp90–p23–GR maturation complex was recently described and was determined at 2.56 Å (PDB 7KRJ) [40]. The Hsp90–p23 components are essentially similar in structure to that previously described for the nucleotide-bound yeast Hsp90–Sba1 structure, except that a single p23 molecule is bound on the same side as the bound GR. the GR is now remodelled from its loading complex and held in an active state conformation. With the loss of Hsp70 and HOP, helix 1 (Leu 532 to Ile 539) and the pre-helix-1 residues (Ala 523 to Thr 531) have retracted back towards the GR LBD (ligan binding domain). The pre-helix-1 is now held within the hydrophobic lumen of Hsp90 (Figure 6A). Leu 525 of the GR faces a hydrophobic pocket lined by Ile 525, Tyr 528, Leu 447 and His 450 and by Leu 619 from the other Hsp90 protomer. Leu 528 of the GR makes a similar set of interactions as Leu 525, but with the symmetry related residues (Ile 525, Tyr 528, Leu 447, His 450 and Leu 619) of the Hsp90 dimer. Some additional polar interactions occur between the carbonyl main-chain of Ala 523 of the GR and the side-chain amide group of His 450 of Hsp90, while the carbonyl main-chain of Thr 529 of the GR makes the symmetry related contact with the side-chain of His 450 in the other Hsp90 protomer (Figure 6A). The residues involved in the pre-helix interactions with Hsp90 were previously identified (HTPG, Glu 466, Trp 467 and Asn 470; Hsp90α, Glu 527, Tyr 528 and Gln 531 and Yeast Hsp90, Glu 507, Tyr 508 and Thr 511) or are close to amino acid residues forming a client-protein binding site, together with residues from an amphipathic helix (HTPG, residues Met 546 to Ala 555; Hsp90α, residues Trp 606 to Lys 615 and Yeast Hsp90, Trp 585 to Lys 594) [37]. The GR LBD also interacts with residues Trp 320 and Phe 349 from the adjacent Hsp90 protomer (Figure 6B). The side-chain of Trp 320 potentially forms a polar interaction with the main-chain carbonyl of Asn 586 and is also shielded by His 588 of the GR. In contrast, Phe 349 points towards a hydrophobic pocket lined by Gly 583, Asn 586, Leu 685, Ile, 689 and Thr 692. Finally, a potential polar interaction between the side-chain oxygen of Asn 586 of the GR and the side-chain of Arg 346 is seen (Figure 6B).

The remodelling of the GR in the Hsp90–GR–p23 complex sees helix 1 packing against the amphipathic helix of Hsp90 (Hsp90α, residues Trp 606 to Lys 615) and helixes 8 and 9 of the GR LBD (Figure 6C). Trp 606 of Hsp90 forms the hub of the hydrophobic interaction with the GR, packing up against Val 538 of helix 1 of the GR and the amphipathic helix residues of Hsp90, Met 610 and 614 (Figure 6C). Met 628 of Hsp90 is also packed between Leu 535 and Val 538 of helix 1 of the GR LBD. Finally, the side-chain carboxyl group Glu 537 from helix 1 forms a bipartite polar interaction with the side-chains of Gln 531 and Lys 534. Collectively, these interactions allow the GR LBD to adopt an active conformation, where helix 12 is in the agonist-bound state [68], and density is visible for an agonist, presumed to be dexamethasone present from the purification of the GR.

As seen with the yeast Hsp90–Sba1 structure [11], the C-terminal tail of p23 interacts with the long helix of the MD of Hsp90 and the catalytic-loop Arg 400 (yeast Hsp90 Arg 380) is in contact with the bound nucleotide (Figure 6D). Specifically, Phe 103 of p23 points towards a hydrophobic pocket lined by Leu 335, Asp 393, Pro 395 and Ile 408 of Hsp90. In contrast, Trp 106 of p23 sits between Leu 335, Lys 407, Ile 408 and Val 411 of Hsp90. In addition, the side-chain of Trp 106 of p23 forms a polar interaction with the side-chain of Gln 334 of Hsp90 (Figure 6D). Finally, the side-chains of Asp 108 and Asp 111 of p23 form salt bridges to the side-chain of Lys 414 of Hsp90. A relay of charged or polar interactions continues between the side-chains of Asp 112, 114 and 116 of p23 with Ser 708, Asn 171 and Lys 695 of the GR, respectively (Figure 6E). The extreme C-terminus of p23 then ends with a helix that interacts with the GR (Figure 6F). The side-chain of Asp 133 of p23 forms a polar interaction with the side-chain of Gln 713 of the GR. A series of hydrophobic residues from p23 (Met 117, Phe 123, Met 126, 127 and 130) are in hydrophobic interaction with Ser 709, Trp 712, Gln 713, Phe 715 and Tyr 716 of the GR (Figure 6F). Phe 123 and Met 127 of p23 also appear to stabilise the C-terminal tail of the GR by interacting with Phe 774 and His 775 (Figure 6G) and potentially helping to stabilise helix 12 of the GR in its agonist binding state. This study ultimately identified a conserved motif in the C-terminal tail of p23, FxxMMNxM, which was also identified in the coactivator 3 (NCoA3), which functions as a co-activator of steroid hormone receptors. In vitro ligand-binding studies showed that deletion of p23 residues beyond Asp 133 did not affect chaperone-mediated ligand binding. However, deletion of residues Ser 113 and beyond resulted in a reduction of such activity [40]. This suggested that other core components of the p23 interaction with Hsp90 are also important for GR activation. In contrast, in vivo studies showed that both the mutants reduced levels of activated GR, which may suggest that p23 has a more dominant downstream function after ligand binding.

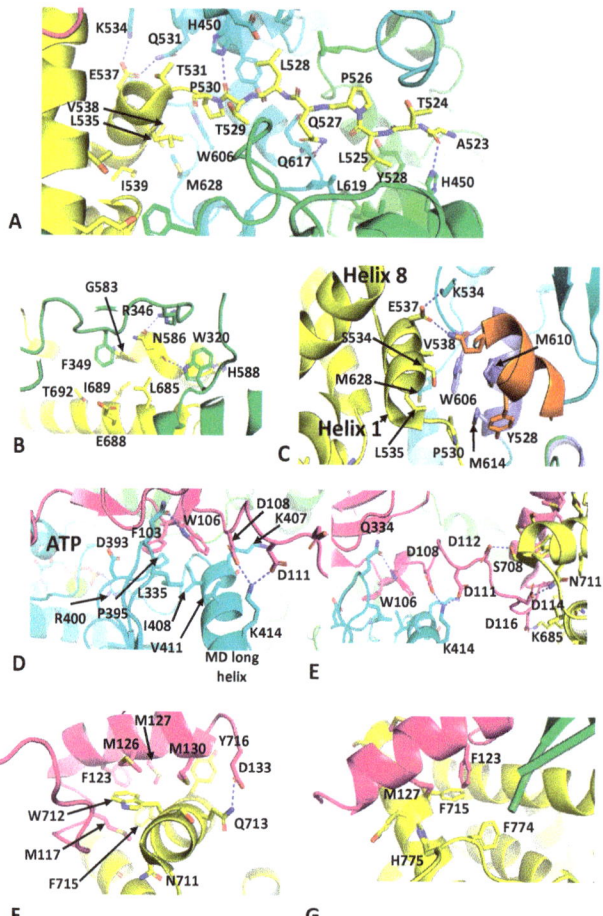

Figure 6. PyMol cartoon of the interactions of the Hsp90-p23-GR complex. (**A**) The pre-helix-1 held within the hydrophobic lumen of Hsp90. Yellow, GR; and cyan and green, Hsp90 dimer. (**B**) GR LBD (yellow) interacts with residues Trp 320 and Phe 349 from the adjacent Hsp90 protomer (green). (**C**) Helix 1 of GR packing against the amphipathic helix of Hsp90. Yellow, GR; cyan, Hsp90; and substrate binding sites of Hsp90 are shown in gold and slate (amphipathic helix). (**D**) The C-terminal tail of p23 (magenta) interacts with the long helix of the MD of Hsp90 (cyan and green) and the catalytic Arg 400 is in contact with the bound nucleotide (stick representation). (**E**) A relay of polar interactions between the C-terminal tail of p23 (magenta) and Hsp90 (cyan and green) and GR (yellow). (**F**,**G**) The extreme C-terminus helix of p23 (magenta) interacts with GR (yellow).

8. The GR Activation Cycle

Collectively, the structures of the loading and maturation complex of the GR, as well as numerous biochemical studies, suggest a series of steps that lead to the activation of the GR [40,62,67,69]. The first step in the activation cycle of the GR is the stabilisation and inactivation of the GR by Hsp70 and capture of the GR is dependent on Hsp40 and ATP hydrolysis by Hsp70 [70–72] (Figure 7). In this state, the ligand bound to the GR would be released. Meanwhile, the binding of HOP to Hsp90 preassembles Hsp90 in order to receive the Hsp70–GR client complex [62,69,73]. The main interaction of HOP is with the MD–CTD junction of Hsp90 and prevents its rotation to a conformation that would allow Hsp90 N-terminal dimerisation [69]. Specifically, the TPR1 domain of HOP sterically blocks the N-terminal dimerisation of Hsp90 by binding between the Hsp90 monomers, while simultaneously interacting with the adjacent MD and CTD of Hsp90. Step 2 of the activation cycle was captured by the cryo-EM structure of the Hsp90–Hsp70–HOP–GR complex [62]. The structure reveals how the Hsp70–GR client complex initially associates with the preassembled Hsp90–HOP complex. In this complex the pre-helix-1 segment of the GR is captured by Hsp70 and helix 1 stabilised by the DP2 domain of HOP (Figure 5E). Interaction with Hsp90 allows the GR post-helix-1 segment to thread through a semi-closed Hsp90. The NTDs of two Hsp70 molecules that were found bound to Hsp90 interact with the NTD of Hsp90, thus providing a link between the ATPase activity of Hsp70 and Hsp90, where the Hsp90 lid-segments are close to the Hsp70 interaction interface with Hsp90. In this state, the GR is held in an inactive conformation (Figure 7). In step 3, ATP binding to Hsp90 and its hydrolysis leads to the release of Hsp70 and HOP from the complex [67]. Evidence suggests that this is a direct result of the hydrolysis of ATP by Hsp90, rather than direct action by a nucleotide exchange factor such as Bag-1 acting on Hsp70. Instead, Bag-1 may play a role in stalled Hsp90–client complexes [67]. It was suggested that during the transition from the Hsp70-present to the Hsp70-absent complex with Hsp90, hormone could bind to the GR LBD. The product of step 3 is captured by the Hsp90–p23–GR cryo-EM structure [40], which is able to bind cortisol. This structure shows how remodelling of the GR allows pre-helix-1, previously held by Hsp70, to move into the lumen of the fully closed Hsp90 molecule and simultaneously may allow helix 1 to associate with the GR LBD and seal the hormone binding pocket. This suggests that the hormone needs to have already bound to the GR. Within this complex, p23, the binding of which is favoured by the fully closed conformation of Hsp90, appears to facilitate the activation of the GR. Firstly, it stabilises the closed conformation of Hsp90, and secondly, it plays a role in stabilising the dynamic helix 12 of the GR in its agonist-binding conformation [40]. In step 4, activated GR must be released from the complex, but it remains unclear what the trigger for this is. However, results show that the activation of the GR is enhanced by the presence of p23 in a fully reconstituted chaperone system that contains Hsp90, Hsp70, Hsp40, HOP and the GR LBD. This suggests that the action of p23 appears to occur prior to the GR–helix 1 capping of hormone access to the LBD of the GR. This may indicate that release of the GR from the Hsp90 complex occurs as a direct result of hormone binding [67]. Clearly, some finer details of the cycle need to be established.

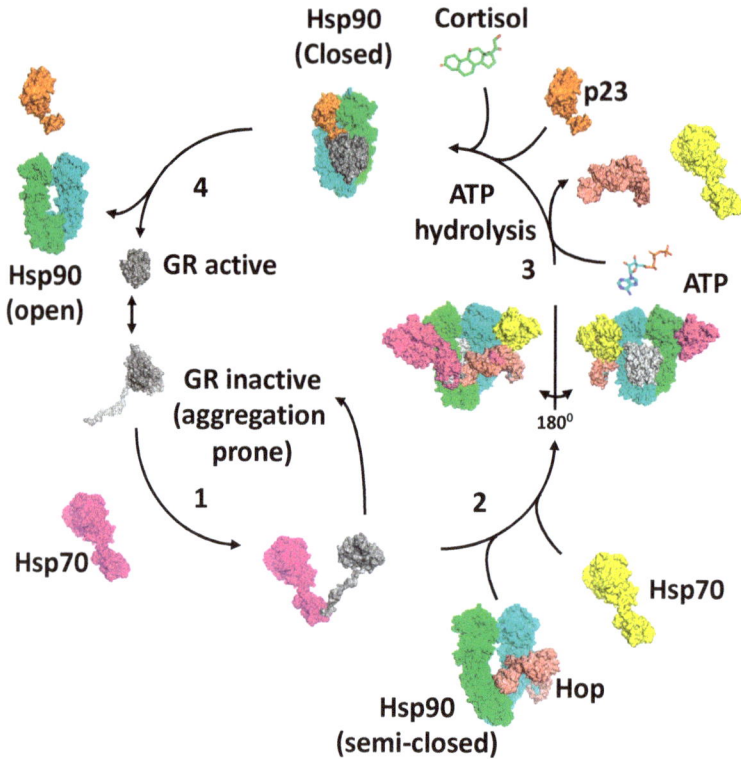

Figure 7. The proposed GR activation cycle. 1 to 4 represents the steps of the cycle. Grey, GR LBD; magenta and yellow, Hsp70; green and cyan, Hsp90 dimer; salmon, HOP; and orange, p23.

9. Hsp90–Tau Complex and Hsp90–FKBP51–Tau Complex

Tau stabilises microtubules that serve as tracks during axonal transport within neurons [74]. Hsp90 can help stabilise and bring about proteasomal degradation of Tau [75]. Unlike CDK4 and the GR LBD, Tau is classified as a partially unfolded protein. Hsc70 can associate with Tau, specifically recognising two motifs (^{275}VQIIN^{279} and ^{306}VQIVY^{310}), and bring about some core domain folding, but significant regions of Tau remain unfolded [76]. Hsp90 has been shown to recognise Tau directly, without co-chaperone delivery [77], which may reflect the fact that Tau is significantly unfolded. The K_D for Hsp90–Tau association was determined to be approximately 4.8 µM and ATPγS did not alter binding affinity [77].

Using an NMR approach, together with small angle scattering, a structural model was obtained for the interaction between Hsp90 and Tau [77]. Hsp90 was found to recognise a broad region of Tau, including its aggregation-prone repeats and the Hsc70 binding motifs. Specifically, regions ^{226}VAVVRT^{231}, ^{244}QTAPV^{248}, ^{275}VQIINK^{280}, ^{306}VQVYK^{311}, ^{340}KSEKL^{344} and ^{377}TRFEN^{381} are bound and, interestingly, these motifs have been implicated in Alzheimer's disease [78]. Collectively, these regions represent hydrophobic centres with a propensity for a positive net charge, although it was also noted that negative charges were not wholly excluded. It was concluded that it is these specific properties of Tau, rather than its unfolded nature, that are the contributing factor for Hsp90 binding [77], although access to such motifs is obviously paramount. The distribution of the hydrophobic Tau residues appears to resemble those of the exposed residues in the intermediates of folding Tau.

By employing specific isotope labelling of isoleucine methyl side-chains and methyl transverse relaxation–optimised spectroscopy (methyl-TROSY) a subset of Hsp90 residues

(Ile, 20, 74, 90, 369 and 440) were implicated in the binding of Tau, indicating a broad Hsp90 binding surface that included both the NTD and MD of Hsp90. Together with Tau, ATPγS was seen to modulate the dynamics of Hsp90 and that the presence of Tau breaks Hsp90 symmetry, as seen with other client protein complexes (CDK4 and the GR). The most intense binding areas of Hsp90 included residues in both the NTDs and MDs of Hsp90, including Leu 24 and 27, Phe 32, Ile 105 and Ala 106 in the NTD and Leu 388, Ile 390, Phe 344, Lys 406 and 410 and Thr 446 in the MD of Hsp90 (Uniprot entry P08238 and numbering from Met 1). These hydrophobic residues compliment interactions between charged residues of Hsp90, including Glu 81 and 393 and Asp 367 and 518 and positive charged segments within Tau. The extensive binding region of Hsp90 appears to allow a high number of low affinity contacts with Tau.

Another methyl-TROSY study looked at the Hsp90–FKBP51–Tau complex [79]. Association of FKBP51 with the Hsp90–Tau complex can promote amorphous aggregation of Tau [80–82]. Hsp90 residues affected by FKBP51 titration appear to include the loop around the catalytic arginine in the MD of Hsp90 but also the residues that appear to line the internal surface of the Hsp90 dimer. This is in contrast to the FKBP51 interactions seen in the closed Hsp90–p23–FKBP51 complex [39]. All domains of FKBP51 were implicated in binding the open conformation of Hsp90. Essentially, Hsp90 and FKBP51 are arranged in a head-to-head topology, where the NTD, MD and CTD of Hsp90 interact with the FK1 domain, the FK1 and FK1-TPR domains and the FK2-TPR domains of FKBP51, respectively. Significantly, the NTD of Hsp90 is rotated away from the catalytic residue of the MD of Hsp90 and the catalytic PPIase pocket of the FK1 domain is solvent accessible. The study also showed that FKBP51 binding helps to stabilise the Hsp90-Tau complex and that Tau's proline-rich region clusters close to the catalytically active FK1 PPIase domain. These proline-rich segments are also sites of Tau phosphorylation, and it was proposed that alteration of the normal proline isomerisation of Tau could lead to enhanced oligomerisation and an increased susceptibility to Alzheimer's disease [80].

10. Concluding Remarks

X-ray crystallography and biochemical studies have identified an Hsp90 ATPase-driven catalytic cycle that is essential for the activation and maturation of client proteins. The role of a variety of co-chaperones was systematically determined and a variety of co-chaperone and client–protein binding sites on Hsp90 were identified, which advanced our understanding of the regulation of the cycle. However, the mechanistic details by which client proteins were activated remain enigmatic due to the structural complexity of Hsp90 client protein complexes. Thus, a unified mechanism of action was not easy to establish.

Recent advances in cryo-EM have now enabled us to understand how Hsp90 recognises client proteins and how it brings about their activation or maturation mechanistically. It appears that clients such as the GR and CDK4 are structurally dynamic and prone to aggregation. These unstable conformations can be captured by Hsp70 or co-chaperones such as Cdc37, stabilising their conformations and allowing their delivery to Hsp90. Other co-chaperones may preassemble Hsp90 so that it is competent for client protein binding and this appears to be a role that HOP plays in the activation of the GR. Other clients, such as Tau, that are inherently unfolded appear to bypass a co-chaperone loading stage, as their binding conformation is accessible to Hsp90. However, this does not necessarily exclude the possibility that Hsp90 might be preassembled for their interaction by a yet undefined co-chaperone. Ultimately, the Hsp90 cycle remodels the client protein towards a state that leads eventually to its activation, either by binding a small molecule hormone, as in the case of the GR, or by refolding, as in the case of kinases.

A series of aromatic residues on Hsp90 appear to play important roles in client protein and co-chaperone recognition that may also be important for communicating the bound state of the Hsp90 complex to features of Hsp90 that carry out ATP hydrolysis. Thus, these aromatic residues may link the presence of client or co-chaperones in the Hsp90 complex to the ATPase activity of Hsp90. Finally, the advances in describing the mechanistic details by which client proteins are activated by Hsp90 will increase our understanding of the underlying mechanisms of disease caused by the dysregulation of the Hsp90 client–protein system. It is clear that we are now entering into a new era for Hsp90 research that will see novel ways of targeting Hsp90-associated disease.

Funding: This research received no external funding.

Institutional Review Board Statement: Not applicable.

Informed Consent Statement: Not applicable.

Data Availability Statement: Not applicable.

Acknowledgments: I would sincerely like to thank the 'Biomolecules' Journal for waiving the publication charges for this review.

Conflicts of Interest: The authors declare no conflict of interest.

References

1. Biebl, M.M.; Buchner, J. Structure, Function, and Regulation of the Hsp90 Machinery. *Cold Spring Harb. Perspect. Biol.* **2019**, *11*, a034017. [CrossRef] [PubMed]
2. Prodromou, C. Mechanisms of Hsp90 regulation. *Biochem. J.* **2016**, *473*, 2439–2452. [CrossRef] [PubMed]
3. Prodromou, C. The "active life" of Hsp90 complexes. *Biochim. Biophys. Acta* **2012**, *1823*, 614–623. [CrossRef] [PubMed]
4. Prodromou, C.; Morgan, R.M.L. Tuning the ATPase Activity of Hsp90. In *Regulation of Ca2+-ATPases, V-ATPases and F-ATPases. Advances in Biochemistry in Health and Disease*; Chakraborti, S., Dhalla, N.S., Eds.; Springer: Cham, Switzerland, 2016; Volume 14, pp. 469–490.
5. Meyer, P.; Prodromou, C.; Liao, C.; Hu, B.; Roe, S.M.; Vaughan, C.K.; Vlasic, I.; Panaretou, B.; Piper, P.W.; Pearl, L.H. Structural basis for recruitment of the ATPase activator Aha1 to the Hsp90 chaperone machinery. *EMBO J.* **2004**, *23*, 1402–1410. [CrossRef] [PubMed]
6. Prodromou, C.; Panaretou, B.; Chohan, S.; Siligardi, G.; O'Brien, R.; Ladbury, J.E.; Roe, S.M.; Piper, P.W.; Pearl, L.H. The ATPase cycle of Hsp90 drives a molecular "clamp" via transient dimerization of the N-terminal domains. *EMBO J.* **2000**, *19*, 4383–4392. [CrossRef]
7. Xu, H. ATP-Driven Nonequilibrium Activation of Kinase Clients by the Molecular Chaperone Hsp90. *Biophys. J.* **2020**, *119*, 1538–1549. [CrossRef]
8. Liu, Y.; Sun, M.; Alexander, G.M.; Elnatan, D.; Delaeter, N.; Nguyenquang, M.; Agard, D.A. Cryo-EM structures reveal a multistep mechanism of Hsp90 activation by co-chaperone Aha1. *bioRxiv* **2020**, in press. [CrossRef]
9. Schulze, A.; Beliu, G.; Helmerich, D.A.; Schubert, J.; Pearl, L.H.; Prodromou, C.; Neuweiler, H. Cooperation of local motions in the Hsp90 molecular chaperone ATPase mechanism. *Nat. Chem. Biol.* **2016**, *12*, 628–635. [CrossRef]
10. Schubert, J.; Schulze, A.; Prodromou, C.; Neuweiler, H. Two-colour single-molecule photoinduced electron transfer fluorescence imaging microscopy of chaperone dynamics. *Nat. Commun.* **2021**, *12*, 6964. [CrossRef]
11. Ali, M.M.; Roe, S.M.; Vaughan, C.K.; Meyer, P.; Panaretou, B.; Piper, P.W.; Prodromou, C.; Pearl, L.H. Crystal structure of an Hsp90-nucleotide-p23/Sba1 closed chaperone complex. *Nature* **2006**, *440*, 1013–1017. [CrossRef]
12. Roe, S.M.; Ali, M.M.; Meyer, P.; Vaughan, C.K.; Panaretou, B.; Piper, P.W.; Prodromou, C.; Pearl, L.H. The Mechanism of Hsp90 Regulation by the Protein Kinase-Specific Cochaperone p50(cdc37). *Cell* **2004**, *116*, 87–98. [CrossRef]
13. Verba, K.A.; Wang, R.Y.; Arakawa, A.; Liu, Y.; Shirouzu, M.; Yokoyama, S.; Agard, D.A. Atomic structure of Hsp90-Cdc37-Cdk4 reveals that Hsp90 traps and stabilizes an unfolded kinase. *Science* **2016**, *352*, 1542–1547. [CrossRef] [PubMed]
14. Li, J.; Buchner, J. Structure, function and regulation of the hsp90 machinery. *Biomed. J.* **2013**, *36*, 106–117. [CrossRef] [PubMed]
15. Hoter, A.; El-Sabban, M.E.; Naim, H.Y. The HSP90 Family: Structure, Regulation, Function, and Implications in Health and Disease. *Int. J. Mol. Sci.* **2018**, *19*, 2560. [CrossRef] [PubMed]
16. Genest, O.; Wickner, S.; Doyle, S.M. Hsp90 and Hsp70 chaperones: Collaborators in protein remodeling. *J. Biol. Chem.* **2019**, *294*, 2109–2120. [CrossRef]
17. Sauer, M.; Neuweiler, H. PET-FCS: Probing rapid structural fluctuations of proteins and nucleic acids by single-molecule fluorescence quenching. *Methods Mol. Biol.* **2014**, *1076*, 597–615. [CrossRef] [PubMed]
18. Hessling, M.; Richter, K.; Buchner, J. Dissection of the ATP-induced conformational cycle of the molecular chaperone Hsp90. *Nat. Struct. Mol. Biol.* **2009**, *16*, 287–293. [CrossRef]
19. Siligardi, G.; Hu, B.; Panaretou, B.; Piper, P.W.; Pearl, L.H.; Prodromou, C. Co-chaperone regulation of conformational switching in the Hsp90 ATPase cycle. *J. Biol. Chem.* **2004**, *279*, 51989–51998. [CrossRef]
20. Li, J.; Richter, K.; Reinstein, J.; Buchner, J. Integration of the accelerator Aha1 in the Hsp90 co-chaperone cycle. *Nat. Struct. Mol. Biol.* **2013**, *20*, 326–331. [CrossRef]
21. Retzlaff, M.; Hagn, F.; Mitschke, L.; Hessling, M.; Gugel, F.; Kessler, H.; Richter, K.; Buchner, J. Asymmetric activation of the hsp90 dimer by its cochaperone aha1. *Mol. Cell* **2010**, *37*, 344–354. [CrossRef]

22. Doose, S.; Neuweiler, H.; Sauer, M. Fluorescence quenching by photoinduced electron transfer: A reporter for conformational dynamics of macromolecules. *Chemphyschem* **2009**, *10*, 1389–1398. [CrossRef] [PubMed]
23. Dollins, D.E.; Warren, J.J.; Immormino, R.M.; Gewirth, D.T. Structures of GRP94-nucleotide complexes reveal mechanistic differences between the hsp90 chaperones. *Mol. Cell* **2007**, *28*, 41–56. [CrossRef] [PubMed]
24. Frey, S.; Leskovar, A.; Reinstein, J.; Buchner, J. The ATPase cycle of the endoplasmic chaperone Grp94. *J. Biol. Chem.* **2007**, *282*, 35612–35620. [CrossRef] [PubMed]
25. McLaughlin, S.H.; Smith, H.W.; Jackson, S.E. Stimulation of the weak ATPase activity of human hsp90 by a client protein. *J. Mol. Biol.* **2002**, *315*, 787–798. [CrossRef] [PubMed]
26. Richter, K.; Soroka, J.; Skalniak, L.; Leskovar, A.; Hessling, M.; Reinstein, J.; Buchner, J. Conserved conformational changes in the ATPase cycle of human Hsp90. *J. Biol. Chem.* **2008**, *283*, 17757–17765. [CrossRef]
27. Cunningham, C.N.; Krukenberg, K.A.; Agard, D.A. Intra- and intermonomer interactions are required to synergistically facilitate ATP hydrolysis in Hsp90. *J. Biol. Chem.* **2008**, *283*, 21170–21178. [CrossRef]
28. Richter, K.; Muschler, P.; Hainzl, O.; Buchner, J. Coordinated ATP hydrolysis by the Hsp90 dimer. *J. Biol. Chem.* **2001**, *276*, 33689–33696. [CrossRef]
29. Elnatan, D.; Betegon, M.; Liu, Y.; Ramelot, T.; Kennedy, M.A.; Agard, D.A. Symmetry broken and rebroken during the ATP hydrolysis cycle of the mitochondrial Hsp90 TRAP1. *Elife* **2017**, *6*, e25235. [CrossRef]
30. Siligardi, G.; Panaretou, B.; Meyer, P.; Singh, S.; Woolfson, D.N.; Piper, P.W.; Pearl, L.H.; Prodromou, C. Regulation of Hsp90 ATPase activity by the co-chaperone Cdc37p/p50cdc37. *J. Biol. Chem.* **2002**, *277*, 20151–20159. [CrossRef]
31. Vaughan, C.K.; Gohlke, U.; Sobott, F.; Good, V.M.; Ali, M.M.; Prodromou, C.; Robinson, C.V.; Saibil, H.R.; Pearl, L.H. Structure of an Hsp90-Cdc37-Cdk4 complex. *Mol. Cell* **2006**, *23*, 697–707. [CrossRef]
32. Meyer, P.; Prodromou, C.; Hu, B.; Vaughan, C.; Roe, S.M.; Panaretou, B.; Piper, P.W.; Pearl, L.H. Structural and functional analysis of the middle segment of hsp90: Implications for ATP hydrolysis and client protein and cochaperone interactions. *Mol. Cell* **2003**, *11*, 647–658. [CrossRef]
33. Keramisanou, D.; Aboalroub, A.; Zhang, Z.; Liu, W.; Marshall, D.; Diviney, A.; Larsen, R.W.; Landgraf, R.; Gelis, I. Molecular Mechanism of Protein Kinase Recognition and Sorting by the Hsp90 Kinome-Specific Cochaperone Cdc37. *Mol. Cell* **2016**, *62*, 260–271. [CrossRef] [PubMed]
34. Vaughan, C.K.; Mollapour, M.; Smith, J.R.; Truman, A.; Hu, B.; Good, V.M.; Panaretou, B.; Neckers, L.; Clarke, P.A.; Workman, P.; et al. Hsp90-dependent activation of protein kinases is regulated by chaperone-targeted dephosphorylation of Cdc37. *Mol. Cell* **2008**, *31*, 886–895. [CrossRef]
35. Panaretou, B.; Siligardi, G.; Meyer, P.; Maloney, A.; Sullivan, J.K.; Singh, S.; Millson, S.H.; Clarke, P.A.; Naaby-Hansen, S.; Stein, R.; et al. Activation of the ATPase activity of hsp90 by the stress-regulated cochaperone aha1. *Mol. Cell* **2002**, *10*, 1307–1318. [CrossRef]
36. Hu, H.; Wang, Q.; Du, J.; Liu, Z.; Ding, Y.; Xue, H.; Zhou, C.; Feng, L.; Zhang, N. Aha1 Exhibits Distinctive Dynamics Behavior and Chaperone-Like Activity. *Molecules* **2021**, *26*, 1943. [CrossRef] [PubMed]
37. Genest, O.; Reidy, M.; Street, T.O.; Hoskins, J.R.; Camberg, J.L.; Agard, D.A.; Masison, D.C.; Wickner, S. Uncovering a region of heat shock protein 90 important for client binding in E. coli and chaperone function in yeast. *Mol. Cell* **2013**, *49*, 464–473. [CrossRef]
38. Mercier, R.; Wolmarans, A.; Schubert, J.; Neuweiler, H.; Johnson, J.L.; LaPointe, P. The conserved NxNNWHW motif in Aha-type co-chaperones modulates the kinetics of Hsp90 ATPase stimulation. *Nat. Commun.* **2019**, *10*, 1273. [CrossRef]
39. Lee, K.; Thwin, A.C.; Nadel, C.M.; Tse, E.; Gates, S.N.; Gestwicki, J.E.; Southworth, D.R. The structure of an Hsp90-immunophilin complex reveals cochaperone recognition of the client maturation state. *Mol. Cell* **2021**, *81*, 3496–3508.e5. [CrossRef]
40. Noddings, C.M.; Wang, R.Y.; Johnson, J.L.; Agard, D.A. Structure of Hsp90-p23-GR reveals the Hsp90 client-remodelling mechanism. *Nature* **2022**, *601*, 465–469. [CrossRef]
41. Zgajnar, N.R.; De Leo, S.A.; Lotufo, C.M.; Erlejman, A.G.; Piwien-Pilipuk, G.; Galigniana, M.D. Biological Actions of the Hsp90-binding Immunophilins FKBP51 and FKBP52. *Biomolecules* **2019**, *9*, 52. [CrossRef]
42. Grad, I.; Picard, D. The glucocorticoid responses are shaped by molecular chaperones. *Mol. Cell Endocrinol.* **2007**, *275*, 2–12. [CrossRef] [PubMed]
43. Pratt, W.B.; Toft, D.O. Steroid receptor interactions with heat shock protein and immunophilin chaperones. *Endocrinol. Rev.* **1997**, *18*, 306–360.
44. Wochnik, G.M.; Ruegg, J.; Abel, G.A.; Schmidt, U.; Holsboer, F.; Rein, T. FK506-binding proteins 51 and 52 differentially regulate dynein interaction and nuclear translocation of the glucocorticoid receptor in mammalian cells. *J. Biol. Chem.* **2005**, *280*, 4609–4616. [CrossRef]
45. Riggs, D.L.; Roberts, P.J.; Chirillo, S.C.; Cheung-Flynn, J.; Prapapanich, V.; Ratajczak, T.; Gaber, R.; Picard, D.; Smith, D.F. The Hsp90-binding peptidylprolyl isomerase FKBP52 potentiates glucocorticoid signaling in vivo. *EMBO J.* **2003**, *22*, 1158–1167. [CrossRef] [PubMed]
46. Storer, C.L.; Dickey, C.A.; Galigniana, M.D.; Rein, T.; Cox, M.B. FKBP51 and FKBP52 in signaling and disease. *Trends Endocrinol. Metab.* **2011**, *22*, 481–490. [CrossRef]
47. Pratt, W.B.; Morishima, Y.; Murphy, M.; Harrell, M. Chaperoning of glucocorticoid receptors. In *Handbook of Experimental Pharmacology*; Springer: Berlin/Heidelberg, Germany, 2006; pp. 111–138.

48. Dittmar, K.D.; Demady, D.R.; Stancato, L.F.; Krishna, P.; Pratt, W.B. Folding of the glucocorticoid receptor by the heat shock protein (hsp) 90-based chaperone machinery. The role of P23 is to stabilize receptor-hsp90 heterocomplexes formed by hsp90-p60-hsp70. *J. Biol. Chem.* **1997**, *272*, 21213–21220. [CrossRef]
49. McLaughlin, S.H.; Sobott, F.; Yao, Z.P.; Zhang, W.; Nielsen, P.R.; Grossmann, J.G.; Laue, E.D.; Robinson, C.V.; Jackson, S.E. The co-chaperone p23 arrests the Hsp90 ATPase cycle to trap client proteins. *J. Mol. Biol.* **2006**, *356*, 746–758. [CrossRef]
50. Morgan, R.M.; Hernandez-Ramirez, L.C.; Trivellin, G.; Zhou, L.; Roe, S.M.; Korbonits, M.; Prodromou, C. Structure of the TPR domain of AIP: Lack of client protein interaction with the C-terminal alpha-7 helix of the TPR domain of AIP is sufficient for pituitary adenoma predisposition. *PLoS ONE* **2012**, *7*, e53339. [CrossRef]
51. Millson, S.H.; Vaughan, C.K.; Zhai, C.; Ali, M.M.; Panaretou, B.; Piper, P.W.; Pearl, L.H.; Prodromou, C. Chaperone ligand-discrimination by the TPR-domain protein Tah1. *Biochem. J.* **2008**, *413*, 261–268. [CrossRef]
52. Blundell, K.L.; Pal, M.; Roe, S.M.; Pearl, L.H.; Prodromou, C. The structure of FKBP38 in complex with the MEEVD tetratricopeptide binding-motif of Hsp90. *PLoS ONE* **2017**, *12*, e0173543. [CrossRef]
53. Scheufler, C.; Brinker, A.; Bourenkov, G.; Pegoraro, S.; Moroder, L.; Bartunik, H.; Hartl, F.U.; Moarefi, I. Structure of TPR domain-peptide complexes: Critical elements in the assembly of the Hsp70-Hsp90 multichaperone machine. *Cell* **2000**, *101*, 199–210. [CrossRef]
54. Sinars, C.R.; Cheung-Flynn, J.; Rimerman, R.A.; Scammell, J.G.; Smith, D.F.; Clardy, J. Structure of the large FK506-binding protein FKBP51, an Hsp90-binding protein and a component of steroid receptor complexes. *Proc. Natl. Acad. Sci. USA* **2003**, *100*, 868–873. [CrossRef] [PubMed]
55. Ruiz-Estevez, M.; Staats, J.; Paatela, E.; Munson, D.; Katoku-Kikyo, N.; Yuan, C.; Asakura, Y.; Hostager, R.; Kobayashi, H.; Asakura, A.; et al. Promotion of Myoblast Differentiation by Fkbp5 via Cdk4 Isomerization. *Cell Rep.* **2018**, *25*, 2537–2551.e8. [CrossRef] [PubMed]
56. Yuan, J.; Ng, W.H.; Lam, P.Y.P.; Wang, Y.; Xia, H.; Yap, J.; Guan, S.P.; Lee, A.S.G.; Wang, M.; Baccarini, M.; et al. The dimer-dependent catalytic activity of RAF family kinases is revealed through characterizing their oncogenic mutants. *Oncogene* **2018**, *37*, 5719–5734. [CrossRef]
57. Gogl, G.; Kornev, A.P.; Remenyi, A.; Taylor, S.S. Disordered Protein Kinase Regions in Regulation of Kinase Domain Cores. *Trends Biochem. Sci.* **2019**, *44*, 300–311. [CrossRef]
58. Desideri, E.; Cavallo, A.L.; Baccarini, M. Alike but Different: RAF Paralogs and Their Signaling Outputs. *Cell* **2015**, *161*, 967–970. [CrossRef]
59. Lavoie, H.; Therrien, M. Regulation of RAF protein kinases in ERK signalling. *Nat. Rev. Mol. Cell Biol.* **2015**, *16*, 281–298. [CrossRef]
60. Roring, M.; Herr, R.; Fiala, G.J.; Heilmann, K.; Braun, S.; Eisenhardt, A.E.; Halbach, S.; Capper, D.; von Deimling, A.; Schamel, W.W.; et al. Distinct requirement for an intact dimer interface in wild-type, V600E and kinase-dead B-Raf signalling. *EMBO J.* **2012**, *31*, 2629–2647. [CrossRef]
61. Kohler, M.; Brummer, T. B-Raf activation loop phosphorylation revisited. *Cell Cycle* **2016**, *15*, 1171–1173. [CrossRef]
62. Wang, R.Y.; Noddings, C.M.; Kirschke, E.; Myasnikov, A.G.; Johnson, J.L.; Agard, D.A. Structure of Hsp90-Hsp70-Hop-GR reveals the Hsp90 client-loading mechanism. *Nature* **2022**, *601*, 460–464. [CrossRef]
63. Arakawa, A.; Handa, N.; Shirouzu, M.; Yokoyama, S. Biochemical and structural studies on the high affinity of Hsp70 for ADP. *Protein Sci.* **2011**, *20*, 1367–1379. [CrossRef] [PubMed]
64. Schmid, A.B.; Lagleder, S.; Grawert, M.A.; Rohl, A.; Hagn, F.; Wandinger, S.K.; Cox, M.B.; Demmer, O.; Richter, K.; Groll, M.; et al. The architecture of functional modules in the Hsp90 co-chaperone Sti1/Hop. *EMBO J.* **2012**, *31*, 1506–1517. [CrossRef] [PubMed]
65. Rohl, A.; Wengler, D.; Madl, T.; Lagleder, S.; Tippel, F.; Herrmann, M.; Hendrix, J.; Richter, K.; Hack, G.; Schmid, A.B.; et al. Hsp90 regulates the dynamics of its cochaperone Sti1 and the transfer of Hsp70 between modules. *Nat. Commun.* **2015**, *6*, 6655. [CrossRef] [PubMed]
66. Reidy, M.; Kumar, S.; Anderson, D.E.; Masison, D.C. Dual Roles for Yeast Sti1/Hop in Regulating the Hsp90 Chaperone Cycle. *Genetics* **2018**, *209*, 1139–1154. [CrossRef]
67. Kirschke, E.; Goswami, D.; Southworth, D.; Griffin, P.R.; Agard, D.A. Glucocorticoid receptor function regulated by coordinated action of the Hsp90 and Hsp70 chaperone cycles. *Cell* **2014**, *157*, 1685–1697. [CrossRef] [PubMed]
68. Bledsoe, R.K.; Montana, V.G.; Stanley, T.B.; Delves, C.J.; Apolito, C.J.; McKee, D.D.; Consler, T.G.; Parks, D.J.; Stewart, E.L.; Willson, T.M.; et al. Crystal structure of the glucocorticoid receptor ligand binding domain reveals a novel mode of receptor dimerization and coactivator recognition. *Cell* **2002**, *110*, 93–105. [CrossRef]
69. Southworth, D.R.; Agard, D.A. Client-loading conformation of the Hsp90 molecular chaperone revealed in the cryo-EM structure of the human Hsp90:Hop complex. *Mol. Cell* **2011**, *42*, 771–781. [CrossRef]
70. Morishima, Y.; Murphy, P.J.; Li, D.P.; Sanchez, E.R.; Pratt, W.B. Stepwise assembly of a glucocorticoid receptor.hsp90 heterocomplex resolves two sequential ATP-dependent events involving first hsp70 and then hsp90 in opening of the steroid binding pocket. *J. Biol. Chem.* **2000**, *275*, 18054–18060. [CrossRef]
71. Smith, D.F.; Stensgard, B.A.; Welch, W.J.; Toft, D.O. Assembly of progesterone receptor with heat shock proteins and receptor activation are ATP mediated events. *J. Biol. Chem.* **1992**, *267*, 1350–1356. [CrossRef]
72. Hernandez, M.P.; Chadli, A.; Toft, D.O. HSP40 binding is the first step in the HSP90 chaperoning pathway for the progesterone receptor. *J. Biol. Chem.* **2002**, *277*, 11873–11881. [CrossRef]

73. Chen, S.; Smith, D.F. Hop as an adaptor in the heat shock protein 70 (Hsp70) and hsp90 chaperone machinery. *J. Biol. Chem.* **1998**, *273*, 35194–35200. [CrossRef] [PubMed]
74. Mandelkow, E.M.; Mandelkow, E. Biochemistry and cell biology of tau protein in neurofibrillary degeneration. *Cold Spring Harb. Perspect. Med.* **2012**, *2*, a006247. [CrossRef]
75. Dickey, C.A.; Kamal, A.; Lundgren, K.; Klosak, N.; Bailey, R.M.; Dunmore, J.; Ash, P.; Shoraka, S.; Zlatkovic, J.; Eckman, C.B.; et al. The high-affinity HSP90-CHIP complex recognizes and selectively degrades phosphorylated tau client proteins. *J. Clin. Investig.* **2007**, *117*, 648–658. [CrossRef]
76. Sarkar, M.; Kuret, J.; Lee, G. Two motifs within the tau microtubule-binding domain mediate its association with the hsc70 molecular chaperone. *J. Neurosci. Res.* **2008**, *86*, 2763–2773. [CrossRef] [PubMed]
77. Karagoz, G.E.; Duarte, A.M.; Akoury, E.; Ippel, H.; Biernat, J.; Moran Luengo, T.; Radli, M.; Didenko, T.; Nordhues, B.A.; Veprintsev, D.B.; et al. Hsp90-Tau complex reveals molecular basis for specificity in chaperone action. *Cell* **2014**, *156*, 963–974. [CrossRef] [PubMed]
78. von Bergen, M.; Friedhoff, P.; Biernat, J.; Heberle, J.; Mandelkow, E.M.; Mandelkow, E. Assembly of tau protein into Alzheimer paired helical filaments depends on a local sequence motif ((306)VQIVYK(311)) forming beta structure. *Proc. Natl. Acad. Sci. USA* **2000**, *97*, 5129–5134. [CrossRef]
79. Oroz, J.; Chang, B.J.; Wysoczanski, P.; Lee, C.T.; Perez-Lara, A.; Chakraborty, P.; Hofele, R.V.; Baker, J.D.; Blair, L.J.; Biernat, J.; et al. Structure and pro-toxic mechanism of the human Hsp90/PPIase/Tau complex. *Nat. Commun.* **2018**, *9*, 4532. [CrossRef]
80. Blair, L.J.; Nordhues, B.A.; Hill, S.E.; Scaglione, K.M.; O'Leary, J.C., III; Fontaine, S.N.; Breydo, L.; Zhang, B.; Li, P.; Wang, L.; et al. Accelerated neurodegeneration through chaperone-mediated oligomerization of tau. *J. Clin. Investig.* **2013**, *123*, 4158–4169. [CrossRef]
81. Cleveland, D.W.; Hwo, S.Y.; Kirschner, M.W. Purification of tau, a microtubule-associated protein that induces assembly of microtubules from purified tubulin. *J. Mol. Biol.* **1977**, *116*, 207–225. [CrossRef]
82. Wang, Y.; Mandelkow, E. Tau in physiology and pathology. *Nat. Rev. Neurosci.* **2016**, *17*, 5–21. [CrossRef]

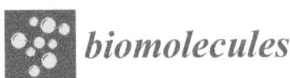

Review

Cytosolic Hsp90 Isoform-Specific Functions and Clinical Significance

Samarpan Maiti and Didier Picard *

Département de Biologie Moléculaire et Cellulaire, Université de Genève, Sciences III, Quai Ernest-Ansermet 30, CH-1211 Geneve, Switzerland
* Correspondence: didier.picard@unige.ch

Abstract: The heat shock protein 90 (Hsp90) is a molecular chaperone and a key regulator of proteostasis under both physiological and stress conditions. In mammals, there are two cytosolic Hsp90 isoforms: Hsp90α and Hsp90β. These two isoforms are 85% identical and encoded by two different genes. Hsp90β is constitutively expressed and essential for early mouse development, while Hsp90α is stress-inducible and not necessary for survivability. These two isoforms are known to have largely overlapping functions and to interact with a large fraction of the proteome. To what extent there are isoform-specific functions at the protein level has only relatively recently begun to emerge. There are studies indicating that one isoform is more involved in the functionality of a specific tissue or cell type. Moreover, in many diseases, functionally altered cells appear to be more dependent on one particular isoform. This leaves space for designing therapeutic strategies in an isoform-specific way, which may overcome the unfavorable outcome of pan-Hsp90 inhibition encountered in previous clinical trials. For this to succeed, isoform-specific functions must be understood in more detail. In this review, we summarize the available information on isoform-specific functions of mammalian Hsp90 and connect it to possible clinical applications.

Keywords: molecular chaperone; paralog; Hsp90 isoforms; Hsp90α; Hsp90β; Hsp90-isoform specific inhibitors; clinical relevance

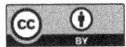

1. Introduction

Heat shock proteins (Hsps) are molecular chaperones which are known for their numerous roles in protein homeostasis (proteostasis), including protein folding and refolding, maturation, disassembly of aggregates, and degradation [1–3]. The term "heat shock" proteins was coined as a legacy of Ritossa's pioneering discovery that heat shock produced chromosomal puffs in the salivary glands of *Drosophila* larvae [4,5]. Later, it was established that the heat-shock response (HSR) is a universal response to an extensive array of stresses [6,7]. HSPs are not only essential during stress, but they are equally crucial in normal conditions to maintain proteostasis [8,9]. The human genome organization (HUGO) gene nomenclature committee recognizes five human HSP families (http://www.genenames.org/data/genegroup/#!/group/582; accessed on 5 August 2022) based on their observed molecular weights: Hsp70, Hsp90, Hsp40, the small HSPs, and chaperonins [10,11]. All Hsp90s consist of three major domains: an N-terminal ATPase domain (NTD), which binds ATP, a middle domain (MD), to which perhaps most clients bind, and a C-terminal dimerization domain (CTD) [12]. In this review, we will focus on mammalian Hsp90 and its cytosolic isoforms.

2. Hsp90 Homologs and Paralogs

Homologous genes or proteins (homologs) are genes or proteins of different species with a common ancestor, whereas paralogs are genes with sequence homology that originate from the intragenomic duplication of an ancestral gene. For the Hsp90 family of proteins, there are homologs in all organisms except in *Archaea* and some bacterial species [13,14]. Hsp90 is conserved from bacteria to humans with a sequence homology of about 53% between *Escherichia coli* (*E. coli*) and humans, which is a strong indication that this protein has remained vital throughout evolution [15]. During evolution, gene duplications allowed the divergence into different paralogous Hsp90 genes, which encode protein isoforms [14,16–18]. These additional isoforms, including organelle-specific ones, with different functional properties evolved as organisms gained more complexity [13,14,16–19]. Bacteria generally have only one isoform, known as the high-temperature protein G (HtpG) [19], but some bacterial species, such as *Streptomyces coelicolor*, contain another paralog, which shares only 30% identity [14]. In some bacteria, HtpG is essential during heat stress [20]. In *E. coli*, although HtpG is not essential, it is relatively abundant under non-stress conditions and further induced during heat stress [21], and indeed, *E. coli htpG* mutants have a growth defect at higher temperatures [22]. During evolution of eukaryotes, Hsp90 gained more importance and became an essential protein for viability [14,18]. Its importance is further emphasized by its abundance. Hsp90 comprises 1–2% of the total cellular protein in unstressed cells and up to 4–6% in the presence of stress [23,24]. The Hsp90 chaperone machinery is a key regulator of proteostasis, both in normal and stress conditions in eukaryotic cells [15,24,25]. In the unicellular eukaryote *Saccharomyces cerevisiae* (*S. cerevisiae*), genome-wide studies suggested that up to 10% of all proteins are directly or indirectly dependent on Hsp90 for function [26,27]. *S. cerevisiae* possesses two cytosolic Hsp90 isoforms encoded by separate genes, which arose from a genome duplication: the cognate Hsc82 and the stress-inducible Hsp82 [28]. Under non-stress conditions, Hsc82 is expressed at tenfold higher levels than Hsp82 [28]. During heat shock, a strong induction of Hsp82 and a merely moderate induction of Hsc82 almost equalize the levels of the two isoforms. Hsp82 and Hsc82 are 709 and 705 amino acids long, respectively, with 96% identity and only 27 amino acid differences [13,29]. In multicellular organisms, there are four different types of Hsp90 paralogs based on their organelle-specific localization. These are the cytosolic Hsp90s [30–33], Trap1 in mitochondria [34,35], Grp94 in the endoplasmic reticulum [36], and chloroplast Hsp90C in plants [37]. Although these paralogs share many highly conserved domains with over 50% sequence identity, they differ in their functions [14,16–18]. In this review, we will focus on the cytosolic Hsp90 isoforms of mammals.

3. Cytosolic Hsp90

In mammals, there are two cytosolic Hsp90 isoforms: Hsp90α and Hsp90β [31]. Human Hsp90α and Hsp90β are encoded by the *HSP90AA1* and *HSP90AB1* genes, respectively [31–33]. Hsp90α was the first Hsp90 to be purified from heat-stressed Hela cells [32]. Later, Hsp90β was cloned based on homology to Hsp90α [33]. Millions of years ago, Hsp90α and Hsp90β originated by gene duplication [38]. These two cytosolic Hsp90 isoforms are highly homologous, with about 84% sequence identity (for 732 and 724 amino acids, respectively) [33]. There are five highly conserved signature sequences. Three are in the N-terminal domain and two are in the middle domain, comprising amino acids 38–59, 106–114, and 130–145, and 360–370 and 387–401, respectively [39]. What makes these two isoforms different in structure is that Hsp90α contains the 9-amino acid extension TQTQDQPME within the very N-terminal residues 4 to 12, which is replaced in Hsp90β by the 4-amino acid segment VHHG [31]. Hsp90β also has the unique signature sequence LKID (residues 71–74), which is not present in any other HSP [14]. Both isoforms function as homodimers [40,41]. Interestingly, the relatively poor dimer formation of human Hsp90β can be mapped to two amino acid differences compared to Hsp90α [42]. While there is evidence for vertebrates that some isoform heterodimers exist as well [43,44], mass spectrometric analysis revealed no α-β heterodimers [45] and sepharose-immobilized Hsp90β pulls out only β [46]. Whereas in *S. cerevisiae*, Hsp90 isoforms readily form heterodimers both in vitro and in vivo [29], this is disfavored in humans [47]. Hence, it remains to be investigated to what extent cytosolic isoform heterodimers exist in multicellular organisms, what regulates the equilibrium between homodimers and heterodimers, and whether they have distinct functions [12,39] (Figure 1).

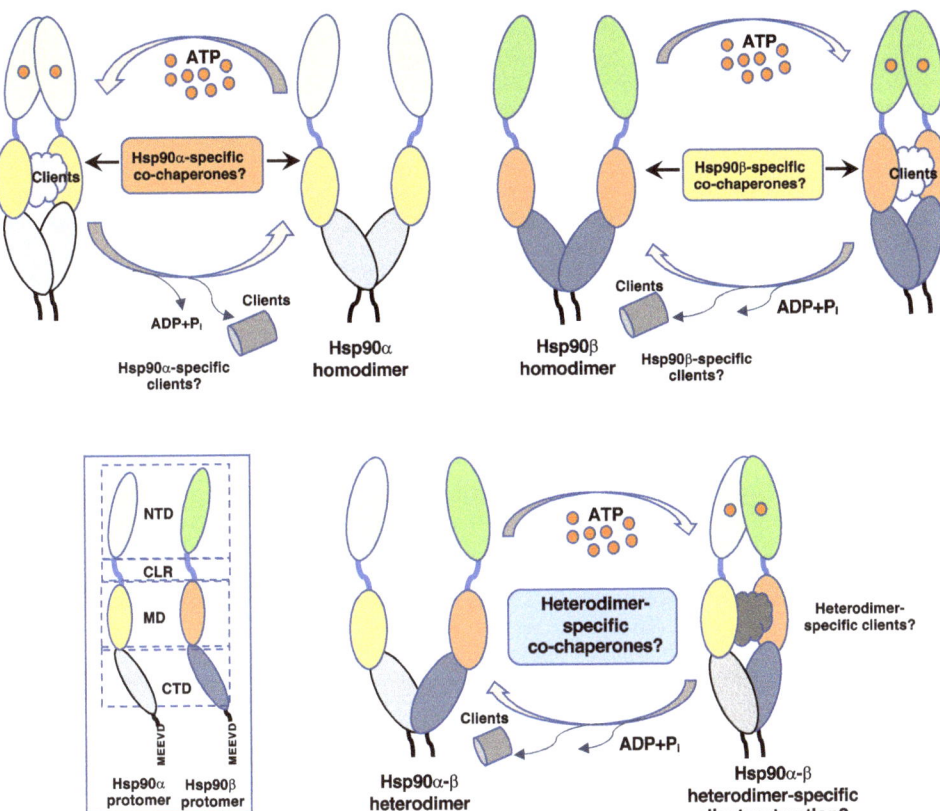

Figure 1. Schematic representation of the molecular chaperone cycle of Hsp90α and Hsp90β, either as isoform homodimers or hypothetically as isoform heterodimers. NTD, MD, and CTD, N-terminal, middle, and C-terminal domains, respectively; CLR, charged linker region.

3.1. Tissue-Specific Expression

The expression levels of the two isoforms varies in a tissue-specific way. In mice, Hsp90β is highly abundant in heart, liver, spleen, lung, intestine, muscle, brain, testis, and kidney. In comparison, the levels of Hsp90α are lower in those tissues. However, in testis, retina, and brain, Hsp90α levels are comparatively higher than Hsp90β, whereas in heart and muscle, Hsp90α is almost absent [48,49]. Indeed, we demonstrated an interesting isoform switch in mouse myoblasts: as they differentiate into myotubes, Hsp90α disappears and only Hsp90β remains [50] (see also chapter 3.2). According to the human protein atlas (https://www.proteinatlas.org; accessed on 5 August 2022), human brain has the highest expression of Hsp90α mRNA, and yet, this is not reflected at the protein level, as it is only moderate. For Hsp90β, there appears to be no such disparities (https://www.proteinatlas.org/search/HSP90AB1; accessed on 5 August 2022). As in mice, human Hsp90β protein is moderately to highly expressed in all the major tissues. Hsp90α protein is more highly expressed in the respiratory system, and in female and male reproductive organs. These differences in tissue distribution patterns suggest that different tissues have distinct isoform-specific functional requirements. It is intriguing to speculate that different tissues might have different intrinsic levels of biophysical stress, due to differences in temperature, osmotic pressure, and oxygen availability, which both affect the differential expression of the two isoforms and impose distinct functional requirements.

3.2. Isoform-Specific Co-Chaperones

During evolution from prokaryotes to eukaryotes, overall proteome complexity dramatically increased without any accompanying gain of core molecular chaperones. To assist the core molecular chaperones and to diversify their functions, a large panel of co-chaperones appeared [16]. Only relatively few co-chaperones are required for core Hsp90 functions (Table 1). These co-chaperones help in the transfer of clients from Hsp70, the N-terminal closure of the client-bound Hsp90 dimer, stimulating/inhibiting the ATPase activity, and the maturation of clients [51,52]. Other co-chaperones have more specialized functions suggesting a correlation between client diversity and the range of available co-chaperones. For now, there is still only limited evidence for isoform specificity of co-chaperones. In a recent review, Dean and Johnson discussed the relative expression of co-chaperones across a wide range of tissues [53]. The results of this survey suggest that some Hsp90 co-chaperones are uniquely required to assist client proteins in certain tissues. For example, the levels of the mRNAs encoding FKBP51, S100A1, ITGB1BP2, Unc45B, Aarsd1, and Harc are elevated in skeletal muscle, and most of them are also elevated in the heart. This correlative observation suggests that these co-chaperones may have muscle-specific functions [53], possibly with a corresponding Hsp90 isoform preference. ITGB1BP2 binds integrin and regulates the interaction between the cytoskeleton and the extracellular matrix, which have cardioprotective effects [54]. Unc45B assists the folding of myosin [55] and S100A1 is a regulator of muscle contractility [56]. FKBP51 functions in myoblast differentiation and in regulating muscle mass [57,58]. We showed that as myoblasts differentiate into myotubes, the co-chaperone p23 is replaced by the muscle-specific co-chaperone Aarsd1, which shares the Hsp90-interacting CS domain with p23, but not all of its activities. We found that the long isoform Aarsd1L interacts exclusively with Hsp90β, the only remaining and functionally important Hsp90 isoform in murine myotubes [50]. An inverse situation may pertain to spermatogenesis where Hsp90α levels are high. This isoform is essential [59], and a subset of co-chaperones have been linked to spermatogenesis. This includes PIH1D1, PIH1D2, PIH1D3, RPAP3, SPAG1, DYX1C1, LRRC6, and NUDCD1 [60,61]. Moreover, loss of FKBP36 results in chromosome mispairing during meiosis and mutations are suspected to cause azoospermia [62,63]. These examples illustrate that expression of Hsp90 isoforms, co-chaperones, and clients, and their respective interactions may have evolved to provide a unique match in certain tissues and cell types.

Table 1. Some co-chaperones of Hsp90α and Hsp90β [1].

Co-Chaperones	Function/Comments
Aha1	Accelerator of Hsp90 ATPase
Hop	Adaptor between Hsp70 and Hsp90; inhibitor of Hsp90 ATPase
p23	Binds closed Hsp90 conformation, inhibits ATPase
Cdc37	Kinase-specific co-chaperone
FKBP51/52	Peptidylprolyl-cis/trans-isomerase; maturation and activation of steroid receptors
Cyp40	Peptidylprolyl-cis/trans-isomerase
PP5	Phosphatase interacting with Hsp90
CHIP	E3 ubiquitine ligase
Pih1	Component of the Rvb1-Rvb2-Tah1-Pih1 (R2TP) complex
Tah1	Component of the Rvb1-Rvb2-Tah1-Pih1 (R2TP) complex
TTC4	Genetic interaction with Cpr7; regulator of protein translation
FKBP8	Peptidylprolyl-cis/trans-isomerase; may preferentially bind Hsp90β
UNC45A	Preferentially binds Hsp90β
Aarsdl1	Competes with p23; only binds Hsp90β

[1] Only some of the most frequently investigated co-chaperones are listed and some of those with reported Hsp90 isoform-selectivity. For full list of co-chaperones and references, see https://www.picard.ch/downloads/Hsp90facts.pdf.

3.3. Isoform-Specific Post-Translational Modifications

Post-translational modifications can have a large impact on the function and regulation of the two isoforms [64]. Both isoforms are modified by phosphorylation, acetylation, S-nitrosylation, oxidation, methylation, sumoylation, and ubiquitination. Many of the modified residues are conserved between Hsp90α and Hsp90β. However, there are a few differences between the two, which allow for specific functions or regulation in an isoform-specific way. We refer the reader to a very recent review on this topic [65].

3.4. Evolutionary Divergence in Gene Expression

HSP90AB1 evolved as the constitutively expressed isoform, while *HSP90AA1* evolved to be inducible in response to different types of stresses. The differential gene expression patterns of mammalian *HSP90AA1* and *HSP90AB1* were first characterized with transformed mouse cells [66]. Ullrich and colleagues showed that *HSP90AB1* is constitutively expressed under normal conditions and has a 2.5-fold higher expression level than *HSP90AA1*. However, upon heat shock, *HSP90AA1* expression increased 7-fold, while *HSP90AB1* increased only 4.5-fold [66]. This suggested that Hsp90β can also be induced when cells are under stress. In a recent study, we observed that Hsp90β expression can be induced by genetic stress as well as by long-term moderate heat stress at the translational level through an IRES in the Hsp90β mRNA [49]. Other studies also showed that Hsp90β can be induced under heat and nutrient stress [67,68]. Heat shock factor 1 (HSF1), which is recruited to DNA through heat shock elements (HSEs) and is the transcriptional master regulator of the response to heat shock and several other stresses, regulates the expression of Hsp90α [69,70]. Upstream of *HSP90AA1*, there are several heat shock elements (HSEs) which enable the stress-mediated expression of Hsp90α [71], and in particular, there is a distal HSE located at −1031 bp from the transcription start site (TSS), which is required for heat-shock induction [26]. Immediately upstream of the TATA box, the proximal HSE located at −96/−60 bp functions as a permissive enhancer. Another HSE is present within the first intron region at +228 bp from the TSS. In contrast, an upstream HSE of located at −648 bp of the TSS of *HSP90AB1* appears not to respond to heat shock [67]. However, HSEs located at +688/733 bp within the first intron are tightly bound by HSF1 and are important for maintaining the high constitutive and heat-shock induced expression levels [67]. In an apparent contradiction, it was observed for mouse oocytes that the basal level of *HSP90AB1* transcripts does not depend on HSF1 since *hsf1* knockout oocytes do not show any reduction in Hsp90β mRNA [72]. The constitutively active core promoter (−36 to +37 bp) of *HSP90AB1* has a CAAT box, a specificity protein 1 (SP1) binding site, and a TATA box (−27 bp) [71]. The promoter of *HSP90AA1* does not contain a CAAT box, but one has been identified far upstream at −1144 bp. The binding of Krüppel-Like-Factor 4 (KLF4) to the promoters of *HSP90AB1* and *HSP90AA1* leads to higher expression of both isoforms [73]. In addition to the activation by HSF1, Hsp90β is upregulated by the signal transducer and activator of transcription (STAT) family transcription factors [74]. Interferon-γ (IFN-γ) activation of STAT1 also induces Hsp90β expression [74]. For the induction of *HSP90AB1* by heat shock, STAT1 phosphorylation by Jak2 and PKC is necessary [75]. However, the activation of these kinases in turn requires the association with Hsp90, establishing a positive auto-regulatory loop. *HSP90AB1* expression is also regulated at the translational level by mTORC1 [76]. This seems to be dependent on a 5′-terminal oligopyrimidine motif in the 5′UTR of the Hsp90β mRNA, but the mechanism is not known. As a general negative feedback mechanism, the Hsp90 complex represses HSF1 activation, thereby inhibiting an over-activation and timely attenuation of the HSF1 response [77,78]. Clearly, there is still much to learn about the tissue- and cell type-specific regulation of the two Hsp90 isoforms, both at the transcriptional and translational levels.

3.5. Functional Specificities of the Two Isoforms

In humans, Hsp90α and Hsp90β together are predicted to interact with more than 2000 proteins [79]. Not quite that many have been experimentally validated, and in the vast majority, isoform specificity has not been thoroughly investigated. Regarding the Hsp90 interactome, we refer the reader to continuously updated resources, which we have been making available as a searchable online database at https://www.picard.ch/Hsp90Int, accessed on 5 August 2022 [79] and a downloadable file at https://www.picard.ch/downloads/Hsp90interactors.pdf, accessed on 5 August 2022. It is natural to assume that highly homologous versions of Hsp90s found in the same cellular compartment would have identical functions. However, these cytosolic Hsp90 isoforms have evolved to have some overlapping, synergistic, and distinct isoform-specific functions. In some contexts, they even have antagonistic functions (see below). Taipale and colleagues systematically characterized the chaperone/co-chaperone/client interaction network in human cells [80]. They provided evidence for both overlapping and distinct client specificities. When they analyzed isoform-specific interactors by gene ontology terms, this again translated to both common and isoform-specific terms. This generally supports the conclusion that isoform-specific interactomes impart isoform-specific functions. It is worth mentioning here that a characterization of the interactomes of the two isoforms of *S. cerevisiae* by immunoprecipitation/mass spectrometry led to globally similar conclusions, except that it was noted that the vast majority of clients are shared by both isoforms [29].

In the next section of the discussion of isoform-specific functions and clinical relevance (Figure 2), we will consider those findings where the involvement of one specific isoform was experimentally validated by using isoform-specific antibodies and genetic or pharmacological inhibition. With many studies, it must be kept in mind, though, that it is not easily possible to exclude the possibility that the observed phenotype is due to reduced total Hsp90 levels or activity. Indeed, we know from our own studies that phenotypes can be due to the latter rather than the loss or inhibition of a specific isoform [49].

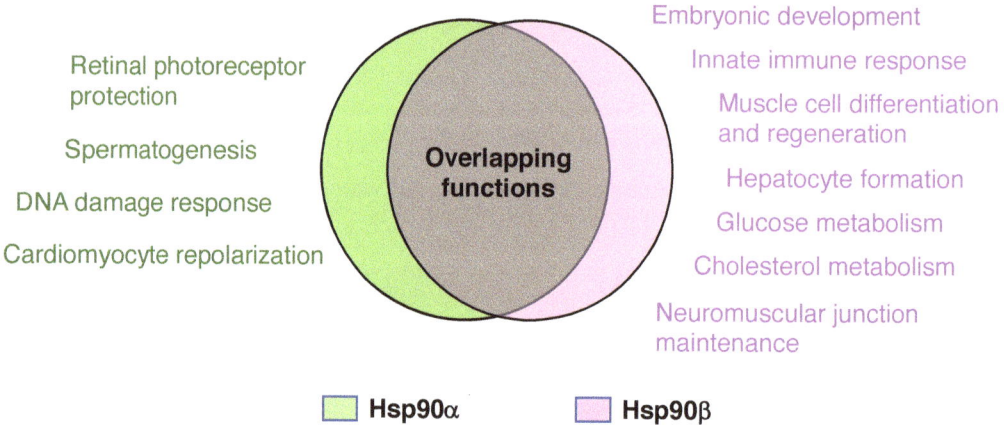

Figure 2. Venn diagram of common and isoform-specific functions of Hsp90. Isoform-specific functions, as discussed in the text, are highlighted in the corresponding colors.

3.6. Hsp90β-Specific Functions

During the course of evolution, the *HSP90AB1* gene has evolved to be expressed more or less constitutively, presumably to support essential cellular housekeeping activities. The embryonic lethality of the mouse knockout may be a reflection of that [81]. Hsp90β was shown to play a role in trophoblast differentiation and that Hsp90β-deficient homozygous mouse embryos with normal expression of Hsp90α failed to differentiate to form placental labyrinths. This resulted in lethality beyond day 9 of embryonic development. While it could be speculated that this indicated a housekeeping role for Hsp90β, it was also suggested that the developmental arrest could be due to a defective critical and potentially Hsp90β-dependent client such as the bone morphogenetic protein receptor. Interestingly,

Hsp90β was demonstrated to regulate the pluripotency of embryonic stem cells via regulating the transcription of Nanog through an interaction with STAT3 [82]. Thus, whether mammalian development truly depends specifically on Hsp90β for the aforementioned reasons or whether it depends on a threshold level of total Hsp90 remains to be determined.

Hsp90β appears to have an exclusive role in muscle cell differentiation and regeneration in the mouse [50,83]. We showed that during skeletal muscle differentiation in the mouse, there is a unique Hsp90 isoform switch [50]. When mouse myoblasts differentiate into myotubes, Hsp90α disappears, and only Hsp90β remains. Hsp90β interacts with the muscle-specific Hsp90 co-chaperone Aarsd1L to support the differentiation of myotubes. As these differentiate, Aarsd1L replaces the ubiquitous cochaperone p23. Later, He and colleagues discovered the importance of Hsp90β in muscle regeneration after tissue injury [83]. They found that in a mouse muscle injury model, the Hsp90β isoform, but not Hsp90α, was strongly elevated during the first few days post injury. Hsp90β expression levels normalized when active myogenesis eventually ceased. Following muscle injury, p53-dependent persistent senescence impairs muscle repair. During regeneration, Hsp90β interacts with the p53-inhibitory protein MDM2 to suppress p53-dependent senescence of the injured muscle. Degeneration of skeletal muscle is one of the features of aging in humans [84]. The reduction of quiescent muscle stem cells through senescence leads to the decline in muscle regeneration in aged mice [85]. Hence, enhancing Hsp90β activity might be protective for muscle fibers during aging.

Hsp90β is involved in controlling the formation of endodermal progenitor cells and development of the liver [86]. For hepatocyte formation, the transcription factor hepatocyte nuclear factor 4 α (HNF4α) is essential [87]. Hsp90β interacts with HNF4α to regulate its half-life and is thus directly linked with the formation of hepatocytes from progenitor cells. The liver is the primary organ involved in the metabolism of nutrients. Not surprisingly, the specific function of Hsp90β in liver formation further connects it to different metabolic disorders. Hsp90β is involved in glucose and cholesterol metabolism [68,88]. In human skeletal muscle myoblasts and in a mouse model of diet-induced obesity, Hsp90β was found to regulate glucose metabolism and insulin signaling. Studies showed that the knockdown of Hsp90β improves glucose tolerance, alters the expression of key metabolic genes, and enhances the activity of the pyruvate dehydrogenase complex. Furthermore, Hsp90β is essential for lipid homeostasis by regulating fatty acid and cholesterol metabolism [88]. Depleting Hsp90β promotes the degradation of mature sterol regulatory element-binding proteins through the Akt-GSK3β-FBW7 pathway, and hence decreases the content of neutral lipids and cholesterol in the body [88,89].

Another important isoform-specific function of Hsp90β is regulating the responsiveness to vitamin D [90]. In the intestine, enterocytes require Hsp90β for optimal vitamin D responsiveness by regulating vitamin D receptor (VDR) signaling. It was observed that knocking down Hsp90β led to reduced vitamin D-mediated transcriptional activity. It is noteworthy that VDR is a member of the nuclear receptor family of transcription factors, which comprises some of the most prototypical Hsp90 clients, such as the steroid receptors.

Hsp90β is necessary for maintaining the neuromuscular junction (NMJ) [91]. Rapsyn, an acetylcholine receptor-interacting protein, is essential for synapse formation [92]. Hsp90β is necessary for rapsyn stabilization and regulating its proteasome-dependent degradation. Luo and colleagues showed that inhibition of Hsp90β activity or expression or disruption of its interaction with rapsyn impairs the development and maintenance of the NMJ.

3.7. Targeting Hsp90β in Different Diseases

As alluded to above, Hsp90β influences pathways regulating insulin resistance [68]. It was observed that when Hsp90β was inhibited, blood glucose levels were reduced. Thus, targeting Hsp90β might help to regulate the blood sugar of patients with type 2 diabetes. In patients with nonalcoholic fatty liver disease (NAFLD), the Hsp90β levels in serum was found to be very high [93]. Balanescu and colleagues conducted a study on overweight and obese children and found serum Hsp90β, but not Hsp90α, to be significantly higher.

This suggests that the ratio of Hsp90α and Hsp90β in blood serum could be a prognostic biomarker for NAFLD. Jing and colleagues found that the novel Hsp90β-selective inhibitor corylin significantly reduced lipid content in both liver cell lines and human primary hepatocytes [88]. In animal models, they observed that corylin ameliorated NAFLD, type 2 diabetes, and atherosclerosis.

Reduced levels of both Hsp90α and Hsp90β are associated with neuronal cell death in patients suffering from Alzheimer's disease (AD) [94]. However, Zhang and colleagues showed that Aβ-induced stress decreased the levels of Hsp90β, but not Hsp90α. Reduced levels of Hsp90β were strongly correlated with reduced abundance of its client and nuclear receptor PPARγ, and down-regulated Aβ clearance-related genes in primary microglia [95]. This exciting observation led them to think about increasing Hsp90β levels in the AD mouse model. Using the natural compound jujuboside A (JuA), they observed that it significantly restored the content and function of PPARγ by enhancing the expression of Hsp90β. JuA-treated AD mice displayed ameliorated cognitive deficiency. In a recent study, Wan and colleagues showed reduced levels of both Hsp90α and Hsp90β levels in the hippocampal CA3 region of the APP/PS1 mouse model of Alzheimer's disease [96]. However, the overexpression of Hsp90β, but not Hsp90α, ameliorated neuronal and synaptic loss, suggesting Hsp90β has a specific neuroprotective role. High-dose preventive treatment with erythropoietin (EPO) attenuated Aβ-induced astrocytosis and increased neovascularization in the hippocampus of the mouse AD model. It reversed dendritic spine loss via upregulation of Hsp90β. Therefore, inducing Hsp90β expression might be explored for the treatment of AD patients.

Hsp90β enhances the innate immune response [97]. Hsp90β interacts with the protein stimulator of interferon genes (STING) and stabilizes STING protein levels in response to microbial infections, allowing the activation of the downstream target TBK1, which is itself an Hsp90 interactor, for inducing IFN responses. This suggests inducing Hsp90β could also be efficient against DNA viruses and microbial infections. Sato and colleagues showed that reduced Hsp90β levels are associated with infections with Herpes simplex virus-1 (HSV-1) and *Listeria monocytogenes*, suggesting that boosting Hsp90β levels and/or activity may protect against pathogenic infections. If so, EPO might also be beneficial against bacterial and viral infections.

Although it is predominantly Hsp90α that is overexpressed in different types of cancer, in some cancers it is Hsp90β, which appears to be responsible for cancer cell survival [98–102]. As discussed above, there are tissues that rely primarily on Hsp90β. It appears that cancers of those tissues often maintain this dependence. For example, hepatocytes primarily require Hsp90β, as do hepatocellular carcinoma cells, notably for vascular endothelial growth factor receptor (VEGFR)-mediated angiogenesis [99,100]. In other cancers, Hsp90α regulates VEGFR-mediated angiogenesis. Meng and colleagues evaluated angiogenesis in hepatocellular carcinoma upon knockdown of Hsp90α or Hsp90β, inhibiting the remaining isoform with an Hsp90 inhibitor. They observed that VEGFR-mediated angiogenesis was inhibited by an Hsp90β inhibitor. Heck and colleagues showed that selective Hsp90β inhibition in human myeloid leukemia cells results in apoptosis [103]. Hsp90β-apoptosome interactions also contribute to chemoresistance in leukemias [104]. Hsp90β inhibition could kill leukemia cells by promoting the degradation of the Hsp90 client HIF1α [103]. Heck and colleagues treated cells with the Hsp90α-selective inhibitor KUNA110, the Hsp90β-selective inhibitor KUNB105, or the pan-Hsp90 inhibitor 17AAG. Inhibition of Hsp90α did not trigger cell death. However, Hsp90β inhibition led to cell death by TNFα- and TRAIL-induced HIF1α degradation. HIF1α is an interactor of both Hsp90 isoforms (see https://www.picard.ch/Hsp90Int, accessed on 5 August 2022), and yet the inhibition of Hsp90β, but not Hsp90α, led to the degradation of HIF1α in leukemia cells. This surprising result illustrated the potential of Hsp90 isoform-specific inhibition for the treatment of certain types of cancer.

In Ewing's sarcoma, it was found that Hsp90β inhibition leads to decreased expression of the multidrug resistance-associated protein 1 associated with mitochondria [105]. In laryngeal carcinoma (LC), Hsp90β directly interacts with Bcl-2 and is involved in the anti-apoptotic progression of LC [101]. In osteosarcoma, extracellular Hsp90β secreted by MG63 cells was found to be associated with cancer cell survival [106]. This could be connected with the observation that muscle cells in the mouse are solely dependent on Hsp90β for differentiation and regeneration. This evidence collectively suggests that sarcoma is mainly dependent on Hsp90β [107]. Not only that, even in the skeletal muscle disorder myotonia congenita, Hsp90β plays an essential role in the quality control of the chloride channel CLC-1 by dynamically coordinating protein folding and degradation. Peng and colleagues showed that by using Hsp90β inhibitors, CLC-1 degradation in myotonia patients can be prevented [108].

Hsp90β plays a role in drug resistance in lung cancer. The P-glycoprotein (P-gp) encoded by the *MDR1* gene is responsible for exporting drugs from cells. Kim and colleagues showed that casein kinase 2 (CK2)-mediated phosphorylation of Hsp90β and the subsequent stabilization of its client PXR, a nuclear receptor, is a key mechanism in the regulation of MDR1 expression [109]. Inhibition of both CK2 and Hsp90β enhances the down-regulation of PXR and P-gp expression. High level expression of Hsp90β is also associated with poor survival in resectable non-small-cell lung cancer patients [98].

Possibly related to the dependence of liver cells on Hsp90β discussed above, Hepatitis B virus (HBV), which causes chronic infection in the liver, evades the immune defense by interaction with Hsp90β [110]. Hsp90β inhibition could also be a useful therapeutic approach in *Helicobacter pylori*-induced gastric injury [111]. Cha and colleagues showed that Hsp90β physically interacts with Rac1, which resulted in the activation of NADPH oxidase. NADPH oxidase activation leads to the production of ROS and increased inflammation in infected cells. Suppression of *H. pylori*-induced translocation of Hsp90β to the membrane may ameliorate gastric injury. Nickel ions-mediated inflammation also occurs through Hsp90β in human B-cells. Nickel ions bind to the linker domain of Hsp90β and reduce its interaction with HIF1α. The released HIF1α then becomes more localized in the nucleus and enhances IL-8 expression [112].

3.8. Hsp90α-Specific Functions

The stress-inducible isoform Hsp90α helps cells adapt to stress [113]. Most of the functions of Hsp90α are thus connected to stress response pathways and proteins. Unlike Hsp90β, Hsp90α is not necessary for viability in the mouse [49,59]. In normal conditions, as discussed above, some organs have a high abundance of Hsp90α, whereas others have negligible expression levels (https://www.proteinatlas.org/search/HSP90AA1; accessed on 5 August 2022). For example, the brain has the highest levels of Hsp90α mRNA expression, which is several folds higher than any other organs. However, the highest levels of mRNA are not translated into proteins as brain expresses only moderate amounts of Hsp90α protein. A recent study says the human brain has a higher temperature than the usual body temperature ranging from 36.1 to 40.9 °C in a circadian way [114]. In addition, the brain temperature varies by age, sex, menstrual cycle, and brain region. It is conceivable that such temperature increases in the brain might trigger a heat-shock response, temporarily generating more Hsp90α protein from the already elevated levels of Hsp90α mRNA. Since brain cells face a substantial temperature fluctuation, proteins may be more prone to misfolding, and brain cells may therefore need higher amounts of Hsp90α under certain circumstances. If we consider reproductive organs, testis and fallopian tube have high levels of Hsp90α expression. At the cellular level, basal prostate cells have the highest amount of Hsp90α mRNA among all cell types. Spermatocytes also have high Hsp90α. This suggests reproductive organs require Hsp90α. Earlier, our lab established that Hsp90α is required for male fertility in mice [59]. Mice without Hsp90α can survive normally but are sterile because of a complete failure to produce sperm. Interestingly, Hsp90α knockout mice develop normal reproductive organs, but spermatogenesis specifically arrests at the pachytene stage of meiosis I. Supporting these findings, Kajiwara and collogues later complemented these findings by demonstrating that spermatogenesis also arrests when the Hsp90α gene is conditionally deleted at the adult stage [115]. Intriguingly, Hsp90α controls the biogenesis of fetal PIWI-interacting RNAs, which act against endogenous transposons during the development of male germ cells in mammals [116]. The Hsp90α knockout causes a reduction of HIF1α levels in the testis, which may also contribute to blocking sperm production and causing infertility [117]. The downregulation of Hsp90β had little effect on the hypoxia-induced accumulation of HIF1α. Thus, HIF1α is required for proper spermiogenesis, and it is the Hsp90α isoform that is needed to keep HIF1α functional, even though both Hsp90α and Hsp90β can interact with HIF1α [118,119]. It remains to be seen whether this unique Hsp90α role has anything to do with the specific physiology and temperature-sensitivity of the testis.

Oogenesis may also be largely dependent on the Hsp90α isoform. Metchat and colleagues showed that extremely low levels of Hsp90α correlate with the developmental defects of *hsf1-/-* oocytes [72]. While *hsf1-/-* females produce oocytes, they do not carry viable embryos. However, later we showed that no difference in embryo production was observed in female mice lacking Hsp90α compared to the wild-type [49,59]. Hence, it is possible that *hsf1-/-* oocytes failed to develop because of some Hsp90α-independent issue.

In the human retina, rod cells have high levels of Hsp90α mRNA expression (https://www.proteinatlas.org; accessed on 5 August 2022), which may be related to elevated local temperatures upon exposure to light. The local rise in temperature of human retina exposed to direct sunlight is about 2 °C [120]. It may even tolerate a local rise of at least 10 °C [121], and yet, intense light causes thermal damage [122]. Wu and colleagues found that Hsp90α deficiency in mice could lead to retinitis pigmentosa [48], a common inherited retinal disease involving progressive photoreceptor degeneration and eventually blindness. They observed that both Hsp90α and Hsp90β were expressed in the developing retina of neonatal mice. Once the retina was fully developed, Hsp90α became the major Hsp90 isoform. In retinal photoreceptors, Hsp90α deficiency caused Golgi apparatus disintegration and impaired intersegmental vesicle trafficking. A proteomic analysis identified the microtubule-associated protein 1B (MAP1B) as an Hsp90α-associated protein in photoreceptors. Hsp90α deficiency increased the degradation of MAP1B by inducing its ubiquitination, causing α-tubulin deacetylation and microtubule destabilization, all potentially contributing to photoreceptor degeneration.

Muscle usually does not have much Hsp90α expression. However, among different type of muscle cells, cardiomyocytes have comparatively high Hsp90α mRNA expression (https://www.proteinatlas.org; accessed on 5 August 2022). Peterson and colleagues showed that the potassium channel hERG, which is critical for cardiac repolarization, solely interacts with Hsp90α and not with Hsp90β [123]. They found a direct relationship between Hsp90α and trafficking of hERG. Hence, the negative impact on hERG and the resulting cardiotoxicity must be considered in the context of treatments with pan-Hsp90 or with Hsp90α-specific inhibitors.

The DNA damage response is assisted by Hsp90α. The DNA-dependent protein kinase (DNA-PK) is a component of the DNA repair machinery, and it is a client of both Hsp90α and Hsp90β [124,125]. However, it was shown that Hsp90α is involved in DNA-PK-mediated DNA repair and apoptosis, but not Hsp90β [126,127]. Hsp90α itself is phosphorylated by DNA-PK at threonines 5 and 7 within its unique N-terminal sequence. Quanz and colleagues found that DNA damage induces the phosphorylation of Hsp90α at the aforementioned sites and its accumulation at sites of DNA double-strand breaks (DSB), where it associates with repair foci and promotes DNA repair [126]. Solier and colleagues showed that phosphorylated Hsp90α is located in the "apoptotic ring" upon induction of apoptosis. Although both phenomena are mediated by DNA-PK, Hsp90α phosphorylation is markedly greater and faster in response to apoptosis than to DNA damage [127]. An additional connection to the DNA damage response comes from the identification of the DNA damage response proteins NBN, and the ataxia-telangiectasia mutated kinase as Hsp90α clients [128]. It is conceivable that Hsp90α-specific inhibition would lead to their destabilization, contributing to defective DNA damage signaling, impaired DNA DSB repair, and increased sensitivity to DNA damage.

Hsp90α controls addictive behavior through the μ opioid receptor (MOR) [129]. Previously, Hsp90 had been found to be required for opioid-induced anti-nociception in the brain by promoting MAPK activation [130]. 17-AAG, a non-selective Hsp90 inhibitor, reduced opioid anti-nociception. In an independent study by Zhang and colleagues, treatment with 17-AAG was observed to reduce morphine analgesia, tolerance, and dependence in mice [131]. Interestingly, Lei and colleagues later found that specific inhibition of Hsp90α with the Hsp90α-selective inhibitor KUNA115 strongly blocked morphine anti-nociception in mice. In contrast, specific inhibition of Hsp90β with the inhibitor KUNB106 did not have any effect on morphine anti-nociception. Their observation suggests that Hsp90β is not involved in regulating opioid anti-nociception in the mouse brain. Surprisingly, Zhang and colleagues demonstrated by co-immunoprecipitation that Hsp90β and not Hsp90α associated with MOR in HEK293T and SH-SY5Y cells [131]. 17-AAG blocked the Hsp90β-MOR interaction and compromised MOR signal transduction in mice. For now, these findings remain contradictory, but if the Hsp90α-specific character of this function could be confirmed, it would suggest the possibility of using Hsp90α inhibitors in psychiatric patients with substance addiction.

Besides functioning as an intracellular molecular chaperone, Hsp90α is also secreted from cells [132–135]. All cells appear to secrete Hsp90α (eHsp90α) in response to environmental stress signals, including heat, hypoxia, inflammatory cytokines, ROS, oxidation agents, and several other stresses [134]. However, normal keratinocytes secrete eHsp90α only in response to tissue injury [136]. When skin is injured, keratinocytes massively release eHsp90α into the wound bed to promote wound repair [135,137]. Cheng and colleagues proposed that eHsp90α drives inward migration of the dermal cells into the wound, which is essential for wound remodeling and formation of new blood vessels [138]. Interestingly, this wound healing activity of eHsp90α does not require dimerization [136] nor ATPase activity, which is, of course, essential for chaperoning [138]. Instead, in this case, only a relatively small portion of eHsp90α is sufficient to elicit the response, essentially as a mitogen, through the LDL-receptor-related protein 1 (LRP1) [139].

3.9. The Clinical Relevance of Targeting Hsp90α

Specifically targeting the Hsp90α isoform could be an attractive therapeutic strategy for treating certain cancers [132,140]. Cancer cells are continuously under replicative, hypoxic, nutrient, and several other stresses [141,142]. Cellular stress leads to the upregulation of the inducible isoform Hsp90α. Hence, in most cancers, Hsp90α is highly upregulated. The knockdown of Hsp90α results in the degradation of several oncogenic client proteins, which suggests that the administration of an Hsp90α-selective inhibitor against Hsp90α-dependent cancers could be beneficial [143]. During cancer progression, many transcription factors encoded by proto-oncogenes are either stabilized by Hsp90α or induce the expression of Hsp90α. For example, the proto-oncogene MYC induces *HSP90AA1* gene expression [144]. The growth hormone prolactin induces *HSP90AA1* expression in breast cancer cells through STAT5 [145]. The nuclear factor-κB (NF-κB) stimulates anti-apoptotic pathways in cancer [146,147]. Ammirante and colleagues showed that two NF-κB putative consensus sequences are present in the *HSP90AA1* 5′ flanking region, and not in that of *HSP90AB1* [148]. This may explain why NF-kB-driven tumorigenic transformation leads to induced *HSP90AA1* expression. In head and neck cancer cells, the transcription factor SOX11 binds to HSP90α [149]. In breast cancer stem cells, Hsp90α and GRP78 interact with PRDM14 [150,151]. As discussed above, *HSP90AB1* is also induced in certain cancers. However, the stress-inducible gene *HSP90AA1* can be expressed several-fold higher than *HSP90AB1*. Thus, the balance of Hsp90α to Hsp90β is specifically shifted towards Hsp90α in cancer cells. It had been found that Hsp90α accounts for 2–3% of total cellular proteins in normal cells, but up to 7% in certain tumor cell lines [152]. Cancer cells may constitutively secrete Hsp90 [153–155], which is essential for enhancing their invasiveness [156]. Although Hsp90β can also be secreted by certain cells, it is eHsp90α and not eHsp90β that is required for invasion in a panel of cancer cell lines. eHsp90α activates matrix metalloproteinase-2, which may be one of the underlying mechanisms explaining enhanced invasiveness and metastasis of cancer cells [132,139,151,157]. The translocation of Hsp90α to the plasma membrane is stimulated by PLCγ1-PKCγ signaling [158], and by mutant p53 via Rab coupling protein-mediated Hsp90α secretion [159]. When Hsp90α is inhibited, the invasiveness of cancer decreases [160–163]. The plasma eHsp90α levels in patients with various cancers correlate with cancer stage [164–166]. For example, plasma Hsp90α levels were increased in patients with thymic epithelial tumor, hepatocellular carcinoma, and colorectal cancer [164–167]. This suggests that serum Hsp90α levels can be a prognostic marker in patients before and during treatment.

Hsp90α plays a significant role in idiopathic pulmonary fibrosis (IPF) [168]. Bellaye and colleagues showed how Hsp90α and Hsp90β synergistically promote myofibroblast persistence in lung fibrosis [169]. Hsp90α, but not Hsp90β, is secreted from IPF lung fibroblasts driven by tissue stiffness and mechanical stretch. Surprisingly, although Hsp90β is not secreted, it binds to LRP1 intracellularly, thus stabilizing the eHsp90 receptor and promoting LRP1 signaling, which feeds forward by inducing the secretion of Hsp90α. Inhibition of eHsp90α, which is increased in serum of patients with IPF, could be beneficial in treating IPF. The non-cell-permeable HSP90 inhibitor HS30 significantly inhibited eHSP90α and LRP1 colocalization, which was significantly increased in patients with moderate and severe IPF. In patients suffering from chronic obstructive pulmonary disease, Hsp90α levels were also found to be elevated in the serum [170], again suggesting that eHsp90α could be used as a biomarker of disease progression. The dysfunction of the airway epithelial barrier is closely related to the pathogenesis of asthma, and eHsp90α participates in the inflammation in asthma [171]. House dust mites (HDM) induce a dysfunction of the airway epithelial barrier. Mice with HDM-induced asthma have high levels of eHsp90α in bronchoalveolar lavage fluid and serum, and eHsp90α can cause the broncial epithelial hyperpermeability. 1G6-D7, a highly selective and inhibitory antibody against Hsp90α, was found to protect against HDM-induced airway epithelial barrier dysfunction. This suggests that eHsp90α-targeted therapy might be a potential asthma treatment.

Wang and colleagues found that HSV-1 survive inside cells using Hsp90α of the host. Hsp90α stabilizes the virion protein 16 (VP16) and promotes VP16-mediated transactivation of HSV-α genes [172]. When Hsp90α was knocked down or inhibited pharmacologically, it resulted in reduced levels of VP16 and of proteins encoded by the HSV-α genes. Considering that Hsp90β may have opposite effects on HSV-1 infections, since they are associated with a drop in Hsp90β levels (see above), careful investigations with highly Hsp90 isoform-selective inhibitors are clearly warranted in order to develop Hsp90-based therapies.

Loss-of-function mutations in the gene encoding the voltage-gated potassium channel KCNQ4 cause DFNA2, a subtype of autosomal dominant non-syndromic deafness characterized by progressive sensorineural hearing loss. The knockdowns of the two Hsp90 isoforms had opposite effects on the total KCNQ4 levels [173,174]. Specifically, the knockdown of Hsp90β led to a dramatic decrease, while the knockdown of Hsp90α resulted in a marked increase. Consistent with these results, overexpression of Hsp90β increased the KCNQ4 levels, whereas up-regulation of Hsp90α expression decreased the total KCNQ4 levels. This suggests that a combination of Hsp90α inhibitor and Hsp90β activator could potentially treat DFNA2.

Hsp90α also has a connection with diabetes. High glucose was shown to induce the translocation of Hsp90α to the outside of aortic endothelial cells [175]. In high glucose conditions, phosphorylation of Hsp90α was increased in a manner dependent on cAMP/protein kinase A, which was responsible for the membrane translocation of Hsp90α and reduced endothelial nitric oxide synthase (eNOS) activity [176]. eNOS is responsible for the production of most of the vascular NO, deficiency in which can promote atherogenesis [177]. Further support for a role of Hsp90α in atherosclerosis and diabetes came from the finding that the levels of eHsp90α were upregulated in patients with aggravated diabetic vascular disease [178]. eHsp90 recruits monocytes through LRP1 activation, which indicates a connection between Hsp90α and inflammatory damage in diabetic vascular complications. These observations suggest that Hsp90α inhibition may be useful in treating patients with type 2 diabetes.

In contrast, the connection of Hsp90 with eNOS was found to be protective against the damages caused by ischemia-reperfusion by reducing the blood flow and glomerular filtration rate [179]. When there is renal ischemia, more Hsp90 is beneficial [179]. Intra-renal transfection of expression plasmids for either Hsp90 isoform was shown to be protective. The protective effect was associated with restoring eNOS–Hsp90 coupling, reestablishing normal PKCα levels, and reducing Rho kinase expression. The transfection events were able to return eNOS phosphorylation to its basal state, restoring NO production and preventing reduced renal blood flow. Hsp90α is also a potential serological biomarker of acute rejection after renal transplantation [180]. Serum Hsp90α levels were significantly higher in kidney recipients upon rejection. In mice receiving a skin transplantation, serum Hsp90α was also found to be elevated when the first graft was rejected, and the levels further increased during more severe rejection of the second graft.

Elevated serum Hsp90α had been found in nonalcoholic steatohepatitis. Serum Hsp90α was increased in patients with metabolic-associated fatty liver disease (MAFLD). A positive correlation was found between age, glycosylated hemoglobin, serum Hsp90α, and grade of steatohepatitis [181]. Xie and colleagues showed that in a MAFLD mouse model, treatment with geranylgeranylacetone leads to decreased Hsp90α levels followed by improvement of steatohepatitis. To the extent that MAFLD may be the same as NAFLD, for which Hsp90β had been pinpointed (see above), here too, a careful classification of MAFLD/NAFLD patients with respect to clinical parameters and Hsp90 levels will be necessary before any Hsp90-based therapy can be considered.

4. Future Perspectives and Conclusions

Overall, Hsp90α-dependent processes contribute to stress adaptation or other specialized functions, while Hsp90β is essential for maintaining standard cellular functions such as cell viability. We recently demonstrated that at cellular and tissue levels, albeit with some exceptions, it is the total Hsp90 levels that matter to sustain essential basic functions, without overt isoform-specific requirements [49]. Pan-Hsp90 inhibitors affect a broad range of key cellular processes, which may have contributed to the failure of several Hsp90 inhibitors in clinical trials [182,183]. However, from the evidence presented in this review, it appears that there are indeed physiological and pathological conditions where one particular isoform is more involved than the other. Hence, targeting only the one critical isoform with isoform-specific inhibitors is the way to go for safer and more efficient treatments (Tables 2–4). Towards reaching that ultimate goal, several major challenges remain. More insights into organ- and cell type-specific functions of the Hsp90 isoforms are needed to stratify patients appropriately for isoform-targeted treatments. Although several groups have begun to report the discovery of isoform-selective inhibitors (Tables 5 and 6), there is still a lot of room for improvement. The ideal Hsp90 isoform-specific inhibitor would have the following features: (i) High isoform-selectivity or even -specificity; (ii) high Hsp90 specificity with limited effects on other biomolecules; (iii) drug-like characteristics, i.e., have favorable pharmacokinetics and pharmacodynamics; (iv) oral availability; (v) for some applications, the ability to cross the blood–brain and blood–testis barriers.

Table 2. Role of specific Hsp90 isoforms in diseases [1].

Expression Levels	Disease
Higher levels of Hsp90α	• Idiopathic pulmonary fibrosis • Asthma • Autosomal dominant non-syndromic deafness • Diabetes type 2 • Nonalcoholic steatohepatitis
Lower levels of Hsp90α	• Male infertility
Higher levels of Hsp90β	• Nonalcoholic fatty liver disease
Lower levels of Hsp90β	• Aβ-induced Alzheimer's disease • DNA viruses and microbial infections

[1] See text for details and references.

Table 3. Cancers with upregulation of specific Hsp90 isoforms [1].

Cancers with Higher Levels of Hsp90β	Cancers with Higher Levels of Hsp90α
Sarcoma	Breast cancer
Hepatocellular carcinoma	Head and neck cancers
Myeloid leukemia	Epithelial cancer
Lung cancer	Colorectal cancer

[1] See text for details and references.

Table 4. Diseases and hypothetical isoform-specific treatments [1].

Diseases	Hypothetical Therapy
Nonalcoholic fatty liver	Hsp90β inhibition
Aβ-induced Alzheimer's disease	Hsp90β induction [2]
Hepatocellular carcinoma	Hsp90β inhibition
Myeloid leukemia cells	Hsp90β inhibition
Ewing's sarcoma	Hsp90β inhibition
Lung cancer	Hsp90β inhibition
Myotonia	Hsp90β inhibition
Hepatitis B virus infection	Hsp90β inhibition
Helicobacter pylori- induced gastric injury	Hsp90β inhibition
Opioid addiction	Hsp90α inhibition
Different cancers	Hsp90α inhibition
Idiopathic pulmonary fibrosis	eHsp90α inhibition
Herpes simplex virus-1 infection	Hsp90α inhibition
Autosomal dominant non-syndromic deafness	Hsp90α inhibitionHsp90β induction
Renal ischemia	Hsp90β/Hsp90α induction

[1] See text for details and references. [2] "Induction" is meant to indicate either increased expression or increased activity.

Table 5. Isoform-specific inhibitors of Hsp90.

Compound	Hsp90 Isoform	Binding Site	References
KUNB31	Hsp90β	N-terminal domain	[184]
Vibsanin B and its derivatives	Hsp90β > Hsp90α	C-terminal domain	[185]
Corylin	Hsp90β	Amino acids 276–602 crucial for corylin binding	[88]
1G6-D7 (antibody)	eHsp90α	Fragment of 115 amino acids encompassing parts of charged and middle domains	[186]
HS30	eHsp90α	N-terminal	[187,188]
KU675	Hsp90α	C-terminal	[189]
NVP-BEP800	Hsp90β > Hsp90α	N-terminal	[190]

Table 6. Inducers of Hsp90β expression.

Compound	References
Jujuboside A	[95]
Erythropoetin	[96]

Author Contributions: S.M. wrote the draft and prepared the Tables and Figures; D.P. edited the draft and figures, and finalized the text for submission. All authors have read and agreed to the published version of the manuscript.

Funding: Work in Didier Picard's laboratory was supported by a grant from the Swiss National Science Foundation and the Canton de Genève.

Institutional Review Board Statement: Not applicable.

Informed Consent Statement: Not applicable.

Data Availability Statement: Not applicable.

Acknowledgments: The authors wish to apologize to all those whose work could not be cited.

Conflicts of Interest: The authors declare no conflict of interest.

References

1. Lindquist, S.; Craig, E.A. The heat-shock proteins. *Annu. Rev. Genet.* **1988**, *22*, 631–677. [CrossRef] [PubMed]
2. Richter, K.; Haslbeck, M.; Buchner, J. The heat shock response: Life on the verge of death. *Mol. Cell* **2010**, *40*, 253–266. [CrossRef] [PubMed]
3. Tissières, A.; Mitchell, H.K.; Tracy, U.M. Protein synthesis in salivary glands of *Drosophila melanogaster*: Relation to chromosome puffs. *J. Mol. Biol.* **1974**, *84*, 389–398. [CrossRef]
4. De Maio, A.; Santoro, M.G.; Tanguay, R.M.; Hightower, L.E. Ferruccio Ritossa's scientific legacy 50 years after his discovery of the heat shock response: A new view of biology, a new society, and a new journal. *Cell Stress Chaperones* **2012**, *17*, 139–143. [CrossRef]
5. Ritossa, F. Discovery of the heat shock response. *Cell Stress Chaperones* **1996**, *1*, 97–98. [CrossRef]
6. Lindquist, S. The heat-shock response. *Annu. Rev. Biochem.* **1986**, *55*, 1151–1191. [CrossRef]
7. Le Breton, L.; Mayer, M.P. A model for handling cell stress. *eLife* **2016**, *5*, e22850. [CrossRef]
8. Whitley, D.; Goldberg, S.P.; Jordan, W.D. Heat shock proteins: A review of the molecular chaperones. *J. Vasc. Surg.* **1999**, *29*, 748–751. [CrossRef]
9. Young, R.A.; Elliott, T.J. Stress proteins, infection, and immune surveillance. *Cell* **1989**, *59*, 5–8. [CrossRef]
10. Jee, H. Size dependent classification of heat shock proteins: A mini-review. *J. Exerc. Rehabil.* **2016**, *12*, 255–259. [CrossRef]
11. Shemesh, N.; Jubran, J.; Dror, S.; Simonovsky, E.; Basha, O.; Argov, C.; Hekselman, I.; Abu-Qarn, M.; Vinogradov, E.; Mauer, O.; et al. The landscape of molecular chaperones across human tissues reveals a layered architecture of core and variable chaperones. *Nat. Commun.* **2021**, *12*, 2180. [CrossRef] [PubMed]
12. Biebl, M.M.; Buchner, J. Structure, function, and regulation of the Hsp90 machinery. *Cold Spring Harb. Perspect. Biol.* **2019**, *11*, a034017. [CrossRef] [PubMed]
13. Stechmann, A.; Cavalier-Smith, T. Evolutionary origins of hsp90 chaperones and a deep paralogy in their bacterial ancestors. *J. Eukaryot. Microbiol.* **2004**, *51*, 364–373. [CrossRef] [PubMed]
14. Chen, B.; Zhong, D.; Monteiro, A. Comparative genomics and evolution of the HSP90 family of genes across all kingdoms of organisms. *BMC Genom.* **2006**, *7*, 156. [CrossRef]
15. Schopf, F.H.; Biebl, M.M.; Buchner, J. The HSP90 chaperone machinery. *Nat. Rev. Mol. Cell. Biol.* **2017**, *18*, 345–360. [CrossRef] [PubMed]
16. Rebeaud, M.E.; Mallik, S.; Goloubinoff, P.; Tawfik, D.S. On the evolution of chaperones and cochaperones and the expansion of proteomes across the Tree of Life. *Proc. Natl. Acad. Sci. USA* **2021**, *118*, e2020885118. [CrossRef]
17. Pantzartzi, C.N.; Drosopoulou, E.; Scouras, Z.G. Assessment and reconstruction of novel HSP90 genes: Duplications, gains and losses in fungal and animal lineages. *PLoS ONE* **2013**, *8*, e73217. [CrossRef]
18. Chen, B.; Piel, W.H.; Gui, L.; Bruford, E.; Monteiro, A. The HSP90 family of genes in the human genome: Insights into their divergence and evolution. *Genomics* **2005**, *86*, 627–637. [CrossRef]
19. Bardwell, J.C.; Craig, E.A. Eukaryotic Mr 83,000 heat shock protein has a homologue in *Escherichia coli*. *Proc. Natl. Acad. Sci. USA* **1987**, *84*, 5177–5181. [CrossRef]
20. Versteeg, S.; Mogk, A.; Schumann, W. The *Bacillus subtilis* htpG gene is not involved in thermal stress management. *Mol. Gen. Genet.* **1999**, *261*, 582–588. [CrossRef]
21. Mason, C.A.; Dunner, J.; Indra, P.; Colangelo, T. Heat-induced expression and chemically induced expression of the *Escherichia coli* stress protein HtpG are affected by the growth environment. *Appl. Environ. Microbiol.* **1999**, *65*, 3433–3440. [CrossRef] [PubMed]

22. Grudniak, A.M.; Pawlak, K.; Bartosik, K.; Wolska, K.I. Physiological consequences of mutations in the *htpG* heat shock gene of *Escherichia coli*. *Mutat. Res.* **2013**, *745–746*, 1–5. [CrossRef] [PubMed]
23. Finka, A.; Goloubinoff, P. Proteomic data from human cell cultures refine mechanisms of chaperone-mediated protein homeostasis. *Cell Stress Chaperones* **2013**, *18*, 591–605. [CrossRef]
24. Picard, D. Heat-shock protein 90, a chaperone for folding and regulation. *Cell. Mol. Life Sci.* **2002**, *59*, 1640–1648. [CrossRef]
25. Bhattacharya, K.; Picard, D. The Hsp70-Hsp90 go-between Hop/Stip1/Sti1 is a proteostatic switch and may be a drug target in cancer and neurodegeneration. *Cell. Mol. Life Sci.* **2021**, *78*, 7257–7273. [CrossRef]
26. Zhao, R.; Davey, M.; Hsu, Y.C.; Kaplanek, P.; Tong, A.; Parsons, A.B.; Krogan, N.; Cagney, G.; Mai, D.; Greenblatt, J.; et al. Navigating the chaperone network: An integrative map of physical and genetic interactions mediated by the hsp90 chaperone. *Cell* **2005**, *120*, 715–727. [CrossRef] [PubMed]
27. McClellan, A.J.; Xia, Y.; Deutschbauer, A.M.; Davis, R.W.; Gerstein, M.; Frydman, J. Diverse cellular functions of the Hsp90 molecular chaperone uncovered using systems approaches. *Cell* **2007**, *131*, 121–135. [CrossRef]
28. Borkovich, K.A.; Farrelly, F.W.; Finkelstein, D.B.; Taulien, J.; Lindquist, S. hsp82 is an essential protein that is required in higher concentrations for growth of cells at higher temperatures. *Mol. Cell. Biol.* **1989**, *9*, 3919–3930. [CrossRef]
29. Girstmair, H.; Tippel, F.; Lopez, A.; Tych, K.; Stein, F.; Haberkant, P.; Schmid, P.W.N.; Helm, D.; Rief, M.; Sattler, M.; et al. The Hsp90 isoforms from *S. cerevisiae* differ in structure, function and client range. *Nat. Commun.* **2019**, *10*, 3626. [CrossRef]
30. Meng, X.; Jerome, V.; Devin, J.; Baulieu, E.E.; Catelli, M.G. Cloning of chicken hsp90β: The only vertebrate hsp90 insensitive to heat shock. *Biochem. Biophys. Res. Commun.* **1993**, *190*, 630–636. [CrossRef]
31. Lees-Miller, S.P.; Anderson, C.W. Two human 90-kDa heat shock proteins are phosphorylated in vivo at conserved serines that are phosphorylated in vitro by casein kinase II. *J. Biol. Chem.* **1989**, *264*, 2431–2437. [CrossRef]
32. Welch, W.J.; Feramisco, J.R. Purification of the major mammalian heat shock proteins. *J. Biol. Chem.* **1982**, *257*, 14949–14959. [CrossRef]
33. Rebbe, N.F.; Ware, J.; Bertina, R.M.; Modrich, P.; Stafford, D.W. Nucleotide sequence of a cDNA for a member of the human 90-kDa heat-shock protein family. *Gene* **1987**, *53*, 235–245. [CrossRef]
34. Song, H.Y.; Dunbar, J.D.; Zhang, Y.X.; Guo, D.; Donner, D.B. Identification of a protein with homology to hsp90 that binds the type 1 tumor necrosis factor receptor. *J. Biol. Chem.* **1995**, *270*, 3574–3581. [CrossRef]
35. Felts, S.J.; Owen, B.A.; Nguyen, P.; Trepel, J.; Donner, D.B.; Toft, D.O. The hsp90-related protein TRAP1 is a mitochondrial protein with distinct functional properties. *J. Biol. Chem.* **2000**, *275*, 3305–3312. [CrossRef]
36. Koch, G.; Smith, M.; Macer, D.; Webster, P.; Mortara, R. Endoplasmic reticulum contains a common, abundant calcium-binding glycoprotein, endoplasmin. *J. Cell Sci.* **1986**, *86*, 217–232. [CrossRef]
37. Krishna, P.; Gloor, G. The Hsp90 family of proteins in *Arabidopsis thaliana*. *Cell Stress Chaperones* **2001**, *6*, 238–246. [CrossRef]
38. Gupta, R.S. Phylogenetic analysis of the 90 kD heat shock family of protein sequences and an examination of the relationship among animals, plants, and fungi species. *Mol. Biol. Evol.* **1995**, *12*, 1063–1073. [CrossRef]
39. Sreedhar, A.S.; Kalmar, E.; Csermely, P.; Shen, Y.F. Hsp90 isoforms: Functions, expression and clinical importance. *FEBS Lett.* **2004**, *562*, 11–15. [CrossRef]
40. Radanyi, C.; Renoir, J.M.; Sabbah, M.; Baulieu, E.E. Chick heat-shock protein of Mr = 90,000, free or released from progesterone receptor, is in a dimeric form. *J. Biol. Chem.* **1989**, *264*, 2568–2573. [CrossRef]
41. Minami, Y.; Kawasaki, H.; Miyata, Y.; Suzuki, K.; Yahara, I. Analysis of native forms and isoform compositions of the mouse 90-kDa heat shock protein, HSP90. *J. Biol. Chem.* **1991**, *266*, 10099–10103. [CrossRef]
42. Kobayakawa, T.; Yamada, S.; Mizuno, A.; Nemoto, T.K. Substitution of only two residues of human Hsp90α causes impeded dimerization of Hsp90β. *Cell Stress Chaperones* **2008**, *13*, 97–104. [CrossRef] [PubMed]
43. Perdew, G.H.; Hord, N.; Hollenback, C.E.; Welsh, M.J. Localization and characterization of the 86- and 84-kDa heat shock proteins in Hepa 1c1c7 cells. *Exp. Cell Res.* **1993**, *209*, 350–356. [CrossRef] [PubMed]
44. Miao, R.Q.; Fontana, J.; Fulton, D.; Lin, M.I.; Harrison, K.D.; Sessa, W.C. Dominant-negative Hsp90 reduces VEGF-stimulated nitric oxide release and migration in endothelial cells. *Arterioscler. Thromb. Vasc. Biol.* **2008**, *28*, 105–111. [CrossRef]
45. Garnier, C.; Lafitte, D.; Jorgensen, T.J.; Jensen, O.N.; Briand, C.; Peyrot, V. Phosphorylation and oligomerization states of native pig brain HSP90 studied by mass spectrometry. *Eur. J. Biochem.* **2001**, *268*, 2402–2407. [CrossRef]
46. Tsaytler, P.A.; Krijgsveld, J.; Goerdayal, S.S.; Rudiger, S.; Egmond, M.R. Novel Hsp90 partners discovered using complementary proteomic approaches. *Cell Stress Chaperones* **2009**, *14*, 629–638. [CrossRef]
47. Richter, K.; Soroka, J.; Skalniak, L.; Leskovar, A.; Hessling, M.; Reinstein, J.; Buchner, J. Conserved conformational changes in the ATPase cycle of human Hsp90. *J. Biol. Chem.* **2008**, *283*, 17757–17765. [CrossRef]
48. Wu, Y.; Zheng, X.; Ding, Y.; Zhou, M.; Wei, Z.; Liu, T.; Liao, K. The molecular chaperone Hsp90α deficiency causes retinal degeneration by disrupting Golgi organization and vesicle transportation in photoreceptors. *J. Mol. Cell. Biol.* **2020**, *12*, 216–229. [CrossRef]
49. Bhattacharya, K.; Maiti, S.; Zahoran, S.; Weidenauer, L.; Hany, D.; Wider, D.; Bernasconi, L.; Quadroni, M.; Collart, M.; Picard, D. Translational reprogramming in response to accumulating stressors ensures critical threshold levels of Hsp90 for mammalian life. *bioRxiv* **2022**. [CrossRef]
50. Echeverria, P.C.; Briand, P.A.; Picard, D. A remodeled Hsp90 molecular chaperone ensemble with the novel cochaperone Aarsd1 is required for muscle differentiation. *Mol. Cell. Biol.* **2016**, *36*, 1310–1321. [CrossRef]

51. Li, J.; Soroka, J.; Buchner, J. The Hsp90 chaperone machinery: Conformational dynamics and regulation by co-chaperones. *Biochim. Biophys. Acta* **2012**, *1823*, 624–635. [CrossRef] [PubMed]
52. Prodromou, C. The 'active life' of Hsp90 complexes. *Biochim. Biophys. Acta* **2012**, *1823*, 614–623. [CrossRef] [PubMed]
53. Dean, M.E.; Johnson, J.L. Human Hsp90 cochaperones: Perspectives on tissue-specific expression and identification of cochaperones with similar in vivo functions. *Cell Stress Chaperones* **2021**, *26*, 3–13. [CrossRef]
54. Tarone, G.; Brancaccio, M. The muscle-specific chaperone protein melusin is a potent cardioprotective agent. *Basic Res. Cardiol.* **2015**, *110*, 10. [CrossRef] [PubMed]
55. Srikakulam, R.; Liu, L.; Winkelmann, D.A. Unc45b forms a cytosolic complex with Hsp90 and targets the unfolded myosin motor domain. *PLoS ONE* **2008**, *3*, e2137. [CrossRef] [PubMed]
56. Most, P.; Bernotat, J.; Ehlermann, P.; Pleger, S.T.; Reppel, M.; Borries, M.; Niroomand, F.; Pieske, B.; Janssen, P.M.; Eschenhagen, T.; et al. S100A1: A regulator of myocardial contractility. *Proc. Natl. Acad. Sci. USA* **2001**, *98*, 13889–13894. [CrossRef]
57. Ruiz-Estevez, M.; Staats, J.; Paatela, E.; Munson, D.; Katoku-Kikyo, N.; Yuan, C.; Asakura, Y.; Hostager, R.; Kobayashi, H.; Asakura, A.; et al. Promotion of myoblast differentiation by Fkbp5 via Cdk4 isomerization. *Cell Rep.* **2018**, *25*, 2537–2551. [CrossRef]
58. Shimoide, T.; Kawao, N.; Tamura, Y.; Morita, H.; Kaji, H. Novel roles of FKBP5 in muscle alteration induced by gravity change in mice. *Biochem. Biophys. Res. Commun.* **2016**, *479*, 602–606. [CrossRef]
59. Grad, I.; Cederroth, C.R.; Walicki, J.; Grey, C.; Barluenga, S.; Winssinger, N.; De Massy, B.; Nef, S.; Picard, D. The molecular chaperone Hsp90α is required for meiotic progression of spermatocytes beyond pachytene in the mouse. *PLoS ONE* **2010**, *5*, e15770. [CrossRef]
60. Fabczak, H.; Osinka, A. Role of the novel Hsp90 co-chaperones in dynein arms' preassembly. *Int. J. Mol. Sci.* **2019**, *20*, 6174. [CrossRef]
61. Wen, Q.; Tang, E.I.; Lui, W.Y.; Lee, W.M.; Wong, C.K.C.; Silvestrini, B.; Cheng, C.Y. Dynein 1 supports spermatid transport and spermiation during spermatogenesis in the rat testis. *Am. J. Physiol. Endocrinol. Metab.* **2018**, *315*, E924–E948. [CrossRef] [PubMed]
62. Crackower, M.A.; Kolas, N.K.; Noguchi, J.; Sarao, R.; Kikuchi, K.; Kaneko, H.; Kobayashi, E.; Kawai, Y.; Kozieradzki, I.; Landers, R.; et al. Essential role of Fkbp6 in male fertility and homologous chromosome pairing in meiosis. *Science* **2003**, *300*, 1291–1295. [CrossRef] [PubMed]
63. Zhang, W.; Zhang, S.; Xiao, C.; Yang, Y.; Zhoucun, A. Mutation screening of the *FKBP6* gene and its association study with spermatogenic impairment in idiopathic infertile men. *Reproduction* **2007**, *133*, 511–516. [CrossRef] [PubMed]
64. Mollapour, M.; Neckers, L. Post-translational modifications of Hsp90 and their contributions to chaperone regulation. *Biochim. Biophys. Acta* **2012**, *1823*, 648–655. [CrossRef]
65. Backe, S.J.; Sager, R.A.; Woodford, M.R.; Makedon, A.M.; Mollapour, M. Post-translational modifications of Hsp90 and translating the chaperone code. *J. Biol. Chem.* **2020**, *295*, 11099–11117. [CrossRef]
66. Ullrich, S.J.; Moore, S.K.; Appella, E. Transcriptional and translational analysis of the murine 84- and 86-kDa heat shock proteins. *J. Biol. Chem.* **1989**, *264*, 6810–6816. [CrossRef]
67. Shen, Y.; Liu, J.; Wang, X.; Cheng, X.; Wang, Y.; Wu, N. Essential role of the first intron in the transcription of hsp90β gene. *FEBS Lett.* **1997**, *413*, 92–98. [CrossRef]
68. Jing, E.; Sundararajan, P.; Majumdar, I.D.; Hazarika, S.; Fowler, S.; Szeto, A.; Gesta, S.; Mendez, A.J.; Vishnudas, V.K.; Sarangarajan, R.; et al. Hsp90β knockdown in DIO mice reverses insulin resistance and improves glucose tolerance. *Nutr. Metab.* **2018**, *15*, 11. [CrossRef]
69. Akerfelt, M.; Morimoto, R.I.; Sistonen, L. Heat shock factors: Integrators of cell stress, development and lifespan. *Nat. Rev. Mol. Cell. Biol.* **2010**, *11*, 545–555. [CrossRef]
70. Prodromou, C. Mechanisms of Hsp90 regulation. *Biochem. J.* **2016**, *473*, 2439–2452. [CrossRef]
71. Zhang, S.L.; Yu, J.; Cheng, X.K.; Ding, L.; Heng, F.Y.; Wu, N.H.; Shen, Y.F. Regulation of human Hsp90α gene expression. *FEBS Lett.* **1999**, *444*, 130–135. [CrossRef]
72. Metchat, A.; Akerfelt, M.; Bierkamp, C.; Delsinne, V.; Sistonen, L.; Alexandre, H.; Christians, E.S. Mammalian heat shock factor 1 is essential for oocyte meiosis and directly regulates Hsp90α expression. *J. Biol. Chem.* **2009**, *284*, 9521–9528. [CrossRef]
73. Liu, Y.; Liu, M.; Liu, J.; Zhang, H.; Tu, Z.; Xiao, X. KLF4 is a novel regulator of the constitutively expressed HSP90. *Cell Stress Chaperones* **2010**, *15*, 211–217. [CrossRef] [PubMed]
74. Stephanou, A.; Latchman, D.S. Transcriptional regulation of the heat shock protein genes by STAT family transcription factors. *Gene Expr.* **1999**, *7*, 311–319.
75. Cheng, M.B.; Zhang, Y.; Zhong, X.; Sutter, B.; Cao, C.Y.; Chen, X.S.; Cheng, X.K.; Zhang, Y.; Xiao, L.; Shen, Y.F. Stat1 mediates an auto-regulation of Hsp90β gene in heat shock response. *Cell. Signal.* **2010**, *22*, 1206–1213. [CrossRef] [PubMed]
76. Thoreen, C.C.; Chantranupong, L.; Keys, H.R.; Wang, T.; Gray, N.S.; Sabatini, D.M. A unifying model for mTORC1-mediated regulation of mRNA translation. *Nature* **2012**, *485*, 109–113. [CrossRef] [PubMed]
77. Zou, J.; Guo, Y.; Guettouche, T.; Smith, D.F.; Voellmy, R. Repression of heat shock transcription factor HSF1 activation by HSP90 (HSP90 complex) that forms a stress-sensitive complex with HSF1. *Cell* **1998**, *94*, 471–480. [CrossRef]
78. Kijima, T.; Prince, T.L.; Tigue, M.L.; Yim, K.H.; Schwartz, H.; Beebe, K.; Lee, S.; Budzynski, M.A.; Williams, H.; Trepel, J.B.; et al. HSP90 inhibitors disrupt a transient HSP90-HSF1 interaction and identify a noncanonical model of HSP90-mediated HSF1 regulation. *Sci. Rep.* **2018**, *8*, 6976. [CrossRef]

79. Echeverria, P.C.; Bernthaler, A.; Dupuis, P.; Mayer, B.; Picard, D. An interaction network predicted from public data as a discovery tool: Application to the Hsp90 molecular chaperone machine. *PLoS ONE* **2011**, *6*, e26044. [CrossRef]
80. Taipale, M.; Tucker, G.; Peng, J.; Krykbaeva, I.; Lin, Z.Y.; Larsen, B.; Choi, H.; Berger, B.; Gingras, A.C.; Lindquist, S. A quantitative chaperone interaction network reveals the architecture of cellular protein homeostasis pathways. *Cell* **2014**, *158*, 434–448. [CrossRef]
81. Voss, A.K.; Thomas, T.; Gruss, P. Mice lacking Hsp90β fail to develop a placental labyrinth. *Development* **2000**, *127*, 1–11. [CrossRef]
82. Okumura, F.; Okumura, A.J.; Matsumoto, M.; Nakayama, K.I.; Hatakeyama, S. TRIM8 regulates Nanog via Hsp90β-mediated nuclear translocation of STAT3 in embryonic stem cells. *Biochim. Biophys. Acta* **2011**, *1813*, 1784–1792. [CrossRef] [PubMed]
83. He, M.Y.; Xu, S.B.; Qu, Z.H.; Guo, Y.M.; Liu, X.C.; Cong, X.X.; Wang, J.F.; Low, B.C.; Li, L.; Wu, Q.; et al. Hsp90β interacts with MDM2 to suppress p53-dependent senescence during skeletal muscle regeneration. *Aging Cell* **2019**, *18*, e13003. [CrossRef] [PubMed]
84. McCormick, R.; Vasilaki, A. Age-related changes in skeletal muscle: Changes to life-style as a therapy. *Biogerontology* **2018**, *19*, 519–536. [CrossRef] [PubMed]
85. Relaix, F.; Bencze, M.; Borok, M.J.; Der Vartanian, A.; Gattazzo, F.; Mademtzoglou, D.; Perez-Diaz, S.; Prola, A.; Reyes-Fernandez, P.C.; Rotini, A.; et al. Perspectives on skeletal muscle stem cells. *Nat. Commun.* **2021**, *12*, 692. [CrossRef] [PubMed]
86. Jing, R.; Duncan, C.B.; Duncan, S.A. A small-molecule screen reveals that HSP90β promotes the conversion of induced pluripotent stem cell-derived endoderm to a hepatic fate and regulates HNF4A turnover. *Development* **2017**, *144*, 1764–1774. [CrossRef] [PubMed]
87. Huck, I.; Gunewardena, S.; Espanol-Suner, R.; Willenbring, H.; Apte, U. Hepatocyte nuclear factor 4 alpha activation is essential for termination of liver regeneration in mice. *Hepatology* **2019**, *70*, 666–681. [CrossRef]
88. Zheng, Z.G.; Zhang, X.; Liu, X.X.; Jin, X.X.; Dai, L.; Cheng, H.M.; Jing, D.; Thu, P.M.; Zhang, M.; Li, H.; et al. Inhibition of HSP90β Improves Lipid Disorders by Promoting Mature SREBPs Degradation via the Ubiquitin-proteasome System. *Theranostics* **2019**, *9*, 5769–5783. [CrossRef]
89. Kuan, Y.C.; Hashidume, T.; Shibata, T.; Uchida, K.; Shimizu, M.; Inoue, J.; Sato, R. Heat shock protein 90 modulates lipid homeostasis by regulating the stability and function of sterol regulatory element-binding protein (SREBP) and SREBP Cleavage-activating Protein. *J. Biol. Chem.* **2017**, *292*, 3016–3028. [CrossRef]
90. Angelo, G.; Lamon-Fava, S.; Sonna, L.A.; Lindauer, M.L.; Wood, R.J. Heat shock protein 90β: A novel mediator of vitamin D action. *Biochem. Biophys. Res. Commun.* **2008**, *367*, 578–583. [CrossRef]
91. Luo, S.; Zhang, B.; Dong, X.P.; Tao, Y.; Ting, A.; Zhou, Z.; Meixiong, J.; Luo, J.; Chiu, F.C.; Xiong, W.C.; et al. Hsp90β regulates rapsyn turnover and subsequent AChR cluster formation and maintenance. *Neuron* **2008**, *60*, 97–110. [CrossRef] [PubMed]
92. Li, L.; Cao, Y.; Wu, H.; Ye, X.; Zhu, Z.; Xing, G.; Shen, C.; Barik, A.; Zhang, B.; Xie, X.; et al. Enzymatic activity of the scaffold protein rapsyn for synapse formation. *Neuron* **2016**, *92*, 1007–1019. [CrossRef] [PubMed]
93. Balanescu, A.; Stan, I.; Codreanu, I.; Comanici, V.; Balanescu, E.; Balanescu, P. Circulating Hsp90 isoform levels in overweight and obese children and the relation to nonalcoholic fatty liver disease: Results from a cross-Sectional study. *Dis. Markers* **2019**, *2019*, 9560247. [CrossRef] [PubMed]
94. Ou, J.R.; Tan, M.S.; Xie, A.M.; Yu, J.T.; Tan, L. Heat shock protein 90 in Alzheimer's disease. *BioMed Res. Int.* **2014**, *2014*, 796869. [CrossRef]
95. Zhang, M.; Qian, C.; Zheng, Z.G.; Qian, F.; Wang, Y.; Thu, P.M.; Zhang, X.; Zhou, Y.; Tu, L.; Liu, Q.; et al. Jujuboside A promotes Aβ clearance and ameliorates cognitive deficiency in Alzheimer's disease through activating Axl/HSP90/PPARγ pathway. *Theranostics* **2018**, *8*, 4262–4278. [CrossRef]
96. Wan, H.L.; Zhang, B.G.; Chen, C.; Liu, Q.; Li, T.; He, Y.; Xie, Y.; Yang, X.; Wang, J.Z.; Liu, G.P. Recombinant human erythropoietin ameliorates cognitive dysfunction of APP/PS1 mice by attenuating neuron apoptosis via HSP90β. *Signal Transduct. Target Ther.* **2022**, *7*, 149. [CrossRef]
97. Sato, S.; Li, K.; Sakurai, N.; Hashizume, M.; Baidya, S.; Nonaka, H.; Noguchi, K.; Ishikawa, K.; Obuse, C.; Takaoka, A. Regulation of an adaptor protein STING by Hsp90β to enhance innate immune responses against microbial infections. *Cell. Immunol.* **2020**, *356*, 104188. [CrossRef]
98. Kim, S.H.; Ji, J.H.; Park, K.T.; Lee, J.H.; Kang, K.W.; Park, J.H.; Hwang, S.W.; Lee, E.H.; Cho, Y.J.; Jeong, Y.Y.; et al. High-level expression of Hsp90β is associated with poor survival in resectable non-small-cell lung cancer patients. *Histopathology* **2015**, *67*, 509–519. [CrossRef]
99. Meng, J.; Liu, Y.; Han, J.; Tan, Q.; Chen, S.; Qiao, K.; Zhou, H.; Sun, T.; Yang, C. Hsp90β promoted endothelial cell-dependent tumor angiogenesis in hepatocellular carcinoma. *Mol. Cancer* **2017**, *16*, 72. [CrossRef]
100. Meng, J.; Chen, S.; Lei, Y.Y.; Han, J.X.; Zhong, W.L.; Wang, X.R.; Liu, Y.R.; Gao, W.F.; Zhang, Q.; Tan, Q.; et al. Hsp90β promotes aggressive vasculogenic mimicry via epithelial-mesenchymal transition in hepatocellular carcinoma. *Oncogene* **2019**, *38*, 228–243. [CrossRef]
101. Li, S.; Li, J.; Hu, T.; Zhang, C.; Lv, X.; He, S.; Yan, H.; Tan, Y.; Wen, M.; Lei, M.; et al. Bcl-2 overexpression contributes to laryngeal carcinoma cell survival by forming a complex with Hsp90β. *Oncol. Rep.* **2017**, *37*, 849–856. [CrossRef] [PubMed]
102. Correia, A.L.; Mori, H.; Chen, E.I.; Schmitt, F.C.; Bissell, M.J. The hemopexin domain of MMP3 is responsible for mammary epithelial invasion and morphogenesis through extracellular interaction with HSP90β. *Genes Dev.* **2013**, *27*, 805–817. [CrossRef] [PubMed]

103. Heck, A.L.; Mishra, S.; Prenzel, T.; Feulner, L.; Achhammer, E.; Sarchen, V.; Blagg, B.S.J.; Schneider-Brachert, W.; Schutze, S.; Fritsch, J. Selective HSP90β inhibition results in TNF and TRAIL mediated HIF1α degradation. *Immunobiology* **2021**, *226*, 152070. [CrossRef] [PubMed]
104. Kurokawa, M.; Zhao, C.; Reya, T.; Kornbluth, S. Inhibition of apoptosome formation by suppression of Hsp90β phosphorylation in tyrosine kinase-induced leukemias. *Mol. Cell. Biol.* **2008**, *28*, 5494–5506. [CrossRef]
105. Roundhill, E.; Turnbull, D.; Burchill, S. Localization of MRP-1 to the outer mitochondrial membrane by the chaperone protein HSP90β. *FASEB J.* **2016**, *30*, 1712–1723. [CrossRef]
106. Suzuki, S.; Kulkarni, A.B. Extracellular heat shock protein Hsp90β secreted by MG63 osteosarcoma cells inhibits activation of latent TGF-β1. *Biochem. Biophys. Res. Commun.* **2010**, *398*, 525–531. [CrossRef]
107. Sousa-Squiavinato, A.C.; Silvestre, R.N.; Elgui De Oliveira, D. Biology and oncogenicity of the Kaposi sarcoma herpesvirus K1 protein. *Rev. Med. Virol.* **2015**, *25*, 273–285. [CrossRef]
108. Peng, Y.J.; Huang, J.J.; Wu, H.H.; Hsieh, H.Y.; Wu, C.Y.; Chen, S.C.; Chen, T.Y.; Tang, C.Y. Regulation of CLC-1 chloride channel biosynthesis by FKBP8 and Hsp90β. *Sci. Rep.* **2016**, *6*, 32444. [CrossRef]
109. Kim, S.W.; Hasanuzzaman, M.; Cho, M.; Heo, Y.R.; Ryu, M.J.; Ha, N.Y.; Park, H.J.; Park, H.Y.; Shin, J.G. Casein kinase 2 (CK2)-mediated phosphorylation of Hsp90β as a novel mechanism of rifampin-induced MDR1 expression. *J. Biol. Chem.* **2015**, *290*, 17029–17040. [CrossRef]
110. Liu, D.; Wu, A.; Cui, L.; Hao, R.; Wang, Y.; He, J.; Guo, D. Hepatitis B virus polymerase suppresses NF-κB signaling by inhibiting the activity of IKKs via interaction with Hsp90β. *PLoS ONE* **2014**, *9*, e91658. [CrossRef]
111. Cha, B.; Lim, J.W.; Kim, K.H.; Kim, H. HSP90β interacts with Rac1 to activate NADPH oxidase in Helicobacter pylori-infected gastric epithelial cells. *Int. J. Biochem. Cell Biol.* **2010**, *42*, 1455–1461. [CrossRef] [PubMed]
112. Asakawa, S.; Onodera, R.; Kasai, K.; Kishimoto, Y.; Sato, T.; Segawa, R.; Mizuno, N.; Ogasawara, K.; Moriya, T.; Hiratsuka, M.; et al. Nickel ions bind to HSP90β and enhance HIF-1α-mediated IL-8 expression. *Toxicology* **2018**, *395*, 45–53. [CrossRef] [PubMed]
113. Zuehlke, A.D.; Beebe, K.; Neckers, L.; Prince, T. Regulation and function of the human *HSP90AA1* gene. *Gene* **2015**, *570*, 8–16. [CrossRef]
114. Rzechorzek, N.M.; Thrippleton, M.J.; Chappell, F.M.; Mair, G.; Ercole, A.; Cabeleira, M.; CENTER-TBI High Resolution ICU (HR ICU) Sub-Study Participants and Investigators; Rhodes, J.; Marshall, I.; O'Neill, J.S. A daily temperature rhythm in the human brain predicts survival after brain injury. *Brain* **2022**, *145*, 2031–2048. [CrossRef]
115. Kajiwara, C.; Kondo, S.; Uda, S.; Dai, L.; Ichiyanagi, T.; Chiba, T.; Ishido, S.; Koji, T.; Udono, H. Spermatogenesis arrest caused by conditional deletion of Hsp90α in adult mice. *Biol. Open* **2012**, *1*, 977–982. [CrossRef]
116. Ichiyanagi, T.; Ichiyanagi, K.; Ogawa, A.; Kuramochi-Miyagawa, S.; Nakano, T.; Chuma, S.; Sasaki, H.; Udono, H. HSP90α plays an important role in piRNA biogenesis and retrotransposon repression in mouse. *Nucleic Acids Res.* **2014**, *42*, 11903–11911. [CrossRef] [PubMed]
117. Tang, X.; Chang, C.; Hao, M.; Chen, M.; Woodley, D.T.; Schonthal, A.H.; Li, W. Heat shock protein-90α (Hsp90α) stabilizes hypoxia-inducible factor-1α (HIF-1α) in support of spermatogenesis and tumorigenesis. *Cancer Gene Ther.* **2021**, *28*, 1058–1070. [CrossRef] [PubMed]
118. Ueda, K.; Xu, J.; Morimoto, H.; Kawabe, A.; Imaoka, S. MafG controls the hypoxic response of cells by accumulating HIF-1α in the nuclei. *FEBS Lett.* **2008**, *582*, 2357–2364. [CrossRef] [PubMed]
119. Hogenesch, J.B.; Chan, W.K.; Jackiw, V.H.; Brown, R.C.; Gu, Y.Z.; Pray-Grant, M.; Perdew, G.H.; Bradfield, C.A. Characterization of a subset of the basic-helix-loop-helix-PAS superfamily that interacts with components of the dioxin signaling pathway. *J. Biol. Chem.* **1997**, *272*, 8581–8593. [CrossRef]
120. Vos, J.J. A theory of retinal burns. *Bull. Math. Biophys.* **1962**, *24*, 115–128. [CrossRef]
121. Van Norren, D.; Vos, J.J. Light damage to the retina: An historical approach. *Eye* **2016**, *30*, 169–172. [CrossRef]
122. Mainster, M.A.; White, T.J.; Tips, J.H.; Wilson, P.W. Retinal-temperature increases produced by intense light sources. *J. Opt. Soc. Am.* **1970**, *60*, 264–270. [CrossRef] [PubMed]
123. Peterson, L.B.; Eskew, J.D.; Vielhauer, G.A.; Blagg, B.S. The hERG channel is dependent upon the Hsp90α isoform for maturation and trafficking. *Mol. Pharm.* **2012**, *9*, 1841–1846. [CrossRef] [PubMed]
124. Falsone, S.F.; Gesslbauer, B.; Tirk, F.; Piccinini, A.M.; Kungl, A.J. A proteomic snapshot of the human heat shock protein 90 interactome. *FEBS Lett.* **2005**, *579*, 6350–6354. [CrossRef] [PubMed]
125. Lees-Miller, S.P.; Anderson, C.W. The human double-stranded DNA-activated protein kinase phosphorylates the 90-kDa heat-shock protein, hsp90α at two NH2-terminal threonine residues. *J. Biol. Chem.* **1989**, *264*, 17275–17280. [CrossRef]
126. Quanz, M.; Herbette, A.; Sayarath, M.; de Koning, L.; Dubois, T.; Sun, J.S.; Dutreix, M. Heat shock protein 90α (Hsp90α) is phosphorylated in response to DNA damage and accumulates in repair foci. *J. Biol. Chem.* **2012**, *287*, 8803–8815. [CrossRef]
127. Solier, S.; Kohn, K.W.; Scroggins, B.; Xu, W.; Trepel, J.; Neckers, L.; Pommier, Y. Heat shock protein 90α (Hsp90α), a substrate and chaperone of DNA-PK necessary for the apoptotic response. *Proc. Natl. Acad. Sci. USA* **2012**, *109*, 12866–12872. [CrossRef]
128. Pennisi, R.; Antoccia, A.; Leone, S.; Ascenzi, P.; di Masi, A. Hsp90α regulates ATM and NBN functions in sensing and repair of DNA double-strand breaks. *FEBS J.* **2017**, *284*, 2378–2395. [CrossRef]
129. Lei, W.; Duron, D.I.; Stine, C.; Mishra, S.; Blagg, B.S.J.; Streicher, J.M. The alpha isoform of heat shock protein 90 and the co-chaperones p23 and Cdc37 promote opioid anti-nociception in the brain. *Front. Mol. Neurosci.* **2019**, *12*, 294. [CrossRef]

130. Lei, W.; Mullen, N.; McCarthy, S.; Brann, C.; Richard, P.; Cormier, J.; Edwards, K.; Bilsky, E.J.; Streicher, J.M. Heat-shock protein 90 (Hsp90) promotes opioid-induced anti-nociception by an ERK mitogen-activated protein kinase (MAPK) mechanism in mouse brain. *J. Biol. Chem.* **2017**, *292*, 10414–10428. [CrossRef]
131. Zhang, Y.; Zhou, P.; Wang, Z.; Chen, M.; Fu, F.; Su, R. Hsp90β positively regulates μ-opioid receptor function. *Life Sci.* **2020**, *252*, 117676. [CrossRef]
132. Eustace, B.K.; Sakurai, T.; Stewart, J.K.; Yimlamai, D.; Unger, C.; Zehetmeier, C.; Lain, B.; Torella, C.; Henning, S.W.; Beste, G.; et al. Functional proteomic screens reveal an essential extracellular role for Hsp90α in cancer cell invasiveness. *Nat. Cell Biol.* **2004**, *6*, 507–514. [CrossRef]
133. Tsutsumi, S.; Neckers, L. Extracellular heat shock protein 90: A role for a molecular chaperone in cell motility and cancer metastasis. *Cancer Sci.* **2007**, *98*, 1536–1539. [CrossRef] [PubMed]
134. Li, W.; Sahu, D.; Tsen, F. Secreted heat shock protein-90 (Hsp90) in wound healing and cancer. *Biochim. Biophys. Acta* **2012**, *1823*, 730–741. [CrossRef] [PubMed]
135. Li, W.; Li, Y.; Guan, S.; Fan, J.; Cheng, C.F.; Bright, A.M.; Chinn, C.; Chen, M.; Woodley, D.T. Extracellular heat shock protein-90α: Linking hypoxia to skin cell motility and wound healing. *EMBO J.* **2007**, *26*, 1221–1233. [CrossRef]
136. Bhatia, A.; O'Brien, K.; Guo, J.; Lincoln, V.; Kajiwara, C.; Chen, M.; Woodley, D.T.; Udono, H.; Li, W. Extracellular and non-chaperone function of heat shock protein-90α is required for skin wound healing. *J. Investig. Dermatol.* **2018**, *138*, 423–433. [CrossRef] [PubMed]
137. Guo, J.; Chang, C.; Li, W. The role of secreted heat shock protein-90 (Hsp90) in wound healing—how could it shape future therapeutics? *Expert Rev. Proteomics* **2017**, *14*, 665–675. [CrossRef] [PubMed]
138. Cheng, C.F.; Sahu, D.; Tsen, F.; Zhao, Z.; Fan, J.; Kim, R.; Wang, X.; O'Brien, K.; Li, Y.; Kuang, Y.; et al. A fragment of secreted Hsp90α carries properties that enable it to accelerate effectively both acute and diabetic wound healing in mice. *J. Clin. Investig.* **2011**, *121*, 4348–4361. [CrossRef] [PubMed]
139. Woodley, D.T.; Fan, J.; Cheng, C.F.; Li, Y.; Chen, M.; Bu, G.; Li, W. Participation of the lipoprotein receptor LRP1 in hypoxia-HSP90α autocrine signaling to promote keratinocyte migration. *J. Cell Sci.* **2009**, *122*, 1495–1498. [CrossRef] [PubMed]
140. Mishra, S.J.; Khandelwal, A.; Banerjee, M.; Balch, M.; Peng, S.; Davis, R.E.; Merfeld, T.; Munthali, V.; Deng, J.; Matts, R.L.; et al. Selective inhibition of the Hsp90α isoform. *Angew. Chem. Int. Ed.* **2021**, *60*, 10547–10551. [CrossRef]
141. Muz, B.; de la Puente, P.; Azab, F.; Azab, A.K. The role of hypoxia in cancer progression, angiogenesis, metastasis, and resistance to therapy. *Hypoxia* **2015**, *3*, 83–92. [CrossRef]
142. Chen, M.; Xie, S. Therapeutic targeting of cellular stress responses in cancer. *Thorac. Cancer* **2018**, *9*, 1575–1582. [CrossRef]
143. Vartholomaiou, E.; Madon-Simon, M.; Hagmann, S.; Muhlebach, G.; Wurst, W.; Floss, T.; Picard, D. Cytosolic Hsp90α and its mitochondrial isoform Trap1 are differentially required in a breast cancer model. *Oncotarget* **2017**, *8*, 17428–17442. [CrossRef]
144. Teng, S.C.; Chen, Y.Y.; Su, Y.N.; Chou, P.C.; Chiang, Y.C.; Tseng, S.F.; Wu, K.J. Direct activation of HSP90A transcription by c-Myc contributes to c-Myc-induced transformation. *J. Biol. Chem.* **2004**, *279*, 14649–14655. [CrossRef] [PubMed]
145. Perotti, C.; Liu, R.; Parusel, C.T.; Bocher, N.; Schultz, J.; Bork, P.; Pfitzner, E.; Groner, B.; Shemanko, C.S. Heat shock protein-90α, a prolactin-STAT5 target gene identified in breast cancer cells, is involved in apoptosis regulation. *Breast Cancer Res.* **2008**, *10*, R94. [CrossRef] [PubMed]
146. Broemer, M.; Krappmann, D.; Scheidereit, C. Requirement of hsp90 activity for IκB kinase (IKK) biosynthesis and for constitutive and inducible IKK and NF-κB activation. *Oncogene* **2004**, *23*, 5378–5386. [CrossRef] [PubMed]
147. Karin, M.; Greten, F.R. NF-κB: Linking inflammation and immunity to cancer development and progression. *Nat. Rev. Immunol.* **2005**, *5*, 749–759. [CrossRef] [PubMed]
148. Ammirante, M.; Rosati, A.; Gentilella, A.; Festa, M.; Petrella, A.; Marzullo, L.; Pascale, M.; Belisario, M.A.; Leone, A.; Turco, M.C. The activity of *hsp90* promoter is regulated by NF-κB transcription factors. *Oncogene* **2008**, *27*, 1175–1178. [CrossRef]
149. Elzakra, N.; Cui, L.; Liu, T.; Li, H.; Huang, J.; Hu, S. Mass spectrometric analysis of SOX11-binding proteins in head and neck cancer cells demonstrates the interaction of SOX11 and HSP90α. *J. Proteome Res.* **2017**, *16*, 3961–3968. [CrossRef]
150. Moriya, C.; Taniguchi, H.; Nagatoishi, S.; Igarashi, H.; Tsumoto, K.; Imai, K. PRDM14 directly interacts with heat shock proteins HSP90α and glucose-regulated protein 78. *Cancer Sci.* **2018**, *109*, 373–383. [CrossRef] [PubMed]
151. Tian, Y.; Wang, C.; Chen, S.; Liu, J.; Fu, Y.; Luo, Y. Extracellular Hsp90α and clusterin synergistically promote breast cancer epithelial-to-mesenchymal transition and metastasis via LRP1. *J. Cell Sci.* **2019**, *132*, jcs228213. [CrossRef] [PubMed]
152. Sahu, D.; Zhao, Z.; Tsen, F.; Cheng, C.F.; Park, R.; Situ, A.J.; Dai, J.; Eginli, A.; Shams, S.; Chen, M.; et al. A potentially common peptide target in secreted heat shock protein-90α for hypoxia-inducible factor-1α-positive tumors. *Mol. Biol. Cell* **2012**, *23*, 602–613. [CrossRef] [PubMed]
153. Song, X.; Luo, Y. The regulatory mechanism of Hsp90α secretion from endothelial cells and its role in angiogenesis during wound healing. *Biochem. Biophys. Res. Commun.* **2010**, *398*, 111–117. [CrossRef] [PubMed]
154. McCready, J.; Sims, J.D.; Chan, D.; Jay, D.G. Secretion of extracellular Hsp90α via exosomes increases cancer cell motility: A role for plasminogen activation. *BMC Cancer* **2010**, *10*, 294. [CrossRef]
155. Wang, X.; Song, X.; Zhuo, W.; Fu, Y.; Shi, H.; Liang, Y.; Tong, M.; Chang, G.; Luo, Y. The regulatory mechanism of Hsp90α secretion and its function in tumor malignancy. *Proc. Natl. Acad. Sci. USA* **2009**, *106*, 21288–21293. [CrossRef]

156. Tang, X.; Chang, C.; Guo, J.; Lincoln, V.; Liang, C.; Chen, M.; Woodley, D.T.; Li, W. Tumour-secreted Hsp90α on external surface of exosomes mediates tumour—Stromal cell communication via autocrine and paracrine mechanisms. *Sci. Rep.* **2019**, *9*, 15108. [CrossRef] [PubMed]
157. Picard, D. Hsp90 invades the outside. *Nat. Cell Biol.* **2004**, *6*, 479–480. [CrossRef]
158. Yang, J.; Song, X.; Chen, Y.; Lu, X.A.; Fu, Y.; Luo, Y. PLCγ1–PKCγ signaling-mediated Hsp90α plasma membrane translocation facilitates tumor metastasis. *Traffic* **2014**, *15*, 861–878. [CrossRef]
159. Zhang, S.; Wang, C.; Ma, B.; Xu, M.; Xu, S.; Liu, J.; Tian, Y.; Fu, Y.; Luo, Y. Mutant p53 drives cancer metastasis via RCP-mediated Hsp90α secretion. *Cell Rep.* **2020**, *32*, 107879. [CrossRef]
160. Yang, Y.; Rao, R.; Shen, J.; Tang, Y.; Fiskus, W.; Nechtman, J.; Atadja, P.; Bhalla, K. Role of acetylation and extracellular location of heat shock protein 90α in tumor cell invasion. *Cancer Res.* **2008**, *68*, 4833–4842. [CrossRef]
161. Rybarczyk, P.; Vanlaeys, A.; Brassart, B.; Dhennin-Duthille, I.; Chatelain, D.; Sevestre, H.; Ouadid-Ahidouch, H.; Gautier, M. The transient receptor potential melastatin 7 channel regulates pancreatic cancer cell invasion through the Hsp90α/uPA/MMP2 pathway. *Neoplasia* **2017**, *19*, 288–300. [CrossRef]
162. Taiyab, A.; Rao Ch, M. HSP90 modulates actin dynamics: Inhibition of HSP90 leads to decreased cell motility and impairs invasion. *Biochim. Biophys. Acta* **2011**, *1813*, 213–221. [CrossRef] [PubMed]
163. Hartmann, S.; Gunther, N.; Biehl, M.; Katzer, A.; Kuger, S.; Worschech, E.; Sukhorukov, V.L.; Krohne, G.; Zimmermann, H.; Flentje, M.; et al. Hsp90 inhibition by NVP-AUY922 and NVP-BEP800 decreases migration and invasion of irradiated normoxic and hypoxic tumor cell lines. *Cancer Lett.* **2013**, *331*, 200–210. [CrossRef] [PubMed]
164. Wei, W.; Liu, M.; Ning, S.; Wei, J.; Zhong, J.; Li, J.; Cai, Z.; Zhang, L. Diagnostic value of plasma HSP90α levels for detection of hepatocellular carcinoma. *BMC Cancer* **2020**, *20*, 6. [CrossRef] [PubMed]
165. Hou, Q.; Chen, S.; An, Q.; Li, B.; Fu, Y.; Luo, Y. Extracellular Hsp90α promotes tumor lymphangiogenesis and lymph node metastasis in breast cancer. *Int. J. Mol. Sci.* **2021**, *22*, 7747. [CrossRef] [PubMed]
166. Dong, H.; Zou, M.; Bhatia, A.; Jayaprakash, P.; Hofman, F.; Ying, Q.; Chen, M.; Woodley, D.T.; Li, W. Breast cancer MDA-MB-231 cells use secreted heat shock protein-90α (Hsp90α) to survive a hostile hypoxic environment. *Sci. Rep.* **2016**, *6*, 20605. [CrossRef]
167. Chen, W.S.; Chen, C.C.; Chen, L.L.; Lee, C.C.; Huang, T.S. Secreted heat shock protein 90α (HSP90α) induces nuclear factor-kappaB-mediated TCF12 protein expression to down-regulate E-cadherin and to enhance colorectal cancer cell migration and invasion. *J. Biol. Chem.* **2013**, *288*, 9001–9010. [CrossRef]
168. Bonniaud, P.; Burgy, O.; Garrido, C. Heat shock protein-90 toward theranostics: A breath of fresh air in idiopathic pulmonary fibrosis. *Eur. Respir. J.* **2018**, *51*, 1702612. [CrossRef]
169. Bellaye, P.S.; Shimbori, C.; Yanagihara, T.; Carlson, D.A.; Hughes, P.; Upagupta, C.; Sato, S.; Wheildon, N.; Haystead, T.; Ask, K.; et al. Synergistic role of HSP90α and HSP90β to promote myofibroblast persistence in lung fibrosis. *Eur. Respir. J.* **2018**, *51*, 1700386. [CrossRef]
170. Hacker, S.; Lambers, C.; Hoetzenecker, K.; Pollreisz, A.; Aigner, C.; Lichtenauer, M.; Mangold, A.; Niederpold, T.; Zimmermann, M.; Taghavi, S.; et al. Elevated HSP27, HSP70 and HSP90α in chronic obstructive pulmonary disease: Markers for immune activation and tissue destruction. *Clin. Lab.* **2009**, *55*, 31–40.
171. Ye, C.; Huang, C.; Zou, M.; Hu, Y.; Luo, L.; Wei, Y.; Wan, X.; Zhao, H.; Li, W.; Cai, S.; et al. The role of secreted Hsp90α in HDM-induced asthmatic airway epithelial barrier dysfunction. *BMC Pulm. Med.* **2019**, *19*, 218. [CrossRef]
172. Wang, Y.; Wang, R.; Li, F.; Wang, Y.; Zhang, Z.; Wang, Q.; Ren, Z.; Jin, F.; Kitazato, K.; Wang, Y. Heat-shock protein 90α is involved in maintaining the stability of VP16 and VP16-mediated transactivation of α genes from herpes simplex virus-1. *Mol. Med.* **2018**, *24*, 65. [CrossRef] [PubMed]
173. Gao, Y.; Yechikov, S.; Vazquez, A.E.; Chen, D.; Nie, L. Impaired surface expression and conductance of the KCNQ4 channel lead to sensorineural hearing loss. *J. Cell. Mol. Med.* **2013**, *17*, 889–900. [CrossRef]
174. Gao, Y.; Yechikov, S.; Vazquez, A.E.; Chen, D.; Nie, L. Distinct roles of molecular chaperones HSP90α and HSP90β in the biogenesis of KCNQ4 channels. *PLoS ONE* **2013**, *8*, e57282. [CrossRef] [PubMed]
175. Lei, H.; Romeo, G.; Kazlauskas, A. Heat shock protein 90α-dependent translocation of annexin II to the surface of endothelial cells modulates plasmin activity in the diabetic rat aorta. *Circ. Res.* **2004**, *94*, 902–909. [CrossRef] [PubMed]
176. Lei, H.; Venkatakrishnan, A.; Yu, S.; Kazlauskas, A. Protein kinase A-dependent translocation of Hsp90α impairs endothelial nitric-oxide synthase activity in high glucose and diabetes. *J. Biol. Chem.* **2007**, *282*, 9364–9371. [CrossRef]
177. Lin, K.Y.; Ito, A.; Asagami, T.; Tsao, P.S.; Adimoolam, S.; Kimoto, M.; Tsuji, H.; Reaven, G.M.; Cooke, J.P. Impaired nitric oxide synthase pathway in diabetes mellitus: Role of asymmetric dimethylarginine and dimethylarginine dimethylaminohydrolase. *Circulation* **2002**, *106*, 987–992. [CrossRef]
178. Ding, X.; Meng, C.; Dong, H.; Zhang, S.; Zhou, H.; Tan, W.; Huang, L.; He, A.; Li, J.; Huang, J.; et al. Extracellular Hsp90α, which participates in vascular inflammation, is a novel serum predictor of atherosclerosis in type 2 diabetes. *BMJ Open Diabetes Res. Care* **2022**, *10*, e002579. [CrossRef]
179. Barrera-Chimal, J.; Perez-Villalva, R.; Ortega, J.A.; Uribe, N.; Gamba, G.; Cortes-Gonzalez, C.; Bobadilla, N.A. Intra-renal transfection of heat shock protein 90 alpha or beta (Hsp90α or Hsp90β) protects against ischemia/reperfusion injury. *Nephrol. Dial. Transplant.* **2014**, *29*, 301–312. [CrossRef]
180. Maehana, T.; Tanaka, T.; Kitamura, H.; Fukuzawa, N.; Ishida, H.; Harada, H.; Tanabe, K.; Masumori, N. Heat shock protein 90α is a potential serological biomarker of acute rejection after renal transplantation. *PLoS ONE* **2016**, *11*, e0162942. [CrossRef]

181. Xie, Y.; Chen, L.; Xu, Z.; Li, C.; Ni, Y.; Hou, M.; Chen, L.; Chang, H.; Yang, Y.; Wang, H.; et al. Predictive modeling of MAFLD based on Hsp90α and the therapeutic application of teprenone in a diet-induced mouse model. *Front. Endocrinol.* **2021**, *12*, 743202. [CrossRef]
182. Yu, J.; Zhang, C.; Song, C. Pan- and isoform-specific inhibition of Hsp90: Design strategy and recent advances. *Eur. J. Med. Chem.* **2022**, *238*, 114516. [CrossRef]
183. Trepel, J.; Mollapour, M.; Giaccone, G.; Neckers, L. Targeting the dynamic HSP90 complex in cancer. *Nat. Rev. Cancer* **2010**, *10*, 537–549. [CrossRef] [PubMed]
184. Khandelwal, A.; Kent, C.N.; Balch, M.; Peng, S.; Mishra, S.J.; Deng, J.; Day, V.W.; Liu, W.; Subramanian, C.; Cohen, M.; et al. Structure-guided design of an Hsp90β N-terminal isoform-selective inhibitor. *Nat. Commun.* **2018**, *9*, 425. [CrossRef] [PubMed]
185. Shao, L.D.; Su, J.; Ye, B.; Liu, J.X.; Zuo, Z.L.; Li, Y.; Wang, Y.Y.; Xia, C.; Zhao, Q.S. Design, synthesis, and biological activities of vibsanin B derivatives: A new class of HSP90 C-terminal inhibitors. *J. Med. Chem.* **2017**, *60*, 9053–9066. [CrossRef] [PubMed]
186. Dong, H.; Luo, L.; Zou, M.; Huang, C.; Wan, X.; Hu, Y.; Le, Y.; Zhao, H.; Li, W.; Zou, F.; et al. Blockade of extracellular heat shock protein 90α by 1G6-D7 attenuates pulmonary fibrosis through inhibiting ERK signaling. *Am. J. Physiol. Lung Cell. Mol. Physiol.* **2017**, *313*, L1006–L1015. [CrossRef]
187. Hughes, P.F.; Barrott, J.J.; Carlson, D.A.; Loiselle, D.R.; Speer, B.L.; Bodoor, K.; Rund, L.A.; Haystead, T.A. A highly selective Hsp90 affinity chromatography resin with a cleavable linker. *Bioorg. Med. Chem.* **2012**, *20*, 3298–3305. [CrossRef]
188. Crowe, L.B.; Hughes, P.F.; Alcorta, D.A.; Osada, T.; Smith, A.P.; Totzke, J.; Loiselle, D.R.; Lutz, I.D.; Gargesha, M.; Roy, D.; et al. A fluorescent Hsp90 probe demonstrates the unique association between extracellular Hsp90 and malignancy in vivo. *ACS Chem. Biol.* **2017**, *12*, 1047–1055. [CrossRef]
189. Liu, W.; Vielhauer, G.A.; Holzbeierlein, J.M.; Zhao, H.; Ghosh, S.; Brown, D.; Lee, E.; Blagg, B.S. KU675, a concomitant heat-shock protein inhibitor of Hsp90 and Hsc70 that manifests isoform selectivity for Hsp90α in prostate cancer cells. *Mol. Pharmacol.* **2015**, *88*, 121–130. [CrossRef]
190. Massey, A.J.; Schoepfer, J.; Brough, P.A.; Brueggen, J.; Chene, P.; Drysdale, M.J.; Pfaar, U.; Radimerski, T.; Ruetz, S.; Schweitzer, A.; et al. Preclinical antitumor activity of the orally available heat shock protein 90 inhibitor NVP-BEP800. *Mol. Cancer Ther.* **2010**, *9*, 906–919. [CrossRef]

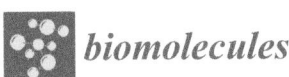

Review

Extracellular Heat Shock Protein-90 (eHsp90): Everything You Need to Know

Daniel Jay [1], Yongzhang Luo [2] and Wei Li [3,*]

1. Department of Developmental Molecular and Chemical Biology, Graduate School of Biomedical Sciences, Tufts University School of Medicine, Boston, MA 02111, USA; daniel.jay@tufts.edu
2. The National Engineering Research Centre for Protein Technology, School of Life Sciences, Tsinghua University, Beijing 100084, China; yluo@mail.tsinghua.edu.cn
3. The Department of Dermatology and the USC-Norris Comprehensive Cancer Centre, The University of Southern California Keck School of Medicine, Los Angeles, CA 90033, USA
* Correspondence: wli@usc.edu

Abstract: "Extracellular" Heat Shock Protein-90 (Hsp90) was initially reported in the 1970s but was not formally recognized until 2008 at the 4th International Conference on The Hsp90 Chaperone Machine (Monastery Seeon, Germany). Studies presented under the topic of "extracellular Hsp90 (eHsp90)" at the conference provided direct evidence for eHsp90's involvement in cancer invasion and skin wound healing. Over the past 15 years, studies have focused on the secretion, action, biological function, therapeutic targeting, preclinical evaluations, and clinical utility of eHsp90 using wound healing, tissue fibrosis, and tumour models both in vitro and in vivo. eHsp90 has emerged as a critical stress-responding molecule targeting each of the pathophysiological conditions. Despite the studies, our current understanding of several fundamental questions remains little beyond speculation. Does eHsp90 indeed originate from purposeful live cell secretion or rather from accidental dead cell leakage? Why did evolution create an intracellular chaperone that also functions as a secreted factor with reported extracellular duties that might be (easily) fulfilled by conventional secreted molecules? Is eHsp90 a safer and more optimal drug target than intracellular Hsp90 chaperone? In this review, we summarize how much we have learned about eHsp90, provide our conceptual views of the findings, and make recommendations on the future studies of eHsp90 for clinical relevance.

Keywords: extracellular Hsp90; stress; mechanism of action; wound healing and cancer

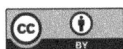

1. Introduction

For decades, the Heat Shock Protein-90 (Hsp90) family proteins have been recognized as ATP binding-dependent molecular chaperones inside almost all types of cells throughout evolution. This understanding has served as an indisputable foundation for both laboratory research and cancer clinical trials targeting the intracellular function of the Hsp90 family proteins [1–6]. Meanwhile, a cell-surface form of Hsp90-related molecule was reported as early as the late 1970s with several publications that appeared to challenge the definition of Hsp90 as an exclusively intracellular chaperone. The question was first raised in the 1990s by Csermely and colleagues, who stated that "the major cellular function of Hsp90 is probably not its chaperone behaviour, but its dynamic participation in the organization and maintenance of the cytoarchitecture" [7], although the exact nature of the dynamic participation was not further elaborated. Throughout the following decade, however, few in the Hsp90 field credited the possible existence of a non-chaperone form of Hsp90 and regarded the reported extracellular or secreted Hsp90 as artifacts, such as leakage by a small number of dying cells in culture. A breakthrough emerged in the 2000s when several laboratories independently demonstrated a critical role for secreted Hsp90 in various pathophysiological processes such as cancer cell invasion and wound healing. Increasing lines of evidence are raising the possibility that cell surface-bound, exosome-anchored, or simply free-secreted Hsp90 may serve as safer and more effective therapeutic targets than their intracellular counterparts in cancer and other inflammatory human disorders. This is especially relevant considering that targeting the intracellular ATP-dependent chaperone function of Hsp90 has encountered setbacks in clinical trials. Several generations of small molecule inhibitors have entered numerous cancer clinical trials since 1999, but to date none have received FDA approval [5,6]. In this review article, we provide a comprehensive walk-through of the discovery, characterization, mechanism of action, and evaluation by animal models and human patients of what is now collectively referred to as "extracellular Hsp90" (eHsp90). More importantly, we offer our answers for the fundamental question of why eHsp90 is chosen by evolution for duties that cannot be served by other conventional extracellular factors.

2. History of eHsp90 Discovery

In the late 1970s, several laboratories independently reported a glucose-regulated 90-kDa protein both on the surface and in the conditioned medium of tumour virus-infected mouse and human fibroblast cells [8–12]. In 1983, Hughes et al. provided direct evidence that Hsp90 protein is located on the external surface of macrophage and mouse embryo 3T3 cells [13]. Srivastava et al. then reported a membrane-associated 96-kDa protein in chemically induced sarcoma cells [14] and Ullrich et al. showed that a Hsp90-related protein was detected on the external surface of both Meth A tumour and NIH3T3 cells using antibody binding to the cells at 4 °C that prevented membrane internalization [15]. A follow-up study by Thangue and Latchman showed cell surface accumulation of Hsp90 in HSV-infected cells [16]. While the findings of these studies were intriguing, they may have not resonated at the time. The observations of extracellular Hsp90 in these studies were thought to be due to intracellular Hsp90 being released non-specifically from dead or dying cells, and there was little preclinical or clinical relevance available. In 1992, Erkeller Yuksel et al. reported that the external surface expression of Hsp90 was a feature of about 20% of the patients with systemic lupus erythematosus (SLE) and it correlated with the severeness of the disease [17]. After the finding, Thomiadou and Patsavoudi reported a 94-kDa "neuron-specific cell surface antigen" recognized by the monoclonal antibody 4C5 [18]. The 94-kDa protein was later identified as an Hsp90-related protein by the same group using mass spectrometry [19]. The take-home message of these studies was the association of the surface or secreted Hsp90 with inflammatory diseases and tissue development. The findings of these earlier studies were, however, largely overlooked by the Hsp90 community due to lack of evidence for active secretion and the undefined function of surface-bound or secreted forms of Hsp90.

In the early 2000s, two laboratories, which had never studied Hsp90 before, were independently searching for secreted proteins that support two distinct and mechanistically related pathophysiological processes, tumour cell invasion and skin wound healing. In 2004, Jay's group at Tufts University first reported the identification of a secreted protein from the conditioned medium of a fibrosarcoma cell line, HT-1080, and showed that the secreted protein promoted tumour cell invasion in vitro by activating the matrix metalloproteinase 2 (MMP2) [20]. In 2007, Li's laboratory at the University of Southern California reported the purification of a secreted protein from the conditioned medium of hypoxia-stressed primary human dermal fibroblasts and keratinocytes through chromatography and showed that this secreted protein strongly stimulated skin cell migration in vitro and promoted wound healing in mice [21,22]. The common protein involved in tumour cell invasion in vitro and wound healing in vivo was identified as the secreted form of Hsp90α. Additional publications on secreted Hsp90α have since emerged and are beginning to receive attention. To provide a common terminology that covers the meanings of "cell surface-bound", "cell-released", "cell-secreted" Hsp90α, Isaacs and colleagues recommended "eHsp90" for extracellular Hsp90 which has since become widely accepted by the Hsp90 community [23]. Over the past 20 years, there have been two dozen excellent review articles on eHsp90, especially eHsp90α [24–41], which we use as the stepping-stones for construction of this article.

3. eHsp90α vs. eHsp90β: Who Calls the Shots and Why?

In comparison to over 70 reports on eHsp90α as of May 2022, several studies in the past have also reported the presence of either eHsp90β alone or the eHsp90α and eHsp90β proteins together in the conditioned medium of various cell types [42,43]. This leads to the question of whether eHsp90β also has extracellular functions. If one only considers the functionality of a protein in its purified form as the ultimate evidence, the answer is negative. Cheng et al. showed that human recombinant Hsp90α (hrHsp90α), but not hrHsp90β, stimulated human keratinocyte migration [22]. Jayaprakash et al. showed that hrHsp90α, but not hrHsp90β, promoted wound healing in pigs [44]. Zou and colleagues demonstrated that the intravenous injection of hrHsp90α, but not hrHsp90β, protein strongly promoted tumour formation and lung metastasis in mice [45].

The human Hsp90α and Hsp90β proteins differ by a total of 100 amino acid residues along their respective 732- (Hsp90α) and 724- (Hsp90β) amino acid sequences, including 58 conservative and 42 non-conservative amino acid substitutions, in addition to 12 amino acid deletions in Hsp90β. The highest variations between Hsp90α and Hsp90β occur within the linker region (LR) and a part of the middle domain (M), with only 61% amino acid identity, the location where Li's group identified the functional "F-5" fragment of eHsp90α that promotes wound healing [46,47]. Mouse genetic studies also showed distinct and non-compensating roles for Hsp90α and Hsp90β during development. Voss et al. reported that Hsp90β gene knockout causes a defect in placental labyrinth formation, resulting in mouse embryonic lethality on E10.5 [48]. In contrast, mice with either chaperone-defective mutations in Hsp90α [49,50] or complete Hsp90α knockout [51] showed indistinguishable difference in their phenotypes from their wild-type counterparts. The straightforward interpretations were that (1) Hsp90β is more critical than Hsp90α during mouse development and (2) Hsp90α is not required under homeostasis.

4. Is eHsp90 Secreted by Living Cells on Purpose or Leaked by Dead Cells by Accident?

While it is technically difficult to prove that eHsp90, specifically eHsp90α, does not result from the leakage of intracellular Hsp90 from a small number of dead cells in culture, several lines of evidence strongly support that eHsp90α is actively secreted. Studies showed that the quantity of eHsp90α was less or undetectable from secreted molecules of normal cells under physiological conditions in vitro, i.e., in serum-containing and pH-balanced medium under normoxia at 37 °C. In comparison, several fold higher eHsp90α proteins became detectable from the conditioned medium of the same cells under a variety of medically-defined stress signals including reactive oxygen species (ROS), heat, hypoxia, gamma-irradiation, UV, and tissue injury [28,52,53]. In contrast, many tumour cells constitutively secrete eHsp90α due to intrinsic oncogenes, such as overexpressing HIF-1α [21], or mutant forms of tumour suppression genes including p53 [42,54]. Eustace et al. showed only Hsp90α and not Hsp90β in the conditioned medium of tumour cells, suggesting a specific secretion of Hsp90α rather than the non-specific release of both forms from dead cells [20]. Cheng and colleagues showed that while both TGFα and EGF bind and signal through EGFR and both promote cell survival and cell growth, only TGFα stimulates the Hsp90α translocation to plasma membrane and secretion to the extracellular environment by primary human keratinocytes, the most critical cell type for skin wound healing [22]. Finally, the stress-induced secretion of Hsp90α was further substantiated by an in vivo observation that skin injury caused up to a 10-fold increase in eHsp90α deposition into the wound bed in a time-dependent fashion. As shown in Figure 1, skin injury in pigs causes an accumulatively increased deposition of eHsp90α into the wound bed in a time-dependent fashion. Since the location with increased anti-Hsp90α antibody staining includes areas in the skin dermis that does not have the continued presence of cells, the massive staining cannot be explained by increased intracellular Hsp90α [55]. This finding provides the first in vivo evidence of biological stress-induced Hsp90α secretion.

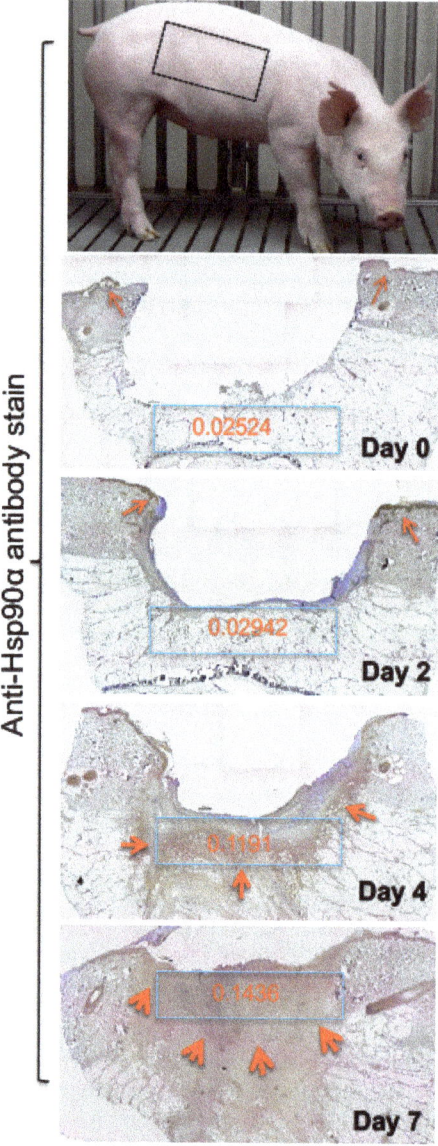

Figure 1. Tissue damage induces massive deposition of eHsp90α into the wound bed. Pig skin is biologically closest to the human skin. 1.5 cm × 1.5 cm full-thickness excision wounds were created in the indicated area of pig torso. Full wedge (2 cm) biopsies cross the wound were made on the indicated days and immediately frozen on dry ice. Sections of the biopsies were stained with an anti-Hsp90α antibody. The red arrows point out the locations of the specific antibody staining (brown). Quantitation of the staining in blue boxes was done using Gabriel Landini's "color deconvolution" and ImageJ analysis. The intensity readings were converted to Optical Density (OD) (The image was taken from reference [55] with permission).

So far, the studies on mechanism(s) of eHsp90α secretion have raised more questions than answers. Two laboratories reported that the secretion can be regulated by either phosphorylation or the C-terminal amino acid EEVD motif of the Hsp90α protein [56,57]. Luo's laboratory further identified a critical role for Rab coupling protein (RCP) in mutp53-induced Hsp90α secretion [54]. Several studies suggested that eHsp90α is secreted via exosomes, based on the observation that DMA (Dimethyl amiloride), an inhibitor of the exosome secretion pathway, blocks Hsp90α secretion both in HIF-1-overexpressing tumour cells and TGFα-stimulated human keratinocytes cells, where Hsp90α was associated with isolated exosome fractions. Therefore, eHsp90α is secreted via the non-classical exosome trafficking pathway [58–61]. Guo and colleagues further identified the proline-rich Akt substrate of 40 kDa (PRAS40) as the unique downstream effector that mediates TGFα-stimulated Hsp90α secretion via exosomes [62]. Tang and colleagues have recently made an interesting observation that eHsp90α is located at the external surface of tumour cell-secreted exosomes [63]. However, recent observations suggest that approximately 90% of both normal and tumour cell- secreted Hsp90α is not associated with secreted exosomes isolated by ultracentrifugation (C. Cheng, X, Tang and W. Li, unpublished; A. Bernstein and D. Jay, unpublished). Taken together, eHsp90α is a secreted protein by cells under either internal or external stress. This general understanding is depicted in Figure 2, where eHsp90α promotes tissue repair under physiological conditions or promotes tumorigenesis under pathological conditions, defined as a "double-edged sword" by Hence and colleagues [30].

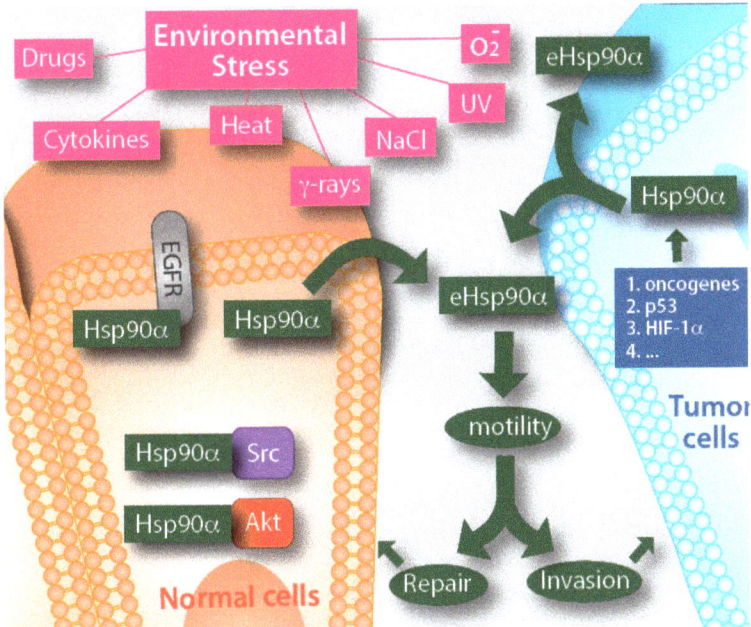

Figure 2. Secretion of eHsp90α by normal cells under medically defined stress and by tumour cells driven by oncogenic signals. Almost all kinds of medically defined stresses have been shown to trigger eHsp90α secretion in a wide variety of cell types. Tumours have either constitutively activated oncogenes or mutant tumour suppressor genes that each triggers eHsp90α secretion even in the absence of environmental stress cues. The mechanisms by which the stress and oncogenic signals cause Hsp90 secretion remain largely unstudied, in which exosome-mediated secretion of Hsp90α only accounts for 10% of the total secreted Hsp90α in both normal and tumour cells. The reported optimal working concentration for the full-length eHsp90α protein was around 3–10 µg/mL.

5. Two Main Biological Functions of eHsp90α

5.1. Promoting Cell Survival under Ischemic Stress

Shortly after tissue injury, the broken blood vessels clot and cells in the injured tissue encounter an ischemic (paucity of nutrient and oxygen) environment. The immediate challenge the cells face is survival, at least temporarily, by adapting a self-supporting mechanism. Similarly, when tumour cells invade surrounding tissues too quickly and temporarily outstrip the nearest blood vessel for 150 mirom or more, they similarly face the stress of ischemia [64]. Under these conditions, the tumour cells must find an autocrine cycle to survive without the help from blood vessels. Bhatia and colleagues showed that topical application of hrHsp90α to burn wounds in pigs prevented heat-induced skin cell apoptosis around the hypoxic wound bed [65]. Dong and colleagues demonstrated that eHsp90α protected tumour cells from hypoxia-triggered apoptosis, whereas neutralizing eHsp90α function with a monoclonal antibody enhanced hypoxia-induced tumour cell apoptosis [66]. Gao and colleagues reported that extracellular supplementation with hrHsp90α (10 μM or ~1 mg/mL) protein promoted rat bone mesenchymal stem cell (MSC) survival and prevented cell apoptosis under ischemic conditions by activating the Akt and ERK kinases [67]. Cheng et al. showed that 10 μg/mL hrHsp90α protein stimulated the maximum migration of primary human skin cells [22] and Dong et al. reported that a similar dosage of hrHsp90α prevented the death of Hsp90α-KO MDA-MB-231 cells under hypoxia [66]. Nonetheless, the conformation and composition of the eHsp90α under the above circumstances is less clear in comparison to its intracellular counterpart.

5.2. Promoting Cell Motility (Not Growth) during Tissue Repair and Tumour Invasion

The initial indication that eHsp90α regulates cell migration was reported in the 1990s by Patsvoudi's group, who showed that a monoclonal antibody against a mouse granule cell surface antigen called 4C5 inhibited the cell migration during cerebellar development [68,69]. The same group later confirmed by immunoprecipitation followed by mass spec that the 4C5 antigen is related to Hsp90 protein [19]. During the same period, Jay's group showed that eHsp90α from the conditioned medium of tumour cells was required for tumour cell invasion via activation of MMP2 in vitro [20]. The direct evidence that eHsp90α protein alone acts as a *bona fide* pro-motility factor came from Li's group that demonstrated hrHsp90α, but not hrHsp90β, stimulated primary human dermal fibroblasts and keratinocyte migration in the total absence of serum factors. Moreover, the pro-motility effect of hrHsp90α could reach approximately 60% of the total pro-motility of 10% FBS-containing medium. Under similar conditions, however, hrHsp90α showed little mitogenic effect on cell growth. More surprisingly, both the wild type and ATPase-defect mutant proteins of Hsp90α bind the cell surface receptor LRP-1 (low-density lipoprotein receptor-related protein 1) and had compatible prom-motility effects on the same cells [21,22].

6. Mechanisms of Action by eHsp90α

By and large, there have been two major parallel mechanisms of action proposed for eHsp90α [28]. The central debate is whether eHsp90α still acts as an ATP-dependent chaperone outside the cell or alternatively acts as a previously unrecognized signalling molecule no longer dependent on ATP hydrolysis. Eustace and colleagues tested DMAG-N-oxide, a cell membrane-impermeable geldanamycin/17-AAG-derived inhibitor that targets the ATPase activity of Hsp90, and showed that it inhibits tumour cell invasion [20]. Similarly, Tsutsumi and colleagues showed that the DMAG-N-oxide inhibitor reduced the invasion of several cancer cell lines in vitro and lung colonization by B16 melanoma cells in mice [70]. Furthermore, Sims et al. showed that blocking ATPase using ATP-gamma S actually increased the ability of hrHsp90α to activate MMP2 in vitro [71]. In particular, a recent elegant study from Bourboulia's group showed that TIMP2 and AHA1 act as a molecular switch for eHsp90α that determines the inhibition or activation of the eHsp90α client protein MMP2 [72]. Song and colleagues showed that Hsp90α, but not Hsp90β, stabilized MMP2 and protected it from degradation in tumour cells in an ATP-independent manner and was mediated by the middle domain of Hsp90α binding to the C-terminal hemopexin domain of MMP2 [73]. Taken together, these studies suggest that the N-terminal ATP-binding domain and the intrinsic ATPase of Hsp90α remain essential for eHsp90α function outside of the cells. Results of other studies from different laboratories also supported the "eHsp90α chaperone mechanism" via their extracellular client proteins, most noticeably MMP2, MMP9, and TLR, just to mention a few. To avoid redundancy in this special issue, we refer readers to two excellent review articles, a prior one by Wong and Jay [32] and the current one in this special issue by Bourboulia and colleagues for more detailed analysis of this mechanism.

On the other hand, the ATPase-independent mechanism has largely focused on the so-called "eHsp90α > LRP-1" signalling pathway [28]. Li's laboratory utilized both deletion and site-directed mutagenesis to narrow down the essential epitope along the 732-amino acid human eHsp90α for supporting the pro-survival, pro-motility, and pro-invasion activity of eHsp90α in vitro and in vivo. First, Cheng and colleagues reported that the ATPase-defective mutants, Hsp90α-E47A (~50% ATPase activity), Hsp90α-E47D (ATPase-defect), and Hsp90α-D93N (ATPase-defect), showed an indistinguishable degree of pro-motility activity from the Hsp90α-wt protein on primary human skin cells in vitro [22]. Second, they narrowed down the pro-motility activity to a 115-amino acid fragment called F-5 (aa-236 to aa-350) between the LR (linker region) and the M (middle domain of human) Hsp90α, as previously mentioned. They demonstrated that the F-5 peptide alone promoted skin cell migration in vitro and wound healing in vivo as effectively as the full-length Hsp90α-wt [46]. Third, they illustrated the so-called "eHsp90α > LRP-1" signalling pathway as: (1) the subdomain II in the extracellular part of the low-density lipoprotein receptor-related protein-1 (LRP-1) that receives the eHsp90α signal; (2) the NPVY, but not NPTY, motif in the cytoplamic tail of LRP-1 that connects the eHsp90α signalling to the serine-473, but not threonine-308, phosphorylation in Akt kinases and (3) activated Akt1 ang Akt2 trigger cell migration [47]. Finally, within the F-5 fragment, Zou and colleagues identified a dual lysine motif (Lys-270/Lys-277) that are evolutionarily conserved in all members of the Hsp90α subfamily but absent in all Hsp90β subfamily members. Mutations at the lysine residues eliminated Hsp90α's ability to promote cell migration in vitro and tumour formation in vivo. Substitutions of the two different amino acids at the corresponding sites in Hsp90β granted Hsp90β with pro-motility activity like Hsp90α [45]. These authors presented an illustration of the F-5 fragment and the dual lysine motif locations in a schematic monomer structure of Hsp90α, as shown in Figure 3, which shows a potential target in eHsp90α for therapeutics. These findings suggest that the N-terminal ATPase domain and the C-terminal dimer-forming and co-factor-binding domain are dispensable for eHsp90α function. More interestingly, Gopal showed a novel crosstalk mechanism involving the eHsp90α-LRP1 dependent regulation of EphA2 function, in which the eHsp90α-LRP1 signalling axis regulates AKT signalling and EphA2 activation during glioblastoma cell invasion [23]. In addition, Tian et al. showed that clusterin served as an eHsp90α modulator to synergistically promote EMT (epithelial-to-mesenchymal transition) and tumour metastasis via LRP1 [74]. Besides binding to MMP2 and LRP-1, Garcia et al. reported that eHsp90α binds to the type I TGFβ receptor to stimulate collagen synthesis, which provides pavement for cell attachment and migration [75]. Nonetheless, the chaperone-dependent mechanism, such as the activation of MMP2, and the chaperone-independent mechanism, such as F-5 binding the LRP-1 receptor, do not necessarily have to be mutually exclusive, as schematically depicted in Figure 4, which may represent two parallel mechanisms of action by eHsp90α. The selectivity and specificity of these two pathways under various pathophysiological conditions remain to be further studied.

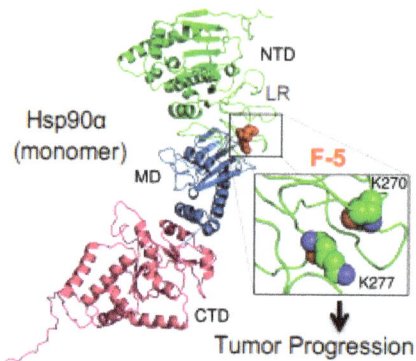

Figure 3. The F-5 fragment is located at the surface of the Hsp90α protein. Based on the previously evaluated crystal structure of a monomer Hsp90α protein with the NTD (green), MD (blue) and CTD (red) domains, the F-5 fragment containing Lysine-270 and lysine-277 is located in the unstructured linker region (LR) between the NTD and MD domains. Inhibitors such as monoclonal antibodies, targeting the dual lysine residues (in enlarged box), are potential anti-tumour therapeutics.

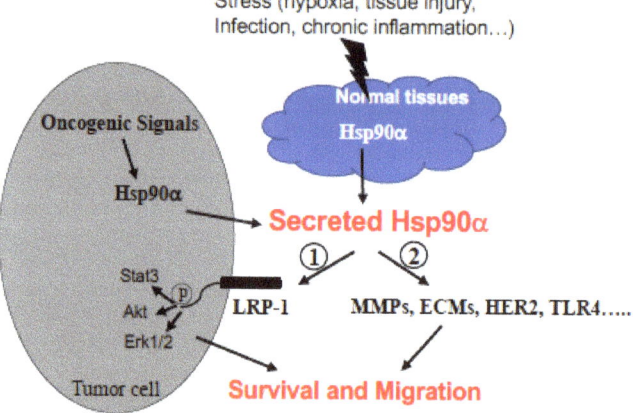

Figure 4. Two proposed mechanisms of action by eHsp90α. eHsp90α acts via an ATPase-dependent or ATPase-independent mechanism, which is determined by different binding partners, as shown. It is possible that the two mechanisms take place in parallel and work synergistically to achieve the ultimate goal under pathophysiological conditions.

7. Preclinical Studies of eHsp90α

eHsp90α has been studied in several human disease models in animals, including cancer, wound healing, idiopathic pulmonary fibrosis (IPF) and wasting syndrome (WS). The implication of eHsp90α in blood circulation supporting tumour metastasis in a number of animal models is especially encouraging considering the long-term and heavy emphasis of Hsp90 on cancer.

7.1. Wound Healing

When tissue is injured and the broken blood vessels clotted, all of the cells surrounding the wound bed face ischemic stress, as previously described. Bhatia and colleagues made full-thickness skin wounds in pigs, biopsied the wounds over time, and immunostained the tissue samples with an anti-Hsp90α antibody. They found a massive, time-dependent increase in the antibody staining in both the epidermis and dermis [56] (see Figure 1). Song and Luo reported that eHsp90α localized on blood vessels in the granulation tissue of wounded skin and promoted angiogenesis during wound healing in mice [76]. A series of studies from Li's group demonstrated that topical application of hrHsp90α, but not hrHsp90β, strongly promoted closure of trauma (excision), burn, and diabetic wounds in mice and pigs. In reserves, topically administered antibodies against eHsp90α blocks wound closure [21,44,55,65,77]. Bhatia and colleagues carried out a clever study by taking advantage of Hsp90α transgenic mice where the Hsp90α's intracellular chaperone function is nullified but the truncated Hsp90α protein still contains the entire F-5 region. They found that these mice heal skin wounds as efficiently as their wild-type counterparts, indicating that the chaperone function of Hsp90α is dispensable. However, topical application of mAb 1G6D7 against eHsp90α inhibited the wound healing, suggesting an essential role for eHsp90α instead [55]. As previous mentioned, the wound healing-promoting effect of the full-length eHsp90α is entirely replicable by the F-5 fragment [46], which is currently undergoing clinical trials for the treatment of diabetic foot ulcers.

7.2. Tissue Fibrosis

While Hsp90α enhances wound healing, excess eHsp90α in the injured lung may do more harm than good [78]. Pulmonary fibrosis is characterized by overactivated lung fibroblasts and massive collagen deposition by the cells at the injured site. Using BLM-induced pulmonary injury and the fibrosis mouse model, which represents failed wound healing, Dong and colleagues showed that mAb 1G6-D7, a monoclonal antibody against eHsp90α, inhibited eHsp90α function and significantly protected against BLM-induced pulmonary fibrosis by ameliorating fibroblast overactivation and ECM production [79]. The same group proposed a possible mechanism by which eHsp90α links the ER stress to the PI-3K-Akt pathway [80]. Ballaye and colleagues reported the significant increase of both eHsp90α and eHsp90β in the circulation of patients with idiopathic pulmonary fibrosis (IPF), and the higher levels correlated with disease severity. They found that eHsp90α signalled through LRP-1 to promote myofibroblast differentiation and persistence in a rat ex vivo model [81]. Together, the above studies argue that the specific inhibition of eHsp90α is a promising therapeutic strategy to reduce pro-fibrotic signalling in IPF.

7.3. Wasting Syndrome

Wasting syndrome (WS) refers to the unwanted weight loss of more than 10 percent of a person's body weight, with diarrhea, weakness, and fever that can last up to 30 days. WS is often a sign of disease, such as cancer, AIDS, heart failure, or advanced chronic obstructive pulmonary disease. "Cachexia", characterized by muscle wasting, is a major contributor to cancer-related mortality. A recent study by Zhang et al. reported elevated serum Hsp70 and Hsp90 in Lewis lung carcinoma (LLC)-bearing mice. The tumour-released and exosome-bound eHsp90 and eHsp70 were both necessary and sufficient to induce muscle wasting in a syngeneic tumour mouse model [82]. These studies may suggest clinical value in inhibiting eHsp90 for WS.

7.4. Tumorigenesis

Given the specific supporting role of eHsp90α in cancer, and the failure of many clinical trials using pan- inhibitors targeting all intracellular Hsp90 chaperone members, several groups have reported on the benefit of selectively inhibiting eHsp90α for reducing tumour metastasis and improving patient survival. Stellas et al. reported that intraperitoneal injection with monoclonal antibody (100–200 μg per mouse daily) against 4C5 antigen (cell surface eHsp90α) into C57BL/6 mice 24 h following tail vein injection with B16-F10 melanoma cells reduced tumour lung colonization and improved the survival of the mice in reference to placebo-treated mice [83]. These authors reported a similar finding using a human breast cancer xenograft model and showed that the antibody disrupted interactions of eHsp90 with MMP2 and MMP9 [84]. Tsutsumi and colleagues showed that DMAG-N-oxide (a membrane-impermeable version of 17-DMAG inhibitor) blocked lung colonization by B16 melanoma cells in nude mice [71]. Results of the study suggest that the N'-terminal ATP-binding of Hsp90α is still required for eHsp90α function. Using a different anti-Hsp90α monoclonal antibody, Song and colleagues showed the dose-dependent inhibition of tumour growth and angiogenesis of B10-F10 cells in nude mice [74]. Using orthotopic breast cancer mouse models, Hou and colleagues showed that the injection of hrHsp90α protein increased primary tumour lymphatic vessel density and sentinel lymph node metastasis. In reverse, injection of another independent anti-Hsp90α neutralizing antibody reduced 70% of lymphatic vessel density and 90% of sentinel lymph node metastasis [85]. Using the well-known human triple negative breast cancer cell line, MDA-MB-231, xenograft mouse model, two laboratories independently reported a critical role for eHsp90α in tumour growth and lung metastasis. Stivarou and colleagues showed that injection with an antibody against 4C5 antigen (Hsp90) inhibited both *de novo* tumour growth and growth of already established mammary tumours [86]. Zou and colleagues demonstrated that injection with hrHsp90α, but not hrHsp90β, protein rescued the tumorigenesis of Hsp90α-knockout MDA-MB-231 cells in nude mice. More interestingly, the authors showed that the ATPase-defective Hsp90α (Hsp90α-D93N) protein showed exactly the same effect as the wild type Hsp90α on tumour formation and lung metastasis. In reverse, injection with the monoclonal antibody mAb1G6-D7, not only blocked de novo tumour formation and lung metastasis, but also significantly reduced (~35%) the continued growth of already formed tumours [45]. Consistently, Secli el al recently reported that "Morgana", a co-chaperone of eHsp90α, induced cancer cell migration through TLR2, TLR4, and LRP1. A monoclonal antibody targeting Morgana inhibited mouse breast cancer cells, EO771, from metastasizing to the lung in C57BL/6 mice [87]. Milani and colleagues established mouse models with human acute lymphoblastic leukemia (ALL) and showed that the background plasma level of eHsp90α was below 1ng/mL blood in healthy mice, whereas the plasma level of eHsp90α was elevated into the 100–150 ng/mL range within two months in a fashion that closely correlated with the increased percentage of hCD45+ cells, a monitoring marker of ALL, in the blood, bone marrow, liver, and spleen of the animals [88]. A recent study by Luo's group showed that PKM2 (pyruvate kinase M2)-like eHsp90α is secreted by lung cancer cells and detected in blood samples of human cancer patients. The injection of mouse recombinant PKM2 protein into blood circulation promoted tumour metastasis to the lung via binding to integrin β1 [89]. Since PKM2 is associated with Hsp90α inside cells [90], it is possible that the secreted PKM2 is in complex with eHsp90α, which remains to be experimentally confirmed.

8. Clinical Studies of eHsp90α in Patients with Cancer and Inflammatory Disorders

Since 2008, close to two dozen clinical studies have compared the eHsp90α levels in blood circulation between healthy humans and patients with various types of cancers and other inflammatory diseases. The cancers from the patients include all of the NCI (National Cancer Institute, USA)-listed major human cancers. Due to space limitations, we are unable to describe each of the individual studies and their findings in detail. Rather, we chose to summarize the common findings of these studies, i.e., elevated plasma eHsp90α in circulation, in Table 1. While the exact amount of plasma/serum eHsp90α markedly vary (from pg/mL to mg/mL) among different reports (though they all used ELISA-based detection methods), a majority of the studies showed a statistically significant increase in cancer patients compared to normal patients in a range of sub μg/mL. More intriguingly, the higher levels of plasma eHsp90α closely correlated with the later stages of the diseases, such as metastasized tumours. These studies raise the possibility of utilizing plasma eHsp90α as a new serum marker for cancer detection and therapeutic targeting, as well as for other chronic inflammatory diseases in humans.

Table 1. Summary of clinical studies on plasma eHsp90 in blood circulation *.

Cancer Type	# of Patients	Plasma eHsp90α	# of Healthy Humans	Plasma eHsp90α	Refs.
Mix of liver, lung, breast, colorectal, stomach, pancreatic, esophagus cancer, and lymphoma.	300	IQR 87.01–235.5 Median 157.80 (ng/mL)	132	IQR 22.87–44.46 Median 31.19 (ng/mL)	[91]
Colon (CRC)	635	51.4 (33.8, 80.3) ng/mL	295	43.7 (34.3, 54.8) ng/mL	[92]
Mix of Breast & Other cancers	85	>50 (ng/mL)	16	50.00 (ng/mL)	[56]
Liver	782	IQR 96.7–246.8 Median 159.9 (ng/mL)	572	IQR 21.1–42.2 Median 30 (ng/mL)	[93]
Lung	1046	Ave. 220.46 (ng/mL)	592	Ave. 48.0 (ng/mL)	[94]
Colon (CRC)	77	135 ± 101.94 (ng/mL)	76	44 ± 15.35 (ng/mL)	[95]
Melanoma	98	Median. 49.76 (ng/mL)	43	Median 25.7 (ng/mL)	[96]
AML	82	Ave. 295 (ng/mL)	20	Ave. 12.1 (ng/mL)	[97]
Pancreas	20	0.57 ± 0.23 (mg/mL)	10	0.18 ± 0.05 (mg/mL)	[98]
Pancreatic ductal adenocarcinoma	114	1 ± 0.86 (mg/mL)	10	0.18 ± 0.05 (mg/mL)	[98]
Hepatocellular carcinoma	76	274 ± 20.3 (µg/mL)	14	186 ± 18.3 (µg/mL)	[99]
Hepatocellular carcinoma	659	144 ± 4.98 (ng/mL)	230	46 ± 1.11 (ng/mL)	[100]
Esophageal squamous cell carcinoma	193	≥82.06 (ng/mL)			[101]
Esophageal squamous cell carcinoma	93	Ave. 85 (ng/mL)	0	0	[102]
Cervical cancer	220	80.6–212.8 (ng/mL)	75	48.6–89.6 (ng/mL)	[103]
Prostate cancer	18	Median 50.7 (25.5–378.1) (ng/mL)	13	Median 27.6 (13.9–46.5) (ng/mL)	[104]
Childhood acute lymphoblastic leukemia	21	1.22–23.85 (ng/mL)	No exact number	3.16–33.58 (ng/mL)	[105]
Gastric cancer	976	Median 64.3 (ng/mL)	100	45.16 (ng/mL)	[106]
Lung cancer	560	97.64 ± 103.36 (ng/mL)	78	38.44 ± 15.4 (ng/mL)	[107]
Mix of Breast, Liver, Lung, Colon, Esophageal, Gastric and Colorectal	370	57.97–294.63 (ng/mL)	Reference range	0~82.06 (ng/mL)	[108]

Table 1. Cont.

Cancer Type	# of Patients	Plasma eHsp90α	# of Healthy Humans	Plasma eHsp90α	Refs.
Non-small-cell lung cancer	60 Pre-chemotherapy	0.29–0.93 (ng/mL)	60 After 4-cycles of chemotherapy	0.12–0.24 (ng/mL)	[109]
Malignant melanoma	60	70.8–140.77 (ng/mL)	60	42.56–61.42 (ng/mL)	[110]
Nasopharyngeal carcinoma	196	212 ± 144.32 (ng/mL)	106	35 ± 17.47 (ng/mL)	[111]
Non-cancer diseases					
Crohn's disease	53	6.4~55.1			[112]
Psoriasis	80	100 ± 193.66 (AU/mL)	80	63 ± 49.71 (AU/mL)	[113]
Chronic glomerulonephritis	32	33.31–77.25 (ng/mL)	10	22.32	[114]
Amyotrophic lateral sclerosis	58	17.02 ± 10.55	85	12.7 ± 9.23	[115]
Overweight and obese children with Nonalcoholic fatty liver disease	26	3.59–119.85 (ng/mL)	Overweight & obese children without Nonalcoholic fatty liver disease	0–105.4 (ng/mL)	[116]
Chronic glomerulonephritis with nephrotic syndrome	21	33.31–77.25 (ng/mL)	10	Approx. 25–30 (ng/mL)	[114]
Systemic sclerosis	92	9.6–17.9 (ng/mL)	92	7.7–12.4 (ng/mL)	[117]
Diabetic lower extremity arterial disease (DLEAD)	46	Ave. 263.88 (pg/mL)			[11]
Idiopathic pulmonary fibrosis (IPF)	31	Ave. 60 (ng/mL)	9	Ave. 35 (ng/mL)	[118]

* Note: The reported original data on plasma Hsp90 from patients varied dramatically from pg/mL to mg/mL, while the reasons remain unclear. Two presentations, "range" and "average", by the original studies were adopted here. Nonetheless, higher plasma Hsp90 levels in patients' blood are evident. IQR: Interquartile range (IQR).

Taking tumorigenesis as an example, the recognized five steps of tumour development include gene mutations, hyperplasia, dysplasia, primary tumour formation, and tumour metastasis [119–122]. The vast majority of the United States Food and Drug Administration (FDA)-approved oncology drugs (>1000 by the end of 2020) target primary tumours, even though cancer patients die predominantly from metastasis [123]. These drugs extend patients' survival for variable periods of time, but many lose efficacy shortly after several months of treatment due to new mutations generated in the tumours. On the other hand, tumour metastasis begins with local expansion and invasion of the tumour at the primary organ driven by oncogenic signals with tumour microenvironmental assistance. Tumour cells migrate away from their origin and infiltrate into new surrounding tissues in which the tumour cells intravasate into the nearest blood circulation or the lymphatic system. After entry into the circulation, the tumour cells become known as circulating tumour cells (CTCs). Continued distal metastasis requires the tumour cells to survive and disseminate via the blood circulation, so-called hematogenous metastasis. Only a small number of CTCs successfully extravasate by crossing the endothelial barrier, leaving the circulation, and entering a distant organ. Thus, identification of a plasma factor that provides critical assistance for CDC to achieve the ultimate success of metastasis could lead to the sought-after target for next generation of anti-tumour therapeutics. If elevated plasma eHsp90α in cancer patients proves to promote CTC survival and dissemination through blood circulation during metastasis, interruption of the plasma eHsp90α function by antibodies that target the F-5 region of eHsp90α, as schematically proposed in Figure 5, would be an attractive approach to slow down tumour metastasis and buy time for patients to eliminate the primary tumours via surgery and the currently available therapies. For the next few years, the potential importance of the plasma eHsp90α reported in human cancer patients must be carefully studied by engineering the pathological plasma eHsp90α levels in Hsp90α-knockout animal models.

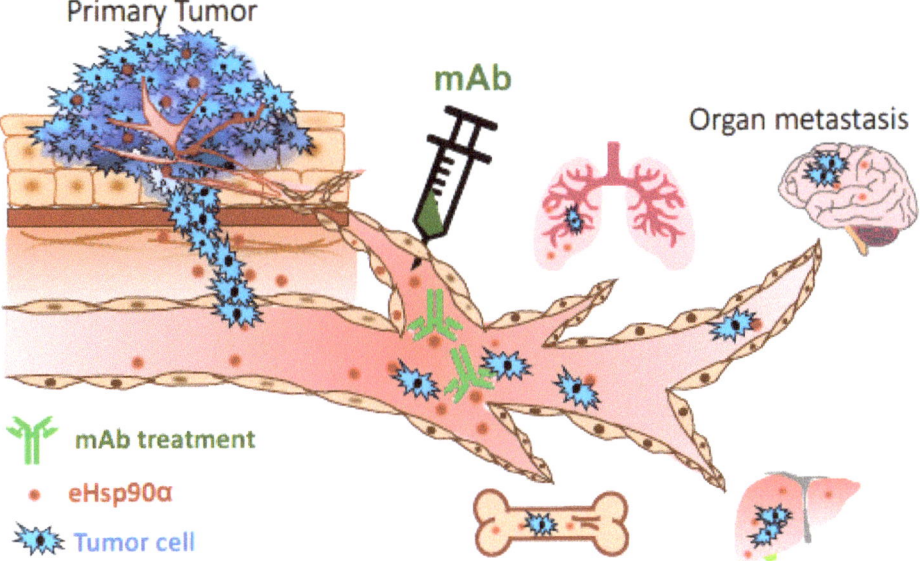

Figure 5. Plasma eHsp90α as a potential target for therapeutics to block tumour metastasis. Findings of the clinical studies shown in Table 1 have raised an exciting possibility that monoclonal antibody therapeutics against plasma eHsp90α block tumour metastasis. Since plasma eHsp90α is low and unessential for homeostasis, targeting plasma eHsp90α in cancer patients may prove to be safer and more effective than targeting the intracellular Hsp90α and Hsp90β.

9. Is eHsp90α a More Effective and Safer Drug Target than Intracellular Hsp90?

As mentioned at the beginning of this article, over the past two decades, intracellular Hsp90 chaperones (Hsp90α, Hsp90β, and possibly other related chaperones) have been targeted by at least 18 small molecule inhibitors binding to the N-terminal ATP/ADP binding site of the proteins in more than 60 cancer clinical trials [4–6]. To date none has received FDA approval for clinical treatment of human cancers due to various speculative reasons [124]. A recent study raised a serious and previously overlooked concern that there might be a complete lack of a druggable window between tumour and normal tissues for ATP-binding inhibitors. Tang and colleagues showed a wide range of Hsp90 expression in different host organs which further exhibited a wide range of toxicity to an ATP-binding inhibitor and heterogenous responses against the conversional theory to the same ATP-binding inhibitor among different tumour cells. These findings could seriously complicate patient and biomarker selections, toxicity readout, and efficacy of the drug candidates for clinical trials [125]. In contrast to the essential role of the intracellular Hsp90, especially Hsp90β for cell and organ homeostasis, the requirement of eHsp90α for life has not been reported. Instead, only when tissue homeostasis is broken, such as during wound healing or disease occurrence such as tumour growth, does eHsp90α then come into the picture. To support this notion, Bhatia and colleagues showed that selectively blocking eHsp90α by antibodies delayed wound healing [55]. Similarly, CRISPR-knockout of the Hsp90α gene selectively eliminated the ability of the MDA-MB-231 tumour cells to invade a Matrigel barrier and form tumours in mice. More remarkably, the defective tumorigenicity of Hsp90α-KO tumour cells could be fully rescued by extracellular supplementation with hrHsp90α proteins in an ATPase-independent fashion [45]. Therefore, in theory, drugs targeting eHsp90 should achieve higher efficacy and pose minimum toxicity to patients. A schematic representation of this simplified thought is depicted in Figure 6.

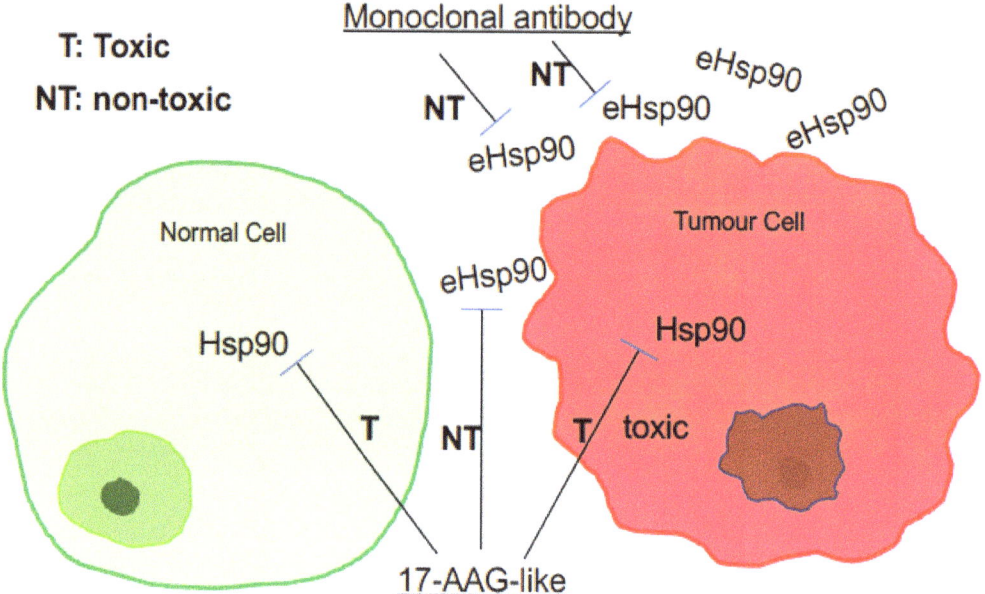

Figure 6. A major difference between targeting eHsp90α and targeting intracellular Hsp90 in cancer. Cytotoxicity and lack of a clear therapeutic window under tolerable dosages have been the major hurdles for ATP-binding inhibitors of Hsp90, especially Hsp90β, in cancer clinical trials. In contrast, selectively targeting eHsp90α with membrane impermeable drug candidates has immerged as a new therapeutic strategy in cancer and beyond.

10. Why Is eHsp90α Co-Opted for Extracellular Duties?

Our current understanding of this fundamental question remains little beyond speculation. An entry point to understand the question is the fact that Hsp90 maintains an unusually high expression level in almost all cell types. Although the statement of "1–2% Hsp90 of total cellular proteins" has been used for decades, this number did not come from direct experimental measurements, but rather from estimations. The first quantitation of the cellular Hsp90 protein was completed by Sahu and colleagues in 2012. Using classical biochemical techniques, these authors demonstrated that Hsp90 accounted for 2–3% of the total cellular proteins among four normal cell lines and 3–7% of the total cellular proteins among four cancer cell lines tested [126]. More surprisingly, a recent study involving 12 (eight tumour and four normal) cell lines reported a much greater variation in the total cellular Hsp90 (α and β) expression, a range of 1.7% to 9% among non-cancer cell lines and different mouse organs and a range of 3 to 7% among the tumour cell lines [125]. If we take the general assumption that a given type of human cell expresses 1/3 of its total 30,000 protein-coding genes, the percentage of the Hsp90 expression is at least several hundred times higher than the rest of the 9999 cellular gene products. The question is why a particular gene product must be given such a spatial privilege. Evolution would not have tolerated such an abundant storage of a protein if functioning as an intracellular chaperone were its sole duty, as Csermely and colleagues have long argued [7]. We speculate that a smaller portion of Hsp90α is required to work with Hsp90β for the intracellular duty of chaperones, such as stabilization of HIF-1α [51], whereas the vast majority of eHsp90α is stockpiled for supply to tolerate environmental insults, such as tissue injuries, that take place all the time. The second possible answer is that eHsp90α provides unique properties that are absent from conventional extracellular factors such as cytokines, growth factors, or ECMs. Li's group showed that topical recombinant eHsp90α protein promoted normal wound healing far more effectively than the (only) FDA-approved growth factor therapy (Raranex^{TM}, PDGF-BB). Their study showed that eHsp90α overrides the inhibitory effect of TGFβ family cytokines, which are abundantly present in fresh wounds. To the best of our knowledge, eHsp90α is the first molecule with this unprecedented property [46]. Third, an effective wound-healing agent is one that must recruit all three types of skin cells (epidermal, dermal, and endothelial) to close the wound. However, all growth factors show selectively targeted cell type(s). This limitation has made any single growth factor therapy less effective in the multi-cell process of wound healing. PDGF-BB only acts on dermal fibroblasts, but not epidermal keratinocytes and dermal microvascular endothelial cells, as the latter do not express either PDGFRα or PDGFRβ [46]. These findings may explain why Raranex has shown limited efficacy in clinic, even with several thousand times higher concentration of PDGF-BB (100 μg/g gel) than found in human circulation (0–15 ng/mL). In contrast, eHsp90α acts as a common pro-motility factor for all three types of skin cells involved in wound healing and shows a far stronger effect than PDGF-BB in wound healing [46,65,78]. For similar reasons, eHsp90α may also have an advantage over conventional extracellular factors in cancer invasion. For instance, Hanahan and Weinberg in their heavily cited review on cancer pointed out that one of the most recognized tumour-suppressing effects comes from the anti-growth signal by TGFβ [127]. To sabotage the inhibitory effect of TGFβ, only a small number of tumours choose to mutate either the type II (TβRII) or type I (TβRI) TGFβ receptor or their downstream effector, Smad4, which forms a complex with activated Smad2/3 to regulate gene expression. How the rest of human tumours bypass the TGFβ's inhibitory signals has never been discussed. We argue that these tumours secrete eHsp90α to override TGFβ inhibition.

11. Conclusions and Perspective

It has been the second decade since the official recognition of eHsp90α as a new research branch of Hsp90 in 2008. Since then, all-round progress, including mechanisms of secretion and action, biological function, therapeutic epitope identification, preclinical evaluation, and clinical relevance of eHsp90α, has been reported around the globe. If we have to provide a single outstanding take-home message to the readers, it would undoubtably be the exciting consensus that eHsp90α is not required for homeostasis but remains an essential player under pathological conditions and crisis. Therapeutically targeting eHsp90α in blood circulation represents a particularly exciting modality due to its ease-of-access, safety, and likely increased efficacy compared to targeting intracellular or nuclear Hsp90. For the next decade, the central challenge is to prove the clinical relevance of eHsp90α, such as in tissue injury, fibrosis, and tumorigenesis, and to concurrently establish the druggable window for targeting eHsp90α in human disorders for therapeutic development.

Funding: This study was supported by NIH grants GM066193 and GM067100 (to W.L.), NIH grant CA183119 (to D.J.) and Self-Topic Fund of Tsinghua University No. 20211080002 (to Y.L.).

Institutional Review Board Statement: Not applicable.

Informed Consent Statement: Not applicable.

Acknowledgments: We thank many of our previous lab colleagues who made contributions to the work described in this review. We apologize if we failed to acknowledge every publication on eHsp90, while this review was being written.

Conflicts of Interest: The authors declare that they have no conflict of interest.

References

1. Young, J.C.; Moarefi, I.; Hartl, F.U. Hsp90: A specialized but essential protein-folding tool. *J. Cell Biol.* **2001**, *154*, 267–273. [CrossRef] [PubMed]
2. Whitesell, L.; Lindquist, S.L. HSP90 and the chaperoning of cancer. *Nat. Rev. Cancer* **2005**, *5*, 761–772. [CrossRef] [PubMed]
3. Trepel, J.; Mollapour, M.; Giaccone, G.; Neckers, L. Targeting the dynamic HSP90 complex in cancer. *Nat. Rev. Cancer* **2010**, *10*, 537–549. [CrossRef] [PubMed]
4. Jhaveri, K.; Taldone, T.; Modi, S.; Chiosis, G. Advances in the clinical development of heat shock protein 90 (Hsp90) inhibitors in cancers. *Biochim. Biophys. Acta Mol.* **2012**, *1823*, 742–755. [CrossRef]
5. Neckers, L.; Blagg, B.; Haystead, T.; Trepel, J.B.; Whitesell, L.; Picard, D. Methods to validate Hsp90 inhibitor specificity, to identify off-target effects, and to rethink approaches for further clinical development. *Cell Stress Chaperones* **2018**, *23*, 467–482. [CrossRef]
6. Sanchez, J.; Carter, T.R.; Cohen, M.S.; Blagg, B.S. Old and new approaches to target the Hsp90 chaperone. *Curr. Cancer Drug Targets* **2020**, *20*, 253–270. [CrossRef]
7. Csermely, P.; Tamás, S.; Csaba, S.; Zoltán, P.; Gábor, N. The 90-kDa molecular chaperone family: Structure, function, and clinical applications. A comprehensive review. *Pharmacol. Ther.* **1998**, *79*, 129–168. [CrossRef]
8. Stone, K.R.; Ralph, E.S.; Wolfgang, K.J. Changes in membrane polypeptides that occur when chick embryo fibroblasts and NRK cells are transformed with avian sarcoma viruses. *Virology* **1974**, *58*, 86–100. [CrossRef]
9. Shiu, R.P.; Pouyssegur, J.; Pastan, I. Glucose depletion accounts for the induction of two transformation-sensitive membrane proteinsin Rous sarcoma virus-transformed chick embryo fibroblasts. *Proc. Natl. Acad. Sci. USA* **1977**, *74*, 3840–3844. [CrossRef]
10. Pouysségur, J.; Shiu, R.P.; Pastan, I. Induction of two transformation-sensitive membrane polypeptides in normal fibroblasts by a block in glycoprotein synthesis or glucose deprivation. *Cell* **1977**, *11*, 941–947. [CrossRef]
11. Pouysségur, J.; Yamada, K.M. Isolation and immunological characterization of a glucose-regulated fibroblast cell surface glycoprotein and its nonglycosylated precursor. *Cell* **1978**, *13*, 139–140. [CrossRef]
12. McCormick, P.J.; Keys, B.J.; Pucci, C.; Millis, A.J. Human fibroblast-conditioned medium contains a 100K dalton glucose-regulated cell surface protein. *Cell* **1979**, *18*, 173–182. [CrossRef]
13. Hughes, E.N.; Colombatti, A.; August, J.T. Murine cell surface glycoproteins. Purification of the polymorphic Pgp-1 antigen and analysis of its expression on macrophages and other myeloid cells. *J. Biol. Chem.* **1983**, *258*, 1014–1021. [CrossRef]
14. Srivastava, P.K.; DeLeo, A.B.; Old, L.J. Tumor rejection antigens of chemically induced sarcomas of inbred mice. *Proc. Natl. Acad. Sci. USA* **1986**, *83*, 3407–3411. [CrossRef] [PubMed]
15. Ullrich, S.J.; Robinson, E.A.; Law, L.W.; Willingham, M.; Appella, E. A mouse tumor-specific transplantation antigen is a heat shock-related protein. *Proc. Natl. Acad. Sci. USA* **1986**, *83*, 3121–3125. [CrossRef]
16. La Thangue, N.B.; Latchman, D.S. A cellular protein related to heat-shock protein 90 accumulates during herpes simplex virus infection and is overexpressed in transformed cells. *Exp. Cell Res.* **1988**, *178*, 169–179. [CrossRef]
17. Erkeller-Yüksel, F.M.; Isenberg, D.A.; Dhillon, V.B.; Latchman, D.S.; Lydyard, P.M. Surface expression of heat shock protein 90 by blood mononuclear cells from patients with systemic lupus erythematosus. *J. Autoimmun.* **1992**, *5*, 803–814. [CrossRef]
18. Thomaidou, D.; Dori, I.; Patsavoudi, E. Developmental expression and functional characterization of the 4C5 antigen in the postnatal cerebellar cortex. *J. Neurochem.* **1995**, *64*, 1937–1944. [CrossRef]
19. Sidera, K.; Samiotaki, M.; Yfanti, E.; Panayotou, G.; Patsavoudi, E. Involvement of cell surface HSP90 in cell migration reveals a novel role in the developing nervous system. *J. Biol. Chem.* **2004**, *279*, 45379–45388. [CrossRef]
20. Eustace, B.K.T.; Sakurai, J.K.; Stewart, D.; Yimlamai, C.; Unger, C.; Zehetmeier, B.; Lain, C.; Torella, S.W.; Henning, G.; Beste, B.T.; et al. Functional proteomic screens reveal an essential extracellular role for hsp90 alpha in cancer cell invasiveness. *Nat. Cell Biol.* **2004**, *6*, 507–514. [CrossRef]
21. Li, W.; Li, Y.; Guan, S.; Fan, J.; Cheng, C.F.; Bright, A.M.; Chinn, C.; Chen, M.; Woodley, D.T. Extracellular heat shock protein-90alpha: Linking hypoxia to skin cell motility and wound healing. *EMBO J.* **2007**, *26*, 1221–1233. [CrossRef]
22. Cheng, C.F.; Fan, J.; Fedesco, M.; Guan, S.; Li, Y.; Bandyopadhyay, B.; Bright, A.M.; Yerushalmi, D.; Liang, M.; Chen, M.; et al. Transforming growth factor alpha (TGFalpha)-stimulated secretion of HSP90alpha: Using the receptor LRP-1/CD91 to promote human skin cell migration against a TGFbeta-rich environment during wound healing. *Mol. Cell. Biol.* **2008**, *28*, 3344–3358. [CrossRef]
23. Gopal, U.; Bohonowych, J.E.; Lema-Tome, C.; Liu, A.; Garrett-Mayer, E.; Wang, B.; Isaacs, J.S. A novel extracellular Hsp90 mediated co-receptor function for LRP1 regulates EphA2 dependent glioblastoma cell invasion. *PLoS ONE* **2011**, *6*, e17649. [CrossRef]
24. Eustace, B.K.; Jay, D.G. Extracellular roles for the molecular chaperone, hsp90. *Cell Cycle* **2004**, *3*, 1098–1100. [CrossRef]
25. Tsutsumi, S.; Neckers, L. Extracellular heat shock protein 90: A role for a molecular chaperone in cell motility and cancer metastasis. *Cancer Sci.* **2007**, *98*, 1536–1539. [CrossRef] [PubMed]

26. Sidera, K.; Patsavoudi, E. Extracellular HSP90: Conquering the cell surface. *Cell Cycle* **2008**, *7*, 1564–1568. [CrossRef] [PubMed]
27. McCready, J.; Sims, J.D.; Chan, D.D.; Jay, D.G. Secretion of extracellular hsp90alpha via exosomes increases cancer cell motility: A role for plasminogen activation. *BMC Cancer* **2010**, *10*, 294–299. [CrossRef] [PubMed]
28. Li, W.; Sahu, D.; Tsen, F. Secreted heat shock protein-90 (Hsp90) in wound healing and cancer. *Biochim. Biophys. Acta* **2012**, *1823*, 730–741. [CrossRef]
29. Li, W.; Tsen, F.; Sahu, D.; Bhatia, A.; Chen, M.; Multhoff, G.; Woodley, D.T. Extracellular Hsp90 (eHsp90) as the actual target in clinical trials: Intentionally or unintentionally. *Int. Rev. Cell Mol. Biol.* **2013**, *303*, 203–235.
30. Hance, M.W.; Nolan, K.D.; Isaacs, J.S. The double-edged sword: Conserved functions of extracellular hsp90 in wound healing and cancer. *Cancers* **2014**, *6*, 1065–1097. [CrossRef]
31. Sidera, K.; Patsavoudi, E. HSP90 inhibitors: Current development and potential in cancer therapy. *Recent Pat. Anticancer Drug Discov.* **2014**, *9*, 1–20. [CrossRef] [PubMed]
32. Wong, D.S.; Jay, D.G. Emerging roles of extracellular Hsp90 in cancer. *Adv. Cancer Res.* **2016**, *129*, 141–163. [PubMed]
33. Kim, H.; Seo, E.H.; Lee, S.H.; Kim, B.J. The telomerase-derived anticancer peptide vaccine GV1001 as an extracellular heat shock protein-mediated cell-penetrating peptide. *Int. J. Mol. Sci.* **2016**, *17*, 2054. [CrossRef] [PubMed]
34. Fernandes, J.C.; Alves, P. Recent patents on heat shock proteins targeting antibodies. *Recent Pat. Anticancer Drug Discov.* **2017**, *12*, 48–54. [CrossRef] [PubMed]
35. Calderwood, S.K. Heat shock proteins and cancer: Intracellular chaperones or extracellularsignalling ligands? *Philos. Trans. R Soc. Lond. B Biol. Sci.* **2018**, *373*, 20160524. [CrossRef] [PubMed]
36. Taha, E.A.; Ono, K.; Eguchi, T. Roles of extracellular HSPs as biomarkers in immune surveillance and immune evasion. *Int. J. Mol. Sci.* **2019**, *20*, 4588. [CrossRef]
37. Calderwood, S.K.; Borges, T.J.; Eguchi, T.; Lang, B.J.; Murshid, A.; Okusha, Y.; Prince, T.L. Extracellular Hsp90 and protection of neuronal cells through Nrf2. *Biochem. Soc. Trans.* **2021**, *49*, 2299–2306. [CrossRef]
38. Birbo, B.; Madu, E.E.; Madu, C.O.; Jain, A.; Lu, Y. Role of HSP90 in cancer. *Int. J. Mol. Sci.* **2021**, *22*, 10317. [CrossRef]
39. Chakraborty, A.; Edkins, A.L. HSP90 as a regulator of extracellular matrix dynamics. *Biochem. Soc. Trans.* **2021**, *49*, 2611–2625. [CrossRef]
40. Poggio, P.; Sorge, M.; Seclì, L.; Brancaccio, M. Extracellular HSP90 machineries build tumor microenvironment and boost cancer progression. *Front. Cell Dev. Biol.* **2021**, *9*, 735529. [CrossRef]
41. Cheng, C.F.; Fan, J.; Zhao, Z.; Woodley, D.T.; Li, W. Secreted heat shock protein-90alpha: A more effective and safer target for anti-cancer drugs? *Curr. Signal Transduct. Ther.* **2010**, *5*, 121–127. [CrossRef]
42. Yu, X.; Harris, S.L.; Levine, A.J. The regulation of exosome secretion: A novel function of the p53 protein. *Cancer Res.* **2006**, *66*, 4795–4801. [CrossRef] [PubMed]
43. Suzuki, S.; Kulkarni, A.B. Extracellular heat shock protein HSP90beta secreted by MG63 osteosarcoma cells inhibits activation of latent TGF-beta1. *Biochem. Biophys. Res. Commun.* **2010**, *398*, 525–5331. [CrossRef] [PubMed]
44. Jayaprakash, P.; Dong, H.; Zou, M.; Bhatia, A.; O'Brien, K.; Chen, M.; Woodley, D.T.; Li, W. Hsp90α and Hsp90β together operate a hypoxia and nutrient paucity stress-response mechanism during wound healing. *J. Cell Sci.* **2015**, *128*, 1475–1480. [PubMed]
45. Zou, M.; Bhatia, A.; Dong, H.; Jayaprakash, P.; Guo, J.; Sahu, D.; Hou, Y.; Tsen, F.; Tong, C.; O'Brien, K. Evolutionarily conserved dual lysine motif determines the non-chaperone function of secreted Hsp90alpha in tumour progression. *Oncogene* **2017**, *36*, 2160–2171. [CrossRef]
46. Cheng, C.F.; Sahu, D.; Tsen, F.; Zhao, Z.; Fan, J.; Kim, R.; Wang, X.; O'Brien, K.; Li, Y.; Kuang, Y.; et al. A fragment of secreted Hsp90α carries properties that enable it to accelerate effectively both acute and diabetic wound healing in mice. *J. Clin. Investig.* **2011**, *121*, 4348–4361. [CrossRef]
47. Tsen, F.; Bhatia, A.; O'Brien, K.; Cheng, C.F.; Chen, M.; Hay, N.; Stiles, B.; Woodley, D.T.; Li, W. Extracellular heat shock protein 90 signals through subdomain II and the NPVY motif of LRP-1 receptor to Akt1 and Akt2: A circuit essential for promoting skin cell migration in vitro and wound healing in vivo. *Mol. Cell. Biol.* **2013**, *33*, 4947–4959. [CrossRef]
48. Voss, A.K.; Thomas, T.; Gruss, P. Mice lacking HSP90beta fail to develop a placental labyrinth. *Development* **2000**, *127*, 1. [CrossRef]
49. Grad, I.; Cederroth, C.R.; Walicki, J.; Grey, C.; Barluenga, S.; Winssinger, N.; De Massy, B.; Nef, S.; Picard, D. The molecular chaperone Hsp90α is required for meiotic progression of spermatocytes beyond pachytene in the mouse. *PLoS ONE* **2010**, *5*, e15770. [CrossRef]
50. Imai, T.; Kato, Y.; Kajiwara, C.; Mizukami, S.; Ishige, I.; Ichiyanagi, T.; Hikida, M.; Wang, J.-Y.; Udono, H. Heat shock protein 90 (HSP90) contributes to cytosolic translocation of extracellular antigen for cross-presentation by dendritic cells. *Proc. Natl. Acad. Sci. USA* **2011**, *108*, 16363–16368. [CrossRef]
51. Tang, X.; Chang CHao, M.; Chen, M.; Woodley, D.T.; Schönthal, A.H.; Li, W. Heat shock protein-90alpha (Hsp90α) stabilizes hypoxia-inducible factor-1α (HIF-1α) in support of spermatogenesis and tumorigenesis. *Cancer Gene Ther.* **2021**, *28*, 1058–1070. [CrossRef] [PubMed]
52. Liao, D.F.; Jin, Z.G.; Baas, A.S.; Daum, G.; Gygi, S.P.; Aebersold, R.; Berk, B.C. Purification and identification of secreted oxidative stress-induced factors from vascular smooth muscle cells. *J. Biol. Chem.* **2000**, *275*, 189–196. [CrossRef] [PubMed]
53. Kuroita, T.; Tachibana, H.; Ohashi, H.; Shirahata, S.; Murakami, H. Growth stimulating activity of heat shock protein 90 alpha to lymphoid cell lines in serum-free medium. *Cytotechnology* **1992**, *8*, 109–117. [CrossRef] [PubMed]

54. Zhang, S.; Wang, C.; Ma, B.; Xu, M.; Xu, S.; Liu, J.; Tian, Y.; Fu, Y.; Luo, Y. Mutant p53 drives cancer metastasis via RCP-mediated Hsp90α secretion. *Cell Rep.* **2020**, *32*, 107879. [CrossRef] [PubMed]
55. Bhatia, A.; O'Brien, K.; Guo, J.; Lincoln, V.; Kajiwara, C.; Chen, M.; Woodley, D.T.; Udono, H.; Li, W. Extracellular and non-chaperone function of heat shock protein−90α is required for skin wound healing. *J. Investig. Dermatol.* **2018**, *138*, 423–433. [CrossRef] [PubMed]
56. Wang, X.; Song, X.; Zhuo, W.; Fu, Y.; Shi, H.; Liang, Y.; Tong, M.; Chang, G.; Luo, Y. The regulatory mechanism of Hsp90α secretion and its function in tumor malignancy. *Proc. Natl. Acad. Sci. USA* **2009**, *106*, 21288–21293. [CrossRef]
57. Tsutsumi, S.; Mollapour, M.; Graf, C.; Lee, C.T.; Scroggins, B.T.; Xu, W.; Haslerova, L.; Hessling, M.; Konstantinova, A.A.; Trepel, J.B.; et al. Neckers Hsp90 charged-linker truncation reverses the functional consequences of weakened hydrophobic contacts in the N domain. *Nat. Struct. Mol. Biol.* **2009**, *16*, 1141–1147. [CrossRef]
58. Lancaster, G.I.; Febbraio, M.A. Exosome-dependent trafficking of HSP70: A novel secretory pathway for cellular stress proteins. *J. Biol. Chem.* **2005**, *280*, 23349–23355. [CrossRef]
59. Savina, A.; Furlan, M.; Vidal, M.; Colombo, M.I. Exosome release is regulated by a calcium-dependent mechanism in K562 cells. *J. Biol. Chem.* **2003**, *278*, 20083–20090. [CrossRef]
60. Mignot, G.; Roux, S.; Thery, C.; Segura, E.; Zitvogel, L. Prospects for exosomes in immunotherapy of cancer. *J. Cell. Mol. Med.* **2006**, *10*, 376–388. [CrossRef]
61. Hegmans, J.P.; Bard, M.P.; Hemmes, A.; Luider, T.M.; Kleijmeer, M.J.; Prins, J.B.; Zitvogel, L.; Burgers, S.A.; Hoogsteden, H.C.; Lambrecht, B.N. Proteomic analysis of exosomes secreted by human mesothelioma cells. *Am. J. Pathol.* **2004**, *164*, 1807–1815. [CrossRef]
62. Guo, J.; Jayaprakash, P.; Dan, J.; Wise, P.; Jang, G.B.; Liang, C.; Chen, M.; Woodley, D.T.; Fabbri, M.; Li, W. PRAS40 connects microenvironmental stress signaling to exosome-mediated secretion. *Mol. Cell. Biol.* **2017**, *37*, e00171-17. [CrossRef] [PubMed]
63. Tang, X.; Chang, C.; Guo, J.; Lincoln, V.; Liang, C.; Chen, M.; Li, W. Tumor-secreted Hsp90α on external surface of exosomes mediates tumor—Stromal cell communication via autocrine and paracrine mechanisms. *Sci. Rep.* **2019**, *9*, 15108. [CrossRef] [PubMed]
64. Bertout, J.; Patel, S.; Simon, M. The impact of O_2 availability on human cancer. *Nat. Rev. Cancer* **2008**, *8*, 967–975. [CrossRef]
65. Bhatia, A.; O'brien, K.; Chen, M.; Wong, A.; Garner, W.; Woodley, D.T.; Li, W. Dual therapeutic functions of F-5 fragment in burn wounds: Preventing wound progression and promoting wound healing in pigs. *Mol. Ther. Methods Clin. Dev.* **2016**, *3*, 16041. [CrossRef]
66. Dong, H.; Zou, M.; Bhatia, A.; Jayaprakash, P.; Hofman, F.; Ying, Q.; Chen, M.; Woodley, D.T.; Li, W. Breast cancer MDA-MB-231 cells use secreted heat shock protein-90alpha (Hsp90α) to survive a hostile hypoxic environment. *Sci. Rep.* **2016**, *6*, 20605. [CrossRef]
67. Gao, F.; Hu, X.Y.; Xie, X.J.; Xu, Q.Y.; Wang, Y.P.; Liu, X.B.; Xiang, M.X.; Sun, Y.; Wang, J.A. Heat shock protein 90 protects rat mesenchymal stem cells against hypoxia and serum deprivation-induced apoptosis via the PI3K/Akt and ERK1/2 pathways. *J. Zhejiang Univ. Sci. B* **2010**, *11*, 608–617. [CrossRef]
68. Thomaidou, D.; Yfanti, E.; Patsavoudi, E.J. Expression of the 4C5 antigen during development and after injury of the rat sciatic nerve. *Neurosci. Res.* **1996**, *46*, 24–33. [CrossRef]
69. Yfanti, E.; Nagata, I.; Patsavoudi, E.J. Migration behavior of rodent granule neurons in the presence of antibody to the 4C5 antigen. *J. Neurochem.* **1998**, *71*, 1381–1389. [CrossRef]
70. Tsutsumi, S.; Scroggins, B.; Koga, F.; Lee, M.J.; Trepel, J.; Felts, S.; Carreras, C.; Neckers, L. A small molecule cell-impermeant Hsp90 antagonist inhibits tumor cell motility and invasion. *Oncogene* **2008**, *27*, 2478–2487. [CrossRef]
71. Sims, J.D.; McCready, J.; Jay, D.G. Extracellular heat shock protein (Hsp)70 and Hsp90a assist in matrix metalloproteinase-2 activation and breast cancer cell migration and invasion. *PLoS ONE* **2011**, *6*, e18848. [CrossRef] [PubMed]
72. Baker-Williams, A.J.; Hashmi, F.; Budzyński, M.A.; Woodford, M.R.; Gleicher, S.; Himanen, S.V.; Makedon, A.M.; Friedman, D.; Cortes, S.; Namek, S.; et al. Co-chaperones TIMP2 and AHA1 competitively regulate extracellular HSP90: Client MMP2 activity and matrix proteolysis. *Cell Rep.* **2019**, *28*, 1894–1906. [CrossRef] [PubMed]
73. Song, X.; Wang, X.; Zhuo, W.; Shi, H.; Feng, D.; Sun, Y.; Liang, Y.; Fu, Y.; Zhou, D.; Luo, Y. The regulatory mechanism of extracellular Hsp90{alpha} on matrix metalloproteinase-2 processing and tumor angiogenesis. *J. Biol. Chem.* **2010**, *285*, 40039–40049. [CrossRef]
74. Tian, Y.; Wang, C.; Chen, S.; Liu, J.; Fu, Y.; Luo, Y. Extracellular Hsp90α and clusterin synergistically promote breast cancer epithelial-to-mesenchymal transition and metastasis via LRP1. *J. Cell Sci.* **2019**, *132*, jcs228213. [CrossRef] [PubMed]
75. García, R.; Merino, D.; Gómez, J.M.; Nistal, J.F.; Hurlé, M.A.; Cortajarena, A.L.; Villar, A.V. Extracellular heat shock protein 90 binding to TGFβ receptor I participates in TGFβ-mediated collagen production in myocardial fibroblasts. *Cell. Signal.* **2016**, *28*, 1563–1579. [CrossRef] [PubMed]
76. Song, X.; Luo, Y. The regulatory mechanism of Hsp90alpha secretion from endothelial cells and its role in angiogenesis during wound healing. *Biochem. Biophys. Res. Commun.* **2010**, *398*, 111–117. [CrossRef]
77. O'Brien, K.; Bhatia, A.; Tsen, F.; Chen, M.; Wong, A.K.; Woodley, D.T.; Li, W. Identification of the critical therapeutic entity in secreted Hsp90α that promotes wound healing in newly re-standardized healthy and diabetic pig models. *PLoS ONE* **2014**, *9*, e113956. [CrossRef]

78. Bellaye, P.S.; Burgy, O.; Causse, S.; Garrido, C.; Bonniaud, P. Heat shock proteins in fibrosis and wound healing: Good or evil? *Pharmacol. Ther.* **2014**, *143*, 119–132. [CrossRef]
79. Dong, H.; Luo, L.; Zou, M.; Huang, C.; Wan, X.; Hu, Y.; Le, Y.; Zhao, H.; Li, W.; Zou, F.; et al. Blockade of extracellular heat shock protein 90a by 1G6-D7 attenuates pulmonary fibrosis through inhibiting ERK signaling. *Am. J. Physiol. Lung Cell. Mol. Physiol.* **2017**, *313*, 1006–1015. [CrossRef]
80. Zhang, J.; Zhong, W.; Liu, Y.; Chen, W.; Lu, Y.; Zeng, Z.; Qiao, Y.; Huang, H.; Wan, X.; Li, W.; et al. Extracellular HSP90α interacts with ER stress to promote fibroblasts activation through PI3K/AKT pathway in pulmonary fibrosis. *Front. Pharmacol.* **2021**, *12*, 708462. [CrossRef]
81. Bellaye, P.S.; Shimbori, C.; Yanagihara, T.; Carlson, D.A.; Hughes, P.; Upagupta, C.; Sato, S.; Wheildon, N.; Haystead, T.; Ask, K.; et al. Synergistic role of HSP90α and HSP90β to promote myofibroblast persistence in lung fibrosis. *Eur. Respir. J.* **2018**, *51*, 1700386. [CrossRef] [PubMed]
82. Zhang, G.; Liu, Z.; Ding, H.; Zhou, Y.; Doan, H.A.; Sin, K.W.T.; Zhu, Z.J.; Flores, R.; Wen, Y.; Gong, X.; et al. Tumor induces muscle wasting in mice through releasing extracellular Hsp70 and Hsp90. *Nat. Commun.* **2017**, *8*, 589. [CrossRef] [PubMed]
83. Stellas, D.; Karameris, A.; Patsavoudi, E. Monoclonal antibody 4C5 immunostains human melanomas and inhibits melanoma cell invasion and metastasis. *Clin. Cancer Res.* **2007**, *13*, 1831–1838. [CrossRef] [PubMed]
84. Stellas, D.; El Hamidieh, A.; Patsavoudi, E. Monoclonal antibody 4C5 prevents activation of MMP2 and MMP9 by disrupting their interaction with extracellular HSP90 and inhibits formation of metastatic breast cancer cell deposits. *BMC Cell Biol.* **2010**, *11*, 51. [CrossRef] [PubMed]
85. Hou, Q.; Chen, S.; An, Q.; Li, B.; Fu, Y.; Luo, Y. Extracellular Hsp90α promotes tumor lymphangiogenesis and lymph node metastasis in breast cancer. *Int. J. Mol. Sci.* **2021**, *22*, 7747. [CrossRef] [PubMed]
86. Stivarou, T.; Stellas, D.; Vartzi, G.; Thomaidou, D.; Patsavoudi, E. Targeting highly expressed extracellular HSP90 in breast cancer stem cells inhibits tumor growth in vitro and in vivo. *Cancer Biol. Ther.* **2016**, *17*, 799–812. [CrossRef]
87. Seclì, L.; Avalle, L.; Poggio, P.; Fragale, G.; Cannata, C.; Conti, L.; Iannucci, A.; Carrà, G.; Rubinetto, C.; Miniscalco, B.; et al. Targeting the extracellular HSP90 co-chaperone morgana inhibits cancer cell migration and promotes anticancer immunity. *Cancer Res.* **2021**, *81*, 4794–4807. [CrossRef]
88. Milani, M.; Laranjeira, A.B.; de Vasconcellos, J.F.; Brandalise, S.R.; Nowill, A.E.; Yunes, J.A. Plasma Hsp90 level as a marker of early acute lymphoblastic Leukemia engraftment and progression in mice. *PLoS ONE* **2015**, *10*, e0129298.
89. Wang, C.; Zhang, S.; Liu, J.; Tian, Y.; Ma, B.; Xu, S.; Fu, Y.; Luo, Y. Secreted pyruvate kinase M2 promotes lung cancer metastasis through activating the integrin Beta1/FAK signaling pathway. *Cell Rep.* **2020**, *30*, 1780–1797. [CrossRef]
90. Xu, Q.; Tu, J.; Dou, C.; Zhang, J.; Yang, L.; Liu, X.; Lei, K.; Liu, Z.; Wang, Y.; Li, L.; et al. HSP90 promotes cell glycolysis, proliferation and inhibits apoptosis by regulating PKM2 abundance via Thr-328 phosphorylation in hepatocellular carcinoma. *Mol. Cancer* **2017**, *16*, 178. [CrossRef]
91. Liu, W.; Li, J.; Zhang, P.; Hou, Q.; Feng, S.; Liu, L.; Cui, D.; Shi, H.; Fu, Y.; Luo, Y. A novel pan-cancer biomarker plasma heat shock protein 90alpha and its diagnosis determinants in clinic. *Cancer Sci.* **2019**, *110*, 2941–2959. [CrossRef] [PubMed]
92. Wei, W.; Zhou, J.H.; Chen, L.P.; Liu, H.Z.; Zhang, F.Y.; Li, J.L.; Ning, S.F.; Li, S.R.; Wang, C.; Huang, Y.; et al. Plasma Levels of Heat Shock Protein 90 Alpha Associated With Colorectal Cancer Development. *Front. Mol. Biosci.* **2021**, *8*, 684836. [CrossRef] [PubMed]
93. Fu, Y.; Xu, X.; Huang, D.; Cui, D.; Liu, L.; Liu, J.; He, Z.; Liu, J.; Zheng, S.; Luo, Y. Plasma heat shock protein 90alpha as a biomarker for the diagnosis of liver cancer: An official, large-scale, and multicenter clinical trial. *EBioMedicine* **2017**, *24*, 56–63. [CrossRef]
94. Shi, Y.; Liu, X.; Lou, J.; Han, X.; Zhang, L.; Wang, Q.; Li, B.; Dong, M.; Zhang, Y. Plasma levels of heat shock protein 90 alpha associated with lung cancer development and treatment responses. *Clin. Cancer Res.* **2014**, *20*, 6016–6022. [CrossRef] [PubMed]
95. Kasanga, M.; Liu, L.; Xue, L.; Song, X. Plasma heat shock protein 90-alpha have an advantage in diagnosis of colorectal cancer at early stage. *Biomark. Med.* **2018**, *12*, 881–890. [CrossRef] [PubMed]
96. Tas, F.; Bilgin, E.; Erturk, K.; Duranyildiz, D. Clinical significance of circulating serum cellular heat shock protein 90 (HSP90) level in patients with cutaneous malignant melanoma. *Asian Pac. J. Cancer Prev.* **2017**, *18*, 599–601.
97. Fredly, H.; Reikvam, H.; Gjertsen, B.T.; Bruserud, O. Disease-stabilizing treatment with all-trans retinoic acid and valproic acid in acute myeloid Leukemia: Serum hsp70 and hsp90 levels and serum cytokine profiles are determined by the disease, patient age, and anti-leukemic treatment. *Am. J. Hematol.* **2012**, *87*, 368–376. [CrossRef]
98. Chen, C.C.; Chen, L.L.; Li, C.P.; Hsu, Y.T.; Jiang, S.S.; Fan, C.S.; Chua, K.V.; Huang, S.X.; Shyr, Y.M.; Chen, L.T.; et al. Myeloid-derived macrophages and secreted HSP90α induce pancreatic ductal adenocarcinoma development. *Oncoimmunology* **2018**, *7*, e1424612. [CrossRef]
99. Zhou, Y.; Deng, X.; Zang, N.; Li, H.; Li, G.; Li, C.; He, M. Transcriptomic and proteomic investigation of HSP90A as a potential biomarker for HCC. *Med. Sci. Monit. Int. Med. J. Exp. Clin. Res.* **2015**, *21*, 4039. [CrossRef]
100. Wei, W.; Liu, M.; Ning, S.; Wei, J.; Zhong, J.; Li, J.; Cai, Z.; Zhang, L. Diagnostic value of plasma HSP90α levels for detection of hepatocellular carcinoma. *BMC Cancer* **2020**, *20*, 6. [CrossRef]
101. Wang, X.T.; An, D.Z.; Wang, X.L.; Liu, X.M.; Li, B.S. Extracellular Hsp90α clinically correlates with tumor malignancy and promotes migration and invasion in esophageal squamous cell carcinoma. *OncoTargets Ther.* **2019**, *12*, 1119–1128. [CrossRef] [PubMed]

102. Zhao, Q.; Miao, C.; Lu, Q.; Wu, W.; He, Y.; Wu, S.; Liu, H.; Lian, C. Clinical significance of monitoring circulating free DNA and plasma heat shock protein 90alpha in patients with esophageal squamous cell carcinoma. *Cancer Manag. Res.* **2021**, *13*, 2223. [CrossRef] [PubMed]
103. Han, S.; Cheng, Z.; Zhao, X.; Huang, Y. Diagnostic value of heat shock protein 90α and squamous cell carcinoma antigen in detection of cervical cancer. *J. Int. Med. Res.* **2019**, *47*, 5518–5525. [CrossRef] [PubMed]
104. Burgess, E.F.; Ham, A.J.L.; Tabb, D.L.; Billheimer, D.; Roth, B.J.; Chang, S.S.; Cookson, M.S.; Hinton, T.J.; Cheek, K.L.; Hill, S.; et al. Prostate cancer serum biomarker discovery through proteomic analysis of alpha-2 macroglobulin protein complexes. *Proteom. Clin. Appl.* **2008**, *2*, 1223–1233. [CrossRef]
105. Pawlik-Gwozdecka, D.; Górska-Ponikowska, M.; Adamkiewicz-Drożyńska, E.; Niedźwiecki, M. Serum heat shock protein 90 as a future predictive biomarker in childhood acute lymphoblastic leukemia. *Central Eur. J. Immunol.* **2021**, *46*, 63. [CrossRef]
106. Liang, X.Q.; Li, K.Z.; Li, Z.; Xie, M.Z.; Tang, Y.P.; Du, J.B.; Huang, Y.; Li, J.L.; Hu, B.L. Diagnostic and prognostic value of plasma heat shock protein 90alpha in gastric cancer. *Int. Immunopharmacol.* **2021**, *90*, 107145. [CrossRef]
107. Yuan, Z.; Hong, S.; Li, L.; He, L.; Xiao, P.; Tang, T.; Shi, C.; Mu, Y.; Sun, C.; Shang, Y.; et al. Diagnostic value of HSP90α and related markers in lung cancer. *J. Clin. Lab. Anal.* **2019**, *36*, e24462. [CrossRef]
108. Fu, M.; Du, F.; Wei, Z.; Xu, C.; Wang, X.; Zhao, X. Hsp90α Is Suitable for Therapy Monitoring in Multiple Cancers. *Res. Sq.* **2021**. [CrossRef]
109. Zhong, B.; Shen, J.; Zhang, C.; Zhou, G.; Yu, Y.; Qin, E.; Tang, J.; Wu, D.; Liang, X. Plasma heat shock protein 90 alpha: A valuable predictor of early chemotherapy effectiveness in advanced non-small-cell lung cancer. *Med. Sci. Monit. Int. Med. J. Exp. Clin. Res.* **2021**, *27*, e924778-1. [CrossRef]
110. Zhang, T.; Li, Q.; Zhang, Y.; Wang, Q.; Wanga, H.; Gua, K. Diagnostic and prognostic value of heat shock protein 90α in malignant melanoma. *Melanoma Res.* **2021**, *31*, 152–161. [CrossRef]
111. Mao, M.; Wang, X.; Sheng, H.; Li, H.; Liu, W.; Han, R.; Wen, W.; Liu, W. Heat shock protein 90α provides an effective and novel diagnosis strategy for nasopharyngeal carcinoma. *Adv. Ther.* **2021**, *38*, 413–422. [CrossRef] [PubMed]
112. Grimstad, T.; Kvivik, I.; Kvaløy, J.T.; Aabakken, L.; Omdal, R. Heat-shock protein 90 α in plasma reflects severity of fatigue in patients with Crohn's disease. *Innate Immune* **2020**, *26*, 146–151. [CrossRef] [PubMed]
113. Damasiewicz-Bodzek, A.; Szumska, M.; Tyrpień-Golder, K. Antibodies to heat shock proteins 90α and 90β in psoriasis. *Arch. Immunol. Ther. Exp.* **2020**, *68*, 9. [CrossRef] [PubMed]
114. Chebotareva, N.; Vinogradov, A.; Gindis, A.; Tao, E.; Moiseev, S. Heat shock protein 90 and NFkB levels in serum and urine in patients with chronic glomerulonephritis. *Cell Stress Chaperones* **2020**, *25*, 495–501. [CrossRef]
115. Miyazaki, D.; Nakamura, A.; Hineno, A.; Kobayashi, C.; Kinoshita, T.; Yoshida, K.; Ikeda, S.I. Elevation of serum heat-shock protein levels in amyotrophic lateral sclerosis. *Neurol. Sci.* **2016**, *37*, 1277–1281. [CrossRef]
116. Bălănescu, A.; Stan, I.; Codreanu, I.; Comănici, V.; Bălănescu, E.; Bălănescu, P. Circulating Hsp90 isoform levels in overweight and obese children and the relation to nonalcoholic fatty liver disease: Results from a cross-sectional study. *Dis. Markers* **2019**, *2019*, 9560247. [CrossRef]
117. Štorkánová, H.; Oreská, S.; Špiritović, M.; Heřmánková, B.; Bubová, K.; Komarc, M.; Pavelka, K.; Vencovský, J.; Distler, J.H.; Šenolt, L.; et al. Plasma Hsp90 levels in patients with systemic sclerosis and relation to lung and skin involvement: A cross-sectional and longitudinal study. *Sci. Rep.* **2021**, *11*, 1. [CrossRef]
118. Ding, X.; Meng, C.; Dong, H.; Zhang, S.; Zhou, H.; Tan, W.; Huang, L.; He, A.; Li, J.; Huang, J.; et al. Extracellular Hsp90α, which participates in vascular inflammation, is a novel serum predictor of atherosclerosis in type 2 diabetes. *BMJ Open Diabetes Res. Care* **2022**, *10*, e002579. [CrossRef]
119. Lambert, A.W.; Pattabiraman, D.R.; Weinberg, R.A. Emerging biological principles of metastasis. *Cell* **2017**, *168*, 670–691. [CrossRef]
120. Massagué, J.; Obenauf, A.C. Metastatic colonization by circulating tumour cells. *Nature* **2016**, *529*, 298–306. [CrossRef]
121. Sethi, N.; Kang, Y. Unravelling the complexity of metastasis—Molecular understanding and targeted therapies. *Nat. Rev. Cancer* **2011**, *11*, 735–748. [CrossRef] [PubMed]
122. Turajlic, S.; Swanton, C. Metastasis as an evolutionary process. *Science* **2016**, *352*, 169–175. [CrossRef] [PubMed]
123. Center Watch. Available online: www.centerwatch.com/directories/1067-fda-approved-drugs/topic/103-oncology (accessed on 17 August 2020).
124. Yuno, A.; Lee, M.J.; Lee, S.; Tomita, Y.; Rekhtman, D.; Moore, B.; Trepel, J.B. Clinical evaluation and biomarker profiling of Hsp90 inhibitors. *Chaperones* **2018**, *1709*, 423–441.
125. Tang, X.; Chang, C.; Mosallaei, D.; Woodley, D.T.; Schönthal, A.H.; Chen, M.; Li, W. Heterogeneous responses and isoform compensation dim the therapeutic window of Hsp90 ATP-binding inhibitors in cancer. *Mol. Cell. Biol.* **2022**, *42*, e0045921. [CrossRef] [PubMed]
126. Sahu, D.; Zhao, Z.; Tsen, F.; Cheng, C.F.; Park, R.; Situ, A.J.; Dai, J.; Eginli, A.; Shams, S.; Chen, M.; et al. A potentially common peptide target in secreted heat shock protein-90α for hypoxia-inducible factor-1α–positive tumors. *Mol. Biol. Cell.* **2012**, *23*, 602–613. [CrossRef]
127. Hanahan, D.; Weinberg, R.A. The hallmarks of cancer. *Cell* **2000**, *100*, 57–70. [CrossRef]

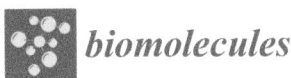

Review

Organismal Roles of Hsp90

Patricija van Oosten-Hawle

Department of Biological Sciences, The University of North Carolina at Charlotte, Charlotte, NC 28223, USA; pvanoost@uncc.edu

Abstract: Heat shock protein 90 (Hsp90) is a highly conserved molecular chaperone that assists in the maturation of many client proteins involved in cellular signal transduction. As a regulator of cellular signaling processes, it is vital for the maintenance of cellular proteostasis and adaptation to environmental stresses. Emerging research shows that Hsp90 function in an organism goes well beyond intracellular proteostasis. In metazoans, Hsp90, as an environmentally responsive chaperone, is involved in inter-tissue stress signaling responses that coordinate and safeguard cell nonautonomous proteostasis and organismal health. In this way, Hsp90 has the capacity to influence evolution and aging, and effect behavioral responses to facilitate tissue-defense systems that ensure organismal survival. In this review, I summarize the literature on the organismal roles of Hsp90 uncovered in multicellular organisms, from plants to invertebrates and mammals.

Keywords: Hsp90; organismal; cell nonautonomous; proteostasis; stress response; inter-tissue stress signaling

1. Introduction

Cellular protein homeostasis depends on the integrity and function of its proteome, of which molecular chaperones play an indispensable role to maintain it. Heat shock protein 90 (Hsp90) is an essential and evolutionary conserved molecular chaperone, that except for archea, is found in all kingdoms of life [1]. Hsp90 is crucial for the viability and growth of eukaryotic cells and organisms, and it is one of the most abundant cellular proteins known to date, representing ~2% of total protein in a cell [2]. This abundance of Hsp90 is required to sustain the wide range of cellular processes it is implicated in, by chaperoning components involved in cellular signal transduction events such as protein kinases and steroid hormone receptors [3–8].

Hsp90 requires ATP function for its activity to help facilitate folding of client proteins, and this function is regulated and controlled by a variety of co-chaperones in a context-specific manner [7,9], as well as post translational modifications [10–13]. Briefly, each Hsp90 dimer binds ATP in its "open conformation", which is followed by dimerization of the N-terminal domains of each protomer, allowing ATP hydrolysis. This subsequently leads to release of the folded and mature client protein, resulting in the open conformation of the Hsp90 dimer [7,8,14]. Each step along the Hsp90 chaperone cycle is finetuned by co-chaperones, such as, e.g., Cdc37/p50, which promote binding to kinase clients [15–17], or Aha1 and p23 that are involved in the regulation of Hsp90 ATP hydrolysis [14,18,19]. For more detailed information on the Hsp90 structure and regulation by co-chaperones, the reader is referred to articles and reviews specifically discussing this topic, including this Special Issue [8,20–22].

Because of its involvement in a wide range of cellular processes, Hsp90 supports an expansive network of more than 300 confirmed client proteins encompassing at least 5% of total proteins in yeast cells, and this number is similarly increased in multicellular organisms and mammals (https://www.picard.ch/downloads/Hsp90interactors.pdf; accessed 20 December 2022). Consequently, it is perhaps not surprising that Hsp90 is involved in almost every cellular process from cell cycle and a multitude of signal transduction

Citation: van Oosten-Hawle, P. Organismal Roles of Hsp90. *Biomolecules* **2023**, *13*, 251. https://doi.org/10.3390/biom13020251

Academic Editor: Chrisostomos Prodromou

Received: 20 December 2022
Revised: 24 January 2023
Accepted: 25 January 2023
Published: 29 January 2023

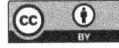

Copyright: © 2023 by the author. Licensee MDPI, Basel, Switzerland. This article is an open access article distributed under the terms and conditions of the Creative Commons Attribution (CC BY) license (https://creativecommons.org/licenses/by/4.0/).

pathways to protein trafficking, transcriptional processes and genomic stability [23–29]. In multicellular organisms, Hsp90's involvement is expanded accordingly, and evidence in the past two decades has shown that Hsp90's role reaches far beyond maintenance of signaling proteins: Its involvement ranges from development and evolution to intercellular stress signaling, aging responses and innate immunity, as well as neuronal function and behavior (Figure 1). In this review, I will highlight these organismal roles of Hsp90 which have been uncovered in different multicellular model systems, including plants, invertebrates and mammals.

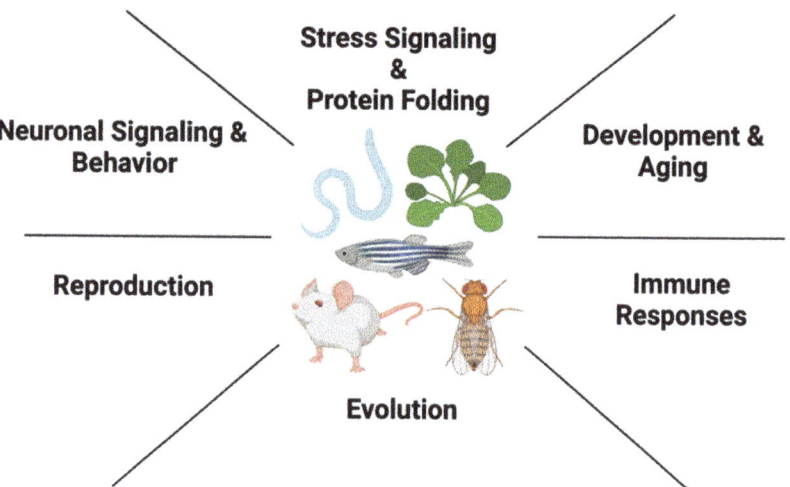

Figure 1. Organismal roles of Hsp90 in different multicellular model systems. In metazoans, such as *C. elegans*, *Mus musculus*, *D. melanogaster*, *Danio rerio* and *A. thaliana*, Hsp90 acts in diverse biological processes to ensure organismal proteostasis.

2. Hsp90 in Organismal Development and Evolution

2.1. Development

The coordination of cell proliferation and differentiation is crucial for proper development. Hsp90's central role in growth and development is profound, as its client proteins regulate almost all phases of the cell cycle. These include PI-3/AKT, NFkB and MAP kinase pathways, which drive progression through G1/S and G2/M checkpoints through transcriptional routes converging on Cyclin D, and Cyclin B and E [30]. Hsp90 also regulates various key cell cycle regulators directly, including Cdk1, Cdk2, Cdk4 and Cdk6 [31–34]. Furthermore, check point kinases Wee-1 and Myt-1 depend on Hsp90 function [35–37]. Later stages of mitosis and cytokinesis also depend on Hsp90 via mitotic regulators Survivin and Aurora B [38,39]. Because of Hsp90 influencing the cell cycle at multiple levels, either directly or indirectly, Hsp90 function is indispensable not only for organismal development but also for tumor cell progression, which was recognized early on through targeted inhibition of Hsp90 function using ansamycin inhibitors such as geldanamycin and 17-AAG [2,40–42]. Due to Hsp90 being involved in signaling pathways promoting cancer cell progression, it has become an attractive and well-established therapeutic cancer target, with Hsp90 inhibitors being continually developed and reviewed in clinical trials in an ongoing basis [43].

Most eukaryotic systems have two different cytosolic Hsp90 isoforms, with the exception of *C. elegans* that has only one cytosolic isoform (HSP-90/DAF-21). In mammals and yeast, the stress-inducible Hsp90α is encoded by the gene HSP90AA1 in humans (HSP82 in yeast), and the constitutively expressed Hsp90β is encoded by HSP90AB1 in humans and HSC82 in yeast. Although both isoforms share extensive sequence identity, their cellular functions are not completely identical and this is also demonstrated in their developmental requirements in an organism. For example, the Hsp90β knockout mouse shows early embryonic lethality [44], whereas this is not the case for mice lacking Hsp90α, which are viable but exhibit a failure of spermatogenesis and become sterile [45]. Moreover, while both isoforms are mutually expressed in most tissues in the mouse, the heart and muscle were found to harbor reduced levels of Hsp90α compared to Hsp90β [45]. Interestingly, zebrafish contains two Hsp90α genes, called Hsp90a1 and Hsp90a2. Hsp90a1 is crucial for myofibril organization in skeletal muscle development, whereas Hsp90a2 has no effect on muscle development [46]. Coherent with observations in vertebrates, the only cytosolic Hsp90 isoform in the invertebrate *C. elegans* (HSP-90) is crucial for myosin folding and muscle development, as RNAi-mediated knockdown leads to disrupted myosin filaments and motility defects [47,48]. Mammals such as mice, however, appear to require higher threshold levels of Hsp90 to promote stress adaptation and survival of the organism compared to yeast. This is accomplished through an internal ribosome entry site (IRES) in the 5′UTR of the Hsp90ab1 mRNA that can reprogram Hsp90 translational levels in stressed conditions [49].

As observed in other multicellular model organisms, depletion of Hsp90 by RNAi in *C. elegans* leads to morphological and transcriptional changes, including developmental changes to the gonad, vulval structures and oocyte development [50]. Indeed, Hsp90 regulates the meiotic prophase to metaphase transition during oocyte development by ensuring *wee-1* kinase functionality, which results in reduced fertility in the worm [51]. Interestingly, besides transcriptional changes that demonstrate induction of the heat shock response, Hsp90 RNAi at the whole animal level also leads to induction of an innate immune response, by altering expression levels of innate immune genes primarily expressed in the intestine [50].

The role of Hsp90 in *C. elegans* development is further highlighted through its involvement in *dauer* formation, TGFβ- and Notch signaling. The *C. elegans* TGF-β pathway regulates a decision between reproductive development and arrest at a larval stage known as *dauer* that is suited for survival under conditions of environmental stress. Hsp90 is implicated in *dauer* formation through its interaction with two components of the TGF-β pathway, TGF-β-RI (DAF-1 in *C. elegans*) and TGF-β-RII (DAF-4 in *C. elegans*) [52]. Hsp90 also regulates the functionality of a DAF-11/guanyl cyclase signaling pathway in sensory ciliae and amphid neurons that controls *dauer* formation in response to environmental cues, in parallel to the TGF-β pathway [53,54], as well as chemosensory behaviors [54,55]. Germline proliferation in *C. elegans* requires signaling from the somatic gonad to the germline, which is mediated by GLP-1 (a Notch orthologue) [56]. If GLP-1/Notch signaling is defective through mutations in the *glp-1* gene, germline stem cells prematurely exit mitosis and enter meiosis to form gametes, resulting in reduced germline proliferation and sterility [57]. Hsp90 has been identified as a regulator of Notch signaling that suppresses defective GLP-1/Notch signaling and promotes germline proliferation [58]. Strikingly, *C. elegans* depleted for Hsp90 by RNA interference or using an HSP-90(I461N) mutant leads to the formation of a proximal germline tumor, despite its reduced function and reduced GLP-1 signaling [57,58]. Further research in solving this paradox will be required to better illuminate the complex tissue-specific and organismal functions of the Hsp90 chaperone system in *C. elegans* and other metazoans.

2.2. Hsp90 as a Capacitor of Organismal Evolution

The physiological requirement of Hsp90 for the growth and development of model organisms was obvious early on using *Saccharomyces cerevisiae* [35,59], but was further highlighted using *Drosophila melanogaster* [60], where point mutations of the *Drosophila* Hsp90 (Hsp83) gene are lethal as homozygotes [61]. Although heterozygous mutant combinations are viable as adults, they are associated with sterility due to defects in microtubule dynamics during spermatogenesis [61]. Further experiments in *Drosophila* designed to identify suppressors of signal transduction *Sevenless* and *Raf* pathway mutants recovered Hsp90 mutants. Progeny of these Hsp90 mutants resulted in developmental abnormalities that, dependent on the genetic background, affected different morphological structures of the fruit fly [60,62]. This discovery led to further demonstration of Hsp90's importance in *Drosophila* spermatogenesis and germline development [61]. It was one of the cornerstones that defined Hsp90's prominent role in evolution, which was established as the "Hsp90 capacitor hypothesis" by the Lindquist lab [63].

The capacitor hypothesis demonstrated that diverse pathways become sensitive to the effects of genetic variation when Hsp90 function is compromised due to environmental stress, pharmacological inhibition or genetic mutation. It showed that Hsp90 functions in a wide variety of morphogenetic processes that are apparent in all model organisms tested, from yeast to vertebrates [63–65]. For example, the diverse phenotypes associated with Hsp90 impairment in *Drosophila* are deformed eye and thickened wing phenotypes [63], whereas in *Arabidopsis thaliana*, this leads to altered leaf and cotyledon shapes [64]. Similar consequences were observed in zebrafish upon reduced Hsp90 expression [66]. In *C. elegans*, the expression level of Hsp90 in particular varies during *C. elegans* embryonic development, causing embryos with stronger induction of Hsp90 to be less affected by mutation, thus buffering genetic variation [67]. However, individuals of a population with increased stress resistance due to higher Hsp90 levels show a "trade-off" with lowered reproductive potential, whereas worms with lower stress resistance are associated with higher reproductive fitness. The reason for this is thought to be a bet-hedging strategy, which is beneficial in ever-changing environments, that ensures survival of the population as a whole [67,68]. The reduced reproductive fitness due to increased Hsp90 expression perhaps highlights the requirement for Hsp90 expression levels to be tightly regulated due to its important role in germline development [57].

Importantly, phenotypic traits revealed upon temporary Hsp90 impairment can be selected for over several generations and become fixed in following generations, establishing Hsp90's crucial role in evolution. An example for this in a natural setting was provided by the cavefish *Asyanax mexicanus*, where cryptic variation in eye size was masked by Hsp90 in the ancestral river but revealed when fish were kept in caves that challenged the Hsp90 system due to low-salinity water [65]. This even plays a role in human disease, as is the case in Fanconi anemia (FA), a complex autosomal recessive human cancer predisposition syndrome that results in point mutations of 19 genes involved in the FA genome maintenance pathway [69]. The function of less severe FANCA mutants was preserved by Hsp90 binding, which maintained FA pathway function but became destabilized and sensitive to genotoxic stress upon Hsp90 impairment [69].

However, while the evolutionary capacitor hypothesis relies on the potential of cytosolic protein instability that can be exposed upon Hsp90 inhibition, other contributions were shown to underlie Hsp90-dependent transcriptional mechanisms and chromatin structure [25–28,70,71]. While these are seemingly different mechanisms leading to the variety of Hsp90 buffered traits, it is perhaps a combination of multiple Hsp90-dependent genetic as well as epigenetic mechanisms working in concert.

3. Hsp90-Dependent Regulation of Organismal Proteostasis, Stress and Aging

3.1. Hsp90 in the Regulation of Cell Nonautonomous Stress Signaling

Hsp90, together with its co-chaperone machinery, is an integral part of the cellular network that safeguards proteostasis. As with other chaperones, Hsp90 expression is regulated by the stress transcription factor Heat Shock Factor 1 (HSF1) and is increased in response to environmental challenges that initiate the cytosolic heat shock response (HSR) [72]. This is accomplished in a negative feedback mechanism, whereby under normal conditions, HSF1 is sequestered by a multichaperone complex including Hsp90 and Hsp70 in an inactive monomeric form [73]. Proteotoxic stress conditions that increase the amount of misfolded proteins in the cell recruit the chaperones away from HSF1 towards the accumulating pool of misfolded proteins and releases HSF1 monomers. This in turn allows HSF1 monomers to form homotrimers that translocate to the nucleus, where they bind to heat shock elements (HSE) that induce molecular chaperones (heat shock proteins), as well as trafficking and proteolytic genes, in order to restore cytosolic proteostasis. Once the levels of Hsp90 and other chaperones have sufficiently increased in the cytosol to refold damaged proteins, they are recruited back to HSF1.

However, expression of Hsp90 can also, directly or indirectly, be regulated by other transcription factors in addition to HSF-1. For example in *C. elegans*, the GATA transcription factor PQM-1 responds to local changes in Hsp90 expression levels as a mediator of transcellular chaperone signaling, but also regulates Hsp90 expression itself [74]. In addition to HSF1, Hsp90 also regulates the function of the FOXO orthologue DAF-16 isoform A by facilitating its translocation into the nucleus upon heat stress and reduced ILS [75].

In metazoans, the stress-dependent induction of HSF-1 transcriptional activity also depends on intercellular stress signaling responses. In *C. elegans*, temperature alterations are sensed by two thermosensory AFD neurons that control temperature-dependent behaviors. This is accomplished through the action of the guanylyl cyclase GCY-8 that is specifically expressed in AFD neurons, and which controls HSF1-dependent induction of the HSR in distal cells in order to restore proteostasis at the organismal level. Neuronal control of proteostasis in response to acute temperature challenges is, however, uncoupled from aging-related responses via a GPCR thermal receptor GTR-1 expressed in chemosensory neurons [76]. The *C. elegans* nervous system relays the signal to distal organs via the neurotransmitter serotonin, thus involving serotonergic neurocircuitry [77,78]. However, astrocyte-like cells in the nervous system can also regulate the cell-nonautonomous HSR in an HSF-1 dependent manner that does not rely on known neurotransmitters but instead requires small clear vesicle release [79]. Non-neuronal tissues such as muscle and gut cells can equally relay information of temperature changes to thermosensory AFD neurons via estrogen signaling through the nuclear hormone receptor NHR-69 [80], an orthologue of the human HNF4 transcription factors that are clients of Hsp90 [81].

Interestingly, heat shock leads to rapid induction of HSF1 activity in the *C. elegans* germline [77,82,83] and HSF1 is required for gametogenesis in invertebrates and vertebrates [72,84]. Like Hsp90, HSF1 is required for germline proliferation and fecundity, relying on Insulin/IGF-1 signaling in the soma that nonautonomously activates HSF-1 in the germline [85], although whether Hsp90 is involved in this regulation is currently unknown.

However, Hsp90 is itself involved in relaying signals from one tissue to another, particularly when its expression levels are altered in the gut or the nervous system, an organismal stress signaling response known as Transcellular Chaperone Signaling (Figure 2) [86,87]. Enhancement of Hsp90 capacity in the gut or the neurons leads to a compensatory transcriptional inter-tissue response, regulated via the transcription factor PQM-1, that induces Hsp90 expression in other distal cell types and primarily muscle cells [74,88]. This protects against the age-associated debilitating consequences of misfolded proteins expressed in muscle cells, including human amyloid beta protein or endogenously expressed metastable myosin [74,88]. How this transcriptional response is relayed from one tissue to another, however, depends on tissue context. Transcellular chaperone signaling from neurons to the muscle requires glutamatergic signaling and relies on the c-type lectin *clec-41* that associates with AMPA receptor in glutamatergic neurons (Figure 2A) [74]. Increased Hsp90 expression in the gut is relayed via the secreted immune peptide *asp-12* which leads to transcriptional upregulation of Hsp90 in muscle cells (Figure 2A) [74].

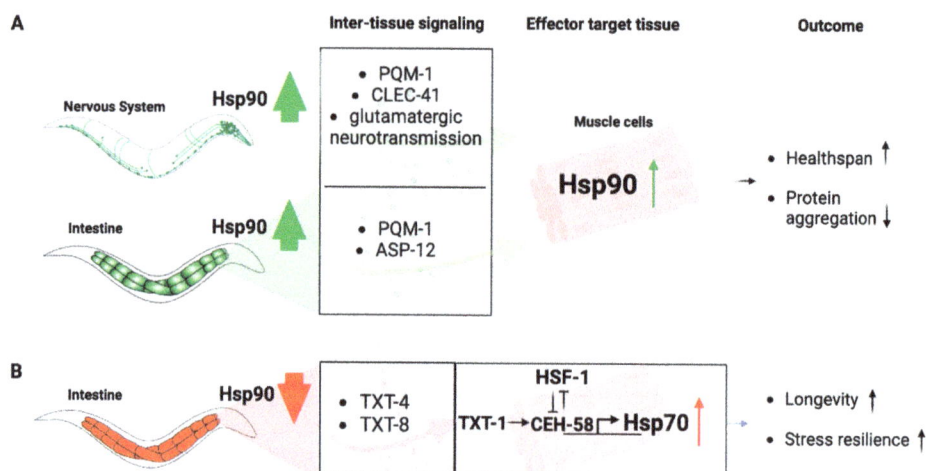

Figure 2. Transcellular chaperone signaling pathways. (**A**) Overexpression of Hsp90 in the nervous system mediates upregulation of Hsp90 in muscle cells via PQM-1, CLEC-41 and glutamatergic neurotransmission. Overexpression of Hsp90 in the intestine relays the signal to upregulate Hsp90 in muscle cells via PQM-1 and ASP-12. The transcription factor regulating Hsp90 in muscle cells in response to TCS has not been determined. The organismal consequences are increased health span and reduced protein aggregation in the muscle tissue. (**B**) Knockdown of Hsp90 in the intestine relays the signal to muscle cells via the secreted lipases TXT-4 and TXT-8. There, TXT-1 signals to the transcription factor CEH-58 to induce Hsp70 expression, resulting in increased longevity and stress resilience. HSF-1 functions as a suppressor of this process.

On the other hand, when Hsp90 levels are reduced by tissue-specific RNA interference in the gut, a compensatory signaling mechanism elevates Hsp70 expression in distant cells (Figure 2B). This is, however, not mediated by a mechanism that relies on HSF1 to activate a canonical HSR, but depends on a homeodomain transcription factor, CEH-58. HSF1 transcriptional activity is suppressed upon gut-specific Hsp90 depletion, and induction of Hsp70 relies on a different intercellular signaling cue involving TXT-1, a membrane-associated guanylate cyclase that relays the signal received from the intestine to the muscle cell nucleus where the homeodomain transcription factor CEH-58 induces Hsp70 expression (Figure 2B) [87]. Thus, there is a difference in intercellular-signaling components which depend on the tissue-type perceiving altered Hsp90 expression levels. This argues for multiple and complex layers of responses that cannot be answered by one particular molecular mechanism, at least not in a multicellular organismal setting [87]. This demonstrates that in metazoans, local Hsp90 capacity can regulate organismal proteostasis and stress resilience via Transcellular Chaperone Signaling.

Comparable organismal effects as a result of local induction of the HSF-1 mediated HSR is also observed in mammals via neuroendocrine signaling. For example, rats undergoing restraint stress have higher cortisol levels secreted by the pituitary gland which signals to activate HSF-1 in the adrenal glands in the kidney to induce Hsp70 expression [89], although how Hsp90 itself could potentially be involved in this response is currently not known and will require further research.

One question that often arises is whether Hsp90 is secreted as part of inter-tissue stress signaling in an organism. Hsp90 secretion has been observed in tissue-culture in response to a variety of stress conditions as well as in cancer cells [90]. Clinically, skin injury promotes Hsp90α secretion and potentiates wound healing in tissue-culture, pigs and dogs [91,92]. However, secreted, extracellular Hsp90 has not been observed as a signaling component itself involved in inter-tissue stress signaling in an organism. In fact, secretion of Hsp90 was not detected in *C. elegans* overexpressing Hsp90 in different cell types [88]. For a more detailed review on the roles of secreted, extracellular Hsp90, the reader is referred to reviews by Li and colleagues [93] in this Special Issue on Hsp90.

3.2. Hsp90-Dependent Regulation of Lifespan and Aging

Consistent with a growth-promoting role, substantial depletion of Hsp90 by RNAi-mediated knockdown can lead to growth defects and larval arrest, and even shorten lifespan [50,75]. The developmental defects associated with Hsp90 RNAi are morphological changes to the gonad and vulva, induction of the HSR and changes to the muscle ultrastructure [50]. Importantly, however, mild impairment of Hsp90 either by RNAi or pharmacological inhibition leads to lifespan extension and enhances health span [94]. This was shown in a pharmacological geroprotector screen using *C. elegans* that identified two Hsp90 inhibitors, Tanespimycin and Monorden, that extended lifespan and improved health of the nematode throughout the course of aging [94]. The study found that both inhibitors acted through HSF1 to induce the age-defying and health span-inducing effects in the worm. This is consistent with HSF1's role in promoting longevity [95–97]. Similar to mild Hsp90 impairment by inhibitors, moderate depletion of Hsp90 RNAi in the gut also enhances lifespan and stress resilience in *C. elegans* without any developmental issues [87]. Similar observations were made in vertebrates, where transient knockdown of Hsp90 during embryonic development in zebrafish results in cold stress resistance in adult animals [98]. Interestingly, the Hs90 co-chaperone p23 acts in key longevity pathways to regulate lifespan in a temperature-dependent manner [99]. At elevated temperatures, p23 mutation extends lifespan through DAF-16 and HSF1 signaling pathways. Short-lived phenotypes depend on the DAF-12 steroid receptor signaling pathway [99], with DAF-12 being a type II nuclear receptor that resembles the human thyroid receptor and is a known client of the p23-HSP90 complex [100]. Apart from being involved in the key longevity pathways, ILS/IGF-1 signaling and HSF-1 signaling pathways, Hsp90 is also involved in the regulation of SIRT1 in both *C. elegans* and mammalian cells [101]. Thus, Hsp90 is unique, as it is a major facilitator that ensures the efficacy of all signaling processes maintaining organismal health and promoting survival.

4. Pathogen Response and Innate Immunity

The involvement of Hsp90 in immune responses is manifold, as it is implicated in the adaptive as well as innate immunity pathways in almost all organisms. In plants, R proteins are client proteins of Hsp90, which is important for the defense response against microbial pathogens [102,103]. The activation of R proteins results in local cell death to limit pathogen proliferation. Because of this, R protein activation also needs to be tightly controlled to avoid tissue damage, which is regulated by Hsp90 [102,103].

In the invertebrate *C. elegans*, which does not have an adaptive immune response, Hsp90 plays an important role in the innate immune response via HSF1. For example, mutant Hsp90, as well as heat shock, causes release of HSF1 from Hsp90, resulting in HSF1 initiating expression of antimicrobial peptide genes [104,105]. Coherently, depletion of Hsp90 by RNA interference also induces an innate immune transcriptional response that was proposed to be similar to the immune response after *C. elegans* exposure to *Pseudomona aeruginosa* [50]. Similarly, pathogen-infected wax moths treated with Hsp90 inhibitor 17-DMAG were protected by an increased immune response [106]. This breadth of Hsp90 being implicated in a process that mediates innate immunity via HSF1 activation demonstrates the importance and conservation of Hsp90 in the innate immune response. In mammals, Hsp90 is implicated in the presentation of antigen to T-cells and activation of macrophages [107]. Hsp90 mediates antigen presentation in target antigen-presenting cells (APC) by facilitating endocytosis of bound polypeptides [108,109]. These generated antigenic peptides are presented to MHC-I/II by Hsp90 [110]. Extracellular Hsp90 can also bind to peptide antigens to facilitate uptake of the Hsp90 antigen complex by endocytosis [107]. After the antigen is internalized, intracellular Hsp90 facilitates further processing of these peptides to the proteasome for degradation [107]. Interestingly, Hsp90 also regulates the reactivation of the human immunodeficiency virus (HIV-1) via regulation of the PKC/ERK MAPK pathways, which influences replication and gene expression of the virus [111]. In the response to pathogens, extracellular Hsp90 can act as a damage-associated molecular pattern (DAMP) signal that regulates the production of cytokines in response to pathogenic infection and inflammation [112]. This involvement of p38 and ERK MAPK pathways in response to pathogens was shown to require Hsp90 for their function through direct interaction of Hsp90 with MAP kinases p38 and ERK in evolutionary diverse organisms [16,113,114]. Hsp90 also plays an important role in growth, development and virulence of parasitic pathogens itself, such as the parasitic protozoa *Plasmodium falciparum* [115] and *Toxoplasma gondii* [116,117]. This makes Hsp90 a high-value drug target to inhibit the parasite's growth and infection cycle in humans [117]. In summary, the role of Hsp90 in the adaptive and innate immune response is vast, and the reader is referred to specialized reviews on this topic for more detailed information (e.g., [110,118]).

5. Neuronal Signaling and Behavior

Considering the wide range of client proteins dependent on Hsp90 function, it is perhaps unsurprising, but nevertheless fascinating, to find it involved in neuronal signaling and function. Some of the first experimental evidence demonstrating a role for Hsp90 in neuronal function stems from research in *C. elegans*. Hsp90 is crucial for the function of specific chemosensory amphid neurons required to sense pheromones and other attractants. It was proposed that Hsp90 accomplishes this through interaction and stabilization of the transmembrane guanylyl cyclase DAF-11, which regulates cGMP levels, a prominent second messenger in *C. elegans* chemosensory transduction [54,55].

In mice, Hsp90 is required for the constitutive trafficking of glutamatergic AMPA-type receptors into synapses during their continuous cycling between synaptic and non-synaptic sites, as well as efficient neurotransmitter release at the presynaptic terminal [119]. In addition to its role in neuronal signaling, Hsp90 chaperones the pro-regenerative dual leucine zipper kinase (DLK), a critical neuronal sensor that drives axon regeneration, degeneration and neurological disease in Drosophila and mammalian neurons [120]. This suggests a vital role for Hsp90 in axon injury signaling, as well as neuronal function that is evolutionary conserved in both vertebrates and invertebrates.

With this importance for neuronal signaling, is it possible that Hsp90 could be involved in the regulation of behavioral responses that facilitate survival during stress conditions? There is at least one example in *C. elegans* that provides direct evidence supporting such a role. Exposure of nematodes to high concentrations of volatile compounds, such as benzaldehyde and diacetyl, induces toxicity and food avoidance behavior [121]. However, preconditioning with benzaldehyde activates stress responses mediated via DAF-16, SKN-1 and HSP-90 in non-neuronal cells that confer increased stress resilience and behavioral tolerance [121]. Another example is provided by the heat stress-induced activation of HSF1, which regulates behavioral responses through estrogen signaling from non-neuronal cells to thermosensory neurons [80]. *hsf-1* mutants are defective in their thermotactic response towards temperature, i.e., migration towards cultivation temperature. Expression of wild type HSF-1 in muscle or intestinal cells rescued this behavioral defect via activation of the NHR-69 nuclear hormone receptor involved in estrogen-like signaling [80], which is a client of Hsp90, as mentioned earlier. Thus, Hsp90, through its role in multiple stress-responsive signaling pathways, may influence behavioral outputs in order to promote survival during environmental stress conditions.

6. Outlook and Conclusions

As a chaperone safeguarding the functionality of clients involved in almost every cellular signaling process, Hsp90 is essential for cellular homeostasis. At the organismal level, intercellular signaling processes that require the involvement of Hsp90 may be underlying the organismal coordination of extra- and intracellular signaling networks between and across different tissues and organs. Especially at the organismal level, many open questions remain to fully comprehend the organismal biology of Hsp90, particularly with regard to intercellular stress signaling.

For example, (1) is there is a tissue map or tissue hierarchy allowing highly coordinated signaling responses to occur? We know that stress signaling can be regulated via both the nervous system and non-neuronal cell types, with, e.g., muscle and gut cells transmitting feedback information to the nervous system or even suppressing stress responses in different cell types and organs. (2) What is the tissue-specific Hsp90 interactome in an organism and how are potential Hsp90 interactors of these tissue-specific networks contributing to intercellular stress signaling? (3) Is there a role of extracellular Hsp90 in intercellular signaling processes? (4) If the tissue-specific expression levels of Hsp90 can affect stress responses in distant tissues, is there a naturally occurring/physiological condition that alters Hsp90 expression levels to induce transcellular chaperone signaling? (5) As Hsp90 function is tightly regulated by co-chaperones and post translational modifications [13], we currently do not know how co-chaperones of the Hsp90 machinery and its PTMs are involved in organismal proteostasis. For example, it can be envisioned that stress responses and intercellular stress signaling pathways are similarly influenced and perhaps finetuned through tissue-specific PTMs and co-chaperone networks. (6) How do the organismal roles of Hsp90 affect diseases, including neurodegenerative diseases and cancer, in a tissue- and disease-specific context?

Thus, the involvement of Hsp90 in almost all aspects of organismal biology, from development to aging, stress adaptation, evolution and different diseases including cancer and neurodegenerative diseases, places it at the nexus of a plethora of cell nonautonomous signaling processes. The challenge for future research will be to navigate through these inter-tissue signaling pathways in a comprehensive manner to understand their increased complexity in the multicellular setting of an organism.

Funding: This work was supported by laboratory start-up funds to P.v.O.-H. from the University of North Carolina at Charlotte.

Institutional Review Board Statement: Not applicable.

Informed Consent Statement: Not applicable.

Data Availability Statement: Not applicable.

Acknowledgments: The Figure was created using Biorender.com.

Conflicts of Interest: The author declares no conflict of interest.

References

1. Johnson, J.L. Evolution and Function of Diverse Hsp90 Homologs and Cochaperone Proteins. *Biochim. Biophys. Acta* **2012**, *1823*, 607–613. [CrossRef] [PubMed]
2. Whitesell, L.; Lindquist, S.L. HSP90 and the Chaperoning of Cancer. *Nat. Rev. Cancer* **2005**, *5*, 761–772. [CrossRef] [PubMed]
3. Picard, D. Chaperoning Steroid Hormone Action. *Trends Endocrinol. Metab.* **2006**, *17*, 229–235. [CrossRef]
4. Picard, D.; Khursheed, B.; Garabedian, M.J.; Fortin, M.G.; Lindquist, S.; Yamamoto, K.R. Reduced Levels of Hsp90 Compromise Steroid Receptor Action in Vivo. *Nature* **1990**, *348*, 166–168. [CrossRef] [PubMed]
5. Echeverria, P.C.; Picard, D. Molecular Chaperones, Essential Partners of Steroid Hormone Receptors for Activity and Mobility. *Biochim. Biophys. Acta* **2010**, *1803*, 641–649. [CrossRef]
6. Riggs, D.L.; Roberts, P.J.; Chirillo, S.C.; Cheung-Flynn, J.; Prapapanich, V.; Ratajczak, T.; Gaber, R.; Picard, D.; Smith, D.F. The Hsp90-Binding Peptidylprolyl Isomerase FKBP52 Potentiates Glucocorticoid Signaling in Vivo. *EMBO J.* **2003**, *22*, 1158–1167. [CrossRef] [PubMed]
7. Sahasrabudhe, P.; Rohrberg, J.; Biebl, M.M.; Rutz, D.A.; Buchner, J. The Plasticity of the Hsp90 Co-Chaperone System. *Mol. Cell* **2017**, *67*, 947–961.e5. [CrossRef] [PubMed]
8. Prodromou, C.; Bjorklund, D.M. Advances towards Understanding the Mechanism of Action of the Hsp90 Complex. *Biomolecules* **2022**, *12*, 600. [CrossRef] [PubMed]
9. Johnson, J.L. Mutations in Hsp90 Cochaperones Result in a Wide Variety of Human Disorders. *Front. Mol. Biosci.* **2021**, *8*, 787260. [CrossRef]

10. Mollapour, M.; Tsutsumi, S.; Truman, A.W.; Xu, W.; Vaughan, C.K.; Beebe, K.; Konstantinova, A.; Vourganti, S.; Panaretou, B.; Piper, P.W.; et al. Threonine 22 Phosphorylation Attenuates Hsp90 Interaction with Cochaperones and Affects Its Chaperone Activity. *Mol. Cell* **2011**, *41*, 672–681. [CrossRef]
11. Woodford, M.R.; Truman, A.W.; Dunn, D.M.; Jensen, S.M.; Cotran, R.; Bullard, R.; Abouelleil, M.; Beebe, K.; Wolfgeher, D.; Wierzbicki, S.; et al. Mps1 Mediated Phosphorylation of Hsp90 Confers Renal Cell Carcinoma Sensitivity and Selectivity to Hsp90 Inhibitors. *Cell Rep.* **2016**, *14*, 872–884. [CrossRef] [PubMed]
12. Mollapour, M.; Bourboulia, D.; Beebe, K.; Woodford, M.R.; Polier, S.; Hoang, A.; Chelluri, R.; Li, Y.; Guo, A.; Lee, M.-J.; et al. Asymmetric Hsp90 N Domain SUMOylation Recruits Aha1 and ATP-Competitive Inhibitors. *Mol. Cell* **2014**, *53*, 317–329. [CrossRef] [PubMed]
13. Backe, S.J.; Sager, R.A.; Woodford, M.R.; Makedon, A.M.; Mollapour, M. Post-Translational Modifications of Hsp90 and Translating the Chaperone Code. *J. Biol. Chem.* **2020**, *295*, 11099–11117. [CrossRef] [PubMed]
14. Ali, M.M.U.; Roe, S.M.; Vaughan, C.K.; Meyer, P.; Panaretou, B.; Piper, P.W.; Prodromou, C.; Pearl, L.H. Crystal Structure of an Hsp90–Nucleotide–P23/Sba1 Closed Chaperone Complex. *Nature* **2006**, *440*, 1013–1017. [CrossRef] [PubMed]
15. Hawle, P.; Siepmann, M.; Harst, A.; Siderius, M.; Reusch, H.P.; Obermann, W.M.J. The Middle Domain of Hsp90 Acts as a Discriminator between Different Types of Client Proteins. *Mol. Cell. Biol.* **2006**, *26*, 8385–8395. [CrossRef]
16. Hawle, P.; Horst, D.; Bebelman, J.P.; Yang, X.X.; Siderius, M.; van der Vies, S.M. Cdc37p Is Required for Stress-Induced High-Osmolarity Glycerol and Protein Kinase C Mitogen-Activated Protein Kinase Pathway Functionality by Interaction with Hog1p and Slt2p (Mpk1p). *Eukaryot. Cell* **2007**, *6*, 521–532. [CrossRef]
17. Vaughan, C.K.; Gohlke, U.; Sobott, F.; Good, V.M.; Ali, M.M.U.; Prodromou, C.; Robinson, C.V.; Saibil, H.R.; Pearl, L.H. Structure of an Hsp90-Cdc37-Cdk4 Complex. *Mol. Cell* **2006**, *23*, 697–707. [CrossRef] [PubMed]
18. Meyer, P.; Prodromou, C.; Liao, C.; Hu, B.; Roe, S.M.; Vaughan, C.K.; Vlasic, I.; Panaretou, B.; Piper, P.W.; Pearl, L.H. Structural Basis for Recruitment of the ATPase Activator Aha1 to the Hsp90 Chaperone Machinery. *EMBO J.* **2004**, *23*, 1402–1410. [CrossRef] [PubMed]
19. Lotz, G.P.; Lin, H.; Harst, A.; Obermann, W.M.J. Aha1 Binds to the Middle Domain of Hsp90, Contributes to Client Protein Activation, and Stimulates the ATPase Activity of the Molecular Chaperone. *J. Biol. Chem.* **2003**, *278*, 17228–17235. [CrossRef]
20. Pearl, L.H.; Prodromou, C. Structure and Mechanism of the Hsp90 Molecular Chaperone Machinery. *Annu. Rev. Biochem.* **2006**, *75*, 271–294. [CrossRef]
21. Maiti, S.; Picard, D. Cytosolic Hsp90 Isoform-Specific Functions and Clinical Significance. *Biomolecules* **2022**, *12*, 1166. [CrossRef] [PubMed]
22. Biebl, M.M.; Buchner, J. Structure, Function, and Regulation of the Hsp90 Machinery. *Cold Spring Harb. Perspect. Biol.* **2019**, *11*, a034017. [CrossRef] [PubMed]
23. Mankovich, A.G.; Freeman, B.C. Regulation of Protein Transport Pathways by the Cytosolic Hsp90s. *Biomolecules* **2022**, *12*, 1077. [CrossRef] [PubMed]
24. McClellan, A.J.; Xia, Y.; Deutschbauer, A.M.; Davis, R.W.; Gerstein, M.; Frydman, J. Diverse Cellular Functions of the Hsp90 Molecular Chaperone Uncovered Using Systems Approaches. *Cell* **2007**, *131*, 121–135. [CrossRef] [PubMed]
25. Echtenkamp, F.J.; Gvozdenov, Z.; Adkins, N.L.; Zhang, Y.; Lynch-Day, M.; Watanabe, S.; Peterson, C.L.; Freeman, B.C. Hsp90 and P23 Molecular Chaperones Control Chromatin Architecture by Maintaining the Functional Pool of the RSC Chromatin Remodeler. *Mol. Cell* **2016**, *64*, 888–899. [CrossRef]
26. DeZwaan, D.C.; Toogun, O.A.; Echtenkamp, F.J.; Freeman, B.C. The Hsp82 Molecular Chaperone Promotes a Switch between Unextendable and Extendable Telomere States. *Nat. Struct. Mol. Biol.* **2009**, *16*, 711–716. [CrossRef]
27. Sawarkar, R.; Paro, R. Hsp90@chromatin.Nucleus: An Emerging Hub of a Networker. *Trends Cell Biol.* **2013**, *23*, 193–201. [CrossRef]
28. Antonova, A.; Hummel, B.; Khavaran, A.; Redhaber, D.M.; Aprile-Garcia, F.; Rawat, P.; Gundel, K.; Schneck, M.; Hansen, E.C.; Mitschke, J.; et al. Heat-Shock Protein 90 Controls the Expression of Cell-Cycle Genes by Stabilizing Metazoan-Specific Host-Cell Factor HCFC1. *Cell Rep.* **2019**, *29*, 1645–1659.e9. [CrossRef]
29. Gvozdenov, Z.; Bendix, L.D.; Kolhe, J.; Freeman, B.C. The Hsp90 Molecular Chaperone Regulates the Transcription Factor Network Controlling Chromatin Accessibility. *J. Mol. Biol.* **2019**, *431*, 4993–5003. [CrossRef]
30. Muise-Helmericks, R.C.; Grimes, H.L.; Bellacosa, A.; Malstrom, S.E.; Tsichlis, P.N.; Rosen, N. Cyclin D Expression Is Controlled Post-Transcriptionally via a Phosphatidylinositol 3-Kinase/Akt-Dependent Pathway *. *J. Biol. Chem.* **1998**, *273*, 29864–29872. [CrossRef]
31. Bedin, M.; Gaben, A.-M.; Saucier, C.; Mester, J. Geldanamycin, an Inhibitor of the Chaperone Activity of HSP90, Induces MAPK-Independent Cell Cycle Arrest. *Int. J. Cancer* **2004**, *109*, 643–652. [CrossRef] [PubMed]
32. Mahony, D.; Parry, D.A.; Lees, E. Active Cdk4 Complexes Are Predominantly Nuclear and Represent Only a Minority of the Cdk6 in T Cells. *Oncogene* **1998**, *16*, 603–611. [CrossRef]
33. Stepanova, L.; Leng, X.; Parker, S.B.; Harper, J.W. Mammalian P50Cdc37 Is a Protein Kinase-Targeting Subunit of Hsp90 That Binds and Stabilizes Cdk4. *Genes Dev.* **1996**, *10*, 1491–1502. [CrossRef] [PubMed]
34. Muñoz, M.J.; Jimenez, J. Genetic Interactions between Hsp90 and the Cdc2 Mitotic Machinery in the Fission Yeast Schizosaccharomyces Pombe. *Mol. Gen. Genet* **1999**, *261*, 242–250. [CrossRef] [PubMed]

35. Aligue, R.; Akhavan-Niak, H.; Russell, P. A Role for Hsp90 in Cell Cycle Control: Wee1 Tyrosine Kinase Activity Requires Interaction with Hsp90. *EMBO J.* **1994**, *13*, 6099–6106. [CrossRef] [PubMed]
36. Goes, F.S.; Martin, J. Hsp90 Chaperone Complexes Are Required for the Activity and Stability of Yeast Protein Kinases Mik1, Wee1 and Swe1. *Eur. J. Biochem.* **2001**, *268*, 2281–2289. [CrossRef] [PubMed]
37. Mollapour, M.; Tsutsumi, S.; Neckers, L. Hsp90 Phosphorylation, Wee1 and the Cell Cycle. *Cell Cycle* **2010**, *9*, 2310–2316. [CrossRef] [PubMed]
38. Fortugno, P.; Beltrami, E.; Plescia, J.; Fontana, J.; Pradhan, D.; Marchisio, P.C.; Sessa, W.C.; Altieri, D.C. Regulation of Survivin Function by Hsp90. *Proc. Natl. Acad. Sci. USA* **2003**, *100*, 13791–13796. [CrossRef]
39. Lange, B.M.H.; Rebollo, E.; Herold, A.; González, C. Cdc37 Is Essential for Chromosome Segregation and Cytokinesis in Higher Eukaryotes. *EMBO J.* **2002**, *21*, 5364–5374. [CrossRef]
40. Jameel, A.; Skilton, R.A.; Campbell, T.A.; Chander, S.K.; Coombes, R.C.; Luqmani, Y.A. Clinical and Biological Significance of HSP89 Alpha in Human Breast Cancer. *Int. J. Cancer* **1992**, *50*, 409–415. [CrossRef]
41. Whitesell, L.; Mimnaugh, E.G.; De Costa, B.; Myers, C.E.; Neckers, L.M. Inhibition of Heat Shock Protein HSP90-Pp60v-Src Heteroprotein Complex Formation by Benzoquinone Ansamycins: Essential Role for Stress Proteins in Oncogenic Transformation. *Proc. Natl. Acad. Sci. USA* **1994**, *91*, 8324–8328. [CrossRef] [PubMed]
42. Neckers, L. Hsp90 Inhibitors as Novel Cancer Chemotherapeutic Agents. *Trends Mol. Med.* **2002**, *8*, S55–S61. [CrossRef] [PubMed]
43. Xiao, Y.; Liu, Y. Recent Advances in the Discovery of Novel HSP90 Inhibitors: An Update from 2014. *Curr. Drug Targets* **2020**, *21*, 302–317. [CrossRef]
44. Voss, A.K.; Thomas, T.; Gruss, P. Mice Lacking HSP90beta Fail to Develop a Placental Labyrinth. *Development* **2000**, *127*, 1–11. [CrossRef] [PubMed]
45. Grad, I.; Cederroth, C.R.; Walicki, J.; Grey, C.; Barluenga, S.; Winssinger, N.; Massy, B.D.; Nef, S.; Picard, D. The Molecular Chaperone Hsp90α Is Required for Meiotic Progression of Spermatocytes beyond Pachytene in the Mouse. *PLoS ONE* **2010**, *5*, e15770. [CrossRef] [PubMed]
46. Du, S.J.; Li, H.; Bian, Y.; Zhong, Y. Heat-Shock Protein 90α1 Is Required for Organized Myofibril Assembly in Skeletal Muscles of Zebrafish Embryos. *Proc. Natl. Acad. Sci. USA* **2008**, *105*, 554–559. [CrossRef] [PubMed]
47. Gaiser, A.M.; Kaiser, C.J.O.; Haslbeck, V.; Richter, K. Downregulation of the Hsp90 System Causes Defects in Muscle Cells of Caenorhabditis Elegans. *PLoS ONE* **2011**, *6*, e25485. [CrossRef]
48. Frumkin, A.; Dror, S.; Pokrzywa, W.; Bar-Lavan, Y.; Karady, I.; Hoppe, T.; Ben-Zvi, A. Challenging Muscle Homeostasis Uncovers Novel Chaperone Interactions in Caenorhabditis Elegans. *Front. Mol. Biosci.* **2014**, *1*, 21. [CrossRef] [PubMed]
49. Bhattacharya, K.; Maiti, S.; Zahoran, S.; Weidenauer, L.; Hany, D.; Wider, D.; Bernasconi, L.; Quadroni, M.; Collart, M.; Picard, D. Translational Reprogramming in Response to Accumulating Stressors Ensures Critical Threshold Levels of Hsp90 for Mammalian Life. *Nat. Commun.* **2022**, *13*, 6271. [CrossRef] [PubMed]
50. Eckl, J.; Sima, S.; Marcus, K.; Lindemann, C.; Richter, K. Hsp90-Downregulation Influences the Heat-Shock Response, Innate Immune Response and Onset of Oocyte Development in Nematodes. *PLoS ONE* **2017**, *12*, e0186386. [CrossRef]
51. Inoue, T.; Hirata, K.; Kuwana, Y.; Fujita, M.; Miwa, J.; Roy, R.; Yamaguchi, Y. Cell Cycle Control by Daf-21/Hsp90 at the First Meiotic Prophase/Metaphase Boundary during Oogenesis in Caenorhabditis Elegans. *Dev. Growth Differ.* **2006**, *48*, 25–32. [CrossRef] [PubMed]
52. Tewari, M.; Hu, P.J.; Ahn, J.S.; Ayivi-Guedehoussou, N.; Vidalain, P.-O.; Li, S.; Milstein, S.; Armstrong, C.M.; Boxem, M.; Butler, M.D.; et al. Systematic Interactome Mapping and Genetic Perturbation Analysis of a C. Elegans TGF-β Signaling Network. *Mol. Cell* **2004**, *13*, 469–482. [CrossRef]
53. Murakami, M.; Koga, M.; Ohshima, Y. DAF-7/TGF-Beta Expression Required for the Normal Larval Development in C. Elegans Is Controlled by a Presumed Guanylyl Cyclase DAF-11. *Mech. Dev.* **2001**, *109*, 27–35. [CrossRef] [PubMed]
54. Birnby, D.A.; Link, E.M.; Vowels, J.J.; Tian, H.; Colacurcio, P.L.; Thomas, J.H. A Transmembrane Guanylyl Cyclase (DAF-11) and Hsp90 (DAF-21) Regulate a Common Set of Chemosensory Behaviors in Caenorhabditis Elegans. *Genetics* **2000**, *155*, 85–104. [CrossRef] [PubMed]
55. Vowels, J.J.; Thomas, J.H. Multiple Chemosensory Defects in Daf-11 and Daf-21 Mutants of Caenorhabditis Elegans. *Genetics* **1994**, *138*, 303–316. [CrossRef]
56. Greenwald, I.; Kovall, R. Notch Signaling: Genetics and Structure. *WormBook* **2013**, 1–28. [CrossRef]
57. Qiao, L.; Lissemore, J.L.; Shu, P.; Smardon, A.; Gelber, M.B.; Maine, E.M. Enhancers of Glp-1, a Gene Required for Cell-Signaling in Caenorhabditis Elegans, Define a Set of Genes Required for Germline Development. *Genetics* **1995**, *141*, 551–569. [CrossRef] [PubMed]
58. Lissemore, J.L.; Connors, E.; Liu, Y.; Qiao, L.; Yang, B.; Edgley, M.L.; Flibotte, S.; Taylor, J.; Au, V.; Moerman, D.G.; et al. The Molecular Chaperone HSP90 Promotes Notch Signaling in the Germline of Caenorhabditis Elegans. *G3 (Bethesda)* **2018**, *8*, 1535–1544. [CrossRef]
59. Borkovich, K.A.; Farrelly, F.W.; Finkelstein, D.B.; Taulien, J.; Lindquist, S. Hsp82 Is an Essential Protein That Is Required in Higher Concentrations for Growth of Cells at Higher Temperatures. *Mol. Cell. Biol.* **1989**, *9*, 3919–3930. [CrossRef]
60. Cutforth, T.; Rubin, G.M. Mutations in Hsp83 and Cdc37 Impair Signaling by the Sevenless Receptor Tyrosine Kinase in Drosophila. *Cell* **1994**, *77*, 1027–1036. [CrossRef]

61. Yue, L.; Karr, T.L.; Nathan, D.F.; Swift, H.; Srinivasan, S.; Lindquist, S. Genetic Analysis of Viable Hsp90 Alleles Reveals a Critical Role in Drosophila Spermatogenesis. *Genetics* **1999**, *151*, 1065–1079. [CrossRef]
62. van der Straten, A.; Rommel, C.; Dickson, B.; Hafen, E. The Heat Shock Protein 83 (Hsp83) Is Required for Raf-Mediated Signalling in Drosophila. *EMBO J.* **1997**, *16*, 1961–1969. [CrossRef] [PubMed]
63. Rutherford, S.L.; Lindquist, S. Hsp90 as a Capacitor for Morphological Evolution. *Nature* **1998**, *396*, 336–342. [CrossRef] [PubMed]
64. Queitsch, C.; Sangster, T.A.; Lindquist, S. Hsp90 as a Capacitor of Phenotypic Variation. *Nature* **2002**, *417*, 618–624. [CrossRef] [PubMed]
65. Rohner, N.; Jarosz, D.F.; Kowalko, J.E.; Yoshizawa, M.; Jeffery, W.R.; Borowsky, R.L.; Lindquist, S.; Tabin, C.J. Cryptic Variation in Morphological Evolution: HSP90 as a Capacitor for Loss of Eyes in Cavefish. *Science* **2013**, *342*, 1372–1375. [CrossRef]
66. Yeyati, P.L.; Bancewicz, R.M.; Maule, J.; van Heyningen, V. Hsp90 Selectively Modulates Phenotype in Vertebrate Development. *PLoS Genet* **2007**, *3*, e43. [CrossRef]
67. Burga, A.; Casanueva, M.O.; Lehner, B. Predicting Mutation Outcome from Early Stochastic Variation in Genetic Interaction Partners. *Nature* **2011**, *480*, 250–253. [CrossRef]
68. Casanueva, M.O.; Burga, A.; Lehner, B. Fitness Trade-Offs and Environmentally Induced Mutation Buffering in Isogenic C. Elegans. *Science* **2012**, *335*, 82–85. [CrossRef]
69. Karras, G.I.; Yi, S.; Sahni, N.; Fischer, M.; Xie, J.; Vidal, M.; D'Andrea, A.D.; Whitesell, L.; Lindquist, S. HSP90 Shapes the Consequences of Human Genetic Variation. *Cell* **2017**, *168*, 856–866.e12. [CrossRef]
70. Hummel, B.; Hansen, E.C.; Yoveva, A.; Aprile-Garcia, F.; Hussong, R.; Sawarkar, R. The Evolutionary Capacitor HSP90 Buffers the Regulatory Effects of Mammalian Endogenous Retroviruses. *Nat. Struct. Mol. Biol.* **2017**, *24*, 234–242. [CrossRef] [PubMed]
71. Sollars, V.; Lu, X.; Xiao, L.; Wang, X.; Garfinkel, M.D.; Ruden, D.M. Evidence for an Epigenetic Mechanism by Which Hsp90 Acts as a Capacitor for Morphological Evolution. *Nat. Genet* **2003**, *33*, 70–74. [CrossRef] [PubMed]
72. Anckar, J.; Sistonen, L. Regulation of HSF1 Function in the Heat Stress Response: Implications in Aging and Disease. *Annu. Rev. Biochem.* **2011**, *80*, 1089–1115. [CrossRef]
73. Zou, L.; Wu, D.; Zang, X.; Wang, Z.; Wu, Z.; Chen, D. Construction of a Germline-Specific RNAi Tool in C. Elegans. *Sci. Rep.* **2019**, *9*, 1–10. [CrossRef] [PubMed]
74. O'Brien, D.; Jones, L.M.; Good, S.; Miles, J.; Vijayabaskar, M.S.; Aston, R.; Smith, C.E.; Westhead, D.R.; van Oosten-Hawle, P. A PQM-1-Mediated Response Triggers Transcellular Chaperone Signaling and Regulates Organismal Proteostasis. *Cell Rep.* **2018**, *23*, 3905–3919. [CrossRef] [PubMed]
75. Somogyvári, M.; Gecse, E.; Sőti, C. DAF-21/Hsp90 Is Required for C. Elegans Longevity by Ensuring DAF-16/FOXO Isoform A Function. *Sci. Rep.* **2018**, *8*, 12048. [CrossRef]
76. Maman, M.; Marques, F.C.; Volovik, Y.; Dubnikov, T.; Bejerano-Sagie, M.; Cohen, E. A Neuronal GPCR Is Critical for the Induction of the Heat Shock Response in the Nematode C. Elegans. *J. Neurosci.* **2013**, *33*, 6102–6111. [CrossRef]
77. Tatum, M.C.; Ooi, F.K.; Chikka, M.R.; Chauve, L.; Martinez-Velazquez, L.A.; Steinbusch, H.W.M.; Morimoto, R.I.; Prahlad, V. Neuronal Serotonin Release Triggers the Heat Shock Response in C. Elegans in the Absence of Temperature Increase. *Curr. Biol.* **2015**, *25*, 163–174. [CrossRef] [PubMed]
78. Prahlad, V.; Cornelius, T.; Morimoto, R.I. Regulation of the Cellular Heat Shock Response in Caenorhabditis Elegans by Thermosensory Neurons. *Science* **2008**, *320*, 811–814. [CrossRef]
79. Gildea, H.K.; Frankino, P.A.; Tronnes, S.U.; Pender, C.L.; Durieux, J.; Dishart, J.G.; Choi, H.O.; Hunter, T.D.; Cheung, S.S.; Frakes, A.E.; et al. Glia of C. Elegans Coordinate a Protective Organismal Heat Shock Response Independent of the Neuronal Thermosensory Circuit. *Sci. Adv.* **2022**, *8*, eabq3970. [CrossRef]
80. Sugi, T.; Nishida, Y.; Mori, I. Regulation of Behavioral Plasticity by Systemic Temperature Signaling in Caenorhabditis Elegans. *Nat. Neurosci.* **2011**, *14*, 984–992. [CrossRef]
81. Jing, R.; Duncan, C.B.; Duncan, S.A. A Small-Molecule Screen Reveals That HSP90β Promotes the Conversion of Induced Pluripotent Stem Cell-Derived Endoderm to a Hepatic Fate and Regulates HNF4A Turnover. *Development* **2017**, *144*, 1764–1774. [CrossRef] [PubMed]
82. Li, J.; Chauve, L.; Phelps, G.; Brielmann, R.M.; Morimoto, R.I. E2F Coregulates an Essential HSF Developmental Program That Is Distinct from the Heat-Shock Response. *Genes Dev.* **2016**, *30*, 2062–2075. [CrossRef]
83. Morton, E.A.; Lamitina, T. Caenorhabditis Elegans HSF-1 Is an Essential Nuclear Protein That Forms Stress Granule-like Structures Following Heat Shock. *Aging Cell* **2013**, *12*, 112–120. [CrossRef] [PubMed]
84. Abane, R.; Mezger, V. Roles of Heat Shock Factors in Gametogenesis and Development. *FEBS J.* **2010**, *277*, 4150–4172. [CrossRef] [PubMed]
85. Edwards, S.L.; Erdenebat, P.; Morphis, A.C.; Kumar, L.; Wang, L.; Chamera, T.; Georgescu, C.; Wren, J.D.; Li, J. Insulin/IGF-1 Signaling and Heat Stress Differentially Regulate HSF1 Activities in Germline Development. *Cell. Rep.* **2021**, *36*, 109623. [CrossRef] [PubMed]
86. Miles, J.; Oosten-Hawle, P. van Tissue-Specific RNAi Tools to Identify Components for Systemic Stress Signaling. *JoVE J. Vis. Exp.* **2020**, *159*, e61257. [CrossRef]
87. Miles, J.; Townend, S.; Smith, W.; Westhead, D.R.; van Oosten-Hawle, P. Transcellular Chaperone Signaling Is an Intercellular Stress-Response Distinct from the HSF-1 Mediated HSR. *bioRxiv* **2022**, 2022.03.17.484707.

88. van Oosten-Hawle, P.; Porter, R.S.; Morimoto, R.I. Regulation of Organismal Proteostasis by Transcellular Chaperone Signaling. *Cell* **2013**, *153*, 1366–1378. [CrossRef]
89. Fawcett, T.W.; Sylvester, S.L.; Sarge, K.D.; Morimoto, R.I.; Holbrook, N.J. Effects of Neurohormonal Stress and Aging on the Activation of Mammalian Heat Shock Factor 1. *J. Biol. Chem.* **1994**, *269*, 32272–32278. [CrossRef] [PubMed]
90. Liao, D.-F.; Jin, Z.-G.; Baas, A.S.; Daum, G.; Gygi, S.P.; Aebersold, R.; Berk, B.C. Purification and Identification of Secreted Oxidative Stress-Induced Factors from Vascular Smooth Muscle Cells *. *J. Biol. Chem.* **2000**, *275*, 189–196. [CrossRef]
91. Bhatia, A.; O'Brien, K.; Guo, J.; Lincoln, V.; Kajiwara, C.; Chen, M.; Woodley, D.T.; Udono, H.; Li, W. Extracellular and Non-Chaperone Function of Heat Shock Protein-90α Is Required for Skin Wound Healing. *J. Invest. Derm.* **2018**, *138*, 423–433. [CrossRef] [PubMed]
92. Li, W.; Sahu, D.; Tsen, F. Secreted Heat Shock Protein-90 (Hsp90) in Wound Healing and Cancer. *Biochim. Et Biophys. Acta (BBA)—Mol. Cell Res.* **2012**, *1823*, 730–741. [CrossRef] [PubMed]
93. Jay, D.; Luo, Y.; Li, W. Extracellular Heat Shock Protein-90 (EHsp90): Everything You Need to Know. *Biomolecules* **2022**, *12*, 911. [CrossRef] [PubMed]
94. Janssens, G.E.; Lin, X.-X.; Millan-Ariño, L.; Kavšek, A.; Sen, I.; Seinstra, R.I.; Stroustrup, N.; Nollen, E.A.A.; Riedel, C.G. Transcriptomics-Based Screening Identifies Pharmacological Inhibition of Hsp90 as a Means to Defer Aging. *Cell Rep.* **2019**, *27*, 467–480.e6. [CrossRef]
95. Hsu, A.-L.; Murphy, C.T.; Kenyon, C. Regulation of Aging and Age-Related Disease by DAF-16 and Heat-Shock Factor. *Science* **2003**, *300*, 1142–1145. [CrossRef]
96. Douglas, P.M.; Baird, N.A.; Simic, M.S.; Uhlein, S.; McCormick, M.A.; Wolff, S.C.; Kennedy, B.K.; Dillin, A. Heterotypic Signals from Neural HSF-1 Separate Thermotolerance from Longevity. *Cell Rep.* **2015**, *12*, 1196–1204. [CrossRef] [PubMed]
97. Morley, J.F.; Morimoto, R.I. Regulation of Longevity in Caenorhabditis Elegans by Heat Shock Factor and Molecular Chaperones. *Mol. Biol. Cell* **2004**, *15*, 657–664. [CrossRef] [PubMed]
98. Han, B.; Luo, J.; Jiang, P.; Li, Y.; Wang, Q.; Bai, Y.; Chen, J.; Wang, J.; Zhang, J. Inhibition of Embryonic HSP 90 Function Promotes Variation of Cold Tolerance in Zebrafish. *Front. Genet.* **2020**, *11*, 541944. [CrossRef] [PubMed]
99. Horikawa, M.; Sural, S.; Hsu, A.-L.; Antebi, A. Co-Chaperone P23 Regulates C. Elegans Lifespan in Response to Temperature. *PLoS Genet* **2015**, *11*, e1005023. [CrossRef] [PubMed]
100. Freeman, B.C.; Felts, S.J.; Toft, D.O.; Yamamoto, K.R. The P23 Molecular Chaperones Act at a Late Step in Intracellular Receptor Action to Differentially Affect Ligand Efficacies. *Genes Dev.* **2000**, *14*, 422–434. [CrossRef]
101. Nguyen, M.T.; Somogyvári, M.; Sőti, C. Hsp90 Stabilizes SIRT1 Orthologs in Mammalian Cells and C. Elegans. *Int. J. Mol. Sci.* **2018**, *19*, 3661. [CrossRef] [PubMed]
102. Hubert, D.A.; Tornero, P.; Belkhadir, Y.; Krishna, P.; Takahashi, A.; Shirasu, K.; Dangl, J.L. Cytosolic HSP90 Associates with and Modulates the Arabidopsis RPM1 Disease Resistance Protein. *EMBO J.* **2003**, *22*, 5679–5689. [CrossRef] [PubMed]
103. Sangster, T.A.; Queitsch, C. The HSP90 Chaperone Complex, an Emerging Force in Plant Development and Phenotypic Plasticity. *Curr. Opin. Plant Biol.* **2005**, *8*, 86–92. [CrossRef] [PubMed]
104. Singh, V.; Aballay, A. Heat-Shock Transcription Factor (HSF)-1 Pathway Required for *Caenorhabditis Elegans* Immunity. *Proc. Natl. Acad. Sci. USA* **2006**, *103*, 13092–13097. [CrossRef]
105. Singh, V.; Aballay, A. Heat Shock and Genetic Activation of HSF-1 Enhance Immunity to Bacteria. *Cell Cycle* **2006**, *5*, 2443–2446. [CrossRef] [PubMed]
106. Wojda, I.; Kowalski, P. Galleria Mellonella Infected with Bacillus Thuringiensis Involves Hsp90. *Open Life Sci.* **2013**, *8*, 561–569. [CrossRef]
107. Oura, J.; Tamura, Y.; Kamiguchi, K.; Kutomi, G.; Sahara, H.; Torigoe, T.; Himi, T.; Sato, N. Extracellular Heat Shock Protein 90 Plays a Role in Translocating Chaperoned Antigen from Endosome to Proteasome for Generating Antigenic Peptide to Be Cross-Presented by Dendritic Cells. *Int. Immunol.* **2011**, *23*, 223–237. [CrossRef]
108. Murshid, A.; Gong, J.; Calderwood, S.K. Heat Shock Protein 90 Mediates Efficient Antigen Cross Presentation through the Scavenger Receptor Expressed by Endothelial Cells-I. *J. Immunol.* **2010**, *185*, 2903–2917. [CrossRef] [PubMed]
109. Murshid, A.; Gong, J.; Calderwood, S.K. Hsp90–Peptide Complexes Stimulate Antigen Presentation through the Class II Pathway after Binding Scavenger Receptor SREC-I. *Immunobiology* **2014**, *219*, 924–931. [CrossRef] [PubMed]
110. Graner, M.W. Chapter Eight - HSP90 and Immune Modulation in Cancer. In *Advances in Cancer Research*; Hsp90 in Cancer: Beyond the Usual Suspects; Isaacs, J., Whitesell, L., Eds.; Academic Press: Cambridge, MA, USA, 2016; Volume 129, pp. 191–224.
111. Anderson, I.; Low, J.S.; Weston, S.; Weinberger, M.; Zhyvoloup, A.; Labokha, A.A.; Corazza, G.; Kitson, R.A.; Moody, C.J.; Marcello, A.; et al. Heat Shock Protein 90 Controls HIV-1 Reactivation from Latency. *Proc. Natl. Acad. Sci. USA* **2014**, *111*, E1528–E1537. [CrossRef]
112. Henderson, B.; Calderwood, S.K.; Coates, A.R.M.; Cohen, I.; van Eden, W.; Lehner, T.; Pockley, A.G. Caught with Their PAMPs Down? The Extracellular Signalling Actions of Molecular Chaperones Are Not Due to Microbial Contaminants. *Cell Stress Chaperones* **2010**, *15*, 123–141. [CrossRef] [PubMed]
113. Kim, D.H.; Feinbaum, R.; Alloing, G.; Emerson, F.E.; Garsin, D.A.; Inoue, H.; Tanaka-Hino, M.; Hisamoto, N.; Matsumoto, K.; Tan, M.-W.; et al. A Conserved P38 MAP Kinase Pathway in Caenorhabditis Elegans Innate Immunity. *Science* **2002**, *297*, 623–626. [CrossRef] [PubMed]

114. Su, B.; Karin, M. Mitogen-Activated Protein Kinase Cascades and Regulation of Gene Expression. *Curr. Opin. Immunol.* **1996**, *8*, 402–411. [CrossRef] [PubMed]
115. Banumathy, G.; Singh, V.; Pavithra, S.R.; Tatu, U. Heat Shock Protein 90 Function Is Essential for Plasmodium Falciparum Growth in Human Erythrocytes. *J. Biol. Chem.* **2003**, *278*, 18336–18345. [CrossRef] [PubMed]
116. Angel, S.O.; Figueras, M.J.; Alomar, M.L.; Echeverria, P.C.; Deng, B. Toxoplasma Gondii Hsp90: Potential Roles in Essential Cellular Processes of the Parasite. *Parasitology* **2014**, *141*, 1138–1147. [CrossRef]
117. Echeverria, P.C.; Matrajt, M.; Harb, O.S.; Zappia, M.P.; Costas, M.A.; Roos, D.S.; Dubremetz, J.F.; Angel, S.O. Toxoplasma Gondii Hsp90 Is a Potential Drug Target Whose Expression and Subcellular Localization Are Developmentally Regulated. *J. Mol. Biol.* **2005**, *350*, 723–734. [CrossRef]
118. Corigliano, M.G.; Sander, V.A.; Sánchez López, E.F.; Ramos Duarte, V.A.; Mendoza Morales, L.F.; Angel, S.O.; Clemente, M. Heat Shock Proteins 90 KDa: Immunomodulators and Adjuvants in Vaccine Design Against Infectious Diseases. *Front. Bioeng. Biotechnol.* **2021**, *8*, 622186. [CrossRef]
119. Gerges, N.Z.; Tran, I.C.; Backos, D.S.; Harrell, J.M.; Chinkers, M.; Pratt, W.B.; Esteban, J.A. Independent Functions of Hsp90 in Neurotransmitter Release and in the Continuous Synaptic Cycling of AMPA Receptors. *J. Neurosci.* **2004**, *24*, 4758–4766. [CrossRef]
120. Karney-Grobe, S.; Russo, A.; Frey, E.; Milbrandt, J.; DiAntonio, A. HSP90 Is a Chaperone for DLK and Is Required for Axon Injury Signaling. *Proc. Natl. Acad. Sci. USA* **2018**, *115*, E9899–E9908. [CrossRef]
121. Hajdú, G.; Gecse, E.; Taisz, I.; Móra, I.; Sőti, C. Toxic Stress-Specific Cytoprotective Responses Regulate Learned Behavioral Decisions in C. Elegans. *BMC Biol.* **2021**, *19*, 26. [CrossRef] [PubMed]

Disclaimer/Publisher's Note: The statements, opinions and data contained in all publications are solely those of the individual author(s) and contributor(s) and not of MDPI and/or the editor(s). MDPI and/or the editor(s) disclaim responsibility for any injury to people or property resulting from any ideas, methods, instructions or products referred to in the content.

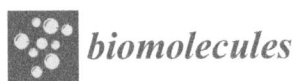

Article

Recognition of BRAF by CDC37 and Re-Evaluation of the Activation Mechanism for the Class 2 BRAF-L597R Mutant

Dennis M. Bjorklund [1], R. Marc L. Morgan [2], Jasmeen Oberoi [3], Katie L. I. M. Day [4], Panagiota A. Galliou [5] and Chrisostomos Prodromou [1,*]

1. Biochemistry and Biomedicine, School of Life Sciences, University of Sussex, Falmer, Brighton BN1 9QG, UK; dennis.bj90@gmail.com
2. Department of Life Sciences, Faculty of Natural Sciences, South Kensington Campus, Imperial College London, London SW7 2AZ, UK; rhodri.morgan@imperial.ac.uk
3. Genome Damage and Stability Centre, School of Life Sciences, University of Sussex, Falmer, Brighton BN1 9RQ, UK; j.oberoi@sussex.ac.uk
4. Domainex, Pampisford, Cambridge CB2 3EG, UK; katie.day@domainex.co.uk
5. Laboratory of Biological Chemistry, Aristotle University of Thessaloniki, 54124 Thessaloniki, Greece; ag.gal.work@gmail.com
* Correspondence: chris.prodromou@sussex.ac.uk

Citation: Bjorklund, D.M.; Morgan, R.M.L.; Oberoi, J.; Day, K.L.I.M.; Galliou, P.A.; Prodromou, C. Recognition of BRAF by CDC37 and Re-Evaluation of the Activation Mechanism for the Class 2 BRAF-L597R Mutant. *Biomolecules* **2022**, *12*, 905. https://doi.org/10.3390/biom12070905

Academic Editor: Mikhail Bogdanov

Received: 6 June 2022
Accepted: 23 June 2022
Published: 28 June 2022

Publisher's Note: MDPI stays neutral with regard to jurisdictional claims in published maps and institutional affiliations.

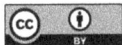

Copyright: © 2022 by the authors. Licensee MDPI, Basel, Switzerland. This article is an open access article distributed under the terms and conditions of the Creative Commons Attribution (CC BY) license (https://creativecommons.org/licenses/by/4.0/).

Abstract: The kinome specific co-chaperone, CDC37 (cell division cycle 37), is responsible for delivering BRAF (B-Rapidly Accelerated Fibrosarcoma) to the Hsp90 (heat shock protein 90) complex, where it is then translocated to the RAS (protooncogene product p21) complex at the plasma membrane for RAS mediated dimerization and subsequent activation. We identify a bipartite interaction between CDC37 and BRAF and delimitate the essential structural elements of CDC37 involved in BRAF recognition. We find an extended and conserved CDC37 motif, ^{20}HPNID—SL–W^{31}, responsible for recognizing the C-lobe of BRAF kinase domain, while the C-terminal domain of CDC37 is responsible for the second of the bipartite interaction with BRAF. We show that dimerization of BRAF, independent of nucleotide binding, can act as a potent signal that prevents CDC37 recognition and discuss the implications of mutations in BRAF and the consequences on signaling in a clinical setting, particularly for class 2 BRAF mutations.

Keywords: Hsp90; CDC37; BRAF; kinase; activation mechanism; chaperone; co-chaperone

1. Introduction

Specific protein kinases are known to exist as an ensemble of conformations due to their metastable state [1,2] and it is this instability that likely defines their dependency on the Hsp90-CDC37 (heat shock protein 90 – cell division cycle 37) complex. CDC37 is a kinase specific co-chaperone that delivers protein kinases, such as BRAF (B-Rapidly Accelerated Fibrosarcoma), to the Hsp90 complex [3]. CDC37 consists of three domains, an N-terminal domain, linked by a beta-strand to the middle domain and finally a small C-terminal helical domain. Several incomplete structures of CDC37 have, to date, been determined [1,4–7]. However, molecular details on how CDC37 recognizes client kinases is still poorly understood. The cryo-EM structure of the Hsp90-CDC37-Cdk4 (Cdk4, cyclindependent kinase 4) complex (PDB 5FWK and EMD-3337), shows that the C-terminal lobe of the Cdk4 kinase domain is engaged with the N-terminal domain of CDC37 and in particular with the base of the C-terminal helix of CDC37 that makes up the helix coiled-coil structure. Specifically, a small loop (HPNI) from CDC37 mimics a similar loop (HPNV in Cdk4 and HVNI in BRAF) found in the N-terminal lobe of kinases [5], which is normally engaged in binding to a helix in the C-terminal lobe of kinase domains. The middle domain of CDC37, as seen in the cryo-EM structure, is also potentially involved in interactions with the N-terminal lobe of kinase domains [5]. Finally, a helix linker leads to the C-terminal domain of CDC37, the function of which is less clear and not visible in the cryo-EM structure of the Hsp90-CDC37-Cdk4 complex [5].

Protein kinases play a central role in regulating eukaryotic signaling pathways in key processes, such as cell survival, metabolism, proliferation, cell migration and differentiation and in the cell cycle [8]. As such, their regulation is of paramount importance, and dysregulation of their activity can lead to cell transformation and cancer [9]. Kinases have been described as molecular switches that can adopt at least two extreme conformations, in which the catalytic machinery through conformational remodeling becomes correctly aligned for catalysis to take place. The maximally active conformation is known as the "on" state, while the inactive state is referred to as the "off" state [9]. In particular, the DFG loop of kinases is conformationally flexible and adopts either an inactive (out) or an active (in) conformation [10], which helps to remodel the rest of the kinase for activity. For example, in the active 'DFG-in' position of epidermal growth factor receptor (EGFR; PDB 5CNO), the phenylalanine residue forms part of the R–(regulatory) spine, which consists of a series of hydrophobic residues that connect essential elements required for catalysis to the F-helix, while the ATP, once bound, helps to complete the C-(catalytic) spine, a series of residues that connect the F-helix to the N-terminal lobe of the kinase domain [11–13]. In the inactive ('out') state of EGFR (PDB 2RF9) the same phenylalanine of the DFG motif is displaced from the R-spine and positions itself so that the C-spine is disrupted [11]. Thus, this phenylalanine is positioned in such a way as to clash with the phosphate groups of the bound ATP. Clearly, the conformational regulation of kinases from their inactive ('out') state to their 'in' or active state is of paramount importance for attaining their enzymatic activity. BRAF mutants that drive oncogenesis consist of three classes [14]. Class 1 BRAF mutants, which consist of Val 600 mutations, signal as RAS (protooncogene product p21)-independent active monomers, where dimerization is disrupted, and are insensitive to ERK1/2 and SOS feedback inhibition. Class 2 mutants function as dimers, but their activation appears to be RAS-independent. Hence, they escape feedback inhibition through the phosphorylation of SOS, a modification that downregulates its activity. Finally, class 3 mutations are kinase impaired but increase signaling through the MAPK (Mitogen-Activated Protein Kinase) pathway, due to enhanced RAS binding and subsequent CRAF activation.

The Hsp90-CDC37 complex is required for the stability of BRAF and, as such, both active (V600E mutant) and inactive forms of the kinase act as clients [15–17]. For wild type BRAF, binding to the Hsp90-CDC37 complex ultimately leads to its delivery at the plasma membrane for interaction with RAS, where BRAF is subsequently activated. This RAS-BRAF complex is more abundant than the Hsp90-CDC37 complex of BRAF [18]. The classical mechanism for BRAF activation occurs by its association with RAS and 14-3-3 at the cellular membrane, together with Hsp90 and CDC37. Activation of BRAF leads to translocation of the cytoplasmic Hsp90-CDC37-Braf complex to the cell membrane [18], while inhibition of Hsp90 by geldanamycin leads to a rapid dissociation of both Hsp90-BRAF and RAS-BRAF multimolecular complexes, increased proteasomal degradation of BRAF and a decrease in translocation of BRAF to the plasma membrane [17,19–21]. In the absence of RAS the most populated state appears to be the autoinhibited form of BRAF that is further stabilized by interaction with 14-3-3, which binds directly to the phosphorylated amino acid residues Ser (pSer) 365 and 729 of BRAF [22]. In the presence of activated RAS, however, there is a shift from the inactive state to an active BRAF signaling complex [23]. The general consensus is that the interaction of RAS with the inactive BRAF-14-3-3 complex displaces 14-3-3 from pSer 365 allowing either homodimerization or heterodimerization of BRAF [24], which remains tethered through the pair of pSer 729 residues of the BRAF dimer to a dimer of 14-3-3. In addition, by RAS promoting dimerization of BRAF this allows the cis- autophosphorylation of Thr 599 and Ser 602 of the BRAF activation loop [24,25]. Such phosphorylation is critical in inducing and stabilizing a conformational change that leads to alignment of the C- and R-hydrophobic spines of the kinase domain, thus promoting ATP uptake and, consequently, MEK (Mitogen-Activated Protein Kinase (MAPK) kinase) phosphorylation [11,26]. In contrast to wild type BRAF, it was recently observed that the

Hsp90-CDC37-BRAF V600E complex was not only more abundant than the 14-3-3 complex, but was shown to be more active [16]. Thus, there appears to be an altered partitioning between the 14-3-3-RAS and the Hsp90-CDC37 complex caused by the V600E mutation in BRAF.

The current work explored the interaction between CDC37 and a variety of BRAF mutants, and defined the CDC37 and BRAF domains involved. We aimed to understand how BRAF mutations cause partitioning between the cytosolic Hsp90-CDC37 complex and the membrane bound 14-3-3—RAS complex. We present evidence that dimerization of BRAF, as seen with the class 2 L597R BRAF mutation [27], severs recognition by the kinome specific CDC37-dependant co-chaperone of Hsp90. We propose that the Hsp90-CDC37 chaperone system may play a regulatory role in maintaining the class 1 BRAF V600E mutant, while the class 2 mutant BRAF L597R assembles into a dimeric structure that is resistant to interaction with CDC37. Consequently, a disequilibrium results to the overall regulatory pathways that tightly govern the normal activity of BRAF and we discuss the consequences of such dysregulation.

2. Material and Methods

2.1. Protein Expression and Purification

Constructs of human C-terminally His-tagged CDC37 cloned in pET28b and N-terminally GST-tagged sBRAF kinase domain (residues 423–723) cloned in p3E (A. W. Oliver, University of Sussex), including mutant forms, were obtained from Genscript for expression in Escherichia coli BL21 (DE3) pLysS by induction at 20 °C with 1 mM isopropyl-1-thio-β-D-galactopyranoside MERCK, catalogue No. I6758, Darmstadt, Germany. CDC37 was expressed as previously described using Talon metal affinity chromatography (Takara Bio company, catalogue No. 635652, Saint-Germain-en-Laye, France), Superdex 75 or 200 PG gel-filtration and Q-sepharose ion-exchange [28]. sBRAF kinase domain constructs were purified using glutathione affinity resin (Genscript, catalogue. No. L00206, Rijswijk, Netherlands), followed by PreScission cleavage overnight, and Superdex 200 gel-filtration. All concentration steps utilized Vivaspin 30 centrifugal concentrators (Sartorius, catalogue number VS2022, Goettingen, Germany). Purified proteins were dialyzed against 20 mm Tris/HCl (MERCK, Calbiochem, catalogue No. 648317, Darmstadt, Germany), pH 7.5, containing 1 mm EDTA (MERCK, Sigma Aldrich, catalogue No. E5134-1KG, Darmstadt, Germany), and 200 mM NaCl (MERCK, Sigma Aldrich,, catalogue No. S9888-5KG, Darmstadt, Germany), in preparation for isothermal titration chromatography (ITC).

2.2. Isothermal Titration Chromatography Kd Determinations

Heat of interaction was measured on an ITC_{200} microcalorimeter (Malvern) under the same buffer conditions (20 mM Tris, pH 7.5, containing 1 mM EDTA and 200 mM NaCl). In most cases, aliquots of sBRAF construct at 350 µM were injected into 30 µM of CDC37 at 20 °C. Heats of dilution were determined by diluting injectant into buffer. Data were fitted using a curve-fitting algorithm (OriginLab Cooperation, Microcal Origin, version 7.0, Northhampton, MA, USA).

2.3. BRAF Kinase Assays

The activity of sBRAF was determined by a MEK phosphorylation assay consisting of 35 µM sBRAF, 6mM $MgCl_2$ (MERCK, CAlbiochem, catalogue No. 442611-M, Darmstadt, Germany), 5 mM ATP (MERCK, Sigma Aldrich, catalogue No. A7699-5G, Darmstadt, Germany), 1 µg inactive MEK1 (C-terminally His-tagged) in a total volume of 40 µL buffer (20 mM Hepes pH 8 (MERCK, Sigma Aldrich, catalogue No. 54457-250G-F, Darmstadt, Germany), 1 mM DTT (MERCK, Sigma Aldrich, catalogue No. D9779-25G, Darmstadt, Germany, 100 mM NaCl). Reactions were incubated at 30 °C for 60–180 min and samples taken for western blot analysis. Phophorylated MEK was detected using anti-phospho MEK 1/2 (residues 218/222 and 222/226, MERCK, catalogue No. 05-747, Darmstadt, Germany) antibody and rabbit secondary HRP (Cyvita, catalogue No. NA934-1ML, Marborough,

MA, USA) both at a 1/5000 dilution. Detection was carried out using a Pierce ECL Western Blotting Substrate (Thermo Fisher Scientific, catalogue No. 32106, Waltham, MA, USA).

2.4. Thermal Shift Assay

Reactions were carried out in triplicate using an Applied Bioscience, StepOnePlus real time PCR system. Experiments were conducted using 2 μM of sBRAF or mutant protein in a total of 20 μL of 20 mM Tris pH 7.5, 1 mM EDTA, 1 mM DTT and 200 mM NaCl containing 2.5 μL of 1/250 diluted SYPRO orange (Applied Biosystems Protein Thermal Shift, Thermo Fisher Scientific, Catalogue No. 2023-08-31, Waltham, MA, USA). The temperature was ramped up from 14 to 90 °C for over 60 min with an integration time of 1 sec. Data was analyzed with the LightCycler 480 Software version 1.5. (Roche, Basel, Switzerland).

2.5. Molecular Mass Determination

Samples of 50 μL of protein were loaded onto a Superdex 200 Increase 10/300 GL gel-filtration column equilibrated in 50 mM HEPES pH 7.5, 300 mM NaCl, 0.5 mM TCEP (MERCK, catalogue No. C4706, Darmstadt, Germany and 1 mM EDTA. The gel-filtration standards used were β-amylase (200 kD), aldolase (158 kD), conalbumin (75 kD), ovalbumin (44 kD) and carbonic anhydrase (29 kD) from a combination of two kits (GE Healthcare, catalogue No. 28-4038-41, Chicago, Illinois, IL, USA and MERCK, Sigma Aldrich, catalogue No. MWGF1000, Darmstadt, Germany).

3. Results

3.1. The Binding of CDC37 to sBRAF and sBRAF V600E Is Essentially Indistinguishable

Many kinases are notoriously difficult to produce in E. coli. In this study, we used a solubilized version of BRAF kinase domain (sBRAF, residues 423-723). This has a series of surface mutations that help to solubilize the kinase and improve yields in E. coli [29]. Previously, work showed that the co-expression of Hsp90, CDC37 and sBRAF in insect cells resulted in a stable Hsp90-CDC37-kinase complex. Such complexes containing sBRAF or sBRAF V600E were indistinguishable from that formed with native (unsolubilized) BRAF kinase domain [17]. Both wild type and sBRAF kinase domains were also shown to bind CDC37 *in vitro*, forming a stable complex in gel-filtration.

We found that both sBRAF and sBRAF V600E bound CDC37 with similar affinities (sBRAF, K_d = 1.0 μM and sBraf V600E K_d = 0.41 μM, Figure 1A,B), confirming earlier studies [17] that the solubilizing mutations on the surface of the kinase, as well as the V600E mutation, did not significantly disrupt the CDC37-BRAF interaction. Since BRAF V600E is more prevalent in Hsp90-CDC37 complexes [16] we chose the sBRAF V600E mutant, which gives reasonable yields following purification from E. coli, to further study CDC37 binding. Binding of sBraf V600E was promoted by an enthalpic change resulting from the interaction (−12,670 cal/mol), which was offset by an unfavorable entropy (−14 cal/mol/°C), indicating some degree of order resulting from the interaction (Figure 1B). This would be consistent with CDC37 stabilizing a dynamically unstable kinase domain.

3.2. Nucleotide Binding Prevents the CDC37-BRAF Interaction

We next tested the effect of the bound nucleotide, which binds deep in a pocket formed by the N- and C-terminal lobes of the kinase domain, on the binding of CDC37 to sBRAF V600E. We found that both AMPPNP and ADP prevented association of CDC37 with the kinase (Figure 1C,D), which was consistent with earlier observations [17]. These results support the idea that the CDC37 interaction with BRAF is focused within the nucleotide binding pocket of the kinase, as observed in the cryo-EM structure of the Hsp90-CDC37-Cdk4 complex [5].

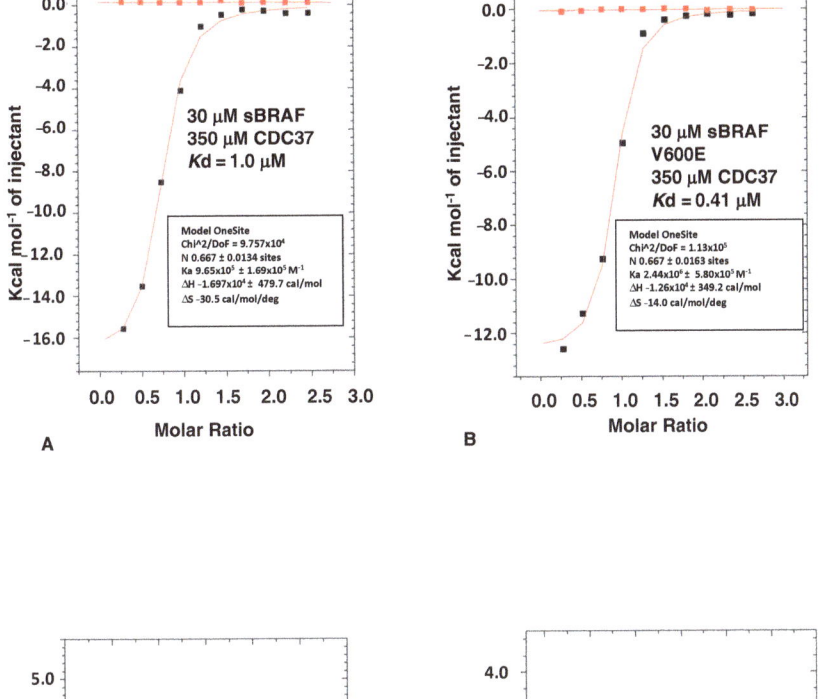

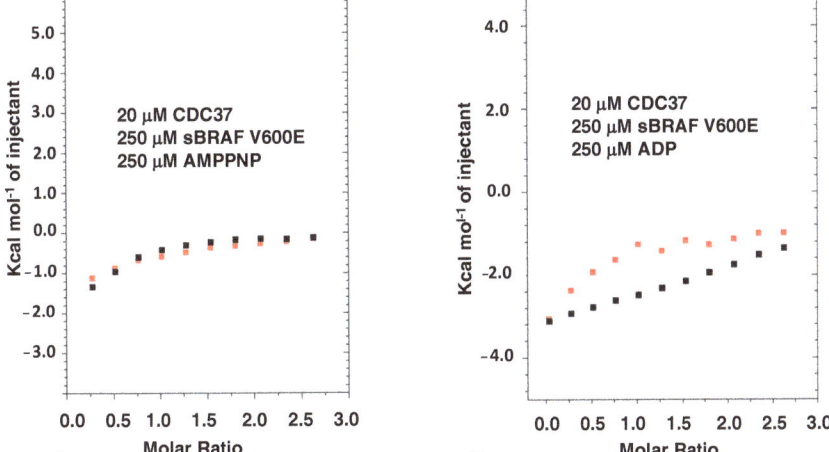

Figure 1. ITC of sBRAF and sBRAF V600E mutant. (**A**) The CDC37 interaction with sBRAF and (**B**) with sBRAF V600E. (**C**) The CDC37 interaction in the presence of AMPPNP with sBRAF V600E and (**D**) ADP with sBRAF V600E. Red markers, represent the heat of dilution and black markers the heat-of-dilution corrected interaction experiment.

3.3. The N-terminal and C-terminal Domains of CDC37 Are Essential for Efficient Bipartite Binding to the Kinase Domain

The interaction between CDC37 and kinases remains enigmatic and we wanted to better understand how kinases are recognized by CDC37. Based on structural studies [4,5] (Figure 2A), three CDC37 constructs, representing the N-terminal-(residues 1–120), the middle-(residues 148 to 269) and the C-terminal-domains (residues 273–353), were expressed and ITC interaction studies conducted to determine which domains of CDC37 were required for the sBRAF V600E interaction. We found that the N-terminal (amino acid residues 1–120) and C-terminal domain (residues 273 to 348) of CDC37 were both compromised in their ability to bind sBRAF V600E (Kd = 278 and 104 µM, respectively; Figure 2B,C) relative to full-length CDC37 (Kd = 0.41 µM; Figure 1B). In contrast, the middle domain failed to interact all together (Figure 2D). This contrasts with the Cryo-EM structure of Hsp90-CDC37-Cdk4, where the C-terminal domain of CDC37 was not visible [5].

3.4. Determining the Minimal CDC37 Structure Required for High-Affinity Binding to sBRAF V600E

In order to delimitate the exact segments that could be deleted from CDC37, but still maintained high affinity binding, we made a series of mutants that lacked structural elements of the CDC37 structure. Figure 2A shows structural elements and sites for CDC37 modification in ITC studies used throughout this study and Supplementary Figure S1 shows a graphical summary of all the constructs made. We first removed a large section of the coiled-coil (CC) structure (residues 44 to 108) from the N-terminal domain of full-length CDC37 and replaced it with a shorter tryptophan zipper (TrpZip) sequence (GSWTWENGKWTWKSG; CDC37-TrpZip) [30]. This sequence allowed the formation of a simple β-hairpin with stable secondary structure and could, therefore, preserve the structure of the remaining N-terminal domain. CDC37-TrpZip was soluble and bound sBRAF V600E with normal affinity (Kd = 0.5 µM, Figure 3A). This suggested that the coiled-coil structure of the N-terminal domain was superfluous for kinase binding by CDC37 alone. We next shortened the remaining coiled-coil region by introduction of a small linker (Gly-Ser-Gly) between residues 41 and 111, and within the same construct deleted the β-strand (βS) immediately following the N-terminal domain, by introducing a Gly-Ser-Gly linker between residues 119 and 140 to create CDC37-Δ(CC-βS). Using ITC, we tested this construct for binding to sBRAF V600E and found that it essentially bound normally (Kd = 0.61 µM, Figure 3B). This suggested that, in addition to the CC region, (residues 42–110), the βS element (residues 120 to 139) that links the N-terminal and middle domains of CDC37 was indispensable for kinase binding. Next, we deleted within the CDC37-Δ(CC-βS) construct the first 7 N-terminal residues and residues 272 to 285, which represent a small piece of helix that joins the middle and C-terminal-domain and terminated the protein at position 348 (to create CDC37-Δ(7-CC-βS-[272-285])). CDC37-Δ(7-CC-βS-[272-285]) bound sBRAF V600E normally (Kd = 1.03 µM; Figure 3C), relative to intact CDC37 (Kd = 0.41 µM; Figure 1B). Next, we created a construct (CDC37-Δ(7-CC-βS-[120-285]-[349-378]); abbreviated N^mC) that essentially linked the N and C-domains of CDC37 together, but maintained the deletions from the previous construct. CDC37-N^mC, resulted in a substantial reduction in affinity for sBRAF V600E (Kd = 145 µM; Figure 3D) to a level previously seen for the individual N- and C-domains of CDC37 (Figure 2B,C). We, therefore, reasoned that the spatial distance between the N- and C-domains was probably the reason for the reduced affinity. Consequently, we reintroduced 14 amino acid residues back into CDC37-N^mC to create CDC37-N^m(+14)-C. Residues 272 to 285 represented a piece of the helix that links the middle- and C-terminal domains of CDC37 and had previously been shown not to be required for direct binding to sBRAF V600E. CDC37-N^m(+14)-C was found to have substantially increased binding affinity to sBRAF V600E (Kd = 8.7 µM; Figure 4A) relative to N^mC (Kd = 145 µM; Figure 3D). Similarly, by reintroducing residues 120-125, representing a piece of the βS that links the N-terminal and middle-domains, into CDC37-N^mC to create CDC37-N^m(+6)-C, some binding affinity was restored (Kd = 18 µM; Figure 4B). It would, thus, appear that the binding affinity of CDC37 and sBRAF V600E was influenced by the spatial separation of the N- and C-terminal domains. We tested this further by then reintroducing residues 245 to 285, which represent a long helix that links the middle and C-domain of CDC37, into CDC37-N^mC to create CDC37-N^m(+41)-C. This construct showed vastly improved binding affinity for sBRAF V600E (Kd = 1.99 µM; Figure 4C) relative to CDC37-N^mC (Kd = 145 µM; Figure 3D). The results suggested that there is a minimal spatial distance between the CDC37 N- and C-terminal domains that is required for efficient kinase binding.

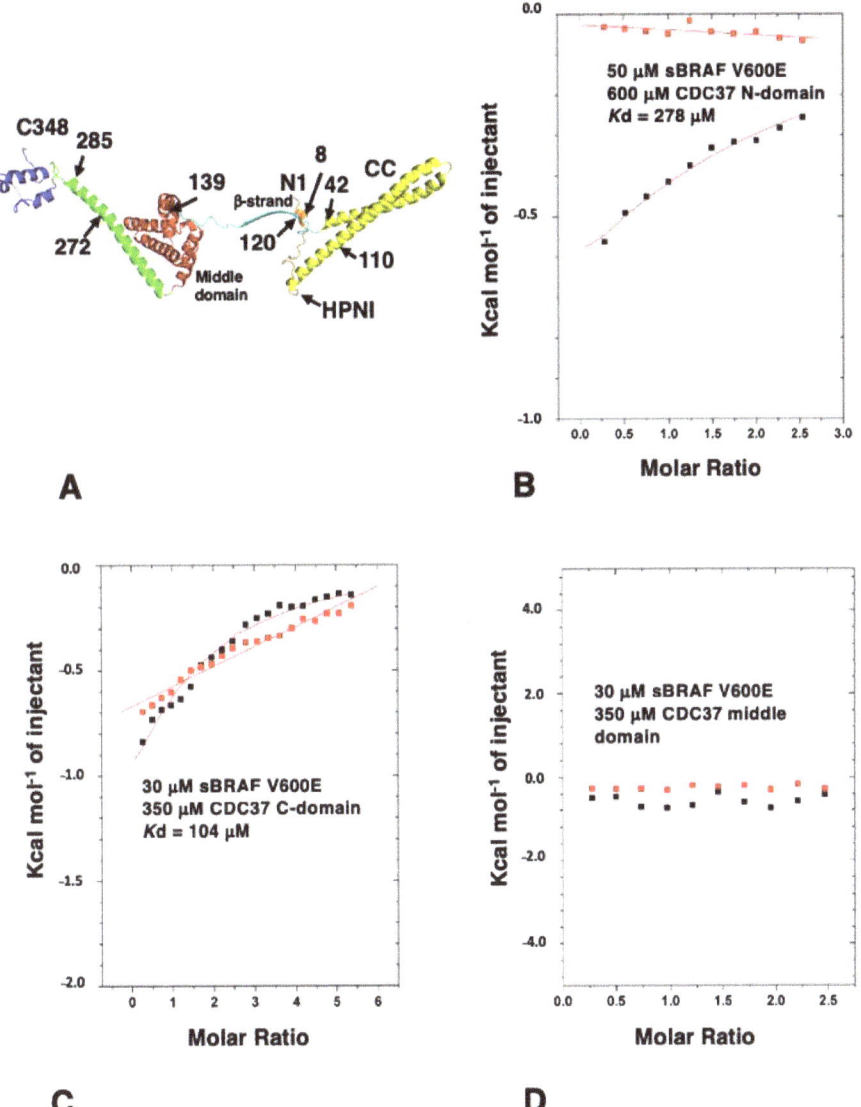

Figure 2. Structure of human CDC37 and ITC using CDC37 domains. (**A**) Individual elements of human CDC37 are colored as follows. orange; residues 1 to 23 including the conserved Ser 13 and HPNI residues; yellow (coiled-coil), residues 24 to 112; cyan, residues 113 to 139 including the beta strand residues 120–129; red, middle domain residues 140–244; green, helix connecting middle- and C-domains residues 245 to 292 and blue, C-terminal domain residues 293 to 348. The structure of residues beyond 348 have not been determined. (**B**) The interaction between sBRAF V600E and the N-terminal domain (residues 1–120), (**C**) with the C-domain (residues 273 to 348) and (**D**) with the middle-domain (residues 148–269) of CDC37. Red markers, represent the heat of dilution and black markers the heat-of-dilution corrected interaction experiment.

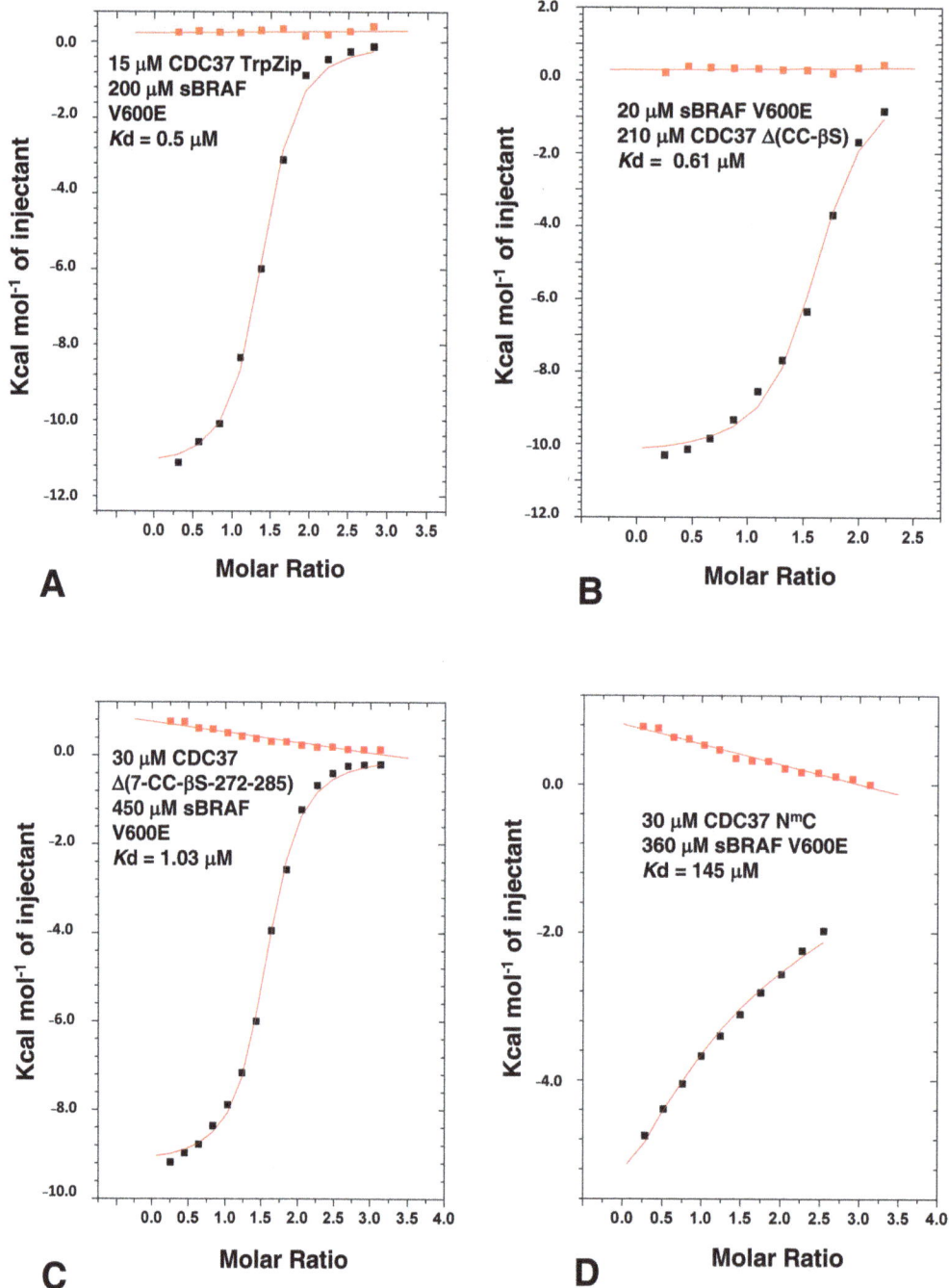

Figure 3. ITC of sBRAF V600E with various CDC37 deletion mutants. (**A**) sBRAF interaction with CDC37 TrpZip, (**B**) with CDC37 Δ(CC-βS), (**C**) with CDC37 Δ(7-CC-βS-272-285) and with (**D**) CDC37 N^{m}C. Red markers, represent the heat of dilution and black markers the heat-of-dilution corrected interaction experiment.

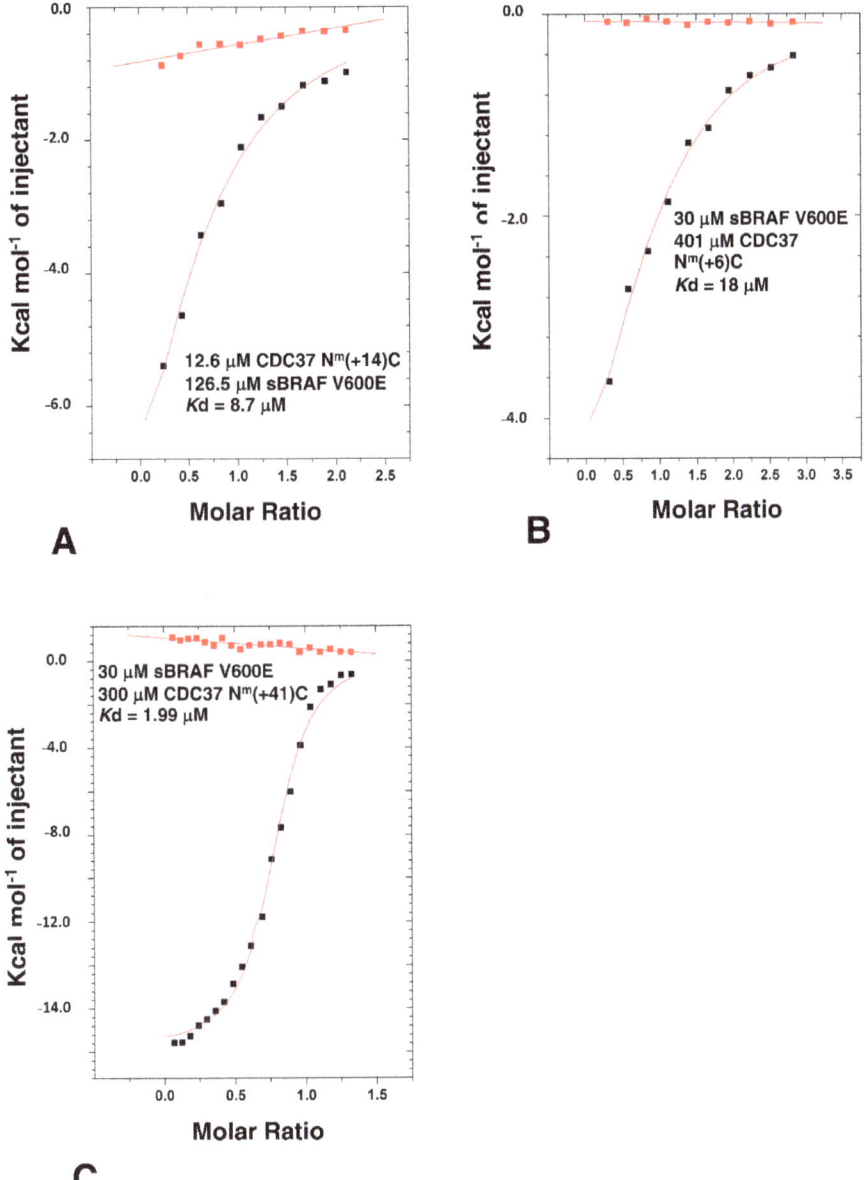

Figure 4. ITC of sBRAF V600E with various CDC37 deletion mutants. (**A**) sBRAF interaction with CDC37 $N^m(+14)C$, (**B**) with CDC37 $N^m(+6)C$ and (**C**) with CDC37 $N^m(+41)C$. Red markers, represent the heat of dilution and black markers the heat-of-dilution corrected interaction experiment.

We next investigated the limits required for binding by the C-terminal domain. The structure of the C-terminal domain of human CDC37 has been previously determined by both X-ray crystallography and by solution NMR [4,6] (PDB, 1US7 and 2N5X, respectively). These structures reveal a small domain that appears to be structurally mobile and Trp 342 is an essential residue of the core required for the folding of the domain. In contrast, valine at position 343 appears not to be fully packed in the core of either structure and its hydrophobic side-chain remains exposed to solvent. CDC37, consisting of residues 1 to 343, bound sBRAF V600E normally (Kd = 0.76 µM; intact CDC37; Kd = 0.41 µM) (Figures 1B and 5A, respectively). Similarly, the V343A and V343R mutants were more or less normal for sBRAF V600E binding (Kd = 0.9 and 1.3 µM, respectively; Figure 5B,C). However, CDC37 1-342 was compromised in its affinity for sBRAF V600E (Kd = 45.7 µM; Figure 5D). This suggests, that Val 343 may aid Trp 342 packing and is essential for folding of the C-terminal domain, but is not, in itself, essential for direct binding of kinases. Consistent with this was that W342A binding to sBRAF V600E was compromised (Kd = 94.3 µM, Figure 5E), whereas, and as expected, the W342R construct failed to bind altogether (Figure 5F), suggesting that Trp 342 is essential for the folding of the C-terminal domain of CDC37.

The results so far suggested that the N-terminal domain (residues 8 to 41, which contains the HPNI motif), residues 111 to 119 (which immediately follow the CC region) and residues 286 to 348 (which represent the C-terminal domain) are the minimal elements required for high affinity binding to kinases, although a non-specific spacer (we used residues 245 to 285) between the N-domain and C-domain elements is also required (Figure 5G). Collectively, the results suggested that the interaction between CDC37 and kinases is bipartite and that the lobes of a kinase domain are probably held in a spatially separated conformation.

3.5. The CDC37 S13E-Phosphomimetic Mutation Does Not Affect Binding to BRAF

It has been reported that phosphorylation of Ser 13 within CDC37 is required for the binding of a kinase and that the S13E mutation can act as a phosphomimetic [31]. However, the cryo-EM structure of Hsp90-CDC37-Cdk4, suggests that Ser 13 is not directly involved in the interaction with the kinase [5]. To test this hypothesis, we compared the binding of sBRAF V600E to CDC37 S13E and CDC37 wild type. We found that the affinity for the binding of the S13E mutant to be similar to unmutated CDC37, (Kd = 0.30 and 0.41 µM, respectively; Figures 1B and 6A). This was consistent with the cryo-EM structure of Hsp90-CDC37-Cdk4 complex that showed that phosphoserine is involved in a serious of contacts involving Lys 406 of Hsp90 and His 33 and Arg 36 of CDC37, but does not contact Cdk4 directly (Figure 6B).

3.6. The CDC37 HPNI Amino Acid Motif Is Essential for High-Affinity Kinase Recognition

Analysis of the Hsp90-CDC37-Cdk4 cryo-EM structure suggests that the C-terminal lobe of Cdk4 is recognized by a conserved amino acid motif, HPNI [5], which mimics the HPNV motif interactions within Cdk4 and HVNI within BRAF. In kinases this motif, present in the N-lobe of these kinases, forms part of the normal packing interactions between the two lobes of the kinase domain. Closer inspection showed that the side-chain of Asn 22, of the CDC37 HPNI motif, may be involved in polar contacts with the side-chains of Thr 153 and Arg 126 and a main-chain carbonyl interaction with Val 154 of Cdk4 (Figure 7A). To test the importance of the HPNI motif we mutated Asn 22 to alanine and arginine. As expected, both the CDC37 N22A and N22R mutants were compromised for binding to sBRAF V600E (Kd = 27.3 and Kd = 14.2 µM, respectively; Figure 7B,C). This confirmed that the HPNI motif of CDC37 is involved in the initial recognition of kinases.

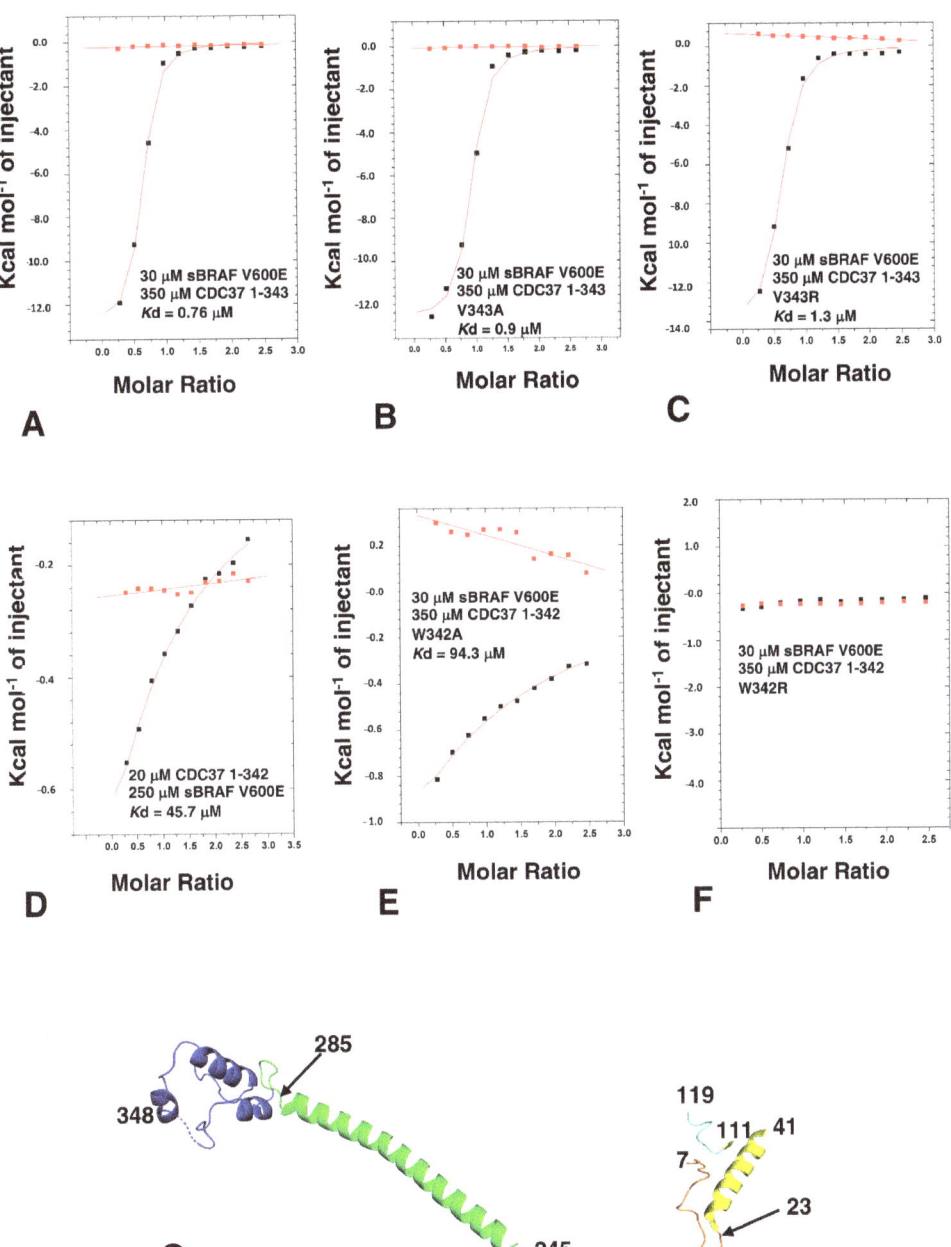

Figure 5. ITC of sBRAF V600E with various CDC37 deletion mutants and the minimal CDC37 elements required for kinase binding. (**A**) sBRAF interaction with CDC37 1–343, (**B**) with CDC37 V343A, (**C**) with CDC37 V343R, (**D**) with CDC37 1–342, (**E**) with CDC37 W342A and (**F**) with CDC37 W342R. Red markers, represent the heat of dilution and black markers the heat-of-dilution corrected interaction experiment. (**G**) Structural elements of CDC37 which can be tethered to approximate towards normal binding with sBRAF. Elements of CDC37 are colored as gold, residues 8–23; yellow, residues 24–41; cyan, 111–119; green, 245–285 and blue, C-terminus residues 286–348.

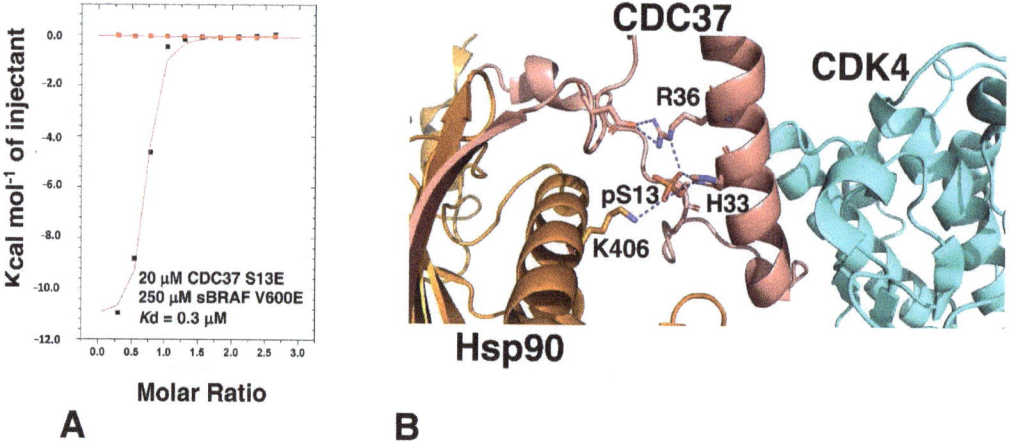

Figure 6. CDC37 pSer 13 is not involved in kinase binding. (**A**) ITC of CDC37-S13E with sBRAF V600E. Red markers, represent the heat of dilution and black markers the heat-of-dilution corrected interaction experiment. (**B**) PyMol cartoon showing the interaction of CDC37 pSER 13 with Hsp90 (gold) and CDC37 (salmon). Direct interactions with Cdk4 (cyan) are not present. Polar interactions are shown by dotted blue lines.

3.7. HPNI Is Part of a More Extensive CDC37 Binding Motif

On closer inspection of the CDC37 structure we noticed that the recognition of the kinase was potentially more extensive and involved a conserved motif consisting of ^{20}HPNID—SL–W–Q^{34}), of which the I—SL–W sequence formed mostly a small hydrophobic patch or pocket that could form interactions with a bound kinase (Figure 8A). In our analysis, amino acid position 23 was generally a conserved Ile or Val, position 24 was a conserved Asp, position 27 was a conserved Ser, position 28 was either a Leu or Phe and position 31 was a conserved Trp. We therefore decided to test whether the mutation of these conserved residues of CDC37 would influence kinase binding. As expected, we found that the L28R mutation completely abolished the interaction with sBRAF V600E (Figure 8B), while the L28A mutant diminished it substantially (Kd = 16.9 µM; Figure 8C), relative to wild type CDC37 (Kd = 0.41 µM; Figure 1B). This was consistent with the L28R mutation causing a steric clash that prevented sBRAF V600E from binding. In contrast, the L28A mutation did not prevent binding, but compromised the strength of the interaction seen. Similarly, the interaction of W31K with CDC37 was abolished. (Figure 8D), but the W31A mutation was well tolerated (Kd = 2.1 µM; Figure 8E). Furthermore, the mutation S27K reduced binding substantially (Kd = 29 µM; Figure 8F), whereas the S27A mutation was well tolerated Kd = 1.6 µM; Figure 8G). In contrast to these mutants, the Q34R and Q34A mutations had very little effect on sBRAF V600E binding (Kd = 0.3 and 0.35 µM, respectively; Figure 8H,I). However, we noted that arginine was found at position Gln 34, in some CDC37 proteins. These results, collectively, suggested that the motif for the recognition of the C-terminal lobe of kinase domains could be extended to include ^{20}HPNID—SL–W^{31}, although experimentally we did not test Asp 24, since the side chain of this amino acid residue is critical for maintaining the structure of the HPNI loop by forming polar interactions with the side-chain of Ser 27 and the main-chain amide of Ala 26 at the base of the proceeding helix.

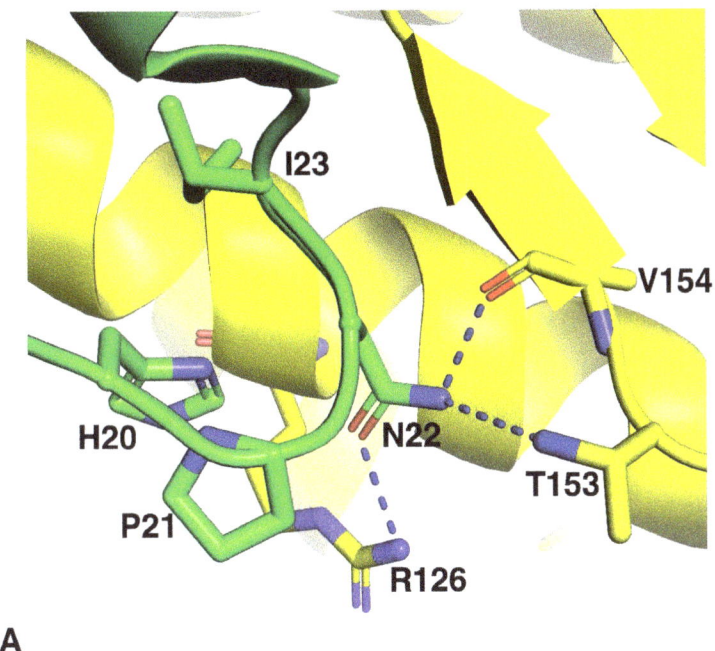

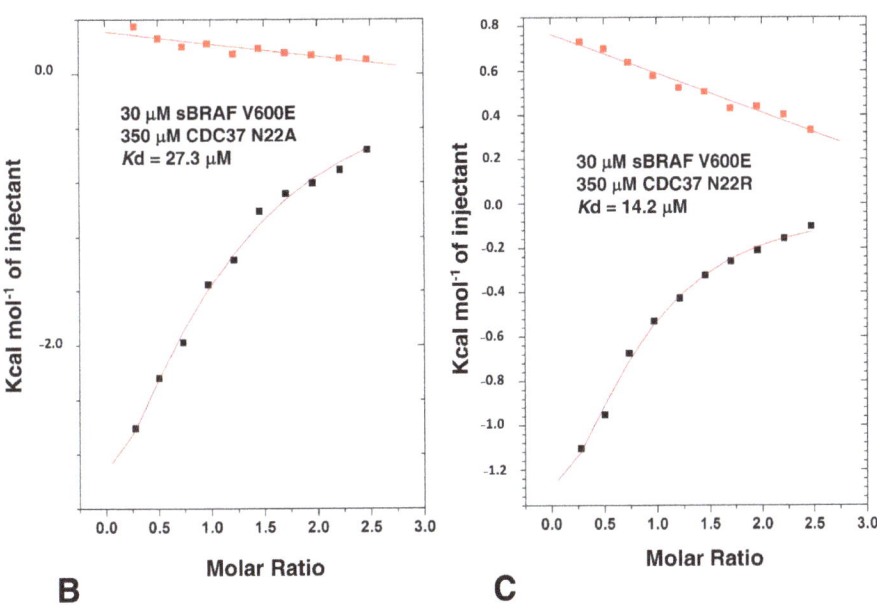

Figure 7. Interaction of CDC37-Asn 22 mutants with Cdk4. (**A**) Possible interaction modelled from the Cryo-EM structure of Hsp90-CDC37-Cdk4 complex. Green, CDC37 and yellow, Cdk4. Polar interactions are shown by dotted blue lines. (**B**) ITC interaction between sBRAF V600E and CDC37 N22A and (**C**) with CDC37 N22R. Red markers, represent the heat of dilution and black markers the heat-of-dilution corrected interaction experiment.

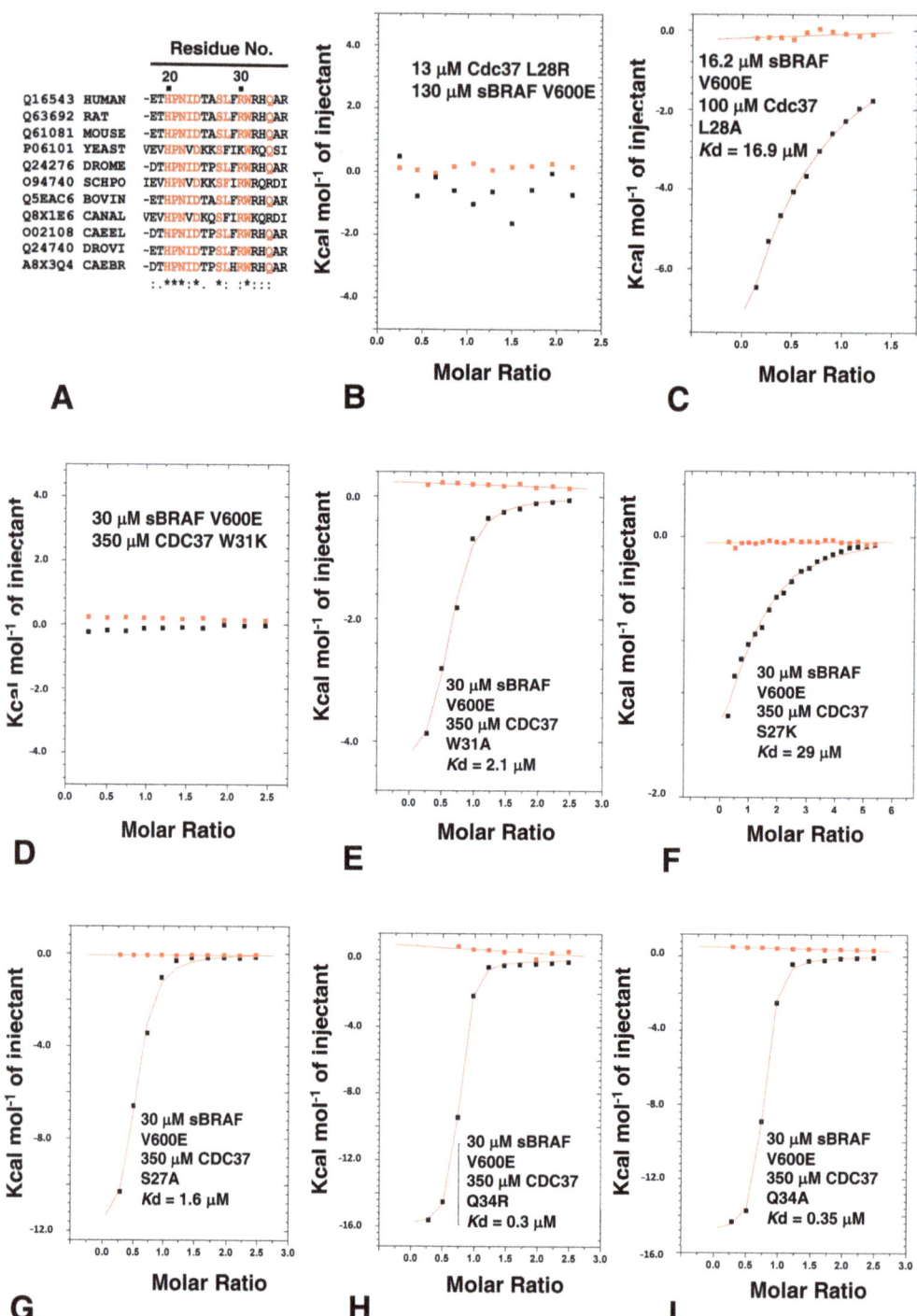

Figure 8. ITC analysis of CDC37 amino acid residues involved in kinase recognition. (**A**) CDC37 alignment with the uniprot accession codes shown together with abbreviation for genus and species.

DROME, Drosophila melanogaster (Fruit fly); SCHPO, Schizosaccharomyces pombe (Fission yeast); CANAL, Candida albicans; CAEEL, Caenorhabditis elegans; DROVI, Drosophila virilis (Fruit fly) and CAEBR, Caenorhabditis briggsae. (.), conservation between groups of weakly similar properties; (:), conservation between groups of strongly similar properties and (*), positions that have a single and fully conserved residue. ITC interactions of sBRAF V600E with (**B**) CDC37 L28R, (**C**) with CDC37 L28A, (**D**) with CDC37 W31K and (**E**) with CDC37 W31A. ITC interaction between sBRAF V600 wild type and (**F**) CDC37 S27K, (**G**) with CDC37 S27A, (**H**) with CDC37 Q34R and (**I**) with CDC37 Q34A. Red markers, represent the heat of dilution and black markers the heat-of-dilution corrected interaction experiment.

3.8. Activation Loop Mutants Do Not Influence BRAF Binding to CDC37

BRAF is activated through phosphorylation of two key residues, T599 and S602 within the activation loop or T loop of kinases. In addition, the V600E mutation is known to constitutively activate BRAF, and is the most prominent mutation in cancer [32]. We have previously seen that the sBRAF V600E mutation does not affect binding to CDC37, but we wondered if the phosphomimetic mutations T599E and S602D would affect Cdc37 binding. The sBRAF T599E-V600E-S602D mutant was previously shown to be catalytically active [17]. Using this active triple mutant in ITC experiments we showed that binding to CDC37 was unaffected (Kd = 0.47 µM; Figure 9A). Furthermore, mutating Thr 599 for a bulky tryptophan, or a positively charged arginine side-chain, did not affect binding to CDC37 (Kd = 0.23 µM; Figure 9B). The results showed that phosphomimetic mutations of the T loop did not influence CDC37 binding.

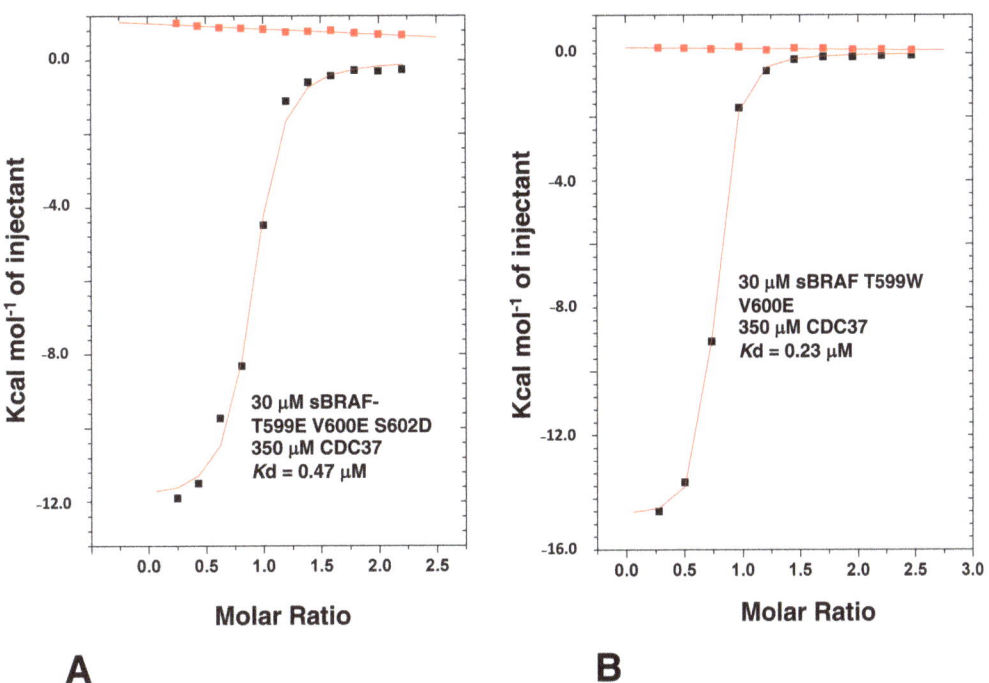

Figure 9. ITC interactions between CDC37 and T-loop mutants of sBRAF. (**A**) Interaction between CDC37 and the triple sBRAF mutant T599E-V600E-S602D and (**B**) with the double mutant T599W-V600E. Red markers, represent the heat of dilution and black markers the corrected interaction experiment.

3.9. The BRAF Mutation L597R Compromises Binding to CDC37

The conformation of the DFG motif of kinases is known to affect kinase activity and numerous mutations have been documented that alter these residues and are associated with oncogenic phenotypes. We, therefore, decided to analyze such oncogenic mutations and their effect on CDC37 binding. Unlike V600E, the F595V mutation in BRAF is inactivating [33] and consequently, to prevent complicated scenarios, we decided to make all activation segment mutants in a V600 background. We found that both the sBRAF F595A and sBRAF F595V mutations did not compromise binding to CDC37 (Kd = 0.5 and 1.4 µM, respectively; Figure 10A,B). Similarly, for sBRAF D594V, where D594V results in impaired kinase activity [34–36], we found this construct bound CDC37 normally (Kd = 1.2 µM; Figure 10C).

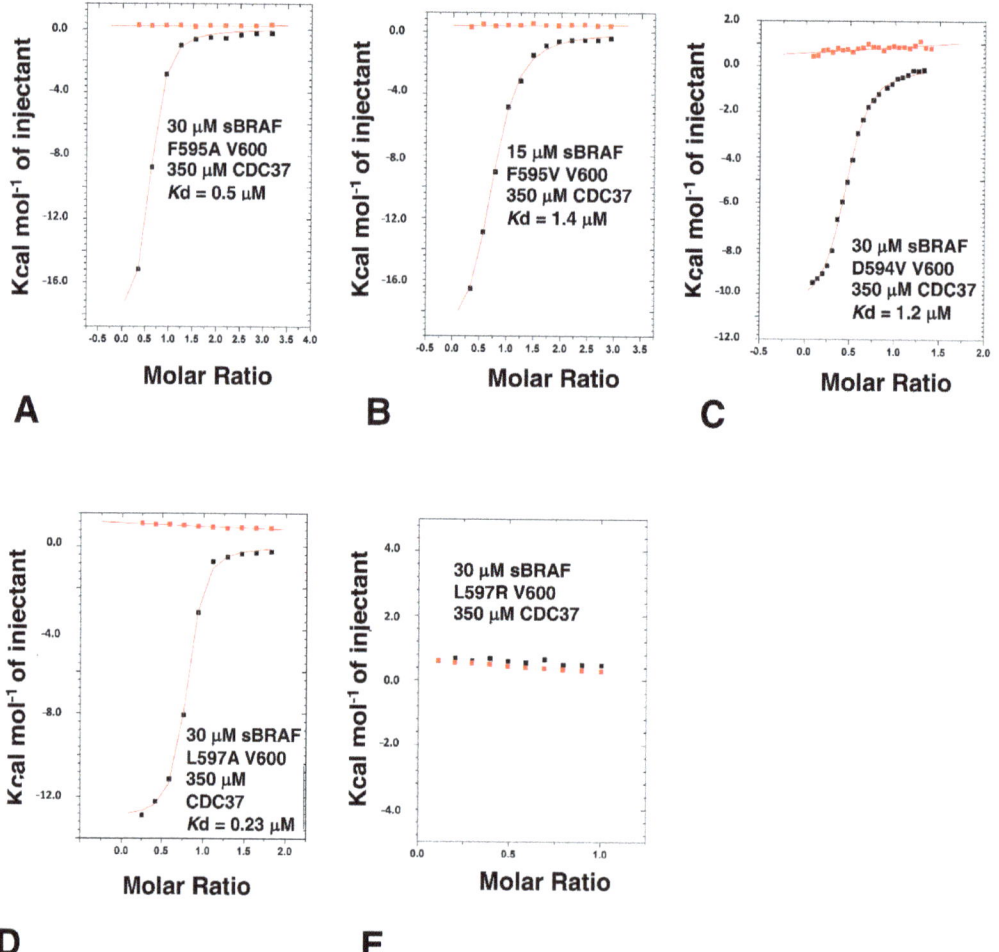

Figure 10. ITC interaction studies with the DFGL mutants of sBRAF. Interactions between CDC37 and (**A**) sBRAF F595A, (**B**) with sBRAF F595V, (**C**) with sBRAF D594V, (**D**) with sBRAF L597A and (**E**) with sBRAF L597R. Red markers, represent the heat of dilution and black markers the heat-of-dilution corrected interaction experiment.

We next tested the binding of sBRAF L597A and sBRAF L597R mutants in a Val 600 background. We found that the L597A mutation did not compromise binding to CDC37 (Kd = 0.23 µM; Figure 10D), whereas we were surprised to find that the L597R mutation abolished binding completely (Figure 10E). In EGFR the equivalent mutation, L858R (L834R in mature EGFR), has been shown to form salt bridges with Glu 758 (BRAF Ala 497) and Glu 762 (BRAF Glu 501) or Glu 761 (BRAF Asn 500), which are found on the dynamic regulatory element, known as the C-helix [26,37]. Another polar residue on the C-helix of BRAF is also found at Gln 496. A structural analysis of the BRAF structure (PDB 4RZV) suggests that L597R may allow salt bridges, among other possible interactions, with the nearly invariant Glu 501, which is located on the C-helix. Glutamate at this position within kinases forms a salt bridge with the invariant Lysine (BRAF Lys 483), which itself becomes coupled to bound ATP. However, a salt bridge between L597R and Glu 501 (or other possible residues) would stabilize the C-helix of sBRAF, which is directly connected, at its C-terminal end, to the αC-β4 loop containing the HPNI residues that CDC37 mimics in binding to kinases. This loop is highly significant as it is the only element from the N-terminal lobe of kinase domain that is functionally and constitutively connected to its C-terminal lobe.

It has been previously shown for the equivalent mutation in EGFR, L858R destabilizes the inactive kinase, but simultaneously stabilizes the C-helix and that this consequently leads to dimerization of the mutant kinase [38–41]. In order to test the stability of the L597R mutation, we conducted a thermal shift assay. We compared the thermal stability of L597R with sBRAF and various other sBRAF mutants (Figure 11A). As expected, we found that inactive sBRAF was the most stabile construct with a Tm = 40 °C and that sBraf V600E was significantly less stabile (Tm = 36.2 °C). However, the L597A mutation destabilized the kinase further (Tm = 35 °C). In contrast, the L597R mutation (Tm = 37.8 °C) was less stable than sBRAF, but more stable than sBRAF V600E. This was in agreement with the destabilizing effect of this mutation on the inactive kinase, whilst simultaneously stabilizing the C-helix, which consequently leads to dimerization of the kinase. The L597R-V600E double mutant Tm (36.8 °C) was found to be in between the V600E Tm (36.2 °C) and the Tm for sBRAF L597R (36.8 °C).

Due to the tendency for EGFR L858R to promote dimerization, we next investigated the oligomeric nature of the equivalent BRAF L597R mutation. It was found that sBRAF had a relative molecular mass of 35.5 kD, as eluted from a Superdex 200 Increase 10/300 GL column, which was similar to its calculated relative molecular mass of 33.4 kD (Figure 11B,C). In contrast, L597R displayed a relative molecular mass of 60.2 kD, which was consistent with a dimeric state for the kinase domain. BRAF V600E eluted with a relative molecular mass of 34.7 kD similar to that of sBRAF, while the double mutant, L597R V600E, reverted the relative molecular mass of L597R back towards the monomeric state (38.9 kD). Collectively, the results suggested that L597R drives BRAF into a dimeric state that is not recognized by CDC37, and that V600E drives the kinase back to a monomeric state.

We next asked whether we could disrupt the potential L597R-Glu 501 salt bridge, as the most likely, but not the only interaction stabilizing the dimerization promoting C-helix conformation. Introducing the E501A mutation into a L597R background we found that the L597R-Glu 501 mutant expressed poorly and was unstable. However, we had previously seen that V600E could disrupt dimerization of L597R and, therefore, further work was conducted with this double mutant, L597R-V600E. We found that introducing the V600E mutation into a L597R background completely restored binding with CDC37 (Kd = 0.34 µM; Figure 11D), suggesting that the V600E mutation had destabilized the L597R dimeric promoting component of the double mutant.

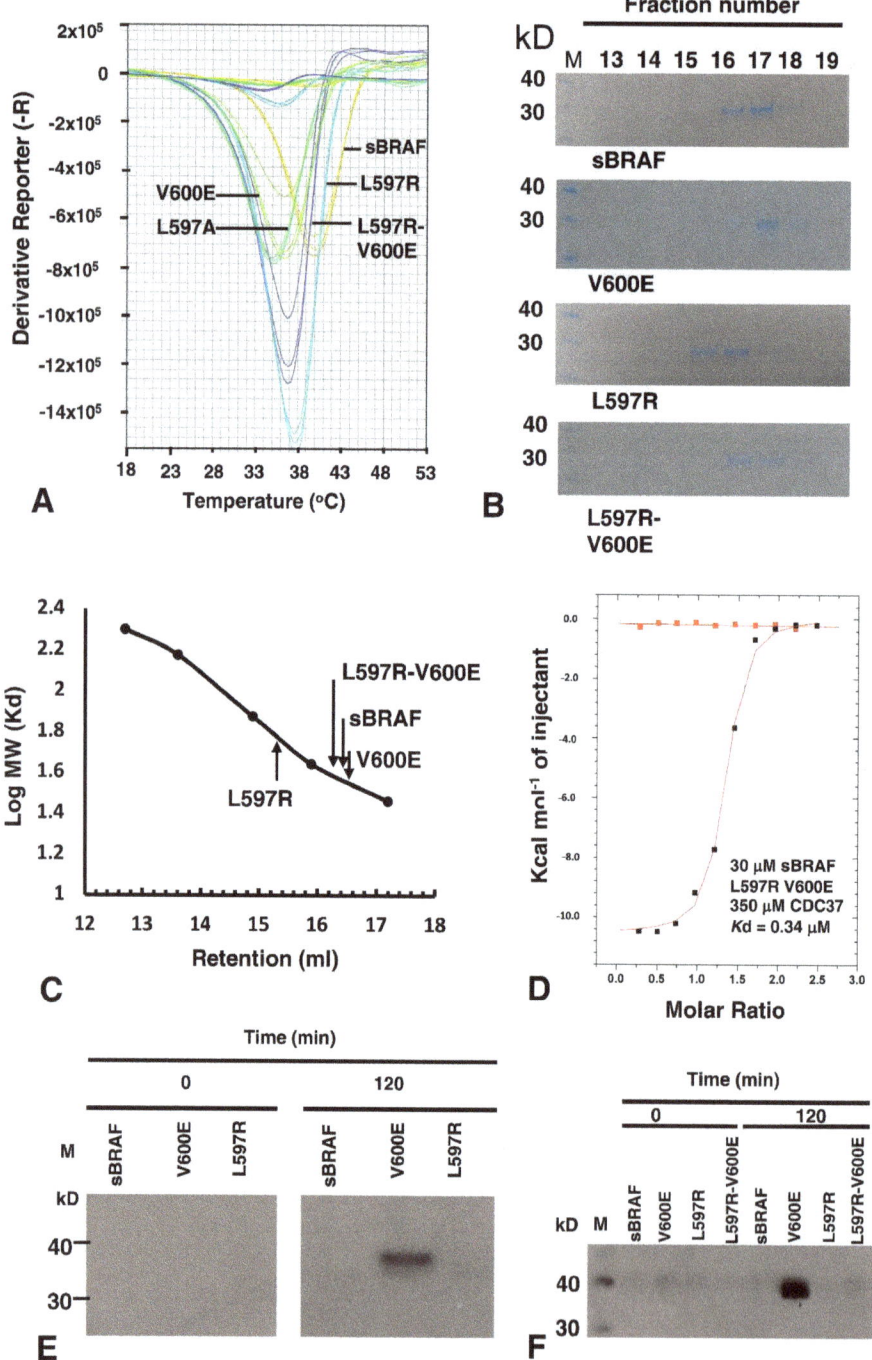

Figure 11. Interaction studies and assays with the L597R mutant of sBRAF. (**A**) Thermal Shift Assay for sBRAF and mutants. In order of decreasing Tm: Orange, sBRAF wild type (Tm = 40 °C); cyan, L587R (Tm = 37.8 °C); blue, L597R-V600E (Tm = 36.8 °C); light green, V600E (Tm = 36.2 °C) and dark

green L597A (Tm = 35 °C). (**B**) Gel-filtration fractions from Superdex 200 Increase 10/300 GL column, showing L597R to have a relative molecular mass equivalent to dimeric sBRAF and that V600E disrupts the dimeric nature of the L597R mutant. M, molecular weight markers (kD). (**C**) Estimation of the relative molecular mass of sBRAF mutants, showing L597R to be dimeric in mass. (**D**) ITC between CDC37 and sBRAF L597R-V600E, showing that the V600E mutation restores binding with CDC37 in the L597R background. Red markers, represent the heat of dilution and black markers the heat-of-dilution corrected interaction experiment. (**E**) MEK phosphorylation assays with L597R and V600E, showing that V600E is active and (**F**) with sBRAF L597R showing that is not activated by a V600E mutation. M, molecular weight markers (kD).

3.10. sBRAF L597R and L597R-V600E Mutant Are Both Inactive

Literature suggests that L597R is an activating mutation [42,43]. However, on closer inspection the results suggested this is inferred indirectly by determining cellular levels of phospho-MEK and phospho-ERK [44,45]. Our *in vitro* MEK phosphorylation assays showed that L597R was inactive relative to V600E (Figure 11E). Thus, it appeared that dimerization alone of L597R was insufficient, under the conditions used, for the activation of its kinase activity. We next assayed the BRAF L597R-V600E mutant for kinase activity. We found that, although V600E restored CDC37 binding, V600E did not activate kinase activity in the double mutant (Figure 11F), which suggested that further mechanisms were required to attain an activated L597R mutant conformation or signaling complex.

4. Discussion

CDC37 is a kinome-specific co-chaperone responsible for delivering protein kinases to Hsp90. The molecular details of how CDC37 recognizes such kinases has remained enigmatic, but recent work suggests that kinases are structurally dynamic and, consequently, require stabilization by CDC37 [1,2]. We have now shown that CDC37 recognizes kinases by a bipartite interaction involving two CDC37 elements, which was recently suggested by NMR and cryo-EM studies [5]. We defined a small N-terminal CDC37 fragment, [20]HPNID—SL–W[31], and its C-terminal domain, as the interaction sites for kinases. The interacting fragments must be connected by a minimal distance, which we achieved by introducing residues 245–285 of the native CDC37 sequence, which normally forms an α-helix, but appeared to be otherwise dispensable for binding. The interaction of the C-terminal domain of CDC37 with the kinase was not observed in the high-resolution cryo-EM structure of Hsp90-CDC37-Cdk4 [5]. This suggested that CDC37-kinase complex may be remodeled after interaction with Hsp90. A bipartite interaction between CDC37 and BRAF was recently reported using NMR [46], but here we more clearly defined residues involved in that interaction. The authors of the NMR study suggested that CDC37 needs to be in a compact form to recognize kinase protein. We found that by replacing the central regions of CDC37 with smaller linkers, which connect the N- and C-terminal domains of CDC37, we could still observe binding between CDC37 and sBRAF. The longest linker, of 41 amino acids, appeared to, more or less, restore full binding, (Kd = 1.99 µM; Figure 4C). However, shorter linkers of 14 and 6 amino acids also displayed significant binding (Kd = 18 and 8.7 µM; Figure 4A,B, respectively). This suggested some flexibility in the exact conformation of CDC37 for its bipartite recognition of the kinase, which might reflect an ensemble of kinase conformations, due to their dynamic instability.

Mutational analyses suggest that the N-terminal domain of CDC37 uses an extended motif ([20]HPNID—SL–W[31]), which incorporates the conserved sequence HPNI, to recognize the C-terminal lobe of kinases. In contrast, mutation of the activation segment residues did not affect CDC37 binding, except for the L597R mutation. The equivalent L858R mutation, in EGFR tyrosine kinase, drives a variety of cancers including non-small-cell lung cancer [47–51]. As with EGFR L858R [37–40], we found L597R also drives dimerization of BRAF.

The Hsp90-CDC37 complex has been reported to be present at the plasma membrane with RAS and, presumably, can deliver BRAF to the RAS complex [18]. The conformation of the kinase, altered by mutation, is likely to influence this process. We suggest that the active class 1 BRAF V600E mutant, although recognized by CDC37, is less able to enter the RAS complex, as entry into this complex normally occurs as a BRAF autoinhibited complex. This could explain why elevated levels of cytoplasmic Hsp90-CDC37-BRAF V600E accumulate above those normally seen for wild type BRAF (Figure 12). In the case for the class 2 BRAF L597R mutant, CDC37 is unable to complex with the already formed dimer of this mutant, which means that elevated levels of BRAF L597R may accumulate in the cytoplasm and enhanced signaling may be established, following activation of such a dimer (Figure 12). In our hands, dimerization of the BRAF L597R mutant was not sufficient to bring about its activation. We also found that the V600E mutation was unable to activate the BRAF L597R mutant. Thus, the activation of BRAF L597R might require other mechanisms that bring about a catalytically active state for this mutant, in whatever form it is signaling.

We propose that the BRAF V600E mutant preferentially partitions to the Hsp90-CDC37 complex and that Hsp90 most likely maintains the cytoplasmic stability of this active mutant by preserving the V600E kinase against proteasomal degradation. It has, of course, been well documented that the V600E mutant is sensitive to Hsp90 inhibition [52]. However, what are the implications of our findings for BRAF L597R signaling? For the L597R mutant, Hsp90-CDC37 may promote dimerization of the kinase by stabilizing initially the monomeric form, soon after translation, which ultimately leads to its dimerization, following the normal cycles of Hsp90 chaperone activity. However, it remains unclear how such a dimer becomes active, as inclusion of V600E in the L597R background failed to activate the double mutant. This raises a number of questions. Firstly, does activation of the L597R mutant require full phosphorylation of the activation loop, where V600E alone is insufficient to bring about activity? Secondly, if phosphorylation alone does not activate L597R, then what does? Thirdly, can the L597R mutant trans-auto-phosphorylate anyway, or is it completely inactive as a L597R mutant homodimer? Certainly, our *in vitro* assays suggest that this might be the case. We speculate that monomeric L597R captured by Hsp90-CDC37, or by 14-3-3, might be transferred to the RAS-14-3-3 complex, where RAS drives the mutant into a stable and active conformation with CRAF. We suggest that L597R is impaired in kinase activity and, consequently, requires an active partner, such as CRAF (Figure 12).

Data suggests that active RAS is able to induce cRAF-BRAF heterodimerization by exposing 14-3-3 binding sites in the C-terminus of CRAF [53]. That CRAF is required for L597R signaling is also supported by the fact that BRAF mutants, with impaired or intermediate kinase activity, were shown to induce strong activation of CRAF. However, only impaired kinase activity mutants, as seen here with L597R, were shown to be dependent on CRAF for ERK activation [35]. We suggest that because of the increased stability of the L597R mutation towards dimerization, perhaps L597R-CRAF activity cannot now be downregulated, whether by RAS or Hsp90-CDC37. Thus, as an overly stable dimer this could lead to enhanced or sustained signaling and apparent RAS independency, in terms of SOS inhibition and down regulation of overall RAF signaling. In fact, it was recently reported that for some class 2 BRAF mutants, there are variable and overlapping levels of enriched RAS alterations [54]. These authors used variation coexistence between activated RAS and BRAF alterations to support *in vivo* RAS dependency and show that class 2 BRAF alterations have a higher frequency of RAS dependency than class 1 mutants, such as V600E. Our findings show that the double mutant, L597R-V600E and the single mutant, L597R, of BRAF are inactive *in vitro*, which suggests that the L597R mutant may require additional factors for attaining an active signaling state. We suggest this probably involves the RAS-14-3-3 complex together with CRAF. However, whatever the scenario, our findings call for reevaluation of RAS dependency for at least some so-called class 2 BRAF mutations and, as such, the exact mechanism for the activation of L597R still needs to be determined. Thus, we find that mutations in BRAF could potentially influence the dynamics of various

BRAF complexes that normally tightly regulate the activity of BRAF. As a result, Hsp90 either preserves V600E kinase domain, by protecting it against proteasomal degradation, or, in the case of L597R, it may promote a dimeric state, probably with CRAF, that is able to signal through MEK in a sustained manner.

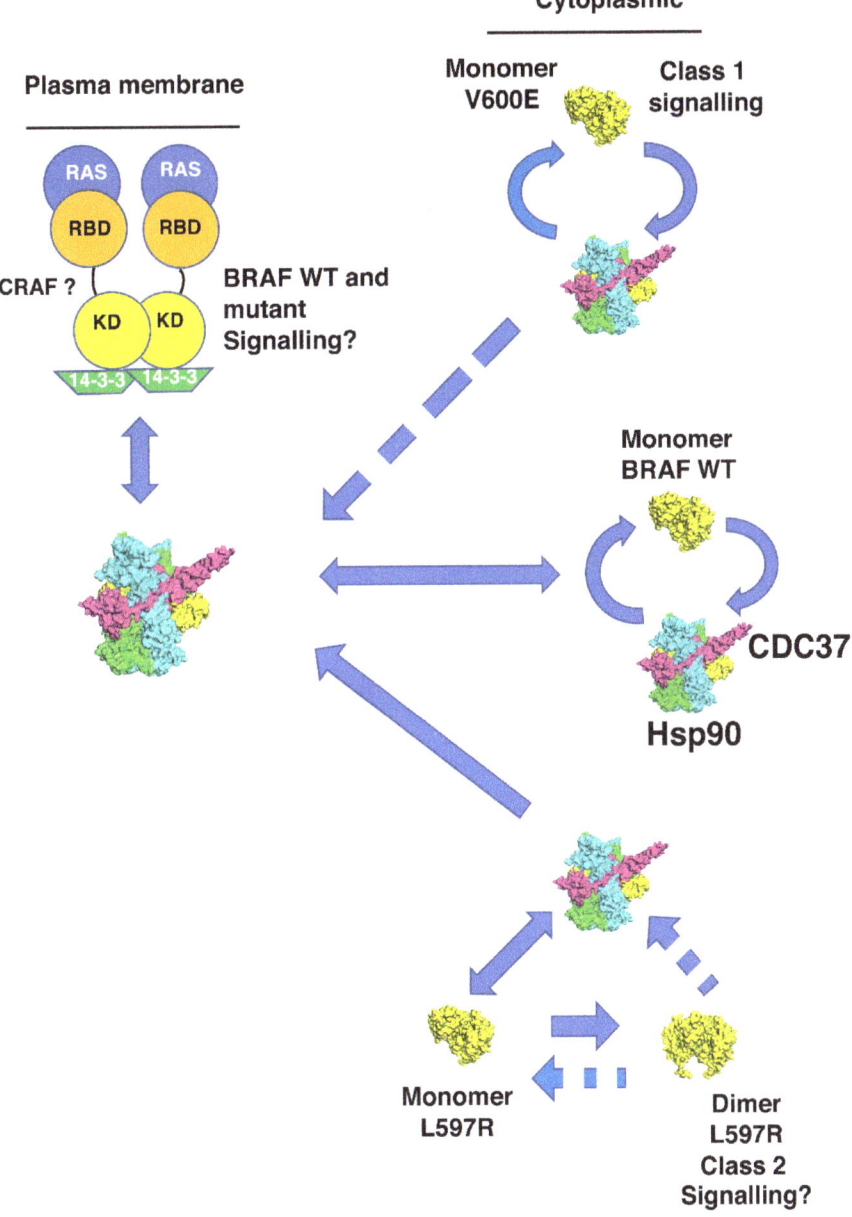

Figure 12. Potential dynamics for the activation of BRAF and the L597R and V600E mutants by Hsp90 and RAS. Wild type (WT) BRAF is transported to the RAS complex by Hsp90-CDC37, where its activity is tightly regulated. V600E is active as a monomer and appears to associate preferentially

with Hsp90 complex, which provides cellular stability. Its active conformation may thus limit its entry to the RAS complex, as early stages of this complex contain BRAF in an autoinhibited conformation. Newly made L597R monomers may be assembled into dimers (perhaps with CRAF) following Hsp90-CDC37 association and activation, where they may then remain resistant to disassembly by the chaperone system. BRAF L597R may also be transferred to the RAS complex where its enhanced stability as a dimer (probably with CRAF) alters the down regulatory mechanism of the BRAF L597R-CRAF kinase heterocomplex. (?—in the figure), represents signaling that needs to be further defined for BRAF L597R kinase. (CRAF?), represents the potential for CRAF replacing one of the BRAF monomers of the dimerized state at the plasma membrane. Solid blue arrows show potential flow of BRAF to the Hsp90 and RAS complex, whereas broken arrows show possible restricted movement relative to wild type BRAF. Delivery of BRAF, its mutants and CRAF could also take place with 14-3-3, but this has been omitted from the figure for clarity. KD, BRAF kinase domain and RBD, RAS binding domain of BRAF. Structural models are represented as green and cyan, Hsp90, magenta, CDC37 and yellow BRAF.

The potentially different signaling complexes of BRAF V600E and BRAF L597R could have clinical implications for how to treat tumors driven by each of these driver mutations. Particularly relevant is the fact that CDC37 protects its clients from inhibitor binding, acting as a competitive inhibitor and altering the structure of the kinase, thus blocking kinase inhibitor binding. However, the Hsp90-CDC37 complex-free V600E is susceptible to inhibitors, such as vemurafenib, but it is likely that elevated levels of Hsp90-Cdc37-BRAF V600E, which are largely insensitive to kinase inhibitor, maintain a reservoir of mutant V600E that re-establishes signaling in the normal course of Hsp90 activity. Thus, the combined use of appropriate inhibitors that target the Hsp90-Cdc37-kinase complex, together with BRAF inhibitor, may be advantageous when targeting V600E-driven tumors. In the case of L597R, Cdc37 appears to act as a competitive inhibitor against non-dimerized L597R mutant, and vemurafenib may effectively inhibit L597R signaling as expected [45]. Furthermore, Hsp90 inhibition is effective against murine lung adenocarcinomas driven by the L858R, the equivalent L597R mutation of EGFR [55]. However, recent findings have also identified a sub-group of melanomas, which are driven by BRAF mutants with low-activity and which consequently rely on CRAF signaling [56]. Such mutant cell lines were particularly sensitive to the CRAF specific inhibitor sorafenib. This is an important consideration in targeting BRAF melanoma, and perhaps tumors driven by L597R, as it has been observed that elevated CRAF levels represent a mechanism for acquired resistance to BRAF inhibition [57]. Furthermore, targeting CRAF in a variety of melanoma cell lines was shown to decrease their viability, which appears to be mediated by Bcl-2 inhibition, rather than MAPK inhibition [58]. This may, therefore, provide a clear rationale for not only targeting non-V600E BRAF-driven tumors with BRAF inhibitors, but also targeting the CRAF-dependency of such cell lines. We, therefore, propose that targeting CRAF in L597R-driven tumors combined with BRAF, and perhaps also Hsp90 inhibition, may have a potential therapeutic benefit.

Supplementary Materials: The following supporting information can be downloaded at: https://www.mdpi.com/article/10.3390/biom12070905/s1, Figure S1: Constructs used in this study.

Author Contributions: Conceptualization, C.P.; methodology, D.M.B., C.P., R.M.L.M., J.O., K.L.I.M.D. and P.A.G.; formal analysis, C.P.; writing—original draft, C.P.; writing—review & editing, C.P., D.M.B., R.M.L.M., J.O., K.L.I.M.D. and P.A.G.; supervision, C.P. All authors have read and agreed to the published version of the manuscript.

Funding: The work was supported by the University of Sussex (RE009-23) and by the Wellcome Trust senior investigator award 095605/Z/11/Z (L.H.P.).

Institutional Review Board Statement: Not applicable.

Informed Consent Statement: Not applicable.

Data Availability Statement: Raw data for ITC and the thermal shift assay can be found at https://doi.org/10.25377/sussex.c.6061241. Constructs used in this study in Supplementary Figure S1.

Acknowledgments: I would like to thank Laurence H. Pearl (university of Sussex) for useful discussions and Emily Outwin (University of Sussex) for proof reading the manuscript.

Conflicts of Interest: The authors declare no conflict of interest.

References

1. Keramisanou, D.; Aboalroub, A.; Zhang, Z.; Liu, W.; Marshall, D.; Diviney, A.; Larsen, R.W.; Landgraf, R.; Gelis, I. Molecular Mechanism of Protein Kinase Recognition and Sorting by the Hsp90 Kinome-Specific Cochaperone Cdc37. *Mol. Cell* **2016**, *62*, 260–271. [CrossRef] [PubMed]
2. Xu, H. ATP-Driven Nonequilibrium Activation of Kinase Clients by the Molecular Chaperone Hsp90. *Biophys. J.* **2020**, *119*, 1538–1549. [CrossRef] [PubMed]
3. Hunter, T.; Poon, R.Y.C. Cdc37: A protein kinase chaperone? *Trends Cell Biol.* **1997**, *7*, 157–161. [CrossRef]
4. Roe, S.M.; Ali, M.M.; Meyer, P.; Vaughan, C.K.; Panaretou, B.; Piper, P.W.; Prodromou, C.; Pearl, L.H. The Mechanism of Hsp90 Regulation by the Protein Kinase-Specific Cochaperone p50(cdc37). *Cell* **2004**, *116*, 87–98. [CrossRef]
5. Verba, K.A.; Wang, R.Y.; Arakawa, A.; Liu, Y.; Shirouzu, M.; Yokoyama, S.; Agard, D.A. Atomic structure of Hsp90-Cdc37-Cdk4 reveals that Hsp90 traps and stabilizes an unfolded kinase. *Science* **2016**, *352*, 1542–1547. [CrossRef] [PubMed]
6. Zhang, Z.; Keramisanou, D.; Dudhat, A.; Pare, M.; Gelis, I. The C-terminal domain of human Cdc37 studied by solution NMR. *J. Biomol. NMR* **2015**, *63*, 315–321. [CrossRef] [PubMed]
7. Sreeramulu, S.; Jonker, H.R.; Langer, T.; Richter, C.; Lancaster, C.R.; Schwalbe, H. The human Cdc37·Hsp90 complex studied by heteronuclear NMR spectroscopy. *J. Biol. Chem.* **2009**, *284*, 3885–3896. [CrossRef]
8. Lemmon, M.A.; Schlessinger, J. Cell signaling by receptor tyrosine kinases. *Cell* **2010**, *141*, 1117–1134. [CrossRef]
9. Huse, M.; Kuriyan, J. The conformational plasticity of protein kinases. *Cell* **2002**, *109*, 275–282. [CrossRef]
10. Meharena, H.S.; Chang, P.; Keshwani, M.M.; Oruganty, K.; Nene, A.K.; Kannan, N.; Taylor, S.S.; Kornev, A.P. Deciphering the structural basis of eukaryotic protein kinase regulation. *PLoS Biol.* **2013**, *11*, e1001680. [CrossRef]
11. Kornev, A.P.; Taylor, S.S.; Ten Eyck, L.F. A helix scaffold for the assembly of active protein kinases. *Proc. Natl. Acad. Sci. USA* **2008**, *105*, 14377–14382. [CrossRef] [PubMed]
12. Hu, J.; Ahuja, L.G.; Meharena, H.S.; Kannan, N.; Kornev, A.P.; Taylor, S.S.; Shaw, A.S. Kinase regulation by hydrophobic spine assembly in cancer. *Mol. Cell. Biol.* **2015**, *35*, 264–276. [CrossRef] [PubMed]
13. Kim, J.; Ahuja, L.G.; Chao, F.A.; Xia, Y.; McClendon, C.L.; Kornev, A.P.; Taylor, S.S.; Veglia, G. A dynamic hydrophobic core orchestrates allostery in protein kinases. *Sci. Adv.* **2017**, *3*, e1600663. [CrossRef] [PubMed]
14. Cook, F.A.; Cook, S.J. Inhibition of RAF dimers: It takes two to tango. *Biochem. Soc. Trans.* **2021**, *49*, 237–251. [CrossRef]
15. Perdew, G.H.; Wiegand, H.; VandenHeuvel, J.P.; Mitchell, C.; Singh, S.S. A 50 kilodalton protein associated with raf and pp(60v-src) protein kinases is a mammalian homolog of the cell cycle control protein cdc37. *Biochemistry* **1997**, *36*, 3600–3607. [CrossRef]
16. Diedrich, B.; Rigbolt, K.T.; Roring, M.; Herr, R.; Kaeser-Pebernard, S.; Gretzmeier, C.; Murphy, R.F.; Brummer, T.; Dengjel, J. Discrete cytosolic macromolecular BRAF complexes exhibit distinct activities and composition. *EMBO J.* **2017**, *36*, 646–663. [CrossRef]
17. Polier, S.; Samant, R.S.; Clarke, P.A.; Workman, P.; Prodromou, C.; Pearl, L.H. ATP-competitive inhibitors block protein kinase recruitment to the Hsp90-Cdc37 system. *Nat. Chem. Biol.* **2013**, *9*, 307–312. [CrossRef]
18. Wartmann, M.; Davis, R.J. The native structure of the activated Raf protein kinase is a membrane-bound multi-subunit complex. *J. Biol. Chem.* **1994**, *269*, 6695–6701. [CrossRef]
19. Grbovic, O.M.; Basso, A.D.; Sawai, A.; Ye, Q.; Friedlander, P.; Solit, D.; Rosen, N. V600E B-Raf requires the Hsp90 chaperone for stability and is degraded in response to Hsp90 inhibitors. *Proc. Natl. Acad. Sci. USA* **2006**, *103*, 57–62. [CrossRef]
20. Sharp, S.; Workman, P. Inhibitors of the HSP90 molecular chaperone: Current status. *Adv. Cancer Res.* **2006**, *95*, 323–348.
21. Schulte, T.W.; Blagosklonny, M.V.; Ingui, C.; Neckers, L. Disruption of the Raf-1-Hsp90 molecular complex results in destabilization of Raf-1 and loss of Raf-1-Ras association. *J. Biol. Chem.* **1995**, *270*, 24585–24588. [CrossRef] [PubMed]
22. Nussinov, R.; Tsai, C.J.; Jang, H. Does Ras Activate Raf and PI3K Allosterically? *Front. Oncol.* **2019**, *9*, 1231. [CrossRef] [PubMed]
23. Kohler, M.; Brummer, T. B-Raf activation loop phosphorylation revisited. *Cell Cycle* **2016**, *15*, 1171–1173. [CrossRef] [PubMed]
24. Lavoie, H.; Therrien, M. Regulation of RAF protein kinases in ERK signalling. *Nat. Rev. Mol. Cell Biol.* **2015**, *16*, 281–298. [CrossRef] [PubMed]
25. Zhang, B.H.; Guan, K.L. Activation of B-Raf kinase requires phosphorylation of the conserved residues Thr598 and Ser601. *EMBO J.* **2000**, *19*, 5429–5439. [CrossRef] [PubMed]
26. Taylor, S.S.; Kornev, A.P. Protein kinases: Evolution of dynamic regulatory proteins. *Trends Biochem. Sci.* **2011**, *36*, 65–77. [CrossRef]
27. Negrao, M.V.; Raymond, V.M.; Lanman, R.B.; Robichaux, J.P.; He, J.; Nilsson, M.B.; Ng, P.K.S.; Amador, B.E.; Roarty, E.B.; Nagy, R.J.; et al. Molecular Landscape of BRAF-Mutant NSCLC Reveals an Association Between Clonality and Driver Mutations and Identifies Targetable Non-V600 Driver Mutations. *J. Thorac. Oncol.* **2020**, *15*, 1611–1623. [CrossRef]

28. Siligardi, G.; Panaretou, B.; Meyer, P.; Singh, S.; Woolfson, D.N.; Piper, P.W.; Pearl, L.H.; Prodromou, C. Regulation of Hsp90 ATPase activity by the co-chaperone Cdc37p/p50^{cdc37}. *J. Biol. Chem.* **2002**, *277*, 20151–20159. [CrossRef]
29. Tsai, J.; Lee, J.T.; Wang, W.; Zhang, J.; Cho, H.; Mamo, S.; Bremer, R.; Gillette, S.; Kong, J.; Haass, N.K.; et al. Discovery of a selective inhibitor of oncogenic B-Raf kinase with potent antimelanoma activity. *Proc. Natl. Acad. Sci. USA* **2008**, *105*, 3041–3046. [CrossRef]
30. Cochran, A.G.; Skelton, N.J.; Starovasnik, M.A. Tryptophan zippers: Stable, monomeric beta-hairpins. *Proc. Natl. Acad. Sci. USA* **2001**, *98*, 5578–5583. [CrossRef]
31. Shao, J.; Prince, T.; Hartson, S.D.; Matts, R.L. Phosphorylation of serine 13 is required for the proper function of the Hsp90 co-chaperone, Cdc37. *J. Biol. Chem.* **2003**, *278*, 38117–38120. [CrossRef] [PubMed]
32. Cantwell-Dorris, E.R.; O'Leary, J.J.; Sheils, O.M. BRAFV600E: Implications for carcinogenesis and molecular therapy. *Mol. Cancer Ther.* **2011**, *10*, 385–394. [CrossRef] [PubMed]
33. Yap, J.; Deepak, R.; Tian, Z.; Ng, W.H.; Goh, K.C.; Foo, A.; Tee, Z.H.; Mohanam, M.P.; Sim, Y.R.M.; Degirmenci, U.; et al. The stability of R-spine defines RAF inhibitor resistance: A comprehensive analysis of oncogenic BRAF mutants with in-frame insertion of alphaC-beta4 loop. *Sci. Adv.* **2021**, *7*, eabg0390. [CrossRef] [PubMed]
34. Noeparast, A.; Teugels, E.; Giron, P.; Verschelden, G.; De Brakeleer, S.; Decoster, L.; De Greve, J. Non-V600 BRAF mutations recurrently found in lung cancer predict sensitivity to the combination of Trametinib and Dabrafenib. *Oncotarget* **2017**, *8*, 60094–60108. [CrossRef]
35. Wan, P.T.; Garnett, M.J.; Roe, S.M.; Lee, S.; Niculescu-Duvaz, D.; Good, V.M.; Jones, C.M.; Marshall, C.J.; Springer, C.J.; Barford, D.; et al. Mechanism of activation of the RAF-ERK signaling pathway by oncogenic mutations of B-RAF. *Cell* **2004**, *116*, 855–867. [CrossRef]
36. Ng, P.K.; Li, J.; Jeong, K.J.; Shao, S.; Chen, H.; Tsang, Y.H.; Sengupta, S.; Wang, Z.; Bhavana, V.H.; Tran, R.; et al. Systematic Functional Annotation of Somatic Mutations in Cancer. *Cancer Cell* **2018**, *33*, 450–462. [CrossRef]
37. Sutto, L.; Gervasio, F.L. Effects of oncogenic mutations on the conformational free-energy landscape of EGFR kinase. *Proc. Natl. Acad. Sci. USA* **2013**, *110*, 10616–10621. [CrossRef]
38. Purba, E.R.; Saita, E.I.; Maruyama, I.N. Activation of the EGF Receptor by Ligand Binding and Oncogenic Mutations: The "Rotation Model". *Cells* **2017**, *6*, 13. [CrossRef]
39. Ruan, Z.; Kannan, N. Altered conformational landscape and dimerization dependency underpins the activation of EGFR by alphaC-beta4 loop insertion mutations. *Proc. Natl. Acad. Sci. USA* **2018**, *115*, E8162–E8171. [CrossRef]
40. Zanetti-Domingues, L.C.; Korovesis, D.; Needham, S.R.; Tynan, C.J.; Sagawa, S.; Roberts, S.K.; Kuzmanic, A.; Ortiz-Zapater, E.; Jain, P.; Roovers, R.C.; et al. The architecture of EGFR's basal complexes reveals autoinhibition mechanisms in dimers and oligomers. *Nat. Commun.* **2018**, *9*, 4325. [CrossRef]
41. Valley, C.C.; Arndt-Jovin, D.J.; Karedla, N.; Steinkamp, M.P.; Chizhik, A.I.; Hlavacek, W.S.; Wilson, B.S.; Lidke, K.A.; Lidke, D.S. Enhanced dimerization drives ligand-independent activity of mutant epidermal growth factor receptor in lung cancer. *Mol. Biol. Cell* **2015**, *26*, 4087–4099. [CrossRef] [PubMed]
42. Taha, T.; Khoury, R.; Brenner, R.; Nasrallah, H.; Shofaniyeh, I.; Yousef, S.; Agbarya, A. Treatment of Rare Mutations in Patients with Lung Cancer. *Biomedicines* **2021**, *9*, 534. [CrossRef] [PubMed]
43. Baik, C.S.; Myall, N.J.; Wakelee, H.A. Targeting BRAF-Mutant Non-Small Cell Lung Cancer: From Molecular Profiling to Rationally Designed Therapy. *Oncologist* **2017**, *22*, 786–796. [CrossRef] [PubMed]
44. Yao, Z.; Torres, N.M.; Tao, A.; Gao, Y.; Luo, L.; Li, Q.; de Stanchina, E.; Abdel-Wahab, O.; Solit, D.B.; Poulikakos, P.I.; et al. BRAF Mutants Evade ERK-Dependent Feedback by Different Mechanisms that Determine Their Sensitivity to Pharmacologic Inhibition. *Cancer Cell* **2015**, *28*, 370–383. [CrossRef] [PubMed]
45. Dahlman, K.B.; Xia, J.; Hutchinson, K.; Ng, C.; Hucks, D.; Jia, P.; Atefi, M.; Su, Z.; Branch, S.; Lyle, P.L.; et al. BRAF(L597) mutations in melanoma are associated with sensitivity to MEK inhibitors. *Cancer Discov.* **2012**, *2*, 791–797. [CrossRef] [PubMed]
46. Keramisanou, D.; Vasantha Kumar, M.V.; Boose, N.; Abzalimov, R.R.; Gelis, I. Assembly mechanism of early Hsp90-Cdc37-kinase complexes. *Sci. Adv.* **2022**, *8*, eabm9294. [CrossRef]
47. Gazdar, A.F.; Shigematsu, H.; Herz, J.; Minna, J.D. Mutations and addiction to EGFR: The Achilles 'heal' of lung cancers? *Trends Mol. Med.* **2004**, *10*, 481–486. [CrossRef]
48. Johnson, B.E.; Janne, P.A. Epidermal growth factor receptor mutations in patients with non-small cell lung cancer. *Cancer Res.* **2005**, *65*, 7525–7529. [CrossRef]
49. Lynch, T.J.; Bell, D.W.; Sordella, R.; Gurubhagavatula, S.; Okimoto, R.A.; Brannigan, B.W.; Harris, P.L.; Haserlat, S.M.; Supko, J.G.; Haluska, F.G.; et al. Activating mutations in the epidermal growth factor receptor underlying responsiveness of non-small-cell lung cancer to gefitinib. *N. Engl. J. Med.* **2004**, *350*, 2129–2139.
50. Paez, J.G.; Janne, P.A.; Lee, J.C.; Tracy, S.; Greulich, H.; Gabriel, S.; Herman, P.; Kaye, F.J.; Lindeman, N.; Boggon, T.J.; et al. EGFR mutations in lung cancer: Correlation with clinical response to gefitinib therapy. *Science* **2004**, *304*, 1497–1500. [CrossRef]
51. Shigematsu, H.; Gazdar, A.F. Somatic mutations of epidermal growth factor receptor signaling pathway in lung cancers. *Int. J. Cancer* **2006**, *118*, 257–262. [CrossRef]
52. Da Rocha Dias, S.; Friedlos, F.; Light, Y.; Springer, C.; Workman, P.; Marais, R. Activated B-RAF is an Hsp90 client protein that is targeted by the anticancer drug 17-allylamino-17-demethoxygeldanamycin. *Cancer Res.* **2005**, *65*, 10686–10691. [CrossRef] [PubMed]

53. Weber, C.K.; Slupsky, J.R.; Kalmes, H.A.; Rapp, U.R. Active Ras induces heterodimerization of cRaf and BRaf. *Cancer Res.* **2001**, *61*, 3595–3598. [PubMed]
54. Zhao, Y.; Yu, H.; Ida, C.M.; Halling, K.C.; Kipp, B.R.; Geiersbach, K.; Rumilla, K.M.; Gupta, S.; Lin, M.T.; Zheng, G. Assessment of RAS Dependency for BRAF Alterations Using Cancer Genomic Databases. *JAMA Netw. Open* **2021**, *4*, e2035479. [CrossRef] [PubMed]
55. Shimamura, T.; Li, D.; Ji, H.; Haringsma, H.J.; Liniker, E.; Borgman, C.L.; Lowell, A.M.; Minami, Y.; McNamara, K.; Perera, S.A.; et al. Hsp90 inhibition suppresses mutant EGFR-T790M signaling and overcomes kinase inhibitor resistance. *Cancer Res.* **2008**, *68*, 5827–5838. [CrossRef]
56. Smalley, K.S.; Xiao, M.; Villanueva, J.; Nguyen, T.K.; Flaherty, K.T.; Letrero, R.; Van Belle, P.; Elder, D.E.; Wang, Y.; Nathanson, K.L.; et al. CRAF inhibition induces apoptosis in melanoma cells with non-V600E BRAF mutations. *Oncogene* **2009**, *28*, 85–94. [CrossRef]
57. Montagut, C.; Sharma, S.V.; Shioda, T.; McDermott, U.; Ulman, M.; Ulkus, L.E.; Dias-Santagata, D.; Stubbs, H.; Lee, D.Y.; Singh, A.; et al. Elevated CRAF as a potential mechanism of acquired resistance to BRAF inhibition in melanoma. *Cancer Res.* **2008**, *68*, 4853–4861. [CrossRef]
58. Jilaveanu, L.B.; Zito, C.R.; Aziz, S.A.; Conrad, P.J.; Schmitz, J.C.; Sznol, M.; Camp, R.L.; Rimm, D.L.; Kluger, H.M. C-Raf is associated with disease progression and cell proliferation in a subset of melanomas. *Clin. Cancer Res.* **2009**, *15*, 5704–5713. [CrossRef]

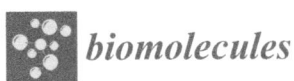 *biomolecules*

Review

Emerging Link between Tsc1 and FNIP Co-Chaperones of Hsp90 and Cancer

Sarah J. Backe [1,2,†], Rebecca A. Sager [1,2,†], Katherine A. Meluni [1,2], Mark R. Woodford [1,2,3], Dimitra Bourboulia [1,2,3] and Mehdi Mollapour [1,2,3,*]

1. Department of Urology, SUNY Upstate Medical University, Syracuse, NY 13210, USA; backes@upstate.edu (S.J.B.); sagerr@upstate.edu (R.A.S.); kam445@cornell.edu (K.A.M.); woodform@upstate.edu (M.R.W.); bourmpod@upstate.edu (D.B.)
2. Upstate Cancer Center, Upstate University Hospital, Syracuse, NY 13210, USA
3. Department of Biochemistry and Molecular Biology, SUNY Upstate Medical University, Syracuse, NY 13210, USA
* Correspondence: mollapom@upstate.edu
† These authors contributed equally to this work.

Abstract: Heat shock protein-90 (Hsp90) is an ATP-dependent molecular chaperone that is tightly regulated by a group of proteins termed co-chaperones. This chaperone system is essential for the stabilization and activation of many key signaling proteins. Recent identification of the co-chaperones FNIP1, FNIP2, and Tsc1 has broadened the spectrum of Hsp90 regulators. These new co-chaperones mediate the stability of critical tumor suppressors FLCN and Tsc2 as well as the various classes of Hsp90 kinase and non-kinase clients. Many early observations of the roles of FNIP1, FNIP2, and Tsc1 suggested functions independent of FLCN and Tsc2 but have not been fully delineated. Given the broad cellular impact of Hsp90-dependent signaling, it is possible to explain the cellular activities of these new co-chaperones by their influence on Hsp90 function. Here, we review the literature on FNIP1, FNIP2, and Tsc1 as co-chaperones and discuss the potential downstream impact of this regulation on normal cellular function and in human diseases.

Keywords: tuberous sclerosis complex (TSC); Tsc1 (hamartin); Tsc2 (tuberin); heat shock protein 90 (Hsp90); FNIP1; FNIP2; co-chaperones; cancer; renal cell carcinoma; kidney cancer

1. Introduction

Heat shock protein-90 (Hsp90) is a molecular chaperone essential for maintaining signaling competence in eukaryotic cells. Hsp90 is comprised of an N-terminal ATP binding domain, a middle domain for binding "client" proteins, and a site of constitutive dimerization at the carboxy-terminus [1–3]. Hsp90 function is coupled to its ability to bind and hydrolyze ATP and undergo a series of conformational changes known as the "chaperone cycle" [4,5]. This cycle facilitates the maturation and activation of more than 300-client proteins, including kinases, and non-kinases such as steroid hormone receptors, transcription factors, and tumor suppressors [6] (https://www.picard.ch/downloads/Hsp90interactors.pdf, accessed on 12 February 2022). A number of these Hsp90 client proteins participate in oncogenesis, and this chaperone machine is often co-opted by cancers to maintain deregulated signaling pathways and buffer the effect of pathogenic mutations [7–11]. The breadth of signaling pathways mediated by its clients makes Hsp90 an attractive therapeutic target and dozens of Hsp90-directed small molecules have been developed. In fact, there are 14-ATP-competitive Hsp90 inhibitors in ongoing clinical trials in various cancers (www.clinicaltrials.gov, accessed on 1 May 2022) [12].

The binding and dissociation of Hsp90-modulating proteins, termed co-chaperones, tailors Hsp90 to particular clients and provides directionality to the chaperone cycle [13–16]. To date, more than 25 Hsp90 co-chaperones with varying characteristics and classifications have been identified. Prior to the recent characterization of the three large co-chaperones Tsc1, FNIP1, and FNIP2 (hereon referred to as FNIP1/2), known Hsp90 regulatory proteins existed within the range of 20–100 kDa [15]. These three large co-chaperones are each approximately 130 kDa [17–21] and were originally identified as stabilizers of specific tumor suppressor proteins implicated in the mTOR pathway [17–19]. The co-chaperone function of FNIP1/2 and Tsc1 gives us an opportunity to reevaluate the previous published work from a new perspective. Here we review the functions and roles of FNIP1/2, and Tsc1 that have been reported, describe their functions as new co-chaperones of Hsp90, and retrospectively evaluate how new functions can help contextualize previous observations. We also review their roles in cancer and cellular response to Hsp90 inhibitors as well as their emerging role in chaperoning of tumor suppressors.

2. FNIP1 and FNIP2
2.1. FNIP1/2 Structure and Function

Folliculin interacting proteins 1 and 2 (FNIP1/2) are named after their first identification in complex with the tumor suppressor folliculin (FLCN) [17,18]. Loss of FLCN function is implicated in Birt-Hogg-Dubé (BHD) syndrome, a hereditary condition characterized by benign fibrofolliculomas, pulmonary cysts, spontaneous pneumothorax, and renal tumors, which are most often of hybrid oncocytic or chromophobe histology [22]. FLCN interacts with FNIP1/2 via its C-terminus, which stabilizes the FLCN protein. This mechanism is supported by the instability of C-terminally truncated FLCN protein products resulting from FLCN mutations identified in BHD [17,18,22,23] and indeed, many of these mutated FLCN proteins fail to associate with FNIPs and are targeted for proteasomal degradation [24]. Recently, portions of the FLCN:FNIP2 structure have been resolved by cryo-EM [25,26]. The structures support previous evidence that FLCN contains a GTPase activating protein (GAP) domain and interacts with FNIP2 through its C-terminal differentially expressed in normal and neoplastic cells (DENN) domain. Additionally, the N-terminal Longin domains of FLCN and FNIP2 proteins also interact, emphasizing the complex nature of the interaction between FLCN and the FNIPs [25,26]. Despite this well-supported finding, the precise mechanism by which FLCN stability is achieved had remained elusive. Our group demonstrated that FLCN is a client of Hsp90 and depends on the co-chaperone activity of FNIP1 and FNIP2 for loading to Hsp90 and thus stability [20].

FNIP1 shares 74% similarity and 49% identity with FNIP2 [18], and the majority of research on FNIPs is exclusive to FNIP1. Initially, FNIP1 was found to be phosphorylated by AMP-activated protein kinase (AMPK) as well as facilitate AMPK-mediated phosphorylation of FLCN [17]. AMPK is a negative regulator of the mTOR nutrient-sensing pathway, and FNIP1 was found to translocate from the cytoplasm to lysosomes under starvation conditions [27], therefore a role for FNIP1 in mTOR signaling was suggested, though direct, mechanistic evidence remains elusive (Figure 1).

2.2. FNIP1 Function in Skeletal Muscle and Adipocytes

One pathway in which the FNIP1-AMPK interaction has been interrogated is skeletal muscle fiber type specification. Broadly, type I muscle fibers are highly aerobic, express elevated levels of myoglobin, and have high mitochondrial function, while type II muscle fibers are comparatively lower in both and favor anaerobic glycolysis [28]. AMPK is known to regulate mitochondrial biogenesis via peroxisome proliferator-activated receptor-γ coactivator-1 α and β (PGC1α/PGC1β) and is activated under low energy conditions to suppress mTOR-dependent ATP utilization [29]. $FNIP1^{-/-}$ mice contain an abundance of type I muscle fibers, similar to mice with gain-of-function mutations in AMPK [30,31]. This suggests that at steady state FNIP1 suppresses AMPK and thus regulates mitochondrial biogenesis. Liu et al. furthered this line of inquiry by demonstrating that miR-499, an intron of the gene encoding the major slow-twitch type I myosin heavy chain (Myh7b), directly targets and inhibits translation of FNIP1 but not FNIP2 [32]. Similar results have been shown for miR-208b [33]. Interestingly, FNIP1-mediated AMPK inhibition can be reversed by the flavonoid dihydromyricetin, which causes a decrease in FNIP1 expression and reactivates AMPK-mediated mitochondrial biogenesis [34]. These data provide a mechanism that explains the FNIP1-dependent regulation of AMPK in skeletal muscle.

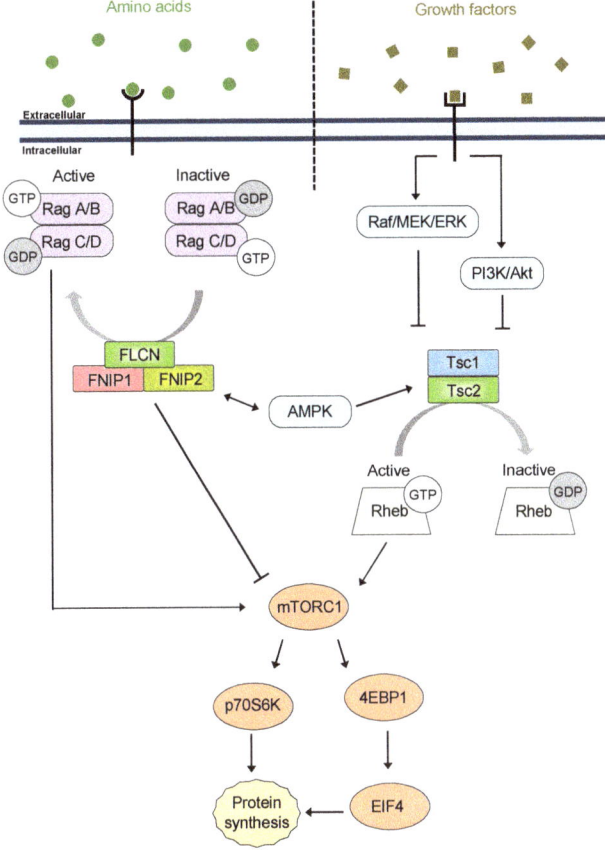

Figure 1. FNIPs and Tsc1 in the mTOR pathway. The mTOR pathway is a cellular signaling hub that integrates signals from several pathways and controls protein synthesis. A simplified schematic representation is shown to highlight the role of the FLCN/FNIPs and TSC complexes as mTOR regulators through GAP activity of RagA/C and Rheb, respectively.

FNIP1 regulation of AMPK may be cell-type dependent however, as recent work has demonstrated that FNIP1 regulates cellular respiration in adipocytes in an AMPK/mTOR independent manner [35]. Specifically, FNIP1 was shown to regulate intracellular Ca^{2+} levels through stabilization of sarcoendoplasmic reticulum calcium transport ATPase (SERCA) and increasing SERCA Ca^{2+} pump activity. This study also suggested a pivotal role for FNIP1 in regulating metabolism and glucose homeostasis in adipocytes, independent of AMPK/mTOR [35].

2.3. FNIP1 in Oxidative Stress

An interesting perspective on FNIP1 regulation of AMPK activity can be gained through an understanding of the factors governing FNIP1 protein dynamics. Recent work has shown that reductive stress promoted the degradation of FNIP1, but not FNIP2 [36]. The mechanism was traced to the chelation of Zn^{2+} by two reduced Cys residues in

FNIP1, which recruits CUL2$^{\text{FEM1B}}$ [36,37], the scaffold and recognition subunits of an E3-ubiquitin ligase complex [38]. Degradation of FNIP1 in this context promotes AMPK-PGC1α-mediated mitochondrial biogenesis to counteract reductive stress [36,37]. Interestingly, loss of FEM1B led to decreased lactate production [36], perhaps as a byproduct of FNIP1-dependent stabilization of FLCN and its recently described tumor suppressive effect on lactate dehydrogenase A [39].

2.4. FNIP1 Function in B-Cell Development

Another striking example of FNIP1 function is in lymphoid differentiation and maturation. Park et al. identified a pre-B cell "checkpoint" where loss of FNIP1 prevents mature B-cell development [40]. These cells were found to be sensitive to nutrient-deprivation-induced apoptosis seemingly due to failure of AMPK to suppress mTOR in the absence of FNIP1 [40]. Interestingly, FNIP1-deficient B-cell progenitors also exhibit elevated TFE3 transcription as well as increased lysosome function and autophagic flux [41]. Similarly, loss of FNIP1 prevents maturation of invariant natural killer T cells and increases their sensitivity to apoptosis [42]. *FNIP1* knockout was again determined to cause downstream mTOR activation, though in this case the effect is definitively indirect, as rapamycin treatment was not able to rescue the phenotype [42]. Concurrent research also found a marked pre-B cell blockade and confirmed that the effect stems from caspase activation and intrinsic apoptosis [43]. This effect was also observed in patients, as *FNIP1* mutation caused a clinically significant reduction in B cell numbers and hypogammaglobulinemia [44,45]. In addition to B-cell deficiency, FNIP1 loss leads to cardiomyopathy, which phenocopies AMPK gain-of-function mutations, consistent with a failure of FNIP1 to regulate AMPK-mediated signaling [46]. Taken together, these data support a role for FNIP1 as an indirect regulator of mTOR through its suppression of AMPK activity, and likely also via its positive regulation of FLCN [47].

2.5. Role of FNIP1/2 in Transcription

Recent work has also demonstrated the impact of the FLCN-FNIP1/2 system on transcriptional reprogramming. It is well established that loss of FLCN induces nuclear localization of the transcription factors TFE3/TFEB and promotes a gene expression program favorable for tumor growth [41,48–51]. Similarly, it was recently shown that simultaneous deletion of *FNIP1/2* in a human renal proximal tubular epithelial cell (RPTEC) line induced a TFE3-mediated gene signature [52]. This is in agreement with previous data showing that *FLCN*-null and *FNIP1/2*-null mice developed phenotypically indistinguishable enlarged polycystic kidneys [53,54]. Additionally, loss of either *FLCN* or *FNIP1/2* induced a STAT2-dependent interferon response transcriptional program, though the impact of interferon signaling in *FLCN*-deficient tumors is unclear [52].

Despite the progress reviewed here, it remains difficult to disentangle the cellular roles of FNIP1/2 in the regulation of AMPK and TFE3 from that of FLCN tumor suppressive function. Given this, it is possible that FNIP1/2-mediated regulation of Hsp90 activity provides a unifying explanation for FNIP-mediated cellular effects.

3. Tsc1

3.1. Structure and Function of the Tsc1/2 Complex

Tuberous Sclerosis Complex (TSC) is an autosomal dominant genetic syndrome caused by mutations in either the *TSC1* or *TSC2* tumor suppressors. In addition to neural associations that include epilepsy, subependymal giant cell astrocytomas (SEGA), intellectual disability, and autism, TSC is also characterized by cutaneous, pulmonary, and renal manifestations, similar to BHD [23,55,56]. These include facial fibrofolliculomas, pulmonary lymphangiomyomatosis, and renal angiomyolipomas (AML). The *TSC2* gene was cloned first in 1993 followed by the non-homologous *TSC1* gene in 1997 [19,57]. The Tsc1 and Tsc2 proteins, also known as hamartin and tuberin, respectively, were then shown to directly interact and form a complex [58]. The 130 kDa Tsc1 and 200 kDa Tsc2 proteins share no homology with each other [59]. Recently, partial structures of this complex were resolved by cryo-EM and revealed an elongated structure with a 2:2 stoichiometry. Further, Tsc1 was consistently found to have a coiled-coil domain which mediated Tsc1 dimerization and interaction with Tsc2 in vitro [60–62]. This is in contrast to a previous study using a yeast two-hybrid system which identified Tsc1 residues 302–430 as the critical region for Tsc2 interaction [63]. Tsc2 interaction with Tsc1 was primarily mediated through the N-terminal Tsc2-HEAT repeat domain, which is consistent with previous findings [60,62,63]. Furthermore, Tsc1 was required for Tsc2 maximal GAP activity likely through proper positioning of the Tsc2 catalytic asparagine-thumb [62].

The Tsc1/2 complex was demonstrated to inhibit mTOR signaling through the GAP activity of Tsc2 towards Rheb [64–66] (Figure 1). The effect of Tsc2 was greatly potentiated by the presence of Tsc1. In this TSC complex, Tsc1 has been shown to be important for the stabilization of Tsc2, preventing its interaction with the HERC1 ubiquitin ligase and its ubiquitination [67,68]. Early identification of Tsc1 and Tsc2 in complex and the role of this complex in the mTOR pathway focused a large portion of the TSC literature on this function and does not address separable functions of Tsc1 and Tsc2.

3.2. Separable Functions of Tsc1 and Tsc2

There are a number of differences in Tsc1 and Tsc2 function that have been identified, as well as mTOR-independent functions. Early reports suggested that although Tsc1 and Tsc2 often co-localize, the subcellular locations as well as tissue and organ expression patterns of Tsc1 and Tsc2 are not identical [69]. Germline mutations in *TSC1* cause a similar but not identical phenotype to *TSC2* mutations in animal models, suggesting commonalities to the pathways involved but some differences as well [70]. Renal tumors developed in heterozygous *TSC1* mice at a slower rate than in $TSC2^{+/-}$ mice. In addition to renal cystadenomas, $TSC1^{+/-}$ mice also develop liver hemangiomas, which are more common and more severe in female mice, demonstrating sex-dependent lethality [71]. Concordantly, an analysis of patients in the TOSCA database (TuberOus SClerosis registry to increase disease Awareness) revealed that female patients were significantly more likely to develop renal AML and experience hemorrhage [72]. Sex-dependent and estrogen linked effects exclusive to Tsc1 can also be seen in mammary development. Conditional Tsc1 loss in mammary epithelium impaired mammary development through suppression of Akt, ER, and cell cycle regulators and did not lead to tissue hyperplasia [73]. Moderate overexpression of Tsc1 also enhances overall health and cardiovascular health in an animal model and improves survival only in female mice [74]. Tsc1 and Tsc2 have also been shown to have separable functions in both cell signaling and cell cycle control [75,76]. Milolaza et al. describe the effect of Tsc1 and Tsc2 on the G1 to S phase transition of the cell cycle. Tsc1 and Tsc2 control cell proliferation independent of each other, and only Tsc2 function is affected by p27 expression [75]. Further evidence for separate functions of Tsc1 and Tsc2 comes from microarray and proteomic approaches, which reveal that each TSC gene triggers substantially different cellular responses [77–82].

3.3. mTOR Independent Functions of Tsc1

While the effects of Tsc1 loss are often ascribed to increased mTOR signaling and are at least partially responsive to rapamycin, there are also mTOR independent functions of Tsc1 that have been reported. Tsc1 haploinsufficiency without mTOR activation was shown to lead to renal cyst formation in $TSC1^{+/-}$ mice [83]. It has also recently been demonstrated that p21 activated kinase 2 (PAK2) is an effector of the Tsc1/Tsc2 complex. Loss of either Tsc1 or Tsc2 promotes hyperactivity of PAK2 downstream of Rheb, but independent of mTOR, as demonstrated by insensitivity to rapamycin treatment [84]. Tsc1 and Tsc2 also differentially modulate the cytoskeleton. $TSC1^{-/-}$ and $TSC2^{-/-}$ MEFs demonstrate rapamycin insensitive increase in number and length of cilia [85] whereas only Tsc2 loss promotes an mTOR-dependent pro-migratory phenotype [86]. On the other hand, Tsc1 loss was shown to dysregulate tight junction development in an mTOR independent manner [87]. Collectively, these studies suggest a role for Tsc1 in cell integrity independent of mTOR.

Furthermore, it has long been observed that clinical features of TSC across multiple organ systems are more severe in patients with mutations in *TSC2* than in patients with *TSC1* mutations [88–90]. There is a higher incidence of intellectual disability in patients with *TSC2* mutations, and it has been suggested that severity of disability may correlate with predicted effects of mutations on Tsc1 and Tsc2 protein [91–93]. Epilepsy generally exhibits an earlier onset and is also more severe as a result of *TSC2* mutations [94,95]. Similarly, the mean age at diagnosis for patients with renal AML was lower in patients with *TSC2* mutations. Additionally, patients with *TSC2* mutations had a higher occurrence of renal AML, multiple renal cysts and polycystic kidney disease compared to patients with *TSC1* mutations [72]. In a mouse model, conditional knockout (CKO) of *TSC2* in GFAP-positive cells also produces a more severe epilepsy phenotype than *TSC1* CKO [96]. Additionally, it has been proposed that perhaps TSC resulting from *TSC1* mutation is not less common than *TSC2* disease but that it is less frequently diagnosed due to the milder clinical features [97].

Collectively, this evidence suggests a role for Tsc1 outside the TSC complex and mTOR signaling. Due to the described role of Tsc1 in stabilizing Tsc2 and protecting it from ubiquitination we questioned whether this protective role involved molecular chaperones and whether Tsc1 was involved in chaperoning Tsc2. In fact, Tsc2 is a client of Hsp90, and Tsc1 is a co-chaperone [21].

4. Regulation of Hsp90 Chaperone Function by Co-Chaperones

The action of co-chaperones towards Hsp90 generally meets one or more of the following criteria: (1) scaffolding of client proteins to Hsp90 (e.g., Hop, p50^{Cdc37}); (2) modulation of Hsp90 ATPase activity (e.g., Aha1); (3) stabilization of specific chaperone complexes (e.g., p23) and are not themselves dependent on Hsp90 for stability [98]. We have shown that the newly identified large co-chaperones FNIP1/2 and Tsc1 are able to satisfy at least two of these observed co-chaperone functions (Figure 2). Indeed, we have a unique opportunity to advance our understanding of the function and effect of these proteins as we reconcile their known functions with their roles as Hsp90 co-chaperones.

Hsp90-dependent maturation and activation of client proteins relies on a continuum of regulated conformational changes of Hsp90 coupled to ATP hydrolysis. As currently understood, there are several "stages" to a generalized chaperone cycle. Initially, immature clients bind to the early chaperone heat shock protein 70 (Hsp70) and the Hsp70-Hsp90 organizing protein (Hop) forms a bridge to the "open" conformation of Hsp90, allowing the transfer of a client protein to Hsp90 [99]. ATP subsequently binds to the amino-terminal nucleotide binding pocket, and concurrent binding of the Activator of Hsp90 ATPase (Aha1) displaces Hop and induces transient N-domain dimerization, forming the "closed 1" state. Aha1 binds to the N-domain as well as the middle domain of Hsp90 and greatly increases the weak intrinsic ATPase activity of Hsp90 [100]. Interaction of the co-chaperone p23 with the N-domain of Hsp90 displaces Aha1 and stabilizes the "closed and twisted" conformation (closed 2). This allows completion of ATP hydrolysis, followed by release of a mature client protein and the return of Hsp90 to the open conformation [101–103].

The complement of co-chaperones that regulate Hsp90 during a single chaperone cycle is largely dependent on the individual requirements of the client protein [104]. For example, kinase clients are loaded to Hsp90 by the co-chaperone Cdc37, a decelerator of Hsp90 ATPase activity, and protein phosphatase 5 (PP5)-mediated dephosphorylation of Cdc37 is required for their release [105,106]. Alternatively, overexpression of Aha1 greatly decreases the folding of CFTR by accelerating the rate of Hsp90 ATP hydrolysis [107–109]. Similarly, steroid hormone receptors prefer a slower chaperone cycle and require the co-chaperone p23, which is known to decelerate the action of Hsp90 [5,110–112]. In fact, GR itself is capable of modulating the conformation of Hsp90 such that Hsp90 ATPase activity decreases [113], demonstrating the degree of specificity that can be achieved by modulation of Hsp90 complexes [15].

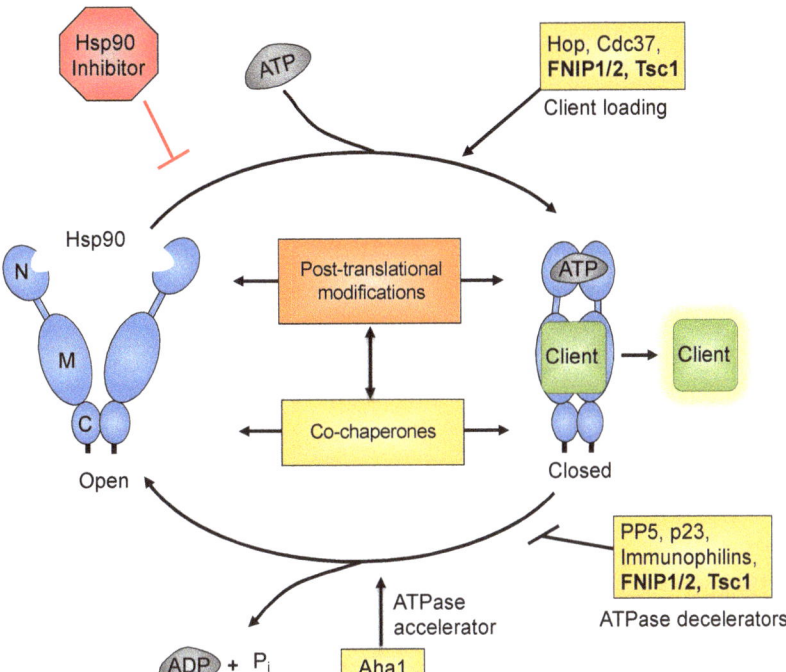

Figure 2. The Hsp90 chaperone cycle. Open Hsp90 is dimerized only through contacts in the CTD. ATP binding and an ordered series of conformational changes allow Hsp90 to adopt a closed conformation, which is N-terminally dimerized. ATP hydrolysis leads Hsp90 to return to the open conformation and begins another chaperone cycle. Throughout the chaperone cycle co-chaperones bind to Hsp90 and regulate its function. PTM of Hsp90 and PTM of co-chaperones provide further regulation of the chaperone cycle.

5. FNIP1/2 and Tsc1: New Co-Chaperones of Hsp90

Recent reports from Mollapour's group demonstrated that the tumor suppressors FLCN and Tsc2 are Hsp90 clients [20,21]. As FNIP1/2 and Tsc1, respectively, have established roles as guardians of these tumor suppressors [17,18,67,68], it follows that there may be a role for molecular chaperones in mediating FLCN and Tsc2 stability. Indeed FNIP1/2 and Tsc1 both interact with Hsp90 and Hsp70, as well as with overlapping complements of Hsp90 co-chaperones including PP5, Cdc37, Hop, and p23 and behave as Hsp90 co-chaperones [20,21] (Figure 3). These reports also demonstrate a role for these new co-chaperones in regulating both kinase and non-kinase clients, as well as provide clues to their chronology in the overall chaperone cycle.

FNIP1 and Tsc1 share a number of striking similarities in their actions as co-chaperones. Both FNIP1 and Tsc1 exhibit complex binding to Hsp90; contacts are made using multiple domains of these co-chaperones as well as multiple domains of Hsp90. The most well characterized interactions thus far however are that of FNIP1 and Tsc1 binding the Hsp90 middle domain via their carboxy-termini. It is through this interaction that they decelerate Hsp90 ATPase activity and compete with the accelerating co-chaperone Aha1 for Hsp90 occupancy. In addition to increasing the dwell time of ATP (and thus client proteins) on Hsp90, interaction with these large co-chaperones also increases Hsp90 binding to its ATP-competitive inhibitors [20,21,114].

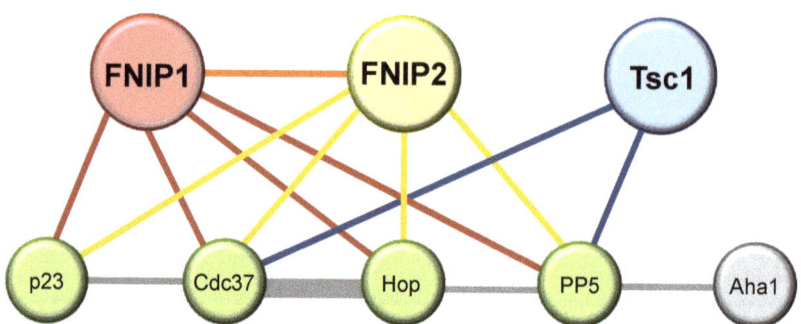

Figure 3. FNIPs and Tsc1 co-chaperone interaction network. Hsp90 co-chaperones are represented by colored circles. Interactions between co-chaperones are denoted by colored lines. FNIP1 interactions are colored red; FNIP2, yellow; Tsc1, blue; other, gray.

While the overall pattern of how FNIP1 and Tsc1 interact with Hsp90 is similar there are key differences between them. The C-terminal fragment of Tsc1 (Tsc1-D) binds to Hsp90 with higher affinity than does the C-terminal fragment of FNIP1 (FNIP1-D). Similarly, Tsc1-D is a potent inhibitor of Hsp90 ATPase activity and very effectively competes with Aha1 for Hsp90 binding as evidenced by in vitro competition experiments. FNIP1 and Tsc1 can also be distinguished by the complement of co-chaperones with which they interact therefore, providing clues to their distinct roles in the chaperone cycle. While neither is found in complex with Aha1, Tsc1 is able to interact with PP5 and Cdc37, whereas FNIP1/2 can additionally be found in complexes containing p23 and Hop (Figure 3). This may demonstrate some promiscuity of FNIPs, but likely reflects the necessity for FNIPs to work in concert with other co-chaperones, while Tsc1 may be capable of modulating Hsp90 independently. This potentially explains the observation that Tsc1 is a much more potent decelerator of Hsp90 ATP hydrolysis than FNIP1/2 [20,21,114]. Interestingly, Tsc1 also inhibits the ATPase activity of another molecular chaperone, Hsp70, in vitro [115]. Whether FNIPs share this function remains unknown.

Despite their shared role in facilitating chaperoning of both kinase and non-kinase clients, FNIP1/2 and Tsc1 over-expression and deletion have different effects. Non-kinase clients are destabilized upon knockdown/knockout of FNIP1/2 or Tsc1 and stabilized with overexpression of the co-chaperones. Interestingly, FNIP1/2 knockdown or overexpression affects the kinase clients in a comparable manner as the non-kinase clients, however overexpression or absence of Tsc1 both negatively affect kinase client stability [20,21]. This may be due to the participation of FNIP1/2 with a variety of chaperone complexes, whereas the semi-exclusive nature of Tsc1 co-chaperone activity disrupts the delicate balance of Hsp90 co-chaperone dynamics.

5.1. FNIP1/2 and Tsc1 in the Chaperone Cycle

This large body of work on co-chaperone dynamics allows us to propose a model of FNIPs and Tsc1 co-chaperones in the Hsp90 chaperone cycle. Our previous work demonstrates that FNIPs and Tsc1 interact with Hsp70 in addition to Hsp90, and FNIP1 and Tsc1 are essential for scaffolding FLCN and Tsc2, respectively, to Hsp90 (Figure 4A,B) [20,21,23]. Subsequent ATP binding triggers conformational changes leading to the N-terminally dimerized 'closed' conformation of Hsp90 (Figure 4C) [116–119]. We have previously shown that Tsc1 and FNIP1 are not found in complex with Aha1 and that phosphorylation of Aha1-Y223 displaces Tsc1 from Hsp90 (Figure 4D) [20,21,109]. p23 is a late-acting co-chaperone that locks Hsp90 in the closed conformation to allow proper client maturation (Figure 4E) [103,120–127]. FNIP1/2, but not Tsc1, are found in complex with p23 (Figure 4F) [20,21]. We propose that p23:FNIP1:FNIP2 holds the matured client in its active conformation until there is a signal for client release, resetting Hsp90 for another cycle (Figure 4G,H).

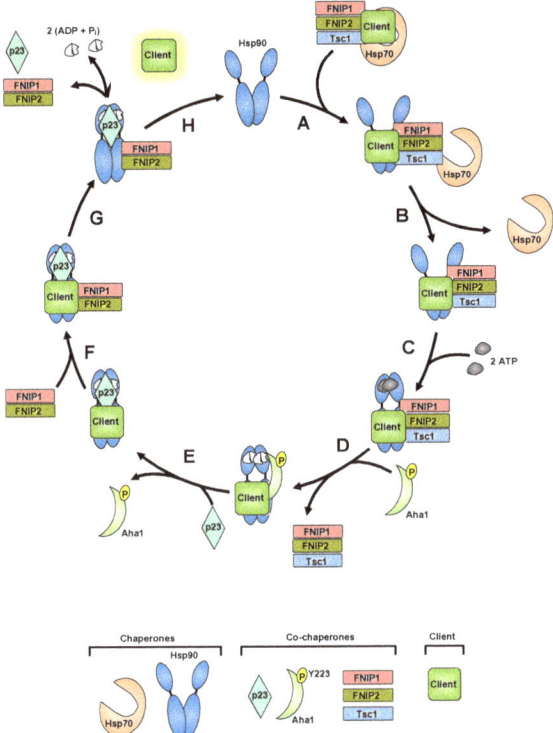

Figure 4. FNIPs and Tsc1 in the Hsp90 chaperone cycle. (A) FNIPs and Tsc1 co-chaperones scaffold a client from Hsp70 to Hsp90. (B) Hsp70 dissociates from the complex. (C) ATP binding triggers Hsp90 conformational rearrangements resulting in the 'closed' conformation. (D) Aha1 phosphorylated at Y223 displaces FNIPs/Tsc1 co-chaperones from the Hsp90 complex and promotes ATP hydrolysis to ADP + Pi. (E) p23 binds and stabilizes the closed conformation of Hsp90. (F) FNIP co-chaperones bind to the Hsp90:client:p23 complex to promote client maturation. (G) The complex dissociates releasing the mature client. (H) Hsp90 is reset to begin another cycle.

5.2. FNIPs, Tsc1 and the Chaperone Code

Hsp90 and its co-chaperones' functions are heavily regulated by post-translational modifications (PTM), collectively known as the 'chaperone code' [128,129]. An additional layer of Hsp90 regulation via FNIP1 is provided through FNIP1 post-translational modification. Recent work by our group identified a series of serine residues (S938, S939, S941, S946, and S948) in the Hsp90-binding region of the FNIP1 carboxy-terminus that are phosphorylated in a relay manner by casein-kinase 2 (CK2) [114]. This sequential phosphorylation promotes FNIP1 interaction with Hsp90 while dephosphorylation of these residues by the Hsp90 co-chaperone PP5 disrupts the Hsp90-FNIP1 complex. Furthermore, stepwise phosphorylation of FNIP1 provides gradual inhibition of Hsp90 ATPase activity and therefore increased activity of a subset of both kinase and non-kinase clients [114].

These new co-chaperones also affect Hsp90 binding to its ATP-competitive inhibitors. Generally, there is an inverse relationship between the rate of ATP hydrolysis and the ability of Hsp90 to bind ATP-competitive inhibitors [20,21,109]. Overexpression of FNIP1/2 or

Tsc1 decreases Hsp90 ATPase activity, thus increasing Hsp90 binding to its inhibitors. As expected, Hsp90 inhibitor binding is decreased upon knockdown of FNIP1/2 or loss of Tsc1 [20,21,114,130]. Interestingly, approximately 15% of bladder cancers have loss-of-function mutations in Tsc1. Tsc1 loss causes hypo-acetylation of Hsp90 on K407 and K419 leading to decreased binding of Hsp90 to its inhibitors, demonstrating another mechanism of Tsc1-mediated regulation of Hsp90 [130]. The precise mechanism of how Tsc1 loss compromises Hsp90 acetylation remains unknown, however it is important to note that Hsp90 acetylation can be restored by histone-deacetylase (HDAC) inhibition, sensitizing *TSC1*-null cells to Hsp90 inhibitors [130].

Targeting Hsp90 in cancer cell lines induces apoptosis, and Hsp90 inhibitors have been found to preferentially accumulate in cancer cells versus normal cells [131–135]. FNIP1/2 were found overexpressed in cancer cell lines originating from several different tissues, and knockdown decreased sensitivity of these cancers to Hsp90 inhibition [20]. This increased expression of FNIP1/2 provides one potential mechanism to explain the tumor selectivity of Hsp90 inhibitors. Similarly, bladder cancer cells lacking functional Tsc1 fail to accumulate Hsp90 inhibitors and are less sensitive to Hsp90 inhibition than those with wild-type Tsc1 [130].

Collectively, these studies provide support for a new functional role for the tumor suppressor Tsc1 and FNIP1/2 as co-chaperones of Hsp90. As Hsp90 co-chaperones the protective function of Tsc1 and the FNIPs goes beyond mediating stability of Tsc2 and FLCN, respectively, and provides insight into a larger role for these proteins in the cellular context.

6. A New Perspective: FNIPs, Tsc1, and mTOR

Early connection of FNIP1/2 and Tsc1 to the mTOR nutrient-sensing pathway has narrowed the focus of research conducted on these proteins. Recent research has demonstrated that FNIP1/2 and Tsc1 act as co-chaperones of Hsp90. This allows us to reevaluate the previous published work with a new perspective.

6.1. FNIP1/2 Co-Chaperone Activity Contributes to mTOR Regulation

As reviewed in this text, FNIP1 negatively regulates AMPK activity. Since the α and γ subunits of AMPK are known clients of Hsp90 [136], the effect of FNIP1 on AMPK could be mediated through the Hsp90 chaperone (Figure 5). In support of this idea, microarray data show that B220$^+$CD43$^+$ pre-B cells from $FNIP1^{-/-}$ mice demonstrate a dramatic increase in expression of AMPK-responsive genes [40]. These data would suggest a role for FNIP1 in activation of mTOR, however we posit that this mechanism may actually be more complicated. First, mTOR is also an Hsp90 client protein [137] and will be subject to the influence of Hsp90 co-chaperones as with any other client protein. Second, it is likely that loss of FLCN is actually responsible for mTOR activation, as is suggested by Baba et al., whose data show that the induction of mTOR is mild in $FNIP1^{-/-}$ mice as compared to $FLCN^{-/-}$ and that $FNIP1$ deletion fails to phenocopy BHD syndrome [17,43,54]. Concordantly, FNIP co-chaperone activity toward FLCN can explain the observation that non-degradable FNIP2 enhances FLCN expression and thus suppresses tumorigenesis in a BHD mouse xenograft model [138]. Together, these data highlight that the co-chaperone activity of FNIP1/2 is essential for FLCN-mediated mTOR suppression, but also underscore our inability to reconcile this observation with the current understanding of FNIP1/2 function.

6.2. Co-Chaperone Activity of Tsc1 in Regulation of mTOR

The newly identified role for Tsc1 as an Hsp90 co-chaperone may help clarify some of the phenotypic differences as a result of Tsc1 versus Tsc2 mutation. Due to its function as a co-chaperone, Tsc1 loss would trigger effects on many cellular pathways, not just mTOR signaling. This could explain the finding of renal cyst formation in $TSC1^{+/-}$ mice, as well as provide insight into the pro-migratory phenotype seen only in $TSC2^{-/-}$ MEFs [83,86]. Furthermore, Tsc1 loss, but not Tsc2 loss, causes hypo-acetylation of Hsp90 further demonstrating a role for Tsc1 independent of both Tsc2 and mTOR [130]. The loss of Tsc1 has a dramatic negative effect on Hsp90 kinase and non-kinase clients, including Tsc2. It is reasonable therefore that loss of Tsc1 co-chaperone activity manifests itself independently of the mTOR pathway.

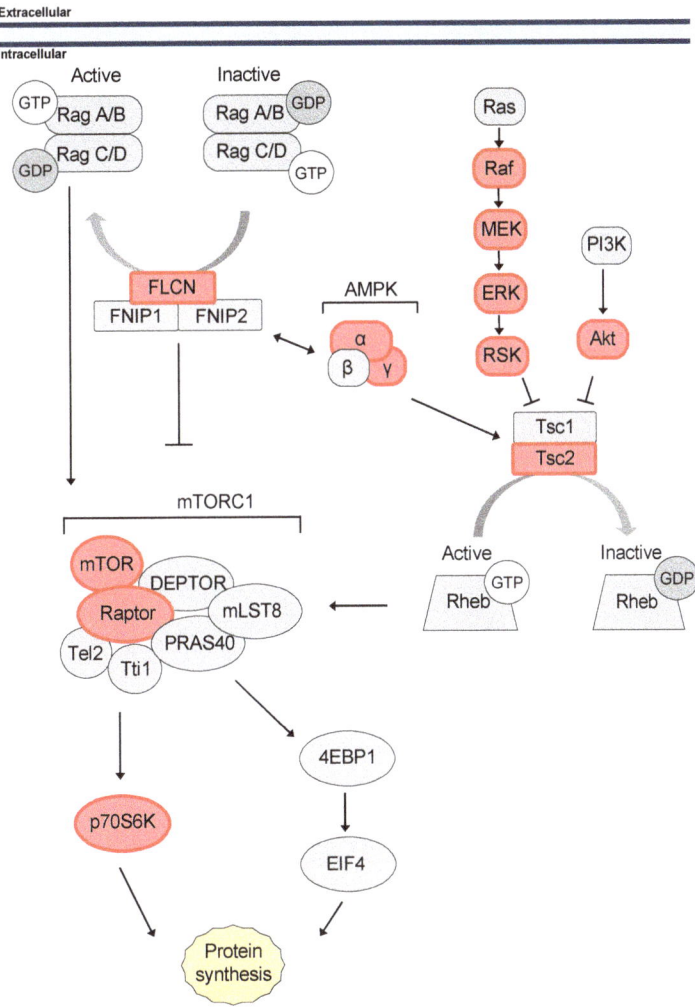

Figure 5. Hsp90 clients in the mTOR pathway. A schematic representation of the mTOR pathway highlighting the components that are Hsp90 clients (red).

As discussed above, Tsc1 loss has long been known to lead to a less severe phenotype than Tsc2 loss both in patients as well as animal models [88–90,94–97]. Canonically, Tsc2 loss leads to upregulation of mTOR signaling due to release of the inhibitory signal from Tsc2-Rheb [139]. Activation and phosphorylation of mTOR and its downstream targets as well as other pathway components such as Akt has been shown to be dependent on Hsp90; in fact, many mTOR pathway components are clients of Hsp90 [140–143] (Figure 5). Activation of the mTOR pathway is therefore dependent on proper function of the Hsp90 chaperone system. Perhaps the milder phenotype seen with Tsc1 loss is a result of the loss of co-chaperone activity toward Hsp90. Upon Tsc1 loss, Tsc2 is destabilized leading to increased mTOR activity; however, the other proteins in the mTOR pathway that are Hsp90 clients would also be destabilized, potentially mitigating the downstream effect.

Rapalogs, such as sirolimus and everolimus, are rapamycin derivatives that are commonly used to treat patients with BHD and TSC. Armed with the information of the role of Hsp90 in BHD and TSC, perhaps preclinical examination of Hsp90 inhibitors in combination with rapalogs is warranted. In fact, Hsp90 inhibitors have been shown to synergize with PI3K/Akt/mTOR inhibitors in preclinical studies for the treatment of various cancers [144–146]. In line with this, Di Nardo et al. identified the heat-shock machinery as an exploitable target in Tsc2-deficient neurons [147]. Accordingly, one study has evaluated mTOR and Hsp90 inhibitors in combination in *TSC1* or *TSC2* deficient cancer models. Unfortunately, the results were inconsistent between cell line and mouse xenograft models, as synergism between Hsp90 inhibitor (GB) and mTOR inhibitors (Torin2, rapamycin) in cell lines did not translate to increased efficacy over monotherapy in xenograft models [148]. Taken together, these studies demonstrate the potential therapeutic benefit of co-targeting Hsp90 and mTOR in BHD and TSC patients. However, further investigation is needed.

7. Specialized Function of FNIP1/2 and Tsc1: Chaperoning Tumor Suppressors

An important and perhaps specialized role for these new Hsp90 co-chaperones is in the chaperoning of tumor suppressors. FLCN and Tsc2 are additions to the growing list of tumor suppressors that interact with Hsp90. The transcription factor p53 was the first reported tumor suppressor client of Hsp90 [149–152]. Since 1996, 17 functional Hsp90 interactions with both kinase and non-kinase tumor suppressors have been discovered (Table 1) [20,21,149,153–163]. Furthermore, several tumor suppressors including, VHL, BDC2, LKB1, p53, FLCN and LATS1/2 were found to interact with Hsp90 co-chaperones including, Hop, p23, Hsp110, Cdc37, PP5, and CHIP [20,23,150,154,159,160,164–167]. As FNIP1/2 and Tsc1 scaffold the tumor suppressors FLCN and Tsc2 to Hsp90, it follows that these co-chaperones may participate in the chaperoning of additional Hsp90-dependent tumor suppressor clients. In line with this notion, Tsc1 was identified as a genetic interactor with VHL in HeLa cells highlighting the need for further exploration in this area [168].

Table 1. Relationships of known tumor suppressor-Hsp90 interactions.

Tumor Suppressor Gene	Relationship to Hsp90	References
ATM Kinase	Client	[153,169]
BMPR1A	Client	[161]
BRCA1/2	Client	[158,170,171]
DBC2	Client	[159]
FBXW7	Interactor	[161]
FLCN	Client	[20,23]
IRF1	Client	[156]
LATS1/2	Client	[162,167,172]
LKB1	Client	[154,173,174]
NDRG2	Interactor	[163]
SYK	Client	[155,175]
TNFAIP3	Interactor	[161,176]
TP53	Client	[8,103,149–152,164–166,177–187]
TSC1	Co-chaperone	[21,130]
TSC2	Client	[21]
VHL	Client	[160,188]
WT1	Client	[157]

Additionally, there is new evidence supporting a compensatory mechanism between FNIP1/2 and Tsc1 co-chaperone activity. FLCN traditionally requires interaction via its C-terminus to FNIP1/2 to mediate its stability. Tsc1, however, is capable of interacting with a truncated FLCN mutant and supporting a low level of expression in the absence of FNIP1/2 binding [23]. Unexpectedly, the truncated FLCN-L460QsX25 was still able to interact with Hsp90 even though it did not bind to its loading co-chaperone FNIP1. Overexpression of Tsc1, but not FNIP1 was capable of stabilizing expression of the mutant FLCN. Notably, Tsc1 interaction with Tsc2 was compromised in this model resulting in loss of Tsc2 tumor suppressive function. Loss of such a compensatory mechanism may also explain why deletion of *FNIP1* synergized with *TSC1* deletion to activate mTOR and subsequently resulted in accelerated renal cyst formation in mice [189]. These findings necessitate investigation into how these large co-chaperones mediate chaperoning of tumor suppressors and the impact of tumor suppressor mutations on this relationship.

8. Conclusions

Hsp90 is an important component of the cellular homeostatic machinery and is regulated by post-translational modification and interaction with co-chaperones. There are more than 25 known co-chaperones that serve several functions including modulating Hsp90 conformations, loading client proteins to Hsp90, and modifying the rate of ATP hydrolysis. New data has identified newly characterized roles for three proteins, FNIP1, FNIP2 and Tsc1, as large co-chaperones of Hsp90. Though these proteins have established roles in the regulation of tumor suppressor proteins FLCN and Tsc2, it seems that many of their other ascribed functions are potentially explained at least in part by their effect on Hsp90. A more thorough understanding of the action and interplay of these new, large co-chaperones may unveil clues that will aid in developing the next generation of cancer therapeutics.

Author Contributions: Conceptualization, M.M.; writing—original draft preparation, S.J.B., R.A.S. and M.R.W.; writing—review and editing, S.J.B., R.A.S., M.R.W., D.B. and M.M.; visualization, S.J.B. and K.A.M.; supervision, M.M.; funding acquisition, M.M. All authors have read and agreed to the published version of the manuscript.

Funding: This work was partly supported with funds from National Institute of General Medical Sciences of the National Institutes of Health under Award Number R35GM139584 (M.M.). The content is solely the responsibility of the authors and does not necessarily represent the official views of the National Institutes of Health. This work was also supported by Carol M. Baldwin Breast Cancer Fund (M.M.), SUNY Upstate Medical University, Upstate Foundation (M.M.).

Institutional Review Board Statement: Not applicable.

Informed Consent Statement: Not applicable.

Data Availability Statement: Not applicable.

Acknowledgments: We are grateful to W. Marston Linehan & Len Neckers (Urologic Oncology Branch, NCI, USA), David J Kwiatkowski (Harvard Medical School, USA) and Chris Prodromou (University of Sussex, UK) for their valuable discussion.

Conflicts of Interest: The authors declare no conflict of interest.

References

1. Prodromou, C.; Roe, S.M.; O'Brien, R.; Ladbury, J.E.; Piper, P.W.; Pearl, L.H. Identification and structural characterization of the ATP/ADP-binding site in the Hsp90 molecular chaperone. *Cell* **1997**, *90*, 65–75. [CrossRef]
2. Wegele, H.; Muschler, P.; Bunck, M.; Reinstein, J.; Buchner, J. Dissection of the contribution of individual domains to the ATPase mechanism of Hsp90. *J. Biol. Chem.* **2003**, *278*, 39303–39310. [CrossRef] [PubMed]
3. Schopf, F.H.; Biebl, M.M.; Buchner, J. The HSP90 chaperone machinery. *Nat. Rev. Mol. Cell Biol.* **2017**, *18*, 345–360. [CrossRef] [PubMed]
4. Panaretou, B.; Prodromou, C.; Roe, S.M.; O'Brien, R.; Ladbury, J.E.; Piper, P.W.; Pearl, L.H. ATP binding and hydrolysis are essential to the function of the Hsp90 molecular chaperone in vivo. *EMBO J.* **1998**, *17*, 4829–4836. [CrossRef] [PubMed]
5. Prodromou, C. The 'active life' of Hsp90 complexes. *Biochim. Biophys. Acta* **2012**, *1823*, 614–623. [CrossRef]
6. Prodromou, C.; Bjorklund, D.M. Advances towards Understanding the Mechanism of Action of the Hsp90 Complex. *Biomolecules* **2022**, *12*, 600. [CrossRef] [PubMed]
7. Tsutsumi, S.; Beebe, K.; Neckers, L. Impact of heat-shock protein 90 on cancer metastasis. *Future Oncol.* **2009**, *5*, 679–688. [CrossRef] [PubMed]
8. Boysen, M.; Kityk, R.; Mayer, M.P. Hsp70- and Hsp90-Mediated Regulation of the Conformation of p53 DNA Binding Domain and p53 Cancer Variants. *Mol. Cell* **2019**, *74*, 831–843. [CrossRef]

9. Calderwood, S.K.; Gong, J. Heat Shock Proteins Promote Cancer: It's a Protection Racket. *Trends Biochem. Sci.* **2016**, *41*, 311–323. [CrossRef]
10. Xu, Y.; Singer, M.A.; Lindquist, S. Maturation of the tyrosine kinase c-src as a kinase and as a substrate depends on the molecular chaperone Hsp90. *Proc. Natl. Acad. Sci. USA* **1999**, *96*, 109–114. [CrossRef] [PubMed]
11. Neckers, L. Hsp90 inhibitors as novel cancer chemotherapeutic agents. *Trends Mol. Med.* **2002**, *8*, S55–S61. [CrossRef]
12. Xiao, Y.; Liu, Y. Recent Advances in the Discovery of Novel HSP90 Inhibitors: An Update from 2014. *Curr. Drug Targets* **2020**, *21*, 302–317. [CrossRef]
13. Cox, M.B.; Johnson, J.L. The Role of p23, Hop, Immunophilins, and Other Co-chaperones in Regulating Hsp90 Function. *Methods Mol. Biol.* **2011**, *787*, 45–66. [CrossRef] [PubMed]
14. Ratzke, C.; Hellenkamp, B.; Hugel, T. Four-colour FRET reveals directionality in the Hsp90 multicomponent machinery. *Nat. Commun.* **2014**, *5*, 4192. [CrossRef] [PubMed]
15. Sahasrabudhe, P.; Rohrberg, J.; Biebl, M.M.; Rutz, D.A.; Buchner, J. The Plasticity of the Hsp90 Co-chaperone System. *Mol. Cell* **2017**, *67*, 947–961.e5. [CrossRef] [PubMed]
16. Dahiya, V.; Rutz, D.A.; Moessmer, P.; Muhlhofer, M.; Lawatscheck, J.; Rief, M.; Buchner, J. The switch from client holding to folding in the Hsp70/Hsp90 chaperone machineries is regulated by a direct interplay between co-chaperones. *Mol. Cell* **2022**. [CrossRef] [PubMed]
17. Baba, M.; Hong, S.B.; Sharma, N.; Warren, M.B.; Nickerson, M.L.; Iwamatsu, A.; Esposito, D.; Gillette, W.K.; Hopkins, R.F., 3rd; Hartley, J.L.; et al. Folliculin encoded by the BHD gene interacts with a binding protein, FNIP1, and AMPK, and is involved in AMPK and mTOR signaling. *Proc. Natl. Acad. Sci. USA* **2006**, *103*, 15552–15557. [CrossRef] [PubMed]
18. Hasumi, H.; Baba, M.; Hong, S.B.; Hasumi, Y.; Huang, Y.; Yao, M.; Valera, V.A.; Linehan, W.M.; Schmidt, L.S. Identification and characterization of a novel folliculin-interacting protein FNIP2. *Gene* **2008**, *415*, 60–67. [CrossRef]
19. van Slegtenhorst, M.; de Hoogt, R.; Hermans, C.; Nellist, M.; Janssen, B.; Verhoef, S.; Lindhout, D.; van den Ouweland, A.; Halley, D.; Young, J.; et al. Identification of the tuberous sclerosis gene TSC1 on chromosome 9q34. *Science* **1997**, *277*, 805–808. [CrossRef] [PubMed]
20. Woodford, M.R.; Dunn, D.M.; Blanden, A.R.; Capriotti, D.; Loiselle, D.; Prodromou, C.; Panaretou, B.; Hughes, P.F.; Smith, A.; Ackerman, V.; et al. The FNIP co-chaperones decelerate the Hsp90 chaperone cycle and enhance drug binding. *Nat. Commun.* **2016**, *7*, 12037. [CrossRef] [PubMed]
21. Woodford, M.R.; Sager, R.A.; Marris, E.; Dunn, D.M.; Blanden, A.R.; Murphy, R.L.; Rensing, N.; Shapiro, O.; Panaretou, B.; Prodromou, C.; et al. Tumor suppressor Tsc1 is a new Hsp90 co-chaperone that facilitates folding of kinase and non-kinase clients. *EMBO J.* **2017**, *36*, 3650–3665. [CrossRef] [PubMed]
22. Schmidt, L.S.; Linehan, W.M. Molecular genetics and clinical features of Birt-Hogg-Dube syndrome. *Nat. Rev. Urol.* **2015**, *12*, 558–569. [CrossRef] [PubMed]
23. Sager, R.A.; Woodford, M.R.; Shapiro, O.; Mollapour, M.; Bratslavsky, G. Sporadic renal angiomyolipoma in a patient with Birt-Hogg-Dube: Chaperones in pathogenesis. *Oncotarget* **2018**, *9*, 22220–22229. [CrossRef] [PubMed]
24. Clausen, L.; Stein, A.; Gronbaek-Thygesen, M.; Nygaard, L.; Soltoft, C.L.; Nielsen, S.V.; Lisby, M.; Ravid, T.; Lindorff-Larsen, K.; Hartmann-Petersen, R. Folliculin variants linked to Birt-Hogg-Dube syndrome are targeted for proteasomal degradation. *PLoS Genet.* **2020**, *16*, e1009187. [CrossRef]
25. Lawrence, R.E.; Fromm, S.A.; Fu, Y.; Yokom, A.L.; Kim, D.J.; Thelen, A.M.; Young, L.N.; Lim, C.Y.; Samelson, A.J.; Hurley, J.H.; et al. Structural mechanism of a Rag GTPase activation checkpoint by the lysosomal folliculin complex. *Science* **2019**, *366*, 971–977. [CrossRef] [PubMed]
26. Shen, K.; Rogala, K.B.; Chou, H.T.; Huang, R.K.; Yu, Z.; Sabatini, D.M. Cryo-EM Structure of the Human FLCN-FNIP2-Rag-Ragulator Complex. *Cell* **2019**, *179*, 1319–1329.e8. [CrossRef] [PubMed]
27. Meng, J.; Ferguson, S.M. GATOR1-dependent recruitment of FLCN-FNIP to lysosomes coordinates Rag GTPase heterodimer nucleotide status in response to amino acids. *J. Cell Biol.* **2018**, *217*, 2765–2776. [CrossRef]
28. Schiaffino, S.; Reggiani, C. Fiber types in mammalian skeletal muscles. *Physiol. Rev.* **2011**, *91*, 1447–1531. [CrossRef]
29. Hardie, D.G. Energy sensing by the AMP-activated protein kinase and its effects on muscle metabolism. *Proc. Nutr. Soc.* **2011**, *70*, 92–99. [CrossRef] [PubMed]
30. Reyes, N.L.; Banks, G.B.; Tsang, M.; Margineantu, D.; Gu, H.; Djukovic, D.; Chan, J.; Torres, M.; Liggitt, H.D.; Hirenallur, S.D.; et al. Fnip1 regulates skeletal muscle fiber type specification, fatigue resistance, and susceptibility to muscular dystrophy. *Proc. Natl. Acad. Sci. USA* **2015**, *112*, 424–429. [CrossRef]
31. Xiao, L.; Liu, J.; Sun, Z.; Yin, Y.; Mao, Y.; Xu, D.; Liu, L.; Xu, Z.; Guo, Q.; Ding, C.; et al. AMPK-dependent and -independent coordination of mitochondrial function and muscle fiber type by FNIP1. *PLoS Genet.* **2021**, *17*, e1009488. [CrossRef] [PubMed]
32. Liu, J.; Liang, X.; Zhou, D.; Lai, L.; Xiao, L.; Liu, L.; Fu, T.; Kong, Y.; Zhou, Q.; Vega, R.B.; et al. Coupling of mitochondrial function and skeletal muscle fiber type by a miR-499/Fnip1/AMPK circuit. *EMBO Mol. Med.* **2016**, *8*, 1212–1228. [CrossRef] [PubMed]
33. Fu, L.; Wang, H.; Liao, Y.; Zhou, P.; Xu, Y.; Zhao, Y.; Xie, S.; Zhao, S.; Li, X. miR-208b modulating skeletal muscle development and energy homoeostasis through targeting distinct targets. *RNA Biol.* **2020**, *17*, 743–754. [CrossRef] [PubMed]
34. Zhou, Q.; Gu, Y.; Lang, H.; Wang, X.; Chen, K.; Gong, X.; Zhou, M.; Ran, L.; Zhu, J.; Mi, M. Dihydromyricetin prevents obesity-induced slow-twitch-fiber reduction partially via FLCN/FNIP1/AMPK pathway. *Biochim. Biophys. Acta Mol. Basis Dis.* **2017**, *1863*, 1282–1291. [CrossRef]

35. Yin, Y.; Xu, D.; Mao, Y.; Xiao, L.; Sun, Z.; Liu, J.; Zhou, D.; Xu, Z.; Liu, L.; Fu, T.; et al. FNIP1 regulates adipocyte browning and systemic glucose homeostasis in mice by shaping intracellular calcium dynamics. *J. Exp. Med.* **2022**, *219*, e20212491. [CrossRef]
36. Manford, A.G.; Rodriguez-Perez, F.; Shih, K.Y.; Shi, Z.; Berdan, C.A.; Choe, M.; Titov, D.V.; Nomura, D.K.; Rape, M. A Cellular Mechanism to Detect and Alleviate Reductive Stress. *Cell* **2020**, *183*, 46–61. [CrossRef]
37. Manford, A.G.; Mena, E.L.; Shih, K.Y.; Gee, C.L.; McMinimy, R.; Martinez-Gonzalez, B.; Sherriff, R.; Lew, B.; Zoltek, M.; Rodriguez-Perez, F.; et al. Structural basis and regulation of the reductive stress response. *Cell* **2021**, *184*, 5375–5390.e16. [CrossRef]
38. Cai, W.; Yang, H. The structure and regulation of Cullin 2 based E3 ubiquitin ligases and their biological functions. *Cell Div.* **2016**, *11*, 7. [CrossRef]
39. Woodford, M.R.; Baker-Williams, A.J.; Sager, R.A.; Backe, S.J.; Blanden, A.R.; Hashmi, F.; Kancherla, P.; Gori, A.; Loiselle, D.R.; Castelli, M.; et al. The tumor suppressor folliculin inhibits lactate dehydrogenase A and regulates the Warburg effect. *Nat. Struct. Mol. Biol.* **2021**, *28*, 662–670. [CrossRef]
40. Park, H.; Staehling, K.; Tsang, M.; Appleby, M.W.; Brunkow, M.E.; Margineantu, D.; Hockenbery, D.M.; Habib, T.; Liggitt, H.D.; Carlson, G.; et al. Disruption of Fnip1 reveals a metabolic checkpoint controlling B lymphocyte development. *Immunity* **2012**, *36*, 769–781. [CrossRef]
41. Ramirez, J.A.; Iwata, T.; Park, H.; Tsang, M.; Kang, J.; Cui, K.; Kwong, W.; James, R.G.; Baba, M.; Schmidt, L.S.; et al. Folliculin Interacting Protein 1 Maintains Metabolic Homeostasis during B Cell Development by Modulating AMPK, mTORC1, and TFE3. *J. Immunol.* **2019**, *203*, 2899–2908. [CrossRef]
42. Park, H.; Tsang, M.; Iritani, B.M.; Bevan, M.J. Metabolic regulator Fnip1 is crucial for iNKT lymphocyte development. *Proc. Natl. Acad. Sci. USA* **2014**, *111*, 7066–7071. [CrossRef]
43. Baba, M.; Keller, J.R.; Sun, H.W.; Resch, W.; Kuchen, S.; Suh, H.C.; Hasumi, H.; Hasumi, Y.; Kieffer-Kwon, K.R.; Gonzalez, C.G.; et al. The folliculin-FNIP1 pathway deleted in human Birt-Hogg-Dube syndrome is required for murine B-cell development. *Blood* **2012**, *120*, 1254–1261. [CrossRef]
44. Niehues, T.; Ozgur, T.T.; Bickes, M.; Waldmann, R.; Schoning, J.; Brasen, J.; Hagel, C.; Ballmaier, M.; Klusmann, J.H.; Niedermayer, A.; et al. Mutations of the gene FNIP1 associated with a syndromic autosomal recessive immunodeficiency with cardiomyopathy and pre-excitation syndrome. *Eur. J. Immunol.* **2020**, *50*, 1078–1080. [CrossRef]
45. Saettini, F.; Poli, C.; Vengoechea, J.; Bonanomi, S.; Orellana, J.C.; Fazio, G.; Rodriguez, F.H.; Noguera, L.P.; Booth, C.; Jarur-Chamy, V.; et al. B cells, agammaglobulinemia, and hypertrophic cardiomyopathy in folliculin-interacting protein 1 deficiency. *Blood* **2021**, *137*, 493–499. [CrossRef]
46. Siggs, O.M.; Stockenhuber, A.; Deobagkar-Lele, M.; Bull, K.R.; Crockford, T.L.; Kingston, B.L.; Crawford, G.; Anzilotti, C.; Steeples, V.; Ghaffari, S.; et al. Mutation of Fnip1 is associated with B-cell deficiency, cardiomyopathy, and elevated AMPK activity. *Proc. Natl. Acad. Sci. USA* **2016**, *113*, E3706–E3715. [CrossRef]
47. Yan, M.; Audet-Walsh, E.; Manteghi, S.; Dufour, C.R.; Walker, B.; Baba, M.; St-Pierre, J.; Giguere, V.; Pause, A. Chronic AMPK activation via loss of FLCN induces functional beige adipose tissue through PGC-1alpha/ERRalpha. *Genes Dev.* **2016**, *30*, 1034–1046. [CrossRef]
48. El-Houjeiri, L.; Possik, E.; Vijayaraghavan, T.; Paquette, M.; Martina, J.A.; Kazan, J.M.; Ma, E.H.; Jones, R.; Blanchette, P.; Puertollano, R.; et al. The Transcription Factors TFEB and TFE3 Link the FLCN-AMPK Signaling Axis to Innate Immune Response and Pathogen Resistance. *Cell Rep.* **2019**, *26*, 3613–3628.e3616. [CrossRef]
49. El-Houjeiri, L.; Biondini, M.; Paquette, M.; Kuasne, H.; Pacis, A.; Park, M.; Siegel, P.M.; Pause, A. Folliculin impairs breast tumor growth by repressing TFE3-dependent induction of the Warburg effect and angiogenesis. *J. Clin. Investig.* **2021**, *131*, e144871. [CrossRef]
50. Endoh, M.; Baba, M.; Endoh, T.; Hirayama, A.; Nakamura-Ishizu, A.; Umemoto, T.; Hashimoto, M.; Nagashima, K.; Soga, T.; Lang, M.; et al. A FLCN-TFE3 Feedback Loop Prevents Excessive Glycogenesis and Phagocyte Activation by Regulating Lysosome Activity. *Cell Rep.* **2020**, *30*, 1823–1834.e1825. [CrossRef]
51. Hong, S.B.; Oh, H.; Valera, V.A.; Baba, M.; Schmidt, L.S.; Linehan, W.M. Inactivation of the FLCN tumor suppressor gene induces TFE3 transcriptional activity by increasing its nuclear localization. *PLoS ONE* **2010**, *5*, e15793. [CrossRef]
52. Glykofridis, I.E.; Knol, J.C.; Balk, J.A.; Westland, D.; Pham, T.V.; Piersma, S.R.; Lougheed, S.M.; Derakhshan, S.; Veen, P.; Rooimans, M.A.; et al. Loss of FLCN-FNIP1/2 induces a non-canonical interferon response in human renal tubular epithelial cells. *eLife* **2021**, *10*, e61630. [CrossRef]
53. Hasumi, H.; Baba, M.; Hasumi, Y.; Lang, M.; Huang, Y.; Oh, H.F.; Matsuo, M.; Merino, M.J.; Yao, M.; Ito, Y.; et al. Folliculin-interacting proteins Fnip1 and Fnip2 play critical roles in kidney tumor suppression in cooperation with Flcn. *Proc. Natl. Acad. Sci. USA* **2015**, *112*, E1624–E1631. [CrossRef]
54. Baba, M.; Furihata, M.; Hong, S.B.; Tessarollo, L.; Haines, D.C.; Southon, E.; Patel, V.; Igarashi, P.; Alvord, W.G.; Leighty, R.; et al. Kidney-targeted Birt-Hogg-Dube gene inactivation in a mouse model: Erk1/2 and Akt-mTOR activation, cell hyperproliferation, and polycystic kidneys. *J. Natl. Cancer Inst.* **2008**, *100*, 140–154. [CrossRef]
55. Henske, E.P.; Jozwiak, S.; Kingswood, J.C.; Sampson, J.R.; Thiele, E.A. Tuberous sclerosis complex. *Nat. Rev. Dis. Primers* **2016**, *2*, 16035. [CrossRef]
56. Woodford, M.R.; Backe, S.J.; Sager, R.A.; Bourboulia, D.; Bratslavsky, G.; Mollapour, M. The Role of Heat Shock Protein-90 in the Pathogenesis of Birt-Hogg-Dube and Tuberous Sclerosis Complex Syndromes. *Urol. Oncol.* **2021**, *39*, 322–326. [CrossRef]

57. European Chromosome 16 Tuberous Sclerosis, C. Identification and characterization of the tuberous sclerosis gene on chromosome 16. *Cell* **1993**, *75*, 1305–1315. [CrossRef]
58. van Slegtenhorst, M.; Nellist, M.; Nagelkerken, B.; Cheadle, J.; Snell, R.; van den Ouweland, A.; Reuser, A.; Sampson, J.; Halley, D.; van der Sluijs, P. Interaction between hamartin and tuberin, the TSC1 and TSC2 gene products. *Hum. Mol. Genet.* **1998**, *7*, 1053–1057. [CrossRef]
59. Huang, J.; Manning, B.D. The TSC1-TSC2 complex: A molecular switchboard controlling cell growth. *Biochem. J.* **2008**, *412*, 179–190. [CrossRef]
60. Ramlaul, K.; Fu, W.; Li, H.; de Martin Garrido, N.; He, L.; Trivedi, M.; Cui, W.; Aylett, C.H.S.; Wu, G. Architecture of the Tuberous Sclerosis Protein Complex. *J. Mol. Biol.* **2021**, *433*, 166743. [CrossRef]
61. Fitzian, K.; Bruckner, A.; Brohee, L.; Zech, R.; Antoni, C.; Kiontke, S.; Gasper, R.; Linard Matos, A.L.; Beel, S.; Wilhelm, S.; et al. TSC1 binding to lysosomal PIPs is required for TSC complex translocation and mTORC1 regulation. *Mol. Cell* **2021**, *81*, 2705–2721.e8. [CrossRef]
62. Yang, H.; Yu, Z.; Chen, X.; Li, J.; Li, N.; Cheng, J.; Gao, N.; Yuan, H.X.; Ye, D.; Guan, K.L.; et al. Structural insights into TSC complex assembly and GAP activity on Rheb. *Nat. Commun.* **2021**, *12*, 339. [CrossRef]
63. Hodges, A.K.; Li, S.; Maynard, J.; Parry, L.; Braverman, R.; Cheadle, J.P.; DeClue, J.E.; Sampson, J.R. Pathological mutations in TSC1 and TSC2 disrupt the interaction between hamartin and tuberin. *Hum. Mol. Genet.* **2001**, *10*, 2899–2905. [CrossRef]
64. Tee, A.R.; Fingar, D.C.; Manning, B.D.; Kwiatkowski, D.J.; Cantley, L.C.; Blenis, J. Tuberous sclerosis complex-1 and -2 gene products function together to inhibit mammalian target of rapamycin (mTOR)-mediated downstream signaling. *Proc. Natl. Acad. Sci. USA* **2002**, *99*, 13571–13576. [CrossRef]
65. Garami, A.; Zwartkruis, F.J.; Nobukuni, T.; Joaquin, M.; Roccio, M.; Stocker, H.; Kozma, S.C.; Hafen, E.; Bos, J.L.; Thomas, G. Insulin activation of Rheb, a mediator of mTOR/S6K/4E-BP signaling, is inhibited by TSC1 and 2. *Mol. Cell* **2003**, *11*, 1457–1466. [CrossRef]
66. Tee, A.R.; Manning, B.D.; Roux, P.P.; Cantley, L.C.; Blenis, J. Tuberous sclerosis complex gene products, Tuberin and Hamartin, control mTOR signaling by acting as a GTPase-activating protein complex toward Rheb. *Curr. Biol.* **2003**, *13*, 1259–1268. [CrossRef]
67. Benvenuto, G.; Li, S.; Brown, S.J.; Braverman, R.; Vass, W.C.; Cheadle, J.P.; Halley, D.J.; Sampson, J.R.; Wienecke, R.; DeClue, J.E. The tuberous sclerosis-1 (TSC1) gene product hamartin suppresses cell growth and augments the expression of the TSC2 product tuberin by inhibiting its ubiquitination. *Oncogene* **2000**, *19*, 6306–6316. [CrossRef]
68. Chong-Kopera, H.; Inoki, K.; Li, Y.; Zhu, T.; Garcia-Gonzalo, F.R.; Rosa, J.L.; Guan, K.L. TSC1 stabilizes TSC2 by inhibiting the interaction between TSC2 and the HERC1 ubiquitin ligase. *J. Biol. Chem.* **2006**, *281*, 8313–8316. [CrossRef]
69. Fukuda, T.; Kobayashi, T.; Momose, S.; Yasui, H.; Hino, O. Distribution of Tsc1 protein detected by immunohistochemistry in various normal rat tissues and the renal carcinomas of Eker rat: Detection of limited colocalization with Tsc1 and Tsc2 gene products in vivo. *Lab. Investig.* **2000**, *80*, 1347–1359. [CrossRef]
70. Kobayashi, T.; Minowa, O.; Sugitani, Y.; Takai, S.; Mitani, H.; Kobayashi, E.; Noda, T.; Hino, O. A germ-line Tsc1 mutation causes tumor development and embryonic lethality that are similar, but not identical to, those caused by Tsc2 mutation in mice. *Proc. Natl. Acad. Sci. USA* **2001**, *98*, 8762–8767. [CrossRef]
71. Kwiatkowski, D.J.; Zhang, H.; Bandura, J.L.; Heiberger, K.M.; Glogauer, M.; el-Hashemite, N.; Onda, H. A mouse model of TSC1 reveals sex-dependent lethality from liver hemangiomas, and up-regulation of p70S6 kinase activity in Tsc1 null cells. *Hum. Mol. Genet.* **2002**, *11*, 525–534. [CrossRef] [PubMed]
72. Kingswood, J.C.; Belousova, E.; Benedik, M.P.; Carter, T.; Cottin, V.; Curatolo, P.; Dahlin, M.; D'Amato, L.; Beaure d'Augeres, G.; de Vries, P.J.; et al. Renal Manifestations of Tuberous Sclerosis Complex: Key Findings from the Final Analysis of the TOSCA Study Focussing Mainly on Renal Angiomyolipomas. *Front. Neurol.* **2020**, *11*, 972. [CrossRef]
73. Qin, Z.; Zheng, H.; Zhou, L.; Ou, Y.; Huang, B.; Yan, B.; Qin, Z.; Yang, C.; Su, Y.; Bai, X.; et al. Tsc1 deficiency impairs mammary development in mice by suppression of AKT, nuclear ERalpha, and cell-cycle-driving proteins. *Sci. Rep.* **2016**, *6*, 19587. [CrossRef]
74. Zhang, H.M.; Diaz, V.; Walsh, M.E.; Zhang, Y. Moderate lifelong overexpression of tuberous sclerosis complex 1 (TSC1) improves health and survival in mice. *Sci. Rep.* **2017**, *7*, 834. [CrossRef]
75. Miloloza, A.; Kubista, M.; Rosner, M.; Hengstschlager, M. Evidence for separable functions of tuberous sclerosis gene products in mammalian cell cycle regulation. *J. Neuropathol. Exp. Neurol.* **2002**, *61*, 154–163. [CrossRef]
76. Thien, A.; Prentzell, M.T.; Holzwarth, B.; Klasener, K.; Kuper, I.; Boehlke, C.; Sonntag, A.G.; Ruf, S.; Maerz, L.; Nitschke, R.; et al. TSC1 activates TGF-beta-Smad2/3 signaling in growth arrest and epithelial-to-mesenchymal transition. *Dev. Cell* **2015**, *32*, 617–630. [CrossRef]
77. Hengstschlager, M.; Rosner, M.; Fountoulakis, M.; Lubec, G. The cellular response to ectopic overexpression of the tuberous sclerosis genes, TSC1 and TSC2: A proteomic approach. *Int. J. Oncol.* **2005**, *27*, 831–838. [CrossRef]
78. Rosner, M.; Freilinger, A.; Lubec, G.; Hengstschlager, M. The tuberous sclerosis genes, TSC1 and TSC2, trigger different gene expression responses. *Int. J. Oncol.* **2005**, *27*, 1411–1424. [CrossRef]
79. Dalal, J.S.; Winden, K.D.; Salussolia, C.L.; Sundberg, M.; Singh, A.; Pham, T.T.; Zhou, P.; Pu, W.T.; Miller, M.T.; Sahin, M. Loss of Tsc1 in cerebellar Purkinje cells induces transcriptional and translation changes in FMRP target transcripts. *eLife* **2021**, *10*, e67399. [CrossRef]

80. Liang, Z.; Zhang, Q.; Zhang, Z.; Sun, L.; Dong, X.; Li, T.; Tan, L.; Xie, X.; Sun, L.; Zhao, Y. The Development and Survival of Thymic Epithelial Cells Require TSC1-Dependent Negative Regulation of mTORC1 Activity. *J. Immunol.* **2021**, *207*, 2039–2050. [CrossRef]
81. Liu, Y.D.; Ma, M.Y.; Hu, X.B.; Yan, H.; Zhang, Y.K.; Yang, H.X.; Feng, J.H.; Wang, L.; Zhang, H.; Zhang, B.; et al. Brain Proteomic Profiling in Intractable Epilepsy Caused by TSC1 Truncating Mutations: A Small Sample Study. *Front. Neurol.* **2020**, *11*, 475. [CrossRef] [PubMed]
82. Kumar, P.; Zadjali, F.; Yao, Y.; Siroky, B.; Astrinidis, A.; Gross, K.W.; Bissler, J.J. Tsc Gene Locus Disruption and Differences in Renal Epithelial Extracellular Vesicles. *Front. Physiol.* **2021**, *12*, 630933. [CrossRef] [PubMed]
83. Wilson, C.; Bonnet, C.; Guy, C.; Idziaszczyk, S.; Colley, J.; Humphreys, V.; Maynard, J.; Sampson, J.R.; Cheadle, J.P. Tsc1 haploinsufficiency without mammalian target of rapamycin activation is sufficient for renal cyst formation in Tsc1$^{+/-}$ mice. *Cancer Res.* **2006**, *66*, 7934–7938. [CrossRef]
84. Alves, M.M.; Fuhler, G.M.; Queiroz, K.C.; Scholma, J.; Goorden, S.; Anink, J.; Spek, C.A.; Hoogeveen-Westerveld, M.; Bruno, M.J.; Nellist, M.; et al. PAK2 is an effector of TSC1/2 signaling independent of mTOR and a potential therapeutic target for Tuberous Sclerosis Complex. *Sci. Rep.* **2015**, *5*, 14534. [CrossRef] [PubMed]
85. Hartman, T.R.; Liu, D.; Zilfou, J.T.; Robb, V.; Morrison, T.; Watnick, T.; Henske, E.P. The tuberous sclerosis proteins regulate formation of the primary cilium via a rapamycin-insensitive and polycystin 1-independent pathway. *Hum. Mol. Genet.* **2009**, *18*, 151–163. [CrossRef]
86. Goncharova, E.A.; James, M.L.; Kudryashova, T.V.; Goncharov, D.A.; Krymskaya, V.P. Tumor suppressors TSC1 and TSC2 differentially modulate actin cytoskeleton and motility of mouse embryonic fibroblasts. *PLoS ONE* **2014**, *9*, e111476. [CrossRef] [PubMed]
87. Lai, M.; Zou, W.; Han, Z.; Zhou, L.; Qiu, Z.; Chen, J.; Zhang, S.; Lai, P.; Li, K.; Zhang, Y.; et al. Tsc1 regulates tight junction independent of mTORC1. *Proc. Natl. Acad. Sci. USA* **2021**, *118*, e2020891118. [CrossRef]
88. Dabora, S.L.; Jozwiak, S.; Franz, D.N.; Roberts, P.S.; Nieto, A.; Chung, J.; Choy, Y.S.; Reeve, M.P.; Thiele, E.; Egelhoff, J.C.; et al. Mutational analysis in a cohort of 224 tuberous sclerosis patients indicates increased severity of TSC2, compared with TSC1, disease in multiple organs. *Am. J. Hum. Genet.* **2001**, *68*, 64–80. [CrossRef]
89. Curatolo, P.; Moavero, R.; Roberto, D.; Graziola, F. Genotype/Phenotype Correlations in Tuberous Sclerosis Complex. *Semin. Pediatr. Neurol.* **2015**, *22*, 259–273. [CrossRef]
90. Sancak, O.; Nellist, M.; Goedbloed, M.; Elfferich, P.; Wouters, C.; Maat-Kievit, A.; Zonnenberg, B.; Verhoef, S.; Halley, D.; van den Ouweland, A. Mutational analysis of the TSC1 and TSC2 genes in a diagnostic setting: Genotype—Phenotype correlations and comparison of diagnostic DNA techniques in Tuberous Sclerosis Complex. *Eur. J. Hum. Genet.* **2005**, *13*, 731–741. [CrossRef]
91. Jones, A.C.; Daniells, C.E.; Snell, R.G.; Tachataki, M.; Idziaszczyk, S.A.; Krawczak, M.; Sampson, J.R.; Cheadle, J.P. Molecular genetic and phenotypic analysis reveals differences between TSC1 and TSC2 associated familial and sporadic tuberous sclerosis. *Hum. Mol. Genet.* **1997**, *6*, 2155–2161. [CrossRef] [PubMed]
92. Niida, Y.; Wakisaka, A.; Tsuji, T.; Yamada, H.; Kuroda, M.; Mitani, Y.; Okumura, A.; Yokoi, A. Mutational analysis of TSC1 and TSC2 in Japanese patients with tuberous sclerosis complex revealed higher incidence of TSC1 patients than previously reported. *J. Hum. Genet.* **2013**, *58*, 216–225. [CrossRef] [PubMed]
93. Wong, H.T.; McCartney, D.L.; Lewis, J.C.; Sampson, J.R.; Howe, C.J.; de Vries, P.J. Intellectual ability in tuberous sclerosis complex correlates with predicted effects of mutations on TSC1 and TSC2 proteins. *J. Med. Genet.* **2015**, *52*, 815–822. [CrossRef] [PubMed]
94. Jansen, F.E.; Braams, O.; Vincken, K.L.; Algra, A.; Anbeek, P.; Jennekens-Schinkel, A.; Halley, D.; Zonnenberg, B.A.; van den Ouweland, A.; van Huffelen, A.C.; et al. Overlapping neurologic and cognitive phenotypes in patients with TSC1 or TSC2 mutations. *Neurology* **2008**, *70*, 908–915. [CrossRef]
95. Kothare, S.V.; Singh, K.; Chalifoux, J.R.; Staley, B.A.; Weiner, H.L.; Menzer, K.; Devinsky, O. Severity of manifestations in tuberous sclerosis complex in relation to genotype. *Epilepsia* **2014**, *55*, 1025–1029. [CrossRef]
96. Zeng, L.H.; Rensing, N.R.; Zhang, B.; Gutmann, D.H.; Gambello, M.J.; Wong, M. Tsc2 gene inactivation causes a more severe epilepsy phenotype than Tsc1 inactivation in a mouse model of tuberous sclerosis complex. *Hum. Mol. Genet.* **2011**, *20*, 445–454. [CrossRef]
97. Langkau, N.; Martin, N.; Brandt, R.; Zugge, K.; Quast, S.; Wiegele, G.; Jauch, A.; Rehm, M.; Kuhl, A.; Mack-Vetter, M.; et al. TSC1 and TSC2 mutations in tuberous sclerosis, the associated phenotypes and a model to explain observed TSC1/TSC2 frequency ratios. *Eur. J. Pediatr.* **2002**, *161*, 393–402. [CrossRef]
98. Dean, M.E.; Johnson, J.L. Human Hsp90 cochaperones: Perspectives on tissue-specific expression and identification of cochaperones with similar in vivo functions. *Cell Stress Chaperones* **2021**, *26*, 3–13. [CrossRef]
99. Wang, R.Y.; Noddings, C.M.; Kirschke, E.; Myasnikov, A.G.; Johnson, J.L.; Agard, D.A. Structure of Hsp90-Hsp70-Hop-GR reveals the Hsp90 client-loading mechanism. *Nature* **2022**, *601*, 460–464. [CrossRef]
100. Li, J.; Richter, K.; Reinstein, J.; Buchner, J. Integration of the accelerator Aha1 in the Hsp90 co-chaperone cycle. *Nat. Struct. Mol. Biol.* **2013**, *20*, 326–331. [CrossRef]
101. Li, J.; Soroka, J.; Buchner, J. The Hsp90 chaperone machinery: Conformational dynamics and regulation by co-chaperones. *Biochim. Biophys. Acta* **2012**, *1823*, 624–635. [CrossRef] [PubMed]
102. Wandinger, S.K.; Richter, K.; Buchner, J. The Hsp90 chaperone machinery. *J. Biol. Chem.* **2008**, *283*, 18473–18477. [CrossRef] [PubMed]

103. Lopez, A.; Dahiya, V.; Delhommel, F.; Freiburger, L.; Stehle, R.; Asami, S.; Rutz, D.; Blair, L.; Buchner, J.; Sattler, M. Client binding shifts the populations of dynamic Hsp90 conformations through an allosteric network. *Sci. Adv.* **2021**, *7*, eabl7295. [CrossRef]
104. Biebl, M.M.; Riedl, M.; Buchner, J. Hsp90 Co-chaperones Form Plastic Genetic Networks Adapted to Client Maturation. *Cell Rep.* **2020**, *32*, 108063. [CrossRef] [PubMed]
105. Vaughan, C.K.; Mollapour, M.; Smith, J.R.; Truman, A.; Hu, B.; Good, V.M.; Panaretou, B.; Neckers, L.; Clarke, P.A.; Workman, P.; et al. Hsp90-dependent activation of protein kinases is regulated by chaperone-targeted dephosphorylation of Cdc37. *Mol. Cell* **2008**, *31*, 886–895. [CrossRef] [PubMed]
106. Sager, R.A.; Dushukyan, N.; Woodford, M.; Mollapour, M. Structure and function of the co-chaperone protein phosphatase 5 in cancer. *Cell Stress Chaperones* **2020**, *25*, 383–394. [CrossRef]
107. Wang, X.; Venable, J.; LaPointe, P.; Hutt, D.M.; Koulov, A.V.; Coppinger, J.; Gurkan, C.; Kellner, W.; Matteson, J.; Plutner, H.; et al. Hsp90 cochaperone Aha1 downregulation rescues misfolding of CFTR in cystic fibrosis. *Cell* **2006**, *127*, 803–815. [CrossRef]
108. Koulov, A.V.; LaPointe, P.; Lu, B.; Razvi, A.; Coppinger, J.; Dong, M.Q.; Matteson, J.; Laister, R.; Arrowsmith, C.; Yates, J.R., 3rd; et al. Biological and structural basis for Aha1 regulation of Hsp90 ATPase activity in maintaining proteostasis in the human disease cystic fibrosis. *Mol. Biol. Cell* **2010**, *21*, 871–884. [CrossRef]
109. Dunn, D.M.; Woodford, M.R.; Truman, A.W.; Jensen, S.M.; Schulman, J.; Caza, T.; Remillard, T.C.; Loiselle, D.; Wolfgeher, D.; Blagg, B.S.; et al. c-Abl Mediated Tyrosine Phosphorylation of Aha1 Activates Its Co-chaperone Function in Cancer Cells. *Cell Rep.* **2015**, *12*, 1006–1018. [CrossRef]
110. Siligardi, G.; Hu, B.; Panaretou, B.; Piper, P.W.; Pearl, L.H.; Prodromou, C. Co-chaperone regulation of conformational switching in the Hsp90 ATPase cycle. *J. Biol. Chem.* **2004**, *279*, 51989–51998. [CrossRef]
111. Rohl, A.; Tippel, F.; Bender, E.; Schmid, A.B.; Richter, K.; Madl, T.; Buchner, J. Hop/Sti1 phosphorylation inhibits its co-chaperone function. *EMBO Rep.* **2015**, *16*, 240–249. [CrossRef] [PubMed]
112. Rohl, A.; Wengler, D.; Madl, T.; Lagleder, S.; Tippel, F.; Herrmann, M.; Hendrix, J.; Richter, K.; Hack, G.; Schmid, A.B.; et al. Hsp90 regulates the dynamics of its cochaperone Sti1 and the transfer of Hsp70 between modules. *Nat. Commun.* **2015**, *6*, 6655. [CrossRef] [PubMed]
113. Lorenz, O.R.; Freiburger, L.; Rutz, D.A.; Krause, M.; Zierer, B.K.; Alvira, S.; Cuellar, J.; Valpuesta, J.M.; Madl, T.; Sattler, M.; et al. Modulation of the Hsp90 chaperone cycle by a stringent client protein. *Mol. Cell* **2014**, *53*, 941–953. [CrossRef]
114. Sager, R.A.; Woodford, M.R.; Backe, S.J.; Makedon, A.M.; Baker-Williams, A.J.; DiGregorio, B.T.; Loiselle, D.R.; Haystead, T.A.; Zachara, N.E.; Prodromou, C.; et al. Post-translational Regulation of FNIP1 Creates a Rheostat for the Molecular Chaperone Hsp90. *Cell Rep.* **2019**, *26*, 1344–1356.e1345. [CrossRef] [PubMed]
115. Natarajan, N.; Shaik, A.; Thiruvenkatam, V. Recombinant Tumor Suppressor TSC1 Differentially Interacts with Escherichia coli DnaK and Human HSP70. *ACS Omega* **2020**, *5*, 19131–19139. [CrossRef] [PubMed]
116. Hessling, M.; Richter, K.; Buchner, J. Dissection of the ATP-induced conformational cycle of the molecular chaperone Hsp90. *Nat. Struct. Mol. Biol.* **2009**, *16*, 287–293. [CrossRef]
117. Mickler, M.; Hessling, M.; Ratzke, C.; Buchner, J.; Hugel, T. The large conformational changes of Hsp90 are only weakly coupled to ATP hydrolysis. *Nat. Struct. Mol. Biol.* **2009**, *16*, 281–286. [CrossRef]
118. Prodromou, C.; Pearl, L.H. Structure and functional relationships of Hsp90. *Curr. Cancer Drug Targets* **2003**, *3*, 301–323. [CrossRef]
119. Shiau, A.K.; Harris, S.F.; Southworth, D.R.; Agard, D.A. Structural Analysis of E. coli hsp90 reveals dramatic nucleotide-dependent conformational rearrangements. *Cell* **2006**, *127*, 329–340. [CrossRef]
120. Noddings, C.M.; Wang, R.Y.; Johnson, J.L.; Agard, D.A. Structure of Hsp90-p23-GR reveals the Hsp90 client-remodelling mechanism. *Nature* **2022**, *601*, 465–469. [CrossRef]
121. Ali, M.M.; Roe, S.M.; Vaughan, C.K.; Meyer, P.; Panaretou, B.; Piper, P.W.; Prodromou, C.; Pearl, L.H. Crystal structure of an Hsp90-nucleotide-p23/Sba1 closed chaperone complex. *Nature* **2006**, *440*, 1013–1017. [CrossRef] [PubMed]
122. Blacklock, K.; Verkhivker, G.M. Differential modulation of functional dynamics and allosteric interactions in the Hsp90-cochaperone complexes with p23 and Aha1: A computational study. *PLoS ONE* **2013**, *8*, e71936. [CrossRef] [PubMed]
123. Cano, L.Q.; Lavery, D.N.; Sin, S.; Spanjaard, E.; Brooke, G.N.; Tilman, J.D.; Abroaf, A.; Gaughan, L.; Robson, C.N.; Heer, R.; et al. The co-chaperone p23 promotes prostate cancer motility and metastasis. *Mol. Oncol.* **2015**, *9*, 295–308. [CrossRef]
124. Martinez-Yamout, M.A.; Venkitakrishnan, R.P.; Preece, N.E.; Kroon, G.; Wright, P.E.; Dyson, H.J. Localization of sites of interaction between p23 and Hsp90 in solution. *J. Biol. Chem.* **2006**, *281*, 14457–14464. [CrossRef]
125. McLaughlin, S.H.; Sobott, F.; Yao, Z.P.; Zhang, W.; Nielsen, P.R.; Grossmann, J.G.; Laue, E.D.; Robinson, C.V.; Jackson, S.E. The co-chaperone p23 arrests the Hsp90 ATPase cycle to trap client proteins. *J. Mol. Biol.* **2006**, *356*, 746–758. [CrossRef] [PubMed]
126. Richter, K.; Walter, S.; Buchner, J. The Co-chaperone Sba1 connects the ATPase reaction of Hsp90 to the progression of the chaperone cycle. *J. Mol. Biol.* **2004**, *342*, 1403–1413. [CrossRef]
127. Woo, S.H.; An, S.; Lee, H.C.; Jin, H.O.; Seo, S.K.; Yoo, D.H.; Lee, K.H.; Rhee, C.H.; Choi, E.J.; Hong, S.I.; et al. A truncated form of p23 down-regulates telomerase activity via disruption of Hsp90 function. *J. Biol. Chem.* **2009**, *284*, 30871–30880. [CrossRef] [PubMed]
128. Backe, S.J.; Sager, R.A.; Woodford, M.R.; Makedon, A.M.; Mollapour, M. Post-translational modifications of Hsp90 and translating the chaperone code. *J. Biol. Chem.* **2020**, *295*, 11099–11117. [CrossRef]
129. Nitika; Porter, C.M.; Truman, A.W.; Truttmann, M.C. Post-translational modifications of Hsp70 family proteins: Expanding the chaperone code. *J. Biol. Chem.* **2020**, *295*, 10689–10708. [CrossRef]

130. Woodford, M.R.; Hughes, M.; Sager, R.A.; Backe, S.J.; Baker-Williams, A.J.; Bratslavsky, M.S.; Jacob, J.M.; Shapiro, O.; Wong, M.; Bratslavsky, G.; et al. Mutation of the co-chaperone Tsc1 in bladder cancer diminishes Hsp90 acetylation and reduces drug sensitivity and selectivity. *Oncotarget* **2019**, *10*, 5824–5834. [CrossRef]
131. Kamal, A.; Thao, L.; Sensintaffar, J.; Zhang, L.; Boehm, M.F.; Fritz, L.C.; Burrows, F.J. A high-affinity conformation of Hsp90 confers tumour selectivity on Hsp90 inhibitors. *Nature* **2003**, *425*, 407–410. [CrossRef] [PubMed]
132. Woodford, M.R.; Truman, A.W.; Dunn, D.M.; Jensen, S.M.; Cotran, R.; Bullard, R.; Abouelleil, M.; Beebe, K.; Wolfgeher, D.; Wierzbicki, S.; et al. Mps1 Mediated Phosphorylation of Hsp90 Confers Renal Cell Carcinoma Sensitivity and Selectivity to Hsp90 Inhibitors. *Cell Rep.* **2016**, *14*, 872–884. [CrossRef] [PubMed]
133. Mollapour, M.; Bourboulia, D.; Beebe, K.; Woodford, M.R.; Polier, S.; Hoang, A.; Chelluri, R.; Li, Y.; Guo, A.; Lee, M.J.; et al. Asymmetric Hsp90 N domain SUMOylation recruits Aha1 and ATP-competitive inhibitors. *Mol. Cell* **2014**, *53*, 317–329. [CrossRef] [PubMed]
134. Bisht, K.S.; Bradbury, C.M.; Mattson, D.; Kaushal, A.; Sowers, A.; Markovina, S.; Ortiz, K.L.; Sieck, L.K.; Isaacs, J.S.; Brechbiel, M.W.; et al. Geldanamycin and 17-allylamino-17-demethoxygeldanamycin potentiate the in vitro and in vivo radiation response of cervical tumor cells via the heat shock protein 90-mediated intracellular signaling and cytotoxicity. *Cancer Res.* **2003**, *63*, 8984–8995.
135. Trepel, J.; Mollapour, M.; Giaccone, G.; Neckers, L. Targeting the dynamic HSP90 complex in cancer. *Nat. Rev. Cancer* **2010**, *10*, 537–549. [CrossRef] [PubMed]
136. Zhang, L.; Yi, Y.; Guo, Q.; Sun, Y.; Ma, S.; Xiao, S.; Geng, J.; Zheng, Z.; Song, S. Hsp90 interacts with AMPK and mediates acetyl-CoA carboxylase phosphorylation. *Cell Signal.* **2012**, *24*, 859–865. [CrossRef]
137. Moulick, K.; Ahn, J.H.; Zong, H.; Rodina, A.; Cerchietti, L.; Gomes DaGama, E.M.; Caldas-Lopes, E.; Beebe, K.; Perna, F.; Hatzi, K.; et al. Affinity-based proteomics reveal cancer-specific networks coordinated by Hsp90. *Nat. Chem. Biol.* **2011**, *7*, 818–826. [CrossRef]
138. Nagashima, K.; Fukushima, H.; Shimizu, K.; Yamada, A.; Hidaka, M.; Hasumi, H.; Ikebe, T.; Fukumoto, S.; Okabe, K.; Inuzuka, H. Nutrient-induced FNIP degradation by SCFbeta-TRCP regulates FLCN complex localization and promotes renal cancer progression. *Oncotarget* **2017**, *8*, 9947–9960. [CrossRef]
139. Inoki, K.; Li, Y.; Xu, T.; Guan, K.L. Rheb GTPase is a direct target of TSC2 GAP activity and regulates mTOR signaling. *Genes Dev.* **2003**, *17*, 1829–1834. [CrossRef]
140. Horejsi, Z.; Takai, H.; Adelman, C.A.; Collis, S.J.; Flynn, H.; Maslen, S.; Skehel, J.M.; de Lange, T.; Boulton, S.J. CK2 phospho-dependent binding of R2TP complex to TEL2 is essential for mTOR and SMG1 stability. *Mol. Cell* **2010**, *39*, 839–850. [CrossRef]
141. Liang, W.; Miao, S.; Zhang, B.; He, S.; Shou, C.; Manivel, P.; Krishna, R.; Chen, Y.; Shi, Y.E. Synuclein gamma protects Akt and mTOR and renders tumor resistance to Hsp90 disruption. *Oncogene* **2015**, *34*, 2398–2405. [CrossRef] [PubMed]
142. Ohji, G.; Hidayat, S.; Nakashima, A.; Tokunaga, C.; Oshiro, N.; Yoshino, K.I.; Yokono, K.; Kikkawa, U.; Yonezawa, K. Suppression of the mTOR-raptor signaling pathway by the inhibitor of heat shock protein 90 geldanamycin. *J. Biochem.* **2006**, *139*, 129–135. [CrossRef] [PubMed]
143. Takai, H.; Xie, Y.; de Lange, T.; Pavletich, N.P. Tel2 structure and function in the Hsp90-dependent maturation of mTOR and ATR complexes. *Genes Dev.* **2010**, *24*, 2019–2030. [CrossRef] [PubMed]
144. Acquaviva, J.; He, S.; Zhang, C.; Jimenez, J.P.; Nagai, M.; Sang, J.; Sequeira, M.; Smith, D.L.; Ogawa, L.S.; Inoue, T.; et al. FGFR3 translocations in bladder cancer: Differential sensitivity to HSP90 inhibition based on drug metabolism. *Mol. Cancer Res.* **2014**, *12*, 1042–1054. [CrossRef]
145. Giulino-Roth, L.; van Besien, H.J.; Dalton, T.; Totonchy, J.E.; Rodina, A.; Taldone, T.; Bolaender, A.; Erdjument-Bromage, H.; Sadek, J.; Chadburn, A.; et al. Inhibition of Hsp90 Suppresses PI3K/AKT/mTOR Signaling and Has Antitumor Activity in Burkitt Lymphoma. *Mol. Cancer Ther.* **2017**, *16*, 1779–1790. [CrossRef]
146. Solarova, Z.; Mojzis, J.; Solar, P. Hsp90 inhibitor as a sensitizer of cancer cells to different therapies (review). *Int. J. Oncol.* **2015**, *46*, 907–926. [CrossRef]
147. Di Nardo, A.; Lenoel, I.; Winden, K.D.; Ruhmkorf, A.; Modi, M.E.; Barrett, L.; Ercan-Herbst, E.; Venugopal, P.; Behne, R.; Lopes, C.A.M.; et al. Phenotypic Screen with TSC-Deficient Neurons Reveals Heat-Shock Machinery as a Druggable Pathway for mTORC1 and Reduced Cilia. *Cell Rep.* **2020**, *31*, 107780. [CrossRef]
148. Mrozek, E.M.; Bajaj, V.; Guo, Y.; Malinowska, I.A.; Zhang, J.; Kwiatkowski, D.J. Evaluation of Hsp90 and mTOR inhibitors as potential drugs for the treatment of TSC1/TSC2 deficient cancer. *PLoS ONE* **2021**, *16*, e0248380. [CrossRef]
149. Blagosklonny, M.V.; Toretsky, J.; Bohen, S.; Neckers, L. Mutant conformation of p53 translated in vitro or in vivo requires functional HSP90. *Proc. Natl. Acad. Sci. USA* **1996**, *93*, 8379–8383. [CrossRef]
150. Whitesell, L.; Sutphin, P.D.; Pulcini, E.J.; Martinez, J.D.; Cook, P.H. The physical association of multiple molecular chaperone proteins with mutant p53 is altered by geldanamycin, an hsp90-binding agent. *Mol. Cell Biol.* **1998**, *18*, 1517–1524. [CrossRef]
151. Muller, L.; Schaupp, A.; Walerych, D.; Wegele, H.; Buchner, J. Hsp90 regulates the activity of wild type p53 under physiological and elevated temperatures. *J. Biol. Chem.* **2004**, *279*, 48846–48854. [CrossRef] [PubMed]
152. Walerych, D.; Kudla, G.; Gutkowska, M.; Wawrzynow, B.; Muller, L.; King, F.W.; Helwak, A.; Boros, J.; Zylicz, A.; Zylicz, M. Hsp90 chaperones wild-type p53 tumor suppressor protein. *J. Biol. Chem.* **2004**, *279*, 48836–48845. [CrossRef] [PubMed]
153. Pennisi, R.; Antoccia, A.; Leone, S.; Ascenzi, P.; di Masi, A. Hsp90alpha regulates ATM and NBN functions in sensing and repair of DNA double-strand breaks. *FEBS J.* **2017**, *284*, 2378–2395. [CrossRef] [PubMed]

154. Boudeau, J.; Deak, M.; Lawlor, M.A.; Morrice, N.A.; Alessi, D.R. Heat-shock protein 90 and Cdc37 interact with LKB1 and regulate its stability. *Biochem. J.* **2003**, *370*, 849–857. [CrossRef]
155. Walter, R.; Pan, K.T.; Doebele, C.; Comoglio, F.; Tomska, K.; Bohnenberger, H.; Young, R.M.; Jacobs, L.; Keller, U.; Bonig, H.; et al. HSP90 promotes Burkitt lymphoma cell survival by maintaining tonic B-cell receptor signaling. *Blood* **2017**, *129*, 598–608. [CrossRef]
156. Narayan, V.; Eckert, M.; Zylicz, A.; Zylicz, M.; Ball, K.L. Cooperative regulation of the interferon regulatory factor-1 tumor suppressor protein by core components of the molecular chaperone machinery. *J. Biol. Chem.* **2009**, *284*, 25889–25899. [CrossRef] [PubMed]
157. Bansal, H.; Bansal, S.; Rao, M.; Foley, K.P.; Sang, J.; Proia, D.A.; Blackman, R.K.; Ying, W.; Barsoum, J.; Baer, M.R.; et al. Heat shock protein 90 regulates the expression of Wilms tumor 1 protein in myeloid leukemias. *Blood* **2010**, *116*, 4591–4599. [CrossRef]
158. Noguchi, M.; Yu, D.; Hirayama, R.; Ninomiya, Y.; Sekine, E.; Kubota, N.; Ando, K.; Okayasu, R. Inhibition of homologous recombination repair in irradiated tumor cells pretreated with Hsp90 inhibitor 17-allylamino-17-demethoxygeldanamycin. *Biochem. Biophys. Res. Commun.* **2006**, *351*, 658–663. [CrossRef]
159. Manjarrez, J.R.; Sun, L.; Prince, T.; Matts, R.L. Hsp90-dependent assembly of the DBC2/RhoBTB2-Cullin3 E3-ligase complex. *PLoS ONE* **2014**, *9*, e90054. [CrossRef]
160. McClellan, A.J.; Scott, M.D.; Frydman, J. Folding and quality control of the VHL tumor suppressor proceed through distinct chaperone pathways. *Cell* **2005**, *121*, 739–748. [CrossRef]
161. Taipale, M.; Krykbaeva, I.; Koeva, M.; Kayatekin, C.; Westover, K.D.; Karras, G.I.; Lindquist, S. Quantitative analysis of HSP90-client interactions reveals principles of substrate recognition. *Cell* **2012**, *150*, 987–1001. [CrossRef] [PubMed]
162. Huntoon, C.J.; Nye, M.D.; Geng, L.; Peterson, K.L.; Flatten, K.S.; Haluska, P.; Kaufmann, S.H.; Karnitz, L.M. Heat shock protein 90 inhibition depletes LATS1 and LATS2, two regulators of the mammalian hippo tumor suppressor pathway. *Cancer Res.* **2010**, *70*, 8642–8650. [CrossRef]
163. Ichikawa, T.; Shanab, O.; Nakahata, S.; Shimosaki, S.; Manachai, N.; Ono, M.; Iha, H.; Shimoda, K.; Morishita, K. Novel PRMT5-mediated arginine methylations of HSP90A are essential for maintenance of HSP90A function in NDRG2(low) ATL and various cancer cells. *Biochim. Biophys. Acta Mol. Cell Res.* **2020**, *1867*, 118615. [CrossRef] [PubMed]
164. King, F.W.; Wawrzynow, A.; Hohfeld, J.; Zylicz, M. Co-chaperones Bag-1, Hop and Hsp40 regulate Hsc70 and Hsp90 interactions with wild-type or mutant p53. *EMBO J.* **2001**, *20*, 6297–6305. [CrossRef] [PubMed]
165. Li, D.; Marchenko, N.D.; Schulz, R.; Fischer, V.; Velasco-Hernandez, T.; Talos, F.; Moll, U.M. Functional inactivation of endogenous MDM2 and CHIP by HSP90 causes aberrant stabilization of mutant p53 in human cancer cells. *Mol. Cancer Res.* **2011**, *9*, 577–588. [CrossRef]
166. Quintana-Gallardo, L.; Martin-Benito, J.; Marcilla, M.; Espadas, G.; Sabido, E.; Valpuesta, J.M. The cochaperone CHIP marks Hsp70- and Hsp90-bound substrates for degradation through a very flexible mechanism. *Sci. Rep.* **2019**, *9*, 5102. [CrossRef]
167. Luo, M.; Meng, Z.; Moroishi, T.; Lin, K.C.; Shen, G.; Mo, F.; Shao, B.; Wei, X.; Zhang, P.; Wei, Y.; et al. Heat stress activates YAP/TAZ to induce the heat shock transcriptome. *Nat. Cell Biol.* **2020**, *22*, 1447–1459. [CrossRef]
168. Shen, J.P.; Zhao, D.; Sasik, R.; Luebeck, J.; Birmingham, A.; Bojorquez-Gomez, A.; Licon, K.; Klepper, K.; Pekin, D.; Beckett, A.N.; et al. Combinatorial CRISPR-Cas9 screens for de novo mapping of genetic interactions. *Nat. Methods* **2017**, *14*, 573–576. [CrossRef]
169. Cheng, A.N.; Fan, C.C.; Lo, Y.K.; Kuo, C.L.; Wang, H.C.; Lien, I.H.; Lin, S.Y.; Chen, C.H.; Jiang, S.S.; Chang, I.S.; et al. Cdc7-Dbf4-mediated phosphorylation of HSP90-S164 stabilizes HSP90-HCLK2-MRN complex to enhance ATR/ATM signaling that overcomes replication stress in cancer. *Sci. Rep.* **2017**, *7*, 17024. [CrossRef]
170. Johnson, N.; Johnson, S.F.; Yao, W.; Li, Y.C.; Choi, Y.E.; Bernhardy, A.J.; Wang, Y.; Capelletti, M.; Sarosiek, K.A.; Moreau, L.A.; et al. Stabilization of mutant BRCA1 protein confers PARP inhibitor and platinum resistance. *Proc. Natl. Acad. Sci. USA* **2013**, *110*, 17041–17046. [CrossRef]
171. Stecklein, S.R.; Kumaraswamy, E.; Behbod, F.; Wang, W.; Chaguturu, V.; Harlan-Williams, L.M.; Jensen, R.A. BRCA1 and HSP90 cooperate in homologous and non-homologous DNA double-strand-break repair and G2/M checkpoint activation. *Proc. Natl. Acad. Sci. USA* **2012**, *109*, 13650–13655. [CrossRef]
172. Nokin, M.J.; Durieux, F.; Peixoto, P.; Chiavarina, B.; Peulen, O.; Blomme, A.; Turtoi, A.; Costanza, B.; Smargiasso, N.; Baiwir, D.; et al. Methylglyoxal, a glycolysis side-product, induces Hsp90 glycation and YAP-mediated tumor growth and metastasis. *eLife* **2016**, *5*, e19375. [CrossRef] [PubMed]
173. Nony, P.; Gaude, H.; Rossel, M.; Fournier, L.; Rouault, J.P.; Billaud, M. Stability of the Peutz-Jeghers syndrome kinase LKB1 requires its binding to the molecular chaperones Hsp90/Cdc37. *Oncogene* **2003**, *22*, 9165–9175. [CrossRef]
174. Gaude, H.; Aznar, N.; Delay, A.; Bres, A.; Buchet-Poyau, K.; Caillat, C.; Vigouroux, A.; Rogon, C.; Woods, A.; Vanacker, J.M.; et al. Molecular chaperone complexes with antagonizing activities regulate stability and activity of the tumor suppressor LKB1. *Oncogene* **2012**, *31*, 1582–1591. [CrossRef] [PubMed]
175. Guo, A.; Lu, P.; Lee, J.; Zhen, C.; Chiosis, G.; Wang, Y.L. HSP90 stabilizes B-cell receptor kinases in a multi-client interactome: PU-H71 induces CLL apoptosis in a cytoprotective microenvironment. *Oncogene* **2017**, *36*, 3441–3449. [CrossRef]
176. Shen, L.J.; Sun, H.W.; Chai, Y.Y.; Jiang, Q.Y.; Zhang, J.; Li, W.M.; Xin, S.J. The Disassociation of the A20/HSP90 Complex via Downregulation of HSP90 Restores the Effect of A20 Enhancing the Sensitivity of Hepatocellular Carcinoma Cells to Molecular Targeted Agents. *Front. Oncol.* **2021**, *11*, 804412. [CrossRef] [PubMed]

177. Dahiya, V.; Agam, G.; Lawatscheck, J.; Rutz, D.A.; Lamb, D.C.; Buchner, J. Coordinated Conformational Processing of the Tumor Suppressor Protein p53 by the Hsp70 and Hsp90 Chaperone Machineries. *Mol. Cell* **2019**, *74*, 816–830.e817. [CrossRef] [PubMed]
178. Fukumoto, R.; Kiang, J.G. Geldanamycin analog 17-DMAG limits apoptosis in human peripheral blood cells by inhibition of p53 activation and its interaction with heat-shock protein 90 kDa after exposure to ionizing radiation. *Radiat. Res.* **2011**, *176*, 333–345. [CrossRef] [PubMed]
179. Giustiniani, J.; Daire, V.; Cantaloube, I.; Durand, G.; Pous, C.; Perdiz, D.; Baillet, A. Tubulin acetylation favors Hsp90 recruitment to microtubules and stimulates the signaling function of the Hsp90 clients Akt/PKB and p53. *Cell Signal.* **2009**, *21*, 529–539. [CrossRef]
180. Hagn, F.; Lagleder, S.; Retzlaff, M.; Rohrberg, J.; Demmer, O.; Richter, K.; Buchner, J.; Kessler, H. Structural analysis of the interaction between Hsp90 and the tumor suppressor protein p53. *Nat. Struct. Mol. Biol.* **2011**, *18*, 1086–1093. [CrossRef]
181. Li, D.; Marchenko, N.D.; Moll, U.M. SAHA shows preferential cytotoxicity in mutant p53 cancer cells by destabilizing mutant p53 through inhibition of the HDAC6-Hsp90 chaperone axis. *Cell Death Differ.* **2011**, *18*, 1904–1913. [CrossRef] [PubMed]
182. Nagata, Y.; Anan, T.; Yoshida, T.; Mizukami, T.; Taya, Y.; Fujiwara, T.; Kato, H.; Saya, H.; Nakao, M. The stabilization mechanism of mutant-type p53 by impaired ubiquitination: The loss of wild-type p53 function and the hsp90 association. *Oncogene* **1999**, *18*, 6037–6049. [CrossRef] [PubMed]
183. Park, S.J.; Borin, B.N.; Martinez-Yamout, M.A.; Dyson, H.J. The client protein p53 adopts a molten globule-like state in the presence of Hsp90. *Nat. Struct. Mol. Biol.* **2011**, *18*, 537–541. [CrossRef] [PubMed]
184. Park, S.J.; Kostic, M.; Dyson, H.J. Dynamic Interaction of Hsp90 with Its Client Protein p53. *J. Mol. Biol.* **2011**, *411*, 158–173. [CrossRef]
185. Rudiger, S.; Freund, S.M.; Veprintsev, D.B.; Fersht, A.R. CRINEPT-TROSY NMR reveals p53 core domain bound in an unfolded form to the chaperone Hsp90. *Proc. Natl. Acad. Sci. USA* **2002**, *99*, 11085–11090. [CrossRef]
186. Walerych, D.; Gutkowska, M.; Klejman, M.P.; Wawrzynow, B.; Tracz, Z.; Wiech, M.; Zylicz, M.; Zylicz, A. ATP binding to Hsp90 is sufficient for effective chaperoning of p53 protein. *J. Biol. Chem.* **2010**, *285*, 32020–32028. [CrossRef]
187. Denney, A.S.; Weems, A.D.; McMurray, M.A. Selective functional inhibition of a tumor-derived p53 mutant by cytosolic chaperones identified using split-YFP in budding yeast. *G3* **2021**, *11*, jkab230. [CrossRef]
188. Woodford, M.R.; Backe, S.J.; Wengert, L.A.; Dunn, D.M.; Bourboulia, D.; Mollapour, M. Hsp90 chaperone code and the tumor suppressor VHL cooperatively regulate the mitotic checkpoint. *Cell Stress Chaperones* **2021**, *26*, 965–971. [CrossRef]
189. Centini, R.; Tsang, M.; Iwata, T.; Park, H.; Delrow, J.; Margineantu, D.; Iritani, B.M.; Gu, H.; Liggitt, H.D.; Kang, J.; et al. Loss of Fnip1 alters kidney developmental transcriptional program and synergizes with TSC1 loss to promote mTORC1 activation and renal cyst formation. *PLoS ONE* **2018**, *13*, e0197973. [CrossRef]

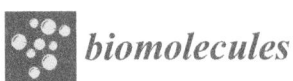

Review

TRAP1 Chaperones the Metabolic Switch in Cancer

Laura A. Wengert [1,2], Sarah J. Backe [1,2], Dimitra Bourboulia [1,2,3], Mehdi Mollapour [1,2,3] and Mark R. Woodford [1,2,3,*]

1. Department of Urology, SUNY Upstate Medical University, Syracuse, NY 13210, USA; wengertl@upstate.edu (L.A.W.); backes@upstate.edu (S.J.B.); bourmpod@upstate.edu (D.B.); mollapom@upstate.edu (M.M.)
2. Upstate Cancer Center, SUNY Upstate Medical University, Syracuse, NY 13210, USA
3. Department of Biochemistry and Molecular Biology, SUNY Upstate Medical University, Syracuse, NY 13210, USA
* Correspondence: woodform@upstate.edu

Abstract: Mitochondrial function is dependent on molecular chaperones, primarily due to their necessity in the formation of respiratory complexes and clearance of misfolded proteins. Heat shock proteins (Hsps) are a subset of molecular chaperones that function in all subcellular compartments, both constitutively and in response to stress. The Hsp90 chaperone TNF-receptor-associated protein-1 (TRAP1) is primarily localized to the mitochondria and controls both cellular metabolic reprogramming and mitochondrial apoptosis. TRAP1 upregulation facilitates the growth and progression of many cancers by promoting glycolytic metabolism and antagonizing the mitochondrial permeability transition that precedes multiple cell death pathways. TRAP1 attenuation induces apoptosis in cellular models of cancer, identifying TRAP1 as a potential therapeutic target in cancer. Similar to cytosolic Hsp90 proteins, TRAP1 is also subject to post-translational modifications (PTM) that regulate its function and mediate its impact on downstream effectors, or 'clients'. However, few effectors have been identified to date. Here, we will discuss the consequence of TRAP1 deregulation in cancer and the impact of post-translational modification on the known functions of TRAP1.

Keywords: TRAP1; Hsp90; chaperone; post-translational modification; cancer; mitochondria; metabolism; Warburg effect

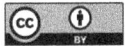

1. Introduction

Molecular chaperones of the heat shock protein-90 (Hsp90) family are involved in signal integration and the cellular stress response. These chaperones mediate cell signaling through the stabilization and activation of their substrate proteins, known as clients (https://www.picard.ch/downloads/Hsp90interactors.pdf, accessed 28 February 2022) [1]. The Hsp90 chaperone function is coupled to the ability to hydrolyze ATP, and chaperone activity can be precisely regulated by a heterogeneous group of proteins known as co-chaperones [2], as well as a diverse array of post-translational modifications (PTM) [3].

TNF-receptor-associated protein-1 (TRAP1) is the mitochondrial-dedicated Hsp90 family member and is localized to the mitochondrial matrix, inner mitochondrial membrane, and the intermembrane space [4–6]. TRAP1 was first identified through its interaction with the intracellular domain of the Type I TNF receptor [7], and early characterization of TRAP1 demonstrated ATP-binding ability and sensitivity to ATP-competitive Hsp90 inhibitors [8]. Despite this, TRAP1 was unable to form complexes with known cytosolic Hsp90 co-chaperones, nor could it promote the maturation of Hsp90 client proteins, suggesting a distinct mechanism of action for TRAP1 [8].

From this time, work has concentrated on the impact of TRAP1 on cellular processes, however identification of TRAP1 effectors and regulatory mechanisms of TRAP1 expression and activity are critical to understanding its biological function. TRAP1 has an established role as a master regulator of metabolic flux, and a large body of evidence has demonstrated that TRAP1 expression serves to suppress oxidative phosphorylation [9–11]. Further, TRAP1 also contributes to cell survival through complex formation with cyclophilin D (CypD), which regulates the opening of the permeability transition pore (PTP) [12]. These two known roles suggest a critical function for TRAP1 in maintaining cellular homeostasis [13]. Despite the critical importance of TRAP1 to these processes, the molecular mechanisms of TRAP1 function remain largely unresolved. Here, we will discuss recent advances in understanding the mechanisms of TRAP1 regulation, the impact of this regulation on TRAP1 function and downstream cellular processes, and the role of TRAP1 in cancer.

2. Structural Basis of TRAP1 Activity

Hsp90 family chaperones are characterized by their dimeric structure. Each of the two protomers are composed of an amino-terminal ATP-binding domain, followed by a middle domain, the primary interface for client interaction, and a C-terminal domain that allows constitutive dimerization of the protomers [14]. Hsp90 chaperone activity is coupled to its ability to hydrolyze ATP [15,16]. The 'chaperone cycle' begins with ATP binding to the 'open' conformation of Hsp90, followed by transient dimerization of the N-terminal domains of each protomer and ATP hydrolysis, and subsequent release of mature client proteins and regeneration of the 'open' Hsp90 dimer [17]. TRAP1 is broadly structurally similar to cytosolic Hsp90, with some notable exceptions, including a cleavable N-terminal mitochondrial localization signal and an N-terminal extension or 'strap' that stabilizes the 'closed' conformation of TRAP1 [18,19]. Asymmetrical post-translational modification and co-chaperone binding are important determinants of Hsp90 molecular chaperone function [18,20–24]. Interestingly, TRAP1 dimers are inherently asymmetric, and uniquely composed of one 'straight' and one 'buckled' protomer, with the buckled protomer demonstrating increased rates of ATP hydrolysis [25] (Figure 1). Recently, structural and cell-based studies have described a tetrameric form of TRAP1 induced in response to dysregulation of oxidative metabolism, although the impact of this TRAP1 state on its activity is as yet unknown [26]. Interestingly, whether TRAP1 ATPase activity is essential for the entire scope of its biological role also remains an open question [26].

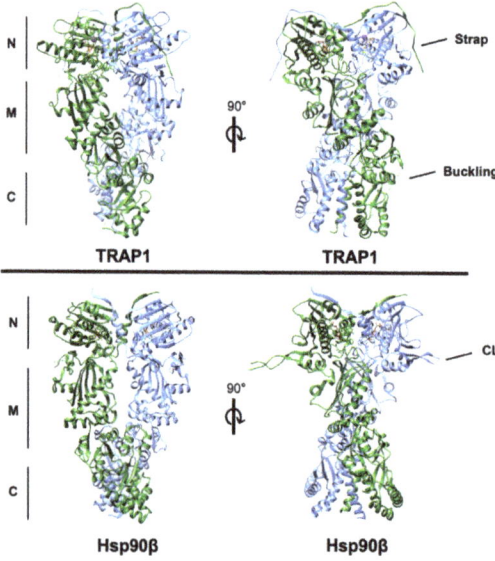

Figure 1. Structures of human TRAP1 (PDB: 6xg6) and human Hsp90β (PDB: 5fwp) bound to nucleotide

with the conserved N-, middle-, and C-domains denoted. One protomer of each is colored blue and the second is colored green. The regulatory N-terminal extension (strap) of each TRAP1 protomer can be observed overlapping the opposite protomer. The region of TRAP1 near the M-C boundary that 'buckles' during conformational rearrangement is incompletely resolved in the structure. Additionally, the resolved residues of the charged linker domain (CL) of cytosolic Hsp90, which is absent in TRAP1, are labeled in the lower right quadrant.

3. Impact of TRAP1 on Cancer Metabolism

Controversially, TRAP1 has alternately been characterized as an oncogene and tumor suppressor, and it has been suggested that TRAP1 is essential for malignant transformation of cells but dispensable at later stages of tumor development [6,27]. Despite this controversy, much of the literature supports the idea that TRAP1 regulates metabolic transformation during tumorigenesis, TRAP1 is overexpressed in many cancers, and TRAP1 attenuation is detrimental to tumor cell survival [28–33]. It may be more appropriate to suggest that, similar to cytosolic Hsp90, many cancers may be 'addicted' to TRAP1 [34–36]. In fact, multiple pathways in which TRAP1 activity can drive tumorigenesis have been described (Figure 2) and will be reviewed in the following section.

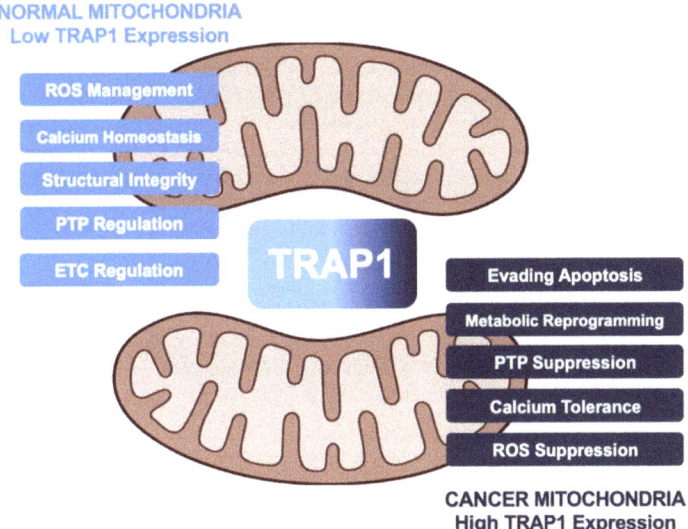

Figure 2. Role of human TRAP1 in mitochondria of normal cells and cancer cells. Normal expression levels (light blue) lead to TRAP1 regulation of ROS and calcium levels, integrity of cristae, function of ETC, and oversight of the PTP. As TRAP1 expression increases (dark blue), mitochondria lose calcium sensitivity, downregulate ROS, and prevent PTP opening, leading to metabolic reprogramming and evasion of apoptosis in cancer.

3.1. Metabolic Regulation

The cellular energy currency adenosine triphosphate (ATP) is generated as a consequence of the complete oxidation of glucose to CO_2 and H_2O, and each molecule of glucose can maximally result in 36–38 ATP molecules [37]. Normal cells produce ATP primarily through cellular respiration, which describes a process in which glucose metabolism by glycolysis is coupled to the tricarboxylic acid cycle (TCA). Concurrent mitochondrial electron transport generates the electrochemical gradient that provides the force by which ATP is disseminated throughout the cell [38]. ATP generation is highly dysregulated in cancers, and many cancer subtypes supplement their ATP supply by upregulating cytosolic glycolysis, simultaneously generating additional ATP driven by the terminal fermentation of pyruvate to lactate [39]. This hyperactive glycolytic phenotype is known as the Warburg effect, and serves to support the accelerated growth of cancers through the increased synthesis of intermediates for anaplerotic metabolism and hypertrophy [40,41]. The phenotypic manifestations of metabolic dysregulation are variable and dependent on cell type and genotype, and many of the details and nuances of this differential regulation remain obscured.

Few specific biological roles and binding partners have been described for TRAP1, despite the broad understanding of its impact on metabolic flux. Two of the few described bona fide clients of TRAP1 however are subunits of electron transport chain (ETC) complexes, Complex II components succinate dehydrogenase subunit A/B (SDHA/B) [42–45], and Complex IV cytochrome *c* oxidase subunit 2 (COXII) [6,46,47]. Complex II/SDH is an iron–sulfur cluster-containing protein complex that functions to transfer electrons from succinate to coenzyme Q10-ubiquinone (Complex III) [48]. In agreement with the understanding of Hsp90 function, TRAP1 maintains SDH in a partially unfolded state [49], and TRAP1 inhibition releases active SDH, leading to an increase in its activity [27,44,50–52]. Further, SDH activity [44,53,54] and the oxygen consumption rate [6,55] are inversely correlated with TRAP1 expression, implicating TRAP1 in promoting the Warburg effect [56]. Notably, SDH also oxidizes succinate to fumarate and thus integrates the TCA cycle and the ETC, indicative of the broad influence of TRAP1 on mitochondrial metabolism [56–58].

Complex IV of the ETC converts molecular oxygen to water, and in doing so enacts the final step in generating the electrochemical gradient that supports ATP production by Complex V (ATP synthase) [59]. COXII is a downstream effector of TRAP1 function in the regulation of apoptosis, and TRAP1 regulates COXII expression [47] and activity [6]. As downregulation or inhibition of TRAP1 has been shown to destabilize COXII [46,50] and deletion of TRAP1 was associated with decreased COXIV subunit levels [60], it is possible that TRAP1 chaperoning of COXII/IV is mechanistically similar to SDHA/B. TRAP1 has also been shown to interact with the Complex V subunit ATPB, although little is known about this interaction [27].

Mitochondrial respiration drives the production of reactive oxygen species (ROS) and is responsible for most cellular ROS (Figure 3) [61]. In considering the role of TRAP1 in chaperoning SDH and COXII, TRAP1-mediated regulation of mitochondrial respiration suppresses ROS production [62], thereby contributing to the regulation of redox homeostasis, metabolic flux, and mitochondrial apoptosis.

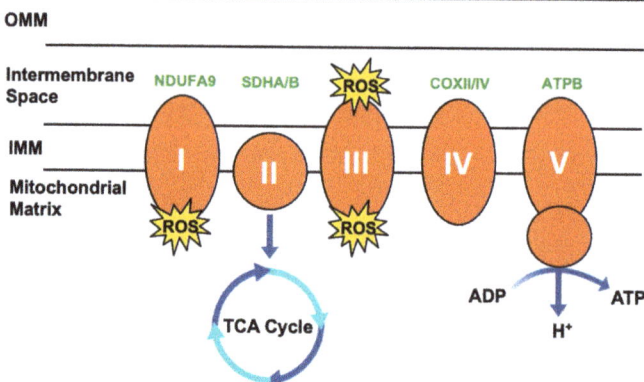

Figure 3. Simplified mitochondrial respiration schematic. Electron transport chain (ETC) complexes (I–V) are represented by orange ovals, and reactive oxygen species (ROS) generated as a byproduct of Complex I and III activity is represented by yellow starbursts. Succinate dehydrogenase (SDH)/Complex II connects the ETC to the tricarboxylic acid (TCA) cycle. TRAP1 interactors involved in this process have been highlighted in green.

3.2. Contribution to Tumorigenesis

Cancer-associated increases in TRAP1 expression suggest a role for TRAP1 in oncogenesis [30,63,64]. Indeed, TRAP1 deletion delayed tumor formation in a mouse model of breast cancer, providing direct evidence of the role of TRAP1 in tumor initiation [65]. Further, TRAP1-mediated SDH inhibition leads to accumulation of the oncometabolite succinate [58]. Increased succinate inhibits the activity of prolyl hydroxylases, which are responsible for the hydroxylation of the transcription factor hypoxia inducible factor (HIF1α), a prerequisite for recognition by the VHL-dependent E3-ubiquitin ligase machinery [66]. Succinate-dependent HIF1α stabilization and activation promotes a well-established glycolytic transcriptional program [67], demonstrating yet another function of TRAP1 in the regulation of cancer-associated metabolic dysregulation.

TRAP1 expression was found to be elevated in aggressive pre-neoplastic lesions in a rat model of hepatocarcinogenesis [68]. The master antioxidant transcription factor NRF2 was also activated in this model, and given the established role of TRAP1 in regulating intracellular ROS, TRAP1 likely participates in NRF2-driven ROS mitigation during tumor development [68]. NRF2 inhibition led to decreased TRAP1 levels independent of TRAP1 transcription [68], suggesting that post-translational regulation is essential for sustained TRAP1 expression in pre-cancerous and cancerous cells. Interestingly, pentose phosphate pathway (PPP) flux was found to be increased in this model, and was determined to be a consequence of elevated citrate synthase activity in aggressive pre-neoplastic lesions [68]. Citrate accumulation inhibits downstream metabolic enzymes phosphofructokinase and SDH and activates the anaplerotic PPP [69]. This increase in citrate synthase activity was alleviated following TRAP1 knockdown or inhibition, suggesting that citrate synthase may also be a TRAP1 client [68].

Cell cycle dysregulation is a well-established driver of tumorigenesis [70]. TRAP1 impacts the cell cycle through regulation of protein quality control in cooperation with the proteasome regulator TBP7 [71,72]. Loss of the TRAP1/TBP7 machinery leads to increased ubiquitination and degradation of the G2-M checkpoint proteins CDK1 and MAD2 and dysregulation of mitotic entry [72]. However, whether TBP7 is a client or perhaps even the first co-chaperone of TRAP1 remains to be seen.

Taken together, these data describe multiple mechanisms through which TRAP1 dysregulation can impact cellular metabolic flux and, potentially, tumorigenesis.

3.3. Evasion of Apoptosis

Mitochondrial involvement in cell death is mediated by the release of cytochrome c [73,74]. Sustained opening of the permeability transition pore (PTP) within the inner mitochondrial membrane (IMM) initiates a series of events that lead to cytochrome c release and apoptosis or necrosis. Upon PTP opening, particles under 1500 Da, such as ions (Ca^{2+}, K^+, and H^+), water, and other solutes, flood the IMM, causing swelling and unfolding of the cristae and eventual outer mitochondrial membrane (OMM) rupture. Subsequent efflux of cytochrome c through the compromised OMM into the cytosol induces the caspase cascade [75,76]. This sustained PTP opening is known as the mitochondrial permeability transition (PT) [77], and it can be triggered by several mechanisms, including elevated ROS, Ca^{2+}, or inorganic phosphate levels, as well as decreased pH or ATP depletion [78]. Interplay between these elements also plays a role in its regulation, as elevated ROS has been shown to decrease the amount of Ca^{2+} required to trigger the PTP [76].

TRAP1 attenuation induces opening of the PTP and release of cytochrome c [47], and expression of TRAP1 likely discourages the initiation of apoptosis through two distinct, but potentially overlapping mechanisms: (1) regulation of triggers that signal into the PTP, and (2) direct disruption of the physical mechanism of PTP opening. TRAP1 knockdown has been shown to lead to increased ROS accumulation under oxidative stress [79] and TRAP1 overexpression insulates cells against iron chelation-mediated ROS production [80]. These effects are likely a consequence of both direct and indirect roles of TRAP1 in minimizing ROS generation. TRAP1 is a direct regulator of oxidative phosphorylation through its chaperoning of Complexes II and IV of the ETC [6,44,46] and has an indirect role in quenching existing ROS, as TRAP1 expression is associated with increased levels of the reduced form of the antioxidant glutathione (GSH) [81]. TRAP1-dependent regulation of ROS generation also results in decreased oxidation of the phospholipid cardiolipin. This phospholipid is responsible for the binding of cytochrome c to the inner folds of cristae, and its oxidation results in an increase of free cytochrome c in the inner membrane space that can potentially escape into the cytosol [78].

Furthermore, TRAP1 has been shown to chaperone the calcium-binding protein Sorcin [82]. TRAP1 is also thought to be responsible for Sorcin translocation into the mitochondria, given that Sorcin lacks its own mitochondrial localization sequence [8,82]. Overexpression of Sorcin in neonatal cardiac myocytes has been shown to increase mitochondrial Ca^{2+} levels, while simultaneously decreasing cytochrome c release, indicating an increase in mitochondrial Ca^{2+} tolerance [83]. Therefore, the chaperoning of Sorcin by TRAP1 is important for desensitizing the PTP to Ca^{2+} levels. Understanding this regulation is particularly important for TRAP1, as Ca^{2+} can replace Mg^{2+} as a co-factor and induce an increased rate of TRAP1 ATP hydrolysis [84]. TRAP1 has also been shown to decrease ubiquitination of the mitochondrial contact site and cristae organizing system subunit 60 (MIC60) under conditions of extracellular acidosis [85]. MIC60 is a critical component of the protein complex MICOS, which is regarded as the master organizer of the IMM through the formation of contact sites with the outer membrane and maintenance of cristae junctions [86,87]. Thus, TRAP1 regulation of MIC60 contributes to its anti-apoptotic function through the preservation of mitochondrial integrity.

Proposals for the structure of the PTP have gone through various iterations, however the prevailing model is that the PTP is formed by coordinated activities of the adenine nucleotide translocator (ANT) and the F-ATP synthase [88–90]. Furthermore, cyclophilin D (CypD) is key to PTP regulation [12,91]. Though its role in this process is controversial, CypD peptidyl-prolyl isomerase activity is required, as is its binding to the mitochondrial peripheral stalk subunit of the F-ATP synthase [63,90,92]. In addition to attenuating the triggers that lead to PTP opening, TRAP1 has been shown to antagonize the opening of the PTP itself. There is a general consensus that TRAP1 accomplishes this by forming a complex with CypD, interfering with the ability of CypD to interact with the PTP [12,63,93] potentially at the peripheral stalk of F-ATP synthase [90].

Further, the mitochondrial chaperones Hsp60 and Hsp90 have been implicated in this process, as their association with CypD also prevents PTP opening; however, the architecture of this complex has yet to be characterized [12,63,93–96].

4. Post-Translational Regulation of TRAP1

Post-translational modification is critically important to mitochondrial function [97] and has previously been shown to regulate TRAP1, though relatively little is known about individual PTM sites (Table 1, Figure 4) [5,6,98,99]. A comprehensive study of cytosolic Hsp90 has demonstrated the importance of post-translational regulation to Hsp90 chaperone activity (reviewed in [3,100]), and in the absence of certain co-chaperone regulatory proteins, specific PTM events have been shown to functionally recapitulate their activity [101]. This phenomenon may be critically important for TRAP1 biology, as TRAP1 is thought to act without the assistance of co-chaperones [8,10].

Table 1. Reported PTMs of TRAP1. Paralog identifies conserved residues in Hsp90α. GSNOR—S-nitrosoglutathione reductase, ERK—extracellular signal-regulated kinase.

Modification	Enzyme	Residue	Paralog	Impact on TRAP1	Reference
S-Nitrosylation	GSNOR	Cys501	Thr495	Decreased activity, proteasomal degradation	[98]
Phosphorylation	ERK1/2	Ser511	Ser505	N/A	[10]
Phosphorylation	ERK1/2	Ser568	Glu562	Increased SDH inhibition	[10]
S/T Phosphorylation	PINK1	N/A	N/A	N/A	[5]
Y Phosphorylation	Unknown, possibly c-Src	N/A	N/A	Disrupts c-Src interaction	[6]
Deacetylation	SIRT3	N/A	N/A	Increased activity	[27]

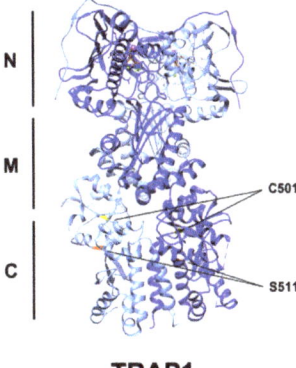

Figure 4. Ribbon structure of human TRAP1 (PDB: 6xg6) with known PTM sites. C501 (yellow) and S511 (red) are highlighted, while S568 is absent.

4.1. Phosphorylation

PINK1 is a mitochondrially targeted serine/threonine kinase whose mutation and inactivation is linked to Parkinson's disease [102]. PINK1 activity has previously been shown to be cytoprotective [103], and when exposed to H_2O_2, cells transfected with siRNA targeting PINK1 showed significant increases in cytochrome *c* release and apoptosis [5]. TRAP1 was shown to be phosphorylated by PINK1 and mediate PINK1 anti-apoptotic activity, as evidenced by the observation that TRAP1 knockdown sensitized cells to PINK1 attenuation [5,104,105]. Interestingly, TRAP1 inhibition leads to activation of PINK1, suggesting a reciprocal regulatory relationship [106].

TRAP1 has also been shown to interact with the mitochondrial serine protease HTRA2 in Parkinson's disease [55]. Canonically, HTRA2 participates in mitochondrial and cellular quality control through inhibition of IAPs (inhibitor of apoptosis proteins) and induction of cell death, while loss of HTRA2 is associated with aberrant mitochondrial function and Parkinson's disease (PD). Overexpression of HTRA2 led to decreased levels of TRAP1, suggesting that HTRA2 may play a role in regulating TRAP1 stability [55]. However, the effect of HTRA2 was independent of its protease activity and the interaction between HTRA2 and TRAP1 was abrogated through treatment with mitochondrial respiratory inhibitors [55]. TRAP1 overexpression is also capable of rescuing mitochondrial dysfunction-associated PINK1 and HTRA2 loss. Interestingly, HTRA2 is also a substrate of PINK1, demonstrating that further work is needed to understand the mechanistic regulation of TRAP1 by HTRA2 and the role of PINK1 in this system.

Neurofibromatosis is caused by mutation and inactivation of the Ras regulatory protein neurofibromin and is characterized by elevated Erk1/2 activity [10]. Active Erk1/2 is associated with TRAP1-SDH in the mitochondria of these cells, and Erk1/2-mediated phosphorylation of TRAP1-S511/S568 strengthens their association, suggestive of a chaperone–client relationship. Association of TRAP1 and SDH decreases SDH activity, leading to accumulation of the oncometabolite succinate [10]. TRAP1 attenuation or loss of phosphorylation at these residues prevents tumor growth, in a succinate-dependent manner [10]. Mitochondrial Erk1/2 was previously shown to antagonize PTP opening [107], perhaps indicating a role for TRAP1 phosphorylation in PTP regulation as well. Taken together, these data suggest that TRAP1 inhibition or combined TRAP1-Erk1/2 targeting may be a viable therapeutic strategy in neurofibromatosis and other cancers.

Interaction with mitochondrially localized c-Src remains the only described TRAP1–tyrosine kinase relationship [6]. Previous work has shown that mitochondrial c-Src is involved in the phosphorylation-mediated activation of ETC Complexes I, II, and IV [108,109]. TRAP1 binds to and maintains c-Src in an inactive state, providing a potential mechanism for TRAP1 suppression of oxidative metabolism and ROS mitigation [6]. Though TRAP1 tyrosine phosphorylation is induced by c-Src expression and abrogated by c-Src inhibition, direct phosphorylation of TRAP1 by c-Src remains to be demonstrated. Taken together, TRAP1 and c-Src play opposing roles in the regulation of mitochondrial metabolism, though the reciprocal impact of c-Src on TRAP1 remains unresolved.

4.2. Acetylation–Deacetylation

Acetylation modulates protein–protein interactions via neutralization of Lys residues and can be reversed by the activity of deacetylases. TRAP1 directly stabilizes one such deacetylase, sirtuin-3 (SIRT3), and augments SIRT3 activity in vitro and in glioma cells [27]. Interestingly, SIRT3 overexpression was also able to rescue the effects of TRAP1 inhibition by the TRAP1 inhibitor gamitrinib [27]. One potential explanation for this observation is that SIRT3-mediated deacetylation of TRAP1 modulates TRAP1 activity or its affinity for gamitrinib, though no direct evidence was reported [27]. SIRT3 knockdown was also shown to increase ROS levels, and SIRT3 overexpression reversed an increase in ROS caused by gamitrinib [27]. Interestingly, attenuation of SIRT3 specifically destabilized TRAP1 substrates NDUFA9 (CI) and SDHB (CII), but not SIRT3 substrates SOD2 and GDH, suggesting that SIRT3-mediated deacetylation of TRAP1 is important for TRAP1 chaperone activity [27]. Interestingly, these interactions were observed in glioblastoma (GBM) cancer stem cells (CSC), which showed a preference for mitochondrial respiration over glycolysis. This work provides a new paradigm for understanding the role of SIRT3 in cancer [110]. Given this context and the known role of both proteins in regulating mitochondrial metabolism, reciprocal regulation of SIRT3 and TRAP1 may provide a positive feedback mechanism that impacts the ability of TRAP1 to chaperone its dependent proteins.

4.3. Nitrosylation

The PTM S-nitrosylation (SNO) is the result of the covalent addition of -NO to the thiol group of cysteine residues [111]. SNO is enzymatically catalyzed by nitrosylases and reversed by the activity of denitrosylases, including S-nitrosoglutathione reductase (GSNOR) [112]. GSNOR is commonly deleted in hepatocellular carcinoma (HCC), and GSNOR-KO mice develop HCC, linking aberrant nitrosylation to cancer [113]. TRAP1-C501-SNO was identified by mass spectrometry [54,114] and this modification was found to decrease TRAP1 ATPase activity, modulate conformational rearrangement, and promote its proteasomal degradation [54,98]. TRAP1 degradation also led to increased SDH activity, in agreement with previous work [44], and sensitized cells to SDH inhibitors, identifying TRAP1-SNO as a predictor of tumor cell response to this class of drugs [54]. It follows that mutation of this residue to TRAP1-C501S provided protection from apoptosis in the presence of nitric oxide donors, demonstrating that disruption of TRAP1-SNO is essential for its anti-apoptotic role [98]. Curiously, however, TRAP1 is overexpressed in many cancers, allowing for the possibility that TRAP1-SNO is context-specific and perhaps also under temporal regulation.

Taken together, PTMs exert influence on TRAP1 through regulating the kinetics of ATP hydrolysis and associated conformational rearrangements, interaction with client proteins, and promoting TRAP1 degradation.

5. Current State of TRAP1 Inhibitor Development

Inhibition of cell metabolism is a re-emerging anti-cancer strategy [115]. TRAP1 control of cellular metabolic flux and mitochondrial apoptosis outlined herein identifies TRAP1 inhibition as a potential anti-cancer therapeutic target. Efforts towards the development of ATP-competitive inhibitors for cytosolic Hsp90 have provided lead compounds for optimization to address the dual challenges of mitochondrial localization and TRAP1 specificity. Conjugation to a chemical scaffold such as the mitochondrial-targeting moiety triphenylphosphonium (TPP) is necessary to provide mitochondrial penetrance [116,117]. Specificity for TRAP1 over Hsp90 may also be a necessary consideration, as well-established Hsp90 ATP-competitive inhibitors cannot differentiate between the ATP-binding pockets, potentially leading to off-target toxicity [33].

5.1. Gamitrinibs

The most widely used mitochondrial Hsp90 inhibitors are gamitrinibs (G), small molecules consisting of the Hsp90 inhibitor 17-allylamino-17-demethoxygeldanamycin (17-AAG) attached to a mitochondrial-targeting moiety such as cyclic guanidinium repeats or TPP (G-G1-4 and G-TPP, respectively) [118]. These gamitrinibs have demonstrably reduced the viability of prostate [91,119–122], colon [119,123], melanoma [119,124], cervix [122,125], ovary [122], breast [118,119,121,124,125], and glioma cancers [126], particularly glioblastomas [120,124,127–129]. Gamitrinibs disrupt the anti-apoptotic effects of TRAP1, as evidenced by decreased mitochondrial membrane potential and increased cytochrome *c* release in G-TPP-treated PC3 prostate cancer cells [119]. Furthermore, the stability of the sensitive cytosolic Hsp90 client proteins Akt and phospho-Y416-Src was impacted by 17-AAG treatment, but unaffected by G-TPP in PC3 cells, demonstrating the selective targeting of gamitrinibs to the mitochondria [119]. A further consideration is the potential for resistance development, as PC3 cells continuously incubated with 17-AAG eventually became resistant to G-TPP, but not G-G4 [118,119]. This finding potentially suggests that the choice of mitochondrial-targeting moiety may be critically important and not necessarily limited simply to drug transport. Overall, selective TRAP1 inhibition with ATP-competitive gamitrinib derivatives remains a challenge. Further, these data emphasize the importance of understanding effectors of TRAP1 for the identification of potential combinatorial therapeutic targets to augment inhibition of TRAP1-mediated signaling pathways.

5.2. Purine-Scaffold Inhibitors

In addition to 17-AAG, mitochondrial targeting of the purine-scaffold Hsp90 inhibitor PU-H71 has also demonstrated efficacy against TRAP1. A TPP-conjugated derivative of PU-H71 (SMTIN-P01) showed a remarkable ability to target mitochondria over non-conjugated PU-H71 and a slight improvement in cytotoxicity over gamitrinibs [130]. Interestingly, adjustments to the length of the TPP resulted in changes in inhibitor behavior. When the TPP was modified to have a 10-length carbon chain (as opposed to the standard 6-length carbon chain), this so-called SMTIN-C10 induced structural changes to TRAP1 and demonstrated increased inhibition of TRAP1 [52]. SMTIN-C10 was found to bind to an allosteric binding site at E115 in the N-terminal domain of TRAP1, in addition to binding to the ATP pocket, resulting in TRAP1 adopting a closed formation [52]. This long linker approach was adapted for other TRAP1 inhibitors as well, including Mitoquinone. TPP-Mitoquinone has shown utility and specificity by targeting the client-binding middle domain of TRAP1 [117]. Mitoquinone has been demonstrated to have protective properties in various animal models of neurological maladies, such as traumatic brain injury [131], Huntington's disease [132], amyotrophic lateral sclerosis (ALS) [133], and Alzheimer's disease [134]. This finding is contradictory to the working model of TRAP1 function, especially considering that TRAP1 downregulation is observed in Alzheimer's disease patients [135] and its overexpression is protective against oxidative stress in ALS [62]. These results highlight the need to understand the disease-specific contexts of TRAP1 function to identify appropriate disease models for the evaluation of TRAP1 inhibitors.

5.3. New Inhibitors

Since their discovery, Hsp90 inhibitors have primarily targeted the ATP-binding pocket (Figure 5). This is the mechanism of the natural product geldanamycin (GA) [136–138] and its derivatives, as well as the first synthetic inhibitor of TRAP1, Shepherdin [139]. Shepherdin was designed by imitating the minimal Hsp90-binding sequence of Survivin (aa 79–87), an anti-apoptotic protein that binds to the N-domain of Hsp90 [140]. Consequently, Shepherdin was also found to disrupt Hsp90-ATP binding with 13 predicted sites of hydrogen bonding in the ATP pocket [139]. Modeling studies based on the structure of Shepherdin identified the small molecule 5-aminoimidazole-4-carboxamide-1-β-D-ribofuranoside (AICAR), a previously characterized AMPK activator [141,142], as a potential Hsp90 inhibitor, though its development as a scaffold for Hsp90 inhibition has not been pursued.

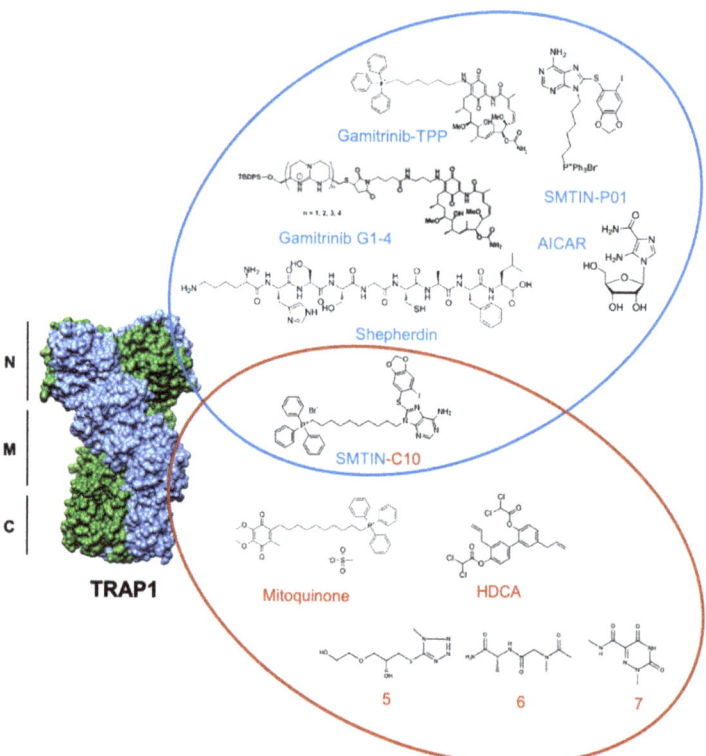

Figure 5. Structures of discussed TRAP1 inhibitors. ATP-competitive small molecules targeting the N-domain of TRAP1 (PDB: 6xg6) are labeled blue, while allosteric inhibitors, primarily targeting the TRAP1 middle domain, are labeled red. SMTIN-C10 is a bifunctional inhibitor, with elements of both ATP-competitive and allosteric inhibition.

Though ATP-competitive Hsp90 inhibitors are still widely used, an alternative approach in hopes of achieving TRAP1 specificity over other Hsp90 family members has emerged through allosteric targeting. One example of this strategy is honokiol bis-dichloroacetate (HDCA), which is able to specifically inhibit TRAP1 by binding to an allosteric pocket within the middle domain. This pocket has a surface landscape defined by a positively charged region sandwiched between two negatively charged regions that are separated from each other by a large hydrophobic area. HDCA binds in this hydrophobic area and allosterically inhibits TRAP1 ATPase activity, but not that of Hsp90 [43].

Further, computational methods by Sanchez-Martin et al. utilized the unique asymmetry of TRAP1 to identify an allosteric pocket on the straight protomer of the TRAP1 dimer that can serve as a TRAP1-specific inhibitor binding surface [42]. Inter-domain communication is essential to the ATPase cycle of TRAP1, and previous work has shown that inhibitor-bound TRAP1 stalls in the NTD dimerized phase [143]. In agreement, the computationally identified compounds (compounds 5–7) were hypothesized to inhibit TRAP1 by reducing the ability of the ATP-binding site to communicate with the client-binding region of the middle domain. In fact, several of these small molecules were shown to decrease TRAP1 ATPase activity to a degree comparable to that of 17-AAG, while not significantly interfering with Hsp90 ATPase activity, demonstrating specificity for TRAP1 [42]. Furthermore, allosterically inhibited TRAP1 bound approximately 30% less SDHA than its control and experienced a significant increase in succinate-coenzyme-Q reductase (SQR) activity. While the tested compound did not alter cell viability, it delayed cell proliferation over a 96 h observation [42]. The successful utilization of TRAP1 asymmetry to identify unique allosteric binding pockets provides a significant starting point for future inhibitor work.

6. Future Perspectives

The function of TRAP1 as a regulator of cellular metabolic flux and mitochondrial apoptosis underscores a duality in which cell fate decisions are determined (Figure 6). Normal cells demonstrate basal TRAP1 expression, facilitating oxidative metabolism and programmed cell death. Dysregulation of TRAP1 expression manifests in noted hallmarks of cancer, including cell death resistance and deregulation of cellular energetics [144]. A thorough delineation of the mechanism of TRAP1 function in these roles is essential to combatting diseases of mitochondrial dysfunction, including cancer and neurodegeneration.

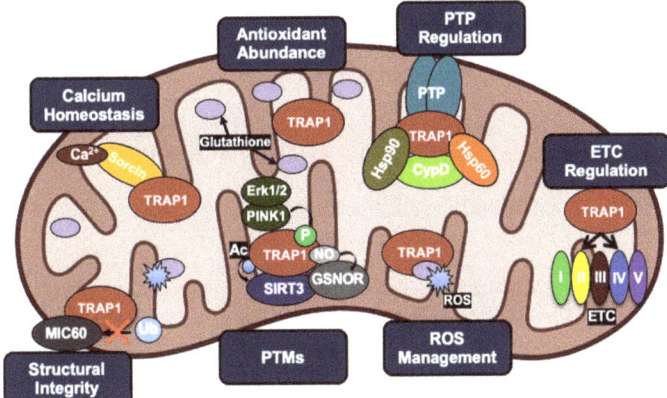

Figure 6. The multiple roles of TRAP1 in cancer cell mitochondria, revolving around evasion of apoptosis and metabolic reprogramming. TRAP1 acts as a chaperone for the Ca^{2+} binding protein Sorcin as well as Complexes II and IV of the ETC. Increased TRAP1 levels are associated with calcium tolerance, increased levels of the antioxidant glutathione, reduced levels of ROS, reduced levels of MIC60 ubiquitination, and in many cases, a shift towards the Warburg effect. TRAP1, along with Hsp90 and Hsp60, can form a complex with CypD to prevent opening of the PTP. TRAP1 is post-translationally modified by PINK1, Erk1/2, GSNOR, and SIRT3.

Though our understanding of the cellular impact of TRAP1 is coming into focus, several outstanding questions remain that are essential to our comprehension of the full scope of TRAP1 biology. (1) Is TRAP1 ATPase activity, and by extension TRAP1 chaperone function, essential for its biological activity? ATP-competitive inhibitors of TRAP1 demonstrate efficacy in cell models of cancer, suggesting that TRAP1 function is coupled to its ATPase activity; however, catalytically inactive TRAP1 mutants are able to complement TRAP1 function and revert metabolic dysfunction [26]. Reconciling these disparate observations is an ongoing challenge. (2) What is the physiological impact of TRAP1 dimeric and tetrameric forms, and is transition between these states essential for its function? Cytosolic Hsp90s are well-established dimers, and though the domain architecture of TRAP1 is similar, it remains unclear whether the TRAP1 dimer is the primary biological unit. (3) Is specific targeting of TRAP1 in cancer essential? Many existing TRAP1 inhibitors are mitochondrially targeted Hsp90 inhibitors. Though strategic inhibition of cytosolic Hsp90 has yet to demonstrate clinical success, perhaps simultaneous disruption of TRAP1 and the mitochondrial Hsp90 pool will prove efficacious [145]. (4) Can TRAP1 be used as a biomarker in cancer? Previous work has demonstrated that circulating Hsp90 can potentially be used as a biomarker in certain conditions, however the presence of circulating TRAP1 has not been evaluated [146–148]. Similarly, TRAP1 expression and activity is dysregulated in cancer, potentially suggesting an ability to serve as a predictive indicator of disease state. (5) TRAP1 mutations have been implicated in several conditions, including congenital anomalies of the kidney and urinary tract (CAKUT), vertebral defects, anal atresia, cardiac defects, tracheo-esophageal fistula, renal anomalies, and limb abnormalities (VACTERL), Parkinson's disease, cardiac hypertrophy, and severe autoinflammation [55,149–151]. What is the structural basis for the impact of these mutations on TRAP1 function? Is mutant-TRAP1 association with these diseases a consequence of its role as a more general regulator of mitochondrial dynamics [152]? (6) Can differential PTM of TRAP1 in normal and disease states predict disease-associated phenotypes? Indeed, it has been shown that PTMs modulate TRAP1, however whether this necessarily predicts TRAP1 behavior in disease states remains to be tested. (7) Do TRAP1 PTMs compensate for a lack of dedicated co-chaperones? In the case of Hsp90, a single phosphorylation can functionally replace the loss of the yeast co-chaperone Hch1 [101]. The relevance of this mechanism for TRAP1 has not yet been investigated, however the reliance of cytosolic Hsp90 on co-chaperone interaction suggests that TRAP1 PTMs can recapitulate some co-chaperone activities. (8) Can these PTMs be specifically manipulated to alter TRAP1 function? Many cancers are associated with increased TRAP1 activity, and decreased TRAP1 activity or loss-of-function mutations contribute to the pathogenesis of some neurodegenerative diseases [153]. Previous work discussed here demonstrates that PTMs play a role in the regulation of TRAP1 stability, and TRAP1 PTMs are dysregulated in disease. High-throughput methods [154] as well as the study of cytosolic Hsp90s suggest that TRAP1 function will be regulated by a constellation of PTMs with differential incidence that correlates with disease state [3].

The literature reviewed here from several experimental systems demonstrates that in cancers that overexpress TRAP1, attenuation of TRAP1 expression or activity is sufficient to slow cell growth, and in some instances, induce apoptosis. Furthermore, nuanced studies of Hsp90 have demonstrated that PTM can modulate the efficacy of Hsp90 inhibitors [3], implying a similar framework for the application of TRAP1 inhibitors. The identification of predictive indicators of response to TRAP1 inhibition and potential targets for anti-cancer therapy in combination with TRAP1 inhibitors are two essential pieces of information that can be gained from decrypting the TRAP1 chaperone code.

Author Contributions: Conceptualization, M.R.W.; writing—original draft preparation, L.A.W. and M.R.W.; writing—review and editing, L.A.W., S.J.B., D.B., M.M. and M.R.W.; visualization, L.A.W., S.J.B. and M.R.W.; supervision, M.R.W.; project administration, M.R.W.; funding acquisition, D.B., M.M. and M.R.W. All authors have read and agreed to the published version of the manuscript.

Funding: This work was partly supported by funds from SUNY Upstate Medical University and The Upstate Foundation (M.M., D.B. and M.R.W.).

Institutional Review Board Statement: Not applicable.

Informed Consent Statement: Not applicable.

Data Availability Statement: Not applicable.

Acknowledgments: We would like to thank Giorgio Colombo and Len Neckers for insightful scientific discussions. The figures were created using elements from Biorender.com on an institutional license from SUNY Upstate Medical University.

Conflicts of Interest: The authors declare no conflict of interest.

Abbreviations

17-AAG, 17-allylamino-17-demethoxygeldanamycin; AICAR, 5-aminoimidazole-4-carboxamide-1-β-D-ribofuranoside; ALS, amyotrophic lateral sclerosis; ANT, adenosine nucleotide translocator; ATP, adenosine triphosphate; ATPB, ATP synthase subunit beta; AMPK, AMP-activated protein kinase; CAKUT, congenital anomalies of the kidney and urinary tract, CDK1, cyclin-dependent kinase 1; COXII/IV, cytochrome c oxidase subunit 2/4; CSC, cancer stem cells; CypD, cyclophilin D; Erk1/2, extracellular signal-regulated kinase 1/2; ETC, electron transport chain; G, gamitrinib; G1-4, cyclic guanidinium 1-4; GA, geldanamycin; GDH, glutamate dehydrogenase; GMB, glioblastoma; GSH, reduced glutathione; GSNOR, S-nitrosoglutathione reductase; HCC, hepatocellular carcinoma; HDCA, honokiol bis-dichloroacetate; HIF1α, hypoxia inducible factor 1α; Hsp, heat shock protein; Hsp60, heat shock protein 60; Hsp90, heat shock protein 90; HTRA2, high-temperature requirement A2; IMM, inner mitochondrial membrane; KO, knockout; MAD2, mitotic arrest deficiency 2; MICOS, mitochondrial contact site and cristae organizing system; NDUFA9, NADH:ubiquinone oxidoreductase subunit A9; NRF2, nuclear factor erythroid 2-related factor 2; NTD, N-terminal domain; OMM, outer mitochondrial membrane; PD, Parkinson's disease; PINK1, phosphatase and tensin homolog (PTEN)-induced kinase 1; PPP, pentose phosphate pathway; PT, mitochondrial permeability transition; PTM, post-translational modification; PTP, permeability transition pore; ROS, reactive oxygen species; SDH, succinate dehydrogenase; SDHA/B, succinate dehydrogenase subunit a/b; SIRT3, sirtuin-3; SNO, S-nitrosylation; SOD2, superoxide dismutase 2; SQR, succinate-coenzyme-Q reductase; TBP7, TATA-Box binding protein 7; TCA, tricarboxylic acid cycle; TPP, triphenylphosphonium; TRAP1, tumor necrosis factor (TNF) receptor-associated protein-1; VACTERL, vertebral defects, anal atresia, cardiac defects, tracheo-esophageal fistula, renal anomalies, and limb abnormalities; VHL, Von Hippel Lindau.

References

1. Prodromou, C.; Bjorklund, D.M. Advances towards Understanding the Mechanism of Action of the Hsp90 Complex. *Biomolecules* **2022**, *12*, 600. [CrossRef] [PubMed]
2. Johnson, J.L. Mutations in Hsp90 Cochaperones Result in a Wide Variety of Human Disorders. *Front. Mol. Biosci.* **2021**, *8*, 787260. [CrossRef] [PubMed]
3. Backe, S.J.; Sager, R.A.; Woodford, M.R.; Makedon, A.M.; Mollapour, M. Post-Translational Modifications of Hsp90 and Translating the Chaperone Code. *J. Biol. Chem.* **2020**, *295*, 11099–11117. [CrossRef] [PubMed]
4. Cechetto, J.D.; Gupta, R.S. Immunoelectron Microscopy Provides Evidence That Tumor Necrosis Factor Receptor-Associated Protein 1 (TRAP-1) Is a Mitochondrial Protein Which Also Localizes at Specific Extramitochondrial Sites. *Exp. Cell Res.* **2000**, *260*, 30–39. [CrossRef]
5. Pridgeon, J.W.; Olzmann, J.A.; Chin, L.-S.; Li, L. PINK1 Protects against Oxidative Stress by Phosphorylating Mitochondrial Chaperone TRAP1. *PLoS Biol.* **2007**, *5*, e172. [CrossRef]
6. Yoshida, S.; Tsutsumi, S.; Muhlebach, G.; Sourbier, C.; Lee, M.-J.; Lee, S.; Vartholomaiou, E.; Tatokoro, M.; Beebe, K.; Miyajima, N.; et al. Molecular Chaperone TRAP1 Regulates a Metabolic Switch between Mitochondrial Respiration and Aerobic Glycolysis. *Proc. Natl. Acad. Sci. USA* **2013**, *110*, E1604–E1612. [CrossRef]
7. Song, H.Y.; Dunbar, J.D.; Zhang, Y.X.; Guo, D.; Donner, D.B. Identification of a Protein with Homology to Hsp90 That Binds the Type 1 Tumor Necrosis Factor Receptor. *J. Biol. Chem.* **1995**, *270*, 3574–3581. [CrossRef]
8. Felts, S.J.; Owen, B.A.L.; Nguyen, P.; Trepel, J.; Donner, D.B.; Toft, D.O. The Hsp90-Related Protein TRAP1 Is a Mitochondrial Protein with Distinct Functional Properties. *J. Biol. Chem.* **2000**, *275*, 3305–3312. [CrossRef]

9. Cannino, G.; Ciscato, F.; Masgras, I.; Sánchez-Martín, C.; Rasola, A. Metabolic Plasticity of Tumor Cell Mitochondria. *Front. Oncol.* **2018**, *8*, 333. [CrossRef]
10. Masgras, I.; Ciscato, F.; Brunati, A.M.; Tibaldi, E.; Indraccolo, S.; Curtarello, M.; Chiara, F.; Cannino, G.; Papaleo, E.; Lambrughi, M.; et al. Absence of Neurofibromin Induces an Oncogenic Metabolic Switch via Mitochondrial ERK-Mediated Phosphorylation of the Chaperone TRAP1. *Cell Rep.* **2017**, *18*, 659–672. [CrossRef]
11. Masgras, I.; Laquatra, C.; Cannino, G.; Serapian, S.A.; Colombo, G.; Rasola, A. The Molecular Chaperone TRAP1 in Cancer: From the Basics of Biology to Pharmacological Targeting. *Semin. Cancer Biol.* **2021**, *76*, 45–53. [CrossRef] [PubMed]
12. Porter, G.A.; Beutner, G. Cyclophilin D, Somehow a Master Regulator of Mitochondrial Function. *Biomolecules* **2018**, *8*, 176. [CrossRef] [PubMed]
13. Altieri, D.C.; Stein, G.S.; Lian, J.B.; Languino, L.R. TRAP-1, the Mitochondrial Hsp90. *Biochim. Et Biophys. Acta (BBA)-Mol. Cell Res.* **2012**, *1823*, 767–773. [CrossRef] [PubMed]
14. Schopf, F.H.; Biebl, M.M.; Buchner, J. The HSP90 Chaperone Machinery. *Nat. Rev. Mol. Cell Biol.* **2017**, *18*, 345–360. [CrossRef] [PubMed]
15. Obermann, W.M.J.; Sondermann, H.; Russo, A.A.; Pavletich, N.P.; Hartl, F.U. In Vivo Function of Hsp90 Is Dependent on ATP Binding and ATP Hydrolysis. *J. Cell Biol.* **1998**, *143*, 901–910. [CrossRef] [PubMed]
16. Panaretou, B. ATP Binding and Hydrolysis Are Essential to the Function of the Hsp90 Molecular Chaperone Invivo. *EMBO J.* **1998**, *17*, 4829–4836. [CrossRef]
17. Sahasrabudhe, P.; Rohrberg, J.; Biebl, M.M.; Rutz, D.A.; Buchner, J. The Plasticity of the Hsp90 Co-Chaperone System. *Mol. Cell* **2017**, *67*, 947–961.e5. [CrossRef]
18. Lavery, L.A.; Partridge, J.R.; Ramelot, T.A.; Elnatan, D.; Kennedy, M.A.; Agard, D.A. Structural Asymmetry in the Closed State of Mitochondrial Hsp90 (TRAP1) Supports a Two-Step ATP Hydrolysis Mechanism. *Mol. Cell* **2014**, *53*, 330–343. [CrossRef]
19. Partridge, J.R.; Lavery, L.A.; Elnatan, D.; Naber, N.; Cooke, R.; Agard, D.A. A Novel N-Terminal Extension in Mitochondrial TRAP1 Serves as a Thermal Regulator of Chaperone Activity. *eLife* **2014**, *3*, e03487. [CrossRef]
20. Ali, M.M.U.; Roe, S.M.; Vaughan, C.K.; Meyer, P.; Panaretou, B.; Piper, P.W.; Prodromou, C.; Pearl, L.H. Crystal Structure of an Hsp90–Nucleotide–P23/Sba1 Closed Chaperone Complex. *Nature* **2006**, *440*, 1013–1017. [CrossRef]
21. Mayer, M.P.; Le Breton, L. Hsp90: Breaking the Symmetry. *Mol. Cell* **2015**, *58*, 8–20. [CrossRef] [PubMed]
22. Mollapour, M.; Bourboulia, D.; Beebe, K.; Woodford, M.R.; Polier, S.; Hoang, A.; Chelluri, R.; Li, Y.; Guo, A.; Lee, M.-J.; et al. Asymmetric Hsp90 N Domain SUMOylation Recruits Aha1 and ATP-Competitive Inhibitors. *Mol. Cell* **2014**, *53*, 317–329. [CrossRef] [PubMed]
23. Retzlaff, M.; Hagn, F.; Mitschke, L.; Hessling, M.; Gugel, F.; Kessler, H.; Richter, K.; Buchner, J. Asymmetric Activation of the Hsp90 Dimer by Its Cochaperone Aha1. *Mol. Cell* **2010**, *37*, 344–354. [CrossRef] [PubMed]
24. Vaughan, C.K.; Gohlke, U.; Sobott, F.; Good, V.M.; Ali, M.M.U.; Prodromou, C.; Robinson, C.V.; Saibil, H.R.; Pearl, L.H. Structure of an Hsp90-Cdc37-Cdk4 Complex. *Mol. Cell* **2006**, *23*, 697–707. [CrossRef]
25. Elnatan, D.; Betegon, M.; Liu, Y.; Ramelot, T.; Kennedy, M.A.; Agard, D.A. Symmetry Broken and Rebroken during the ATP Hydrolysis Cycle of the Mitochondrial TRAP1. *eLife* **2017**, *6*, e25235. [CrossRef]
26. Joshi, A.; Dai, L.; Liu, Y.; Lee, J.; Ghahhari, N.M.; Segala, G.; Beebe, K.; Jenkins, L.M.; Lyons, G.C.; Bernasconi, L.; et al. The Mitochondrial HSP90 Paralog TRAP1 Forms an OXPHOS-Regulated Tetramer and Is Involved in Mitochondrial Metabolic Homeostasis. *BMC Biol.* **2020**, *18*, 10. [CrossRef]
27. Park, H.-K.; Hong, J.-H.; Oh, Y.T.; Kim, S.S.; Yin, J.; Lee, A.-J.; Chae, Y.C.; Kim, J.H.; Park, S.-H.; Park, C.-K.; et al. Interplay between TRAP1 and Sirtuin-3 Modulates Mitochondrial Respiration and Oxidative Stress to Maintain Stemness of Glioma Stem Cells. *Cancer Res* **2019**, *79*, 1369–1382. [CrossRef]
28. Lisanti, S.; Garlick, D.S.; Bryant, K.G.; Tavecchio, M.; Mills, G.B.; Lu, Y.; Kossenkov, A.V.; Showe, L.C.; Languino, L.R.; Altieri, D.C. Transgenic Expression of the Mitochondrial Chaperone TNFR-Associated Protein 1 (TRAP1) Accelerates Prostate Cancer Development. *J. Biol. Chem.* **2016**, *291*, 25247–25254. [CrossRef]
29. Ramkumar, B.; Dharaskar, S.P.; Mounika, G.; Paithankar, K.; Sreedhar, A.S. Mitochondrial Chaperone, TRAP1 as a Potential Pharmacological Target to Combat Cancer Metabolism. *Mitochondrion* **2020**, *50*, 42–50. [CrossRef]
30. Si, T.; Yang, G.; Qiu, X.; Luo, Y.; Liu, B.; Wang, B. Expression of Tumor Necrosis Factor Receptor-Associated. *Int. J. Clin. Exp. Pathol.* **2015**, *8*, 13090–13095.
31. Zhang, B.; Wang, J.; Huang, Z.; Wei, P.; Liu, Y.; Hao, J.; Zhao, L.; Zhang, F.; Tu, Y.; Wei, T. Aberrantly Upregulated TRAP1 Is Required for Tumorigenesis of Breast Cancer. *Oncotarget* **2015**, *6*, 44495–44508. [CrossRef] [PubMed]
32. Xie, S. The Mitochondrial Chaperone TRAP1 as a Candidate Target of Oncotherapy. *Front. Oncol.* **2021**, *10*, 11.
33. Serapian, S.A.; Sanchez-Martín, C.; Moroni, E.; Rasola, A.; Colombo, G. Targeting the Mitochondrial Chaperone TRAP1: Strategies and Therapeutic Perspectives. *Trends Pharmacol. Sci.* **2021**, *42*, 566–576. [CrossRef] [PubMed]
34. Miyata, Y.; Nakamoto, H.; Neckers, L. The Therapeutic Target Hsp90 and Cancer Hallmarks. *Curr. Pharm. Des.* **2013**, *19*, 347–365. [CrossRef] [PubMed]
35. Trepel, J.; Mollapour, M.; Giaccone, G.; Neckers, L. Targeting the Dynamic HSP90 Complex in Cancer. *Nat. Rev. Cancer* **2010**, *10*, 537–549. [CrossRef]

36. Zong, H.; Gozman, A.; Caldas-Lopes, E.; Taldone, T.; Sturgill, E.; Brennan, S.; Ochiana, S.O.; Gomes-DaGama, E.M.; Sen, S.; Rodina, A.; et al. A Hyperactive Signalosome in Acute Myeloid Leukemia Drives Addiction to a Tumor-Specific Hsp90 Species. *Cell Rep.* **2015**, *13*, 2159–2173. [CrossRef]
37. Vander Heiden, M.G.; Cantley, L.C.; Thompson, C.B. Understanding the Warburg Effect: The Metabolic Requirements of Cell Proliferation. *Science* **2009**, *324*, 1029–1033. [CrossRef]
38. Martínez-Reyes, I.; Chandel, N.S. Mitochondrial TCA Cycle Metabolites Control Physiology and Disease. *Nat. Commun.* **2020**, *11*, 102. [CrossRef]
39. Woodford, M.R.; Baker-Williams, A.J.; Sager, R.A.; Backe, S.J.; Blanden, A.R.; Hashmi, F.; Kancherla, P.; Gori, A.; Loiselle, D.R.; Castelli, M.; et al. The Tumor Suppressor Folliculin Inhibits Lactate Dehydrogenase A and Regulates the Warburg Effect. *Nat. Struct. Mol. Biol.* **2021**, *28*, 662–670. [CrossRef]
40. DeBerardinis, R.J.; Chandel, N.S. We Need to Talk about the Warburg Effect. *Nat. Metab.* **2020**, *2*, 127–129. [CrossRef]
41. Warburg, O. The Metabolism of Carcinoma Cells. *J. Cancer Res.* **1925**, *9*, 148–163. [CrossRef]
42. Sanchez-Martin, C.; Moroni, E.; Ferraro, M.; Laquatra, C.; Cannino, G.; Masgras, I.; Negro, A.; Quadrelli, P.; Rasola, A.; Colombo, G. Rational Design of Allosteric and Selective Inhibitors of the Molecular Chaperone TRAP1. *Cell Rep.* **2020**, *31*, 107531. [CrossRef] [PubMed]
43. Sanchez-Martin, C.; Menon, D.; Moroni, E.; Ferraro, M.; Masgras, I.; Elsey, J.; Arbiser, J.L.; Colombo, G.; Rasola, A. Honokiol Bis-Dichloroacetate Is a Selective Allosteric Inhibitor of the Mitochondrial Chaperone TRAP1. *Antioxid. Redox Signal.* **2021**, *34*, 505–516. [CrossRef] [PubMed]
44. Sciacovelli, M.; Guzzo, G.; Morello, V.; Frezza, C.; Zheng, L.; Nannini, N.; Calabrese, F.; Laudiero, G.; Esposito, F.; Landriscina, M.; et al. The Mitochondrial Chaperone TRAP1 Promotes Neoplastic Growth by Inhibiting Succinate Dehydrogenase. *Cell Metab.* **2013**, *17*, 988–999. [CrossRef]
45. Serapian, S.A.; Moroni, E.; Ferraro, M.; Colombo, G. Atomistic Simulations of the Mechanisms of the Poorly Catalytic Mitochondrial Chaperone Trap1: Insights into the Effects of Structural Asymmetry on Reactivity. *ACS Catal.* **2021**, *11*, 8605–8620. [CrossRef]
46. Xiang, F.; Ma, S.; Lv, Y.; Zhang, D.; Song, H.; Huang, Y. Tumor Necrosis Factor Receptor-Associated Protein 1 Regulates Hypoxia-Induced Apoptosis through a Mitochondria-Dependent Pathway Mediated by Cytochrome c Oxidase Subunit II. *Burn. Trauma* **2019**, *7*, s41038-019-0154-3s41038–s019. [CrossRef]
47. Xiang, F.; Ma, S.-Y.; Zhang, D.-X.; Zhang, Q.; Huang, Y.-S. Tumor Necrosis Factor Receptor-Associated Protein 1 Improves Hypoxia-Impaired Energy Production in Cardiomyocytes through Increasing Activity of Cytochrome c Oxidase Subunit II. *Int. J. Biochem. Cell Biol.* **2016**, *79*, 239–248. [CrossRef]
48. Bezawork-Geleta, A.; Rohlena, J.; Dong, L.; Pacak, K.; Neuzil, J. Mitochondrial Complex II: At the Crossroads. *Trends Biochem. Sci.* **2017**, *42*, 312–325. [CrossRef]
49. Liu, Y.; Elnatan, D.; Sun, M.; Myasnikov, A.G.; Agard, D.A. Cryo-EM Reveals the Dynamic Interplay between Mitochondrial Hsp90 and SdhB Folding Intermediates. *bioRxiv* **2020**. [CrossRef]
50. Agarwal, E.; Altman, B.J.; Seo, J.H.; Ghosh, J.C.; Kossenkov, A.V.; Tang, H.-Y.; Krishn, S.R.; Languino, L.R.; Gabrilovich, D.I.; Speicher, D.W.; et al. Myc-Mediated Transcriptional Regulation of the Mitochondrial Chaperone TRAP1 Controls Primary and Metastatic Tumor Growth. *J. Biol. Chem.* **2019**, *294*, 10407–10414. [CrossRef]
51. Chae, Y.C.; Angelin, A.; Lisanti, S.; Kossenkov, A.V.; Speicher, K.D.; Wang, H.; Powers, J.F.; Tischler, A.S.; Pacak, K.; Fliedner, S.; et al. Landscape of the Mitochondrial Hsp90 Metabolome in Tumours. *Nat. Commun.* **2013**, *4*, 2139. [CrossRef] [PubMed]
52. Hu, S.; Ferraro, M.; Thomas, A.P.; Chung, J.M.; Yoon, N.G.; Seol, J.-H.; Kim, S.; Kim, H.; An, M.Y.; Ok, H.; et al. Dual Binding to Orthosteric and Allosteric Sites Enhances the Anticancer Activity of a TRAP1-Targeting Drug. *J. Med. Chem.* **2020**, *63*, 2930–2940. [CrossRef] [PubMed]
53. Masgras, I.; Sanchez-Martin, C.; Colombo, G.; Rasola, A. The Chaperone TRAP1 As a Modulator of the Mitochondrial Adaptations in Cancer Cells. *Front. Oncol.* **2017**, *7*, 58. [CrossRef]
54. Rizza, S.; Montagna, C.; Cardaci, S.; Maiani, E.; Di Giacomo, G.; Sanchez-Quiles, V.; Blagoev, B.; Rasola, A.; De Zio, D.; Stamler, J.S.; et al. S-Nitrosylation of the Mitochondrial Chaperone TRAP1 Sensitizes Hepatocellular Carcinoma Cells to Inhibitors of Succinate Dehydrogenase. *Cancer Res.* **2016**, *76*, 4170–4182. [CrossRef] [PubMed]
55. Fitzgerald, J.C.; Zimprich, A.; Carvajal Berrio, D.A.; Schindler, K.M.; Maurer, B.; Schulte, C.; Bus, C.; Hauser, A.-K.; Kübler, M.; Lewin, R.; et al. Metformin Reverses TRAP1 Mutation-Associated Alterations in Mitochondrial Function in Parkinson's Disease. *Brain* **2017**, *140*, 2444–2459. [CrossRef]
56. Guzzo, G.; Sciacovelli, M.; Bernardi, P.; Rasola, A. Inhibition of Succinate Dehydrogenase by the Mitochondrial Chaperone TRAP1 Has Anti-Oxidant and Anti-Apoptotic Effects on Tumor Cells. *Oncotarget* **2014**, *5*, 11897–11908. [CrossRef] [PubMed]
57. Hsu, C.-C.; Tseng, L.-M.; Lee, H.-C. Role of Mitochondrial Dysfunction in Cancer Progression. *Exp. Biol. Med.* **2016**, *241*, 1281–1295. [CrossRef] [PubMed]
58. Selak, M.A.; Armour, S.M.; MacKenzie, E.D.; Boulahbel, H.; Watson, D.G.; Mansfield, K.D.; Pan, Y.; Simon, M.C.; Thompson, C.B.; Gottlieb, E. Succinate Links TCA Cycle Dysfunction to Oncogenesis by Inhibiting HIF-α Prolyl Hydroxylase. *Cancer Cell* **2005**, *7*, 77–85. [CrossRef]

59. Zong, S.; Wu, M.; Gu, J.; Liu, T.; Guo, R.; Yang, M. Structure of the Intact 14-Subunit Human Cytochrome *c* Oxidase. *Cell Res.* **2018**, *28*, 1026–1034. [CrossRef]
60. Lisanti, S.; Tavecchio, M.; Chae, Y.C.; Liu, Q.; Brice, A.K.; Thakur, M.L.; Languino, L.R.; Altieri, D.C. Deletion of the Mitochondrial Chaperone TRAP-1 Uncovers Global Reprogramming of Metabolic Networks. *Cell Rep.* **2014**, *8*, 671–677. [CrossRef]
61. Sullivan, L.B.; Chandel, N.S. Mitochondrial Reactive Oxygen Species and Cancer. *Cancer Metab.* **2014**, *2*, 17. [CrossRef] [PubMed]
62. Clarke, B.E.; Kalmar, B.; Greensmith, L. Enhanced Expression of TRAP1 Protects Mitochondrial Function in Motor Neurons under Conditions of Oxidative Stress. *Int. J. Mol. Sci.* **2022**, *23*, 1789. [CrossRef] [PubMed]
63. Kang, B.H.; Plescia, J.; Dohi, T.; Rosa, J.; Doxsey, S.J.; Altieri, D.C. Regulation of Tumor Cell Mitochondrial Homeostasis by an Organelle-Specific Hsp90 Chaperone Network. *Cell* **2007**, *131*, 257–270. [CrossRef] [PubMed]
64. Leav, I.; Plescia, J.; Goel, H.L.; Li, J.; Jiang, Z.; Cohen, R.J.; Languino, L.R.; Altieri, D.C. Cytoprotective Mitochondrial Chaperone TRAP-1 As a Novel Molecular Target in Localized and Metastatic Prostate Cancer. *Am. J. Pathol.* **2010**, *176*, 393–401. [CrossRef] [PubMed]
65. Vartholomaiou, E.; Madon-Simon, M.; Hagmann, S.; Mühlebach, G.; Wurst, W.; Floss, T.; Picard, D. Cytosolic Hsp90α and Its Mitochondrial Isoform Trap1 Are Differentially Required in a Breast Cancer Model. *Oncotarget* **2017**, *8*, 17428–17442. [CrossRef] [PubMed]
66. Linehan, W.M.; Schmidt, L.S.; Crooks, D.R.; Wei, D.; Srinivasan, R.; Lang, M.; Ricketts, C.J. The Metabolic Basis of Kidney Cancer. *Cancer Discov.* **2019**, *9*, 1006–1021. [CrossRef] [PubMed]
67. Semenza, G.L. HIF-1: Upstream and Downstream of Cancer Metabolism. *Curr. Opin. Genet. Dev.* **2010**, *20*, 51–56. [CrossRef]
68. Kowalik, M.A.; Guzzo, G.; Morandi, A.; Perra, A.; Menegon, S.; Masgras, I.; Trevisan, E.; Angioni, M.M.; Fornari, F.; Quagliata, L.; et al. Metabolic Reprogramming Identifies the Most Aggressive Lesions at Early Phases of Hepatic Carcinogenesis. *Oncotarget* **2016**, *7*, 32375–32393. [CrossRef]
69. Iacobazzi, V.; Infantino, V. Citrate—New Functions for an Old Metabolite. *Biol. Chem.* **2014**, *395*, 387–399. [CrossRef]
70. Liu, J.; Peng, Y.; Wei, W. Cell Cycle on the Crossroad of Tumorigenesis and Cancer Therapy. *Trends Cell Biol.* **2022**, *32*, 30–44. [CrossRef]
71. Amoroso, M.R.; Matassa, D.S.; Laudiero, G.; Egorova, A.V.; Polishchuk, R.S.; Maddalena, F.; Piscazzi, A.; Paladino, S.; Sarnataro, D.; Garbi, C.; et al. TRAP1 and the Proteasome Regulatory Particle TBP7/Rpt3 Interact in the Endoplasmic Reticulum and Control Cellular Ubiquitination of Specific Mitochondrial Proteins. *Cell Death Differ.* **2012**, *19*, 592–604. [CrossRef] [PubMed]
72. Sisinni, L.; Maddalena, F.; Condelli, V.; Pannone, G.; Simeon, V.; Li Bergolis, V.; Lopes, E.; Piscazzi, A.; Matassa, D.S.; Mazzoccoli, C.; et al. TRAP1 Controls Cell Cycle G2-M Transition through the Regulation of CDK1 and MAD2 Expression/Ubiquitination: TRAP1 Regulates Mitotic Entry through CDK1 Quality Control. *J. Pathol.* **2017**, *243*, 123–134. [CrossRef] [PubMed]
73. Liu, X.; Kim, C.N.; Yang, J.; Jemmerson, R.; Wang, X. Induction of Apoptotic Program in Cell-Free Extracts: Requirement for DATP and Cytochrome *c*. *Cell* **1996**, *86*, 147–157. [CrossRef]
74. Li, P.; Nijhawan, D.; Budihardjo, I.; Srinivasula, S.M.; Ahmad, M.; Alnemri, E.S.; Wang, X. Cytochrome *c* and DATP-Dependent Formation of Apaf-1/Caspase-9 Complex Initiates an Apoptotic Protease Cascade. *Cell* **1997**, *91*, 479–489. [CrossRef]
75. Javadov, S.; Chapa-Dubocq, X.; Makarov, V. Different Approaches to Modeling Analysis of Mitochondrial Swelling. *Mitochondrion* **2018**, *38*, 58–70. [CrossRef]
76. Orrenius, S.; Gogvadze, V.; Zhivotovsky, B. Calcium and Mitochondria in the Regulation of Cell Death. *Biochem. Biophys. Res. Commun.* **2015**, *460*, 72–81. [CrossRef]
77. Bernardi, P.; Rasola, A.; Forte, M.; Lippe, G. The Mitochondrial Permeability Transition Pore: Channel Formation by F-ATP Synthase, Integration in Signal Transduction, and Role in Pathophysiology. *Physiol. Rev.* **2015**, *95*, 1111–1155. [CrossRef]
78. Redza-Dutordoir, M.; Averill-Bates, D.A. Activation of Apoptosis Signalling Pathways by Reactive Oxygen Species. *Biochim. Et Biophys. Acta (BBA)-Mol. Cell Res.* **2016**, *1863*, 2977–2992. [CrossRef]
79. Hua, G.; Zhang, Q.; Fan, Z. Heat Shock Protein 75 (TRAP1) Antagonizes Reactive Oxygen Species Generation and Protects Cells from Granzyme M-Mediated Apoptosis. *J. Biol. Chem.* **2007**, *282*, 20553–20560. [CrossRef]
80. Im, C.-N.; Lee, J.-S.; Zheng, Y.; Seo, J.-S. Iron Chelation Study in a Normal Human Hepatocyte Cell Line Suggests That Tumor Necrosis Factor Receptor-Associated Protein 1 (TRAP1) Regulates Production of Reactive Oxygen Species. *J. Cell. Biochem.* **2007**, *100*, 474–486. [CrossRef]
81. Costantino, E.; Maddalena, F.; Calise, S.; Piscazzi, A.; Tirino, V.; Fersini, A.; Ambrosi, A.; Neri, V.; Esposito, F.; Landriscina, M. TRAP1, a Novel Mitochondrial Chaperone Responsible for Multi-Drug Resistance and Protection from Apoptotis in Human Colorectal Carcinoma Cells. *Cancer Lett.* **2009**, *279*, 39–46. [CrossRef] [PubMed]
82. Landriscina, M.; Laudiero, G.; Maddalena, F.; Amoroso, M.R.; Piscazzi, A.; Cozzolino, F.; Monti, M.; Garbi, C.; Fersini, A.; Pucci, P.; et al. Mitochondrial Chaperone Trap1 and the Calcium Binding Protein Sorcin Interact and Protect Cells against Apoptosis Induced by Antiblastic Agents. *Cancer Res.* **2010**, *70*, 6577–6586. [CrossRef] [PubMed]
83. Suarez, J.; McDonough, P.M.; Scott, B.T.; Suarez-Ramirez, A.; Wang, H.; Fricovsky, E.S.; Dillmann, W.H. Sorcin Modulates Mitochondrial Ca2+ Handling and Reduces Apoptosis in Neonatal Rat Cardiac Myocytes. *Am. J. Physiol. -Cell Physiol.* **2013**, *304*, C248–C256. [CrossRef] [PubMed]
84. Elnatan, D.; Agard, D.A. Calcium Binding to a Remote Site Can Replace Magnesium as Cofactor for Mitochondrial Hsp90 (TRAP1) ATPase Activity. *J. Biol. Chem.* **2018**, *293*, 13717–13724. [CrossRef]

85. Zhang, L.; Su, N.; Luo, Y.; Chen, S.; Zhao, T. TRAP1 Inhibits MIC60 Ubiquitination to Mitigate the Injury of Cardiomyocytes and Protect Mitochondria in Extracellular Acidosis. *Cell Death Discov.* **2021**, *7*, 389. [CrossRef]
86. Friedman, J.R.; Mourier, A.; Yamada, J.; McCaffery, J.M.; Nunnari, J. MICOS Coordinates with Respiratory Complexes and Lipids to Establish Mitochondrial Inner Membrane Architecture. *eLife* **2015**, *4*, e07739. [CrossRef]
87. Rampelt, H.; Zerbes, R.M.; van der Laan, M.; Pfanner, N. Role of the Mitochondrial Contact Site and Cristae Organizing System in Membrane Architecture and Dynamics. *Biochim. Et Biophys. Acta (BBA)-Mol. Cell Res.* **2017**, *1864*, 737–746. [CrossRef]
88. Baines, C.P.; Gutiérrez-Aguilar, M. The Mitochondrial Permeability Transition Pore: Is It Formed by the ATP Synthase, Adenine Nucleotide Translocators or Both? *Biochim. Et Biophys. Acta (BBA)-Bioenerg.* **2020**, *1861*, 148249. [CrossRef]
89. Carrer, A.; Tommasin, L.; Šileikytė, J.; Ciscato, F.; Filadi, R.; Urbani, A.; Forte, M.; Rasola, A.; Szabò, I.; Carraro, M.; et al. Defining the Molecular Mechanisms of the Mitochondrial Permeability Transition through Genetic Manipulation of F-ATP Synthase. *Nat. Commun.* **2021**, *12*, 4835. [CrossRef]
90. Giorgio, V.; von Stockum, S.; Antoniel, M.; Fabbro, A.; Fogolari, F.; Forte, M.; Glick, G.D.; Petronilli, V.; Zoratti, M.; Szabó, I.; et al. Dimers of Mitochondrial ATP Synthase Form the Permeability Transition Pore. *Proc. Natl. Acad. Sci. USA* **2013**, *110*, 5887–5892. [CrossRef]
91. Kang, B.H.; Tavecchio, M.; Goel, H.L.; Hsieh, C.-C.; Garlick, D.S.; Raskett, C.M.; Lian, J.B.; Stein, G.S.; Languino, L.R.; Altieri, D.C. Targeted Inhibition of Mitochondrial Hsp90 Suppresses Localised and Metastatic Prostate Cancer Growth in a Genetic Mouse Model of Disease. *Br. J. Cancer* **2011**, *104*, 629–634. [CrossRef] [PubMed]
92. Baines, C.P.; Kaiser, R.A.; Purcell, N.H.; Blair, N.S.; Osinska, H.; Hambleton, M.A.; Brunskill, E.W.; Sayen, M.R.; Gottlieb, R.A.; Dorn, G.W.; et al. Loss of Cyclophilin D Reveals a Critical Role for Mitochondrial Permeability Transition in Cell Death. *Nature* **2005**, *434*, 658–662. [CrossRef] [PubMed]
93. Matassa, D.S.; Amoroso, M.R.; Maddalena, F.; Landriscina, M. New Insights into TRAP1 Pathway. *Am. J. Cancer Res.* **2012**, *2*, 235–248. [PubMed]
94. Ghosh, J.C.; Siegelin, M.D.; Dohi, T.; Altieri, D.C. Heat Shock Protein 60 Regulation of the Mitochondrial Permeability Transition Pore in Tumor Cells. *Cancer Res.* **2010**, *70*, 8988–8993. [CrossRef] [PubMed]
95. Lebedev, I.; Nemajerova, A.; Foda, Z.H.; Kornaj, M.; Tong, M.; Moll, U.M.; Seeliger, M.A. A Novel In Vitro CypD-Mediated P53 Aggregation Assay Suggests a Model for Mitochondrial Permeability Transition by Chaperone Systems. *J. Mol. Biol.* **2016**, *428*, 4154–4167. [CrossRef] [PubMed]
96. Sinha, D.; D'Silva, P. Chaperoning Mitochondrial Permeability Transition: Regulation of Transition Pore Complex by a J-Protein, DnaJC15. *Cell Death Dis.* **2014**, *5*, e1101. [CrossRef]
97. Niemi, N.M.; Pagliarini, D.J. The Extensive and Functionally Uncharacterized Mitochondrial Phosphoproteome. *J. Biol. Chem.* **2021**, *297*, 100880. [CrossRef]
98. Faienza, F.; Lambrughi, M.; Rizza, S.; Pecorari, C.; Giglio, P.; Salamanca Viloria, J.; Allega, M.F.; Chiappetta, G.; Vinh, J.; Pacello, F.; et al. S-Nitrosylation Affects TRAP1 Structure and ATPase Activity and Modulates Cell Response to Apoptotic Stimuli. *Biochem. Pharmacol.* **2020**, *176*, 113869. [CrossRef]
99. Rasola, A.; Neckers, L.; Picard, D. Mitochondrial Oxidative Phosphorylation TRAP(1)Ped in Tumor Cells. *Trends Cell Biol.* **2014**, *24*, 455–463. [CrossRef]
100. Cloutier, P.; Coulombe, B. Regulation of Molecular Chaperones through Post-Translational Modifications: Decrypting the Chaperone Code. *Biochim. Biophys. Acta (BBA)-Gene Regul. Mech.* **2013**, *1829*, 443–454. [CrossRef]
101. Zuehlke, A.D.; Reidy, M.; Lin, C.; LaPointe, P.; Alsomairy, S.; Lee, D.J.; Rivera-Marquez, G.M.; Beebe, K.; Prince, T.; Lee, S.; et al. An Hsp90 Co-Chaperone Protein in Yeast Is Functionally Replaced by Site-Specific Posttranslational Modification in Humans. *Nat. Commun.* **2017**, *8*, 15328. [CrossRef] [PubMed]
102. Quinn, P.M.J.; Moreira, P.I.; Ambrósio, A.F.; Alves, C.H. PINK1/PARKIN Signalling in Neurodegeneration and Neuroinflammation. *Acta Neuropathol. Commun.* **2020**, *8*, 189. [CrossRef] [PubMed]
103. Arena, G.; Gelmetti, V.; Torosantucci, L.; Vignone, D.; Lamorte, G.; De Rosa, P.; Cilia, E.; Jonas, E.A.; Valente, E.M. PINK1 Protects against Cell Death Induced by Mitochondrial Depolarization, by Phosphorylating Bcl-XL and Impairing Its pro-Apoptotic Cleavage. *Cell Death Differ.* **2013**, *20*, 920–930. [CrossRef] [PubMed]
104. Costa, A.C.; Loh, S.H.Y.; Martins, L.M. Drosophila Trap1 Protects against Mitochondrial Dysfunction in a PINK1/Parkin Model of Parkinson's Disease. *Cell Death Dis.* **2013**, *4*, e467. [CrossRef]
105. Zhang, L.; Karsten, P.; Hamm, S.; Pogson, J.H.; Müller-Rischart, A.K.; Exner, N.; Haass, C.; Whitworth, A.J.; Winklhofer, K.F.; Schulz, J.B.; et al. TRAP1 Rescues PINK1 Loss-of-Function Phenotypes. *Hum. Mol. Genet.* **2013**, *22*, 2829–2841. [CrossRef]
106. Fiesel, F.C.; James, E.D.; Hudec, R.; Springer, W. Mitochondrial Targeted HSP90 Inhibitor Gamitrinib-TPP (G-TPP) Induces PINK1/Parkin-Dependent Mitophagy. *Oncotarget* **2017**, *8*, 106233–106248. [CrossRef]
107. Rasola, A.; Sciacovelli, M.; Chiara, F.; Pantic, B.; Brusilow, W.S.; Bernardi, P. Activation of Mitochondrial ERK Protects Cancer Cells from Death through Inhibition of the Permeability Transition. *Proc. Natl. Acad. Sci. USA* **2010**, *107*, 726–731. [CrossRef]
108. Miyazaki, T.; Neff, L.; Tanaka, S.; Horne, W.C.; Baron, R. Regulation of Cytochrome c Oxidase Activity by C-Src in Osteoclasts. *J. Cell Biol.* **2003**, *160*, 709–718. [CrossRef]
109. Ogura, M.; Yamaki, J.; Homma, M.K.; Homma, Y. Mitochondrial C-Src Regulates Cell Survival through Phosphorylation of Respiratory Chain Components. *Biochem. J.* **2012**, *447*, 281–289. [CrossRef]

110. George, J.; Ahmad, N. Mitochondrial Sirtuins in Cancer: Emerging Roles and Therapeutic Potential. *Cancer Res.* **2016**, *76*, 2500–2506. [CrossRef]
111. Stomberski, C.T.; Hess, D.T.; Stamler, J.S. Protein S-Nitrosylation: Determinants of Specificity and Enzymatic Regulation of S-Nitrosothiol-Based Signaling. *Antioxid. Redox Signal.* **2019**, *30*, 1331–1351. [CrossRef] [PubMed]
112. Liu, L.; Hausladen, A.; Zeng, M.; Que, L.; Heitman, J.; Stamler, J.S. A Metabolic Enzyme for S-Nitrosothiol Conserved from Bacteria to Humans. *Nature* **2001**, *410*, 490–494. [CrossRef] [PubMed]
113. Wei, W.; Yang, Z.; Tang, C.-H.; Liu, L. Targeted Deletion of GSNOR in Hepatocytes of Mice Causes Nitrosative Inactivation of O6-Alkylguanine-DNA Alkyltransferase and Increased Sensitivity to Genotoxic Diethylnitrosamine. *Carcinogenesis* **2011**, *32*, 973–977. [CrossRef] [PubMed]
114. Forrester, M.T.; Thompson, J.W.; Foster, M.W.; Nogueira, L.; Moseley, M.A.; Stamler, J.S. Proteomic Analysis of S-Nitrosylation and Denitrosylation by Resin-Assisted Capture. *Nat. Biotechnol.* **2009**, *27*, 557–559. [CrossRef]
115. Stine, Z.E.; Schug, Z.T.; Salvino, J.M.; Dang, C.V. Targeting Cancer Metabolism in the Era of Precision Oncology. *Nat. Rev. Drug Discov.* **2022**, *21*, 141–162. [CrossRef]
116. Bryant, K.G.; Chae, Y.C.; Martinez, R.L.; Gordon, J.C.; Elokely, K.M.; Kossenkov, A.V.; Grant, S.; Childers, W.E.; Abou-Gharbia, M.; Altieri, D.C. A Mitochondrial-Targeted Purine-Based HSP90 Antagonist for Leukemia Therapy. *Oncotarget* **2017**, *8*, 112184–112198. [CrossRef]
117. Yoon, N.G.; Lee, H.; Kim, S.-Y.; Hu, S.; Kim, D.; Yang, S.; Hong, K.B.; Lee, J.H.; Kang, S.; Kim, B.-G.; et al. Mitoquinone Inactivates Mitochondrial Chaperone TRAP1 by Blocking the Client Binding Site. *J. Am. Chem. Soc.* **2021**, *143*, 19684–19696. [CrossRef]
118. Kang, B.H.; Plescia, J.; Song, H.Y.; Meli, M.; Colombo, G.; Beebe, K.; Scroggins, B.; Neckers, L.; Altieri, D.C. Combinatorial Drug Design Targeting Multiple Cancer Signaling Networks Controlled by Mitochondrial Hsp90. *J. Clin. Investig.* **2009**, *119*, 454–464. [CrossRef]
119. Kang, B.H.; Siegelin, M.D.; Plescia, J.; Raskett, C.M.; Garlick, D.S.; Dohi, T.; Lian, J.B.; Stein, G.S.; Languino, L.R.; Altieri, D.C. Preclinical Characterization of Mitochondria-Targeted Small Molecule Hsp90 Inhibitors, Gamitrinibs, in Advanced Prostate Cancer. *Clin. Cancer Res.* **2010**, *16*, 4779–4788. [CrossRef]
120. Chae, Y.C.; Caino, M.C.; Lisanti, S.; Ghosh, J.C.; Dohi, T.; Danial, N.N.; Villanueva, J.; Ferrero, S.; Vaira, V.; Santambrogio, L.; et al. Control of Tumor Bioenergetics and Survival Stress Signaling by Mitochondrial HSP90s. *Cancer Cell* **2012**, *22*, 331–344. [CrossRef]
121. Caino, M.C.; Chae, Y.C.; Vaira, V.; Ferrero, S.; Nosotti, M.; Martin, N.M.; Weeraratna, A.; O'Connell, M.; Jernigan, D.; Fatatis, A.; et al. Metabolic Stress Regulates Cytoskeletal Dynamics and Metastasis of Cancer Cells. *J. Clin. Investig.* **2013**, *123*, 2907–2920. [CrossRef] [PubMed]
122. Park, H.-K.; Lee, J.-E.; Lim, J.; Jo, D.-E.; Park, S.-A.; Suh, P.-G.; Kang, B.H. Combination Treatment with Doxorubicin and Gamitrinib Synergistically Augments Anticancer Activity through Enhanced Activation of Bim. *BMC Cancer* **2014**, *14*, 431. [CrossRef] [PubMed]
123. Condelli, V.; Maddalena, F.; Sisinni, L.; Lettini, G.; Matassa, D.S.; Piscazzi, A.; Palladino, G.; Amoroso, M.R.; Esposito, F.; Landriscina, M. Targeting TRAP1 as a Downstream Effector of BRAF Cytoprotective Pathway: A Novel Strategy for Human BRAF-Driven Colorectal Carcinoma. *Oncotarget* **2015**, *6*, 22298–22309. [CrossRef]
124. Karpel-Massler, G.; Ishida, C.T.; Bianchetti, E.; Shu, C.; Perez-Lorenzo, R.; Horst, B.; Banu, M.; Roth, K.A.; Bruce, J.N.; Canoll, P.; et al. Inhibition of Mitochondrial Matrix Chaperones and Antiapoptotic Bcl-2 Family Proteins Empower Antitumor Therapeutic Responses. *Cancer Res.* **2017**, *77*, 3513–3526. [CrossRef] [PubMed]
125. Kim, H.; Yang, J.; Kim, M.J.; Choi, S.; Chung, J.-R.; Kim, J.-M.; Yoo, Y.H.; Chung, J.; Koh, H. Tumor Necrosis Factor Receptor-Associated Protein 1 (TRAP1) Mutation and TRAP1 Inhibitor Gamitrinib-Triphenylphosphonium (G-TPP) Induce a Forkhead Box O (FOXO)-Dependent Cell Protective Signal from Mitochondria. *J. Biol. Chem.* **2016**, *291*, 1841–1853. [CrossRef]
126. Wei, S.; Yin, D.; Yu, S.; Lin, X.; Savani, M.R.; Du, K.; Ku, Y.; Wu, D.; Li, S.; Liu, H.; et al. Anti-Tumor Activity of a Mitochondrial Targeted HSP90 Inhibitor in Gliomas. *Clin. Cancer Res. Off. J. Am. Assoc. Cancer Res.* **2022**, *28*, 2180–2195. [CrossRef] [PubMed]
127. Nguyen, T.T.T.; Ishida, C.T.; Shang, E.; Shu, C.; Bianchetti, E.; Karpel-Massler, G.; Siegelin, M.D. Activation of LXR Receptors and Inhibition of TRAP1 Causes Synthetic Lethality in Solid Tumors. *Cancers* **2019**, *11*, 788. [CrossRef]
128. Nguyen, T.T.T.; Zhang, Y.; Shang, E.; Shu, C.; Quinzii, C.M.; Westhoff, M.-A.; Karpel-Massler, G.; Siegelin, M.D. Inhibition of HDAC1/2 Along with TRAP1 Causes Synthetic Lethality in Glioblastoma Model Systems. *Cells* **2020**, *9*, 1661. [CrossRef]
129. Wang, N.; Zhu, P.; Huang, R.; Sun, L.; Dong, D.; Gao, Y. Suppressing TRAP1 Sensitizes Glioblastoma Multiforme Cells to Temozolomide. *Exp. Ther. Med.* **2021**, *22*, 1246. [CrossRef]
130. Lee, C.; Park, H.-K.; Jeong, H.; Lim, J.; Lee, A.-J.; Cheon, K.Y.; Kim, C.-S.; Thomas, A.P.; Bae, B.; Kim, N.D.; et al. Development of a Mitochondria-Targeted Hsp90 Inhibitor Based on the Crystal Structures of Human TRAP1. *J. Am. Chem. Soc.* **2015**, *137*, 4358–4367. [CrossRef]
131. Haidar, M.A.; Shakkour, Z.; Barsa, C.; Tabet, M.; Mekhjian, S.; Darwish, H.; Goli, M.; Shear, D.; Pandya, J.D.; Mechref, Y.; et al. Mitoquinone Helps Combat the Neurological, Cognitive, and Molecular Consequences of Open Head Traumatic Brain Injury at Chronic Time Point. *Biomedicines* **2022**, *10*, 250. [CrossRef] [PubMed]
132. Pinho, B.R.; Duarte, A.I.; Canas, P.M.; Moreira, P.I.; Murphy, M.P.; Oliveira, J.M.A. The Interplay between Redox Signalling and Proteostasis in Neurodegeneration: In Vivo Effects of a Mitochondria-Targeted Antioxidant in Huntington's Disease Mice. *Free Radic. Biol. Med.* **2020**, *146*, 372–382. [CrossRef] [PubMed]

133. Miquel, E.; Cassina, A.; Martínez-Palma, L.; Souza, J.M.; Bolatto, C.; Rodríguez-Bottero, S.; Logan, A.; Smith, R.A.J.; Murphy, M.P.; Barbeito, L.; et al. Neuroprotective Effects of the Mitochondria-Targeted Antioxidant MitoQ in a Model of Inherited Amyotrophic Lateral Sclerosis. *Free Radic. Biol. Med.* **2014**, *70*, 204–213. [CrossRef] [PubMed]
134. McManus, M.J.; Murphy, M.P.; Franklin, J.L. The Mitochondria-Targeted Antioxidant MitoQ Prevents Loss of Spatial Memory Retention and Early Neuropathology in a Transgenic Mouse Model of Alzheimer's Disease. *J. Neurosci.* **2011**, *31*, 15703–15715. [CrossRef] [PubMed]
135. Koopman, M.B.; Rüdiger, S.G.D. Alzheimer Cells on Their Way to Derailment Show Selective Changes in Protein Quality Control Network. *Front. Mol. Biosci.* **2020**, *7*, 214. [CrossRef]
136. DeBoer, C.; Meulman, P.A.; Wnuk, R.J.; Peterson, D.H. Geldanamycin, a New Antibiotic. *J. Antibiot.* **2006**, *23*, 442–447. [CrossRef]
137. Grenert, J.P.; Sullivan, W.P.; Fadden, P.; Haystead, T.A.J.; Clark, J.; Mimnaugh, E.; Krutzsch, H.; Ochel, H.-J.; Schulte, T.W.; Sausville, E.; et al. The Amino-Terminal Domain of Heat Shock Protein 90 (Hsp90) That Binds Geldanamycin Is an ATP/ADP Switch Domain That Regulates Hsp90 Conformation*. *J. Biol. Chem.* **1997**, *272*, 23843–23850. [CrossRef]
138. Prodromou, C.; Roe, S.M.; O'Brien, R.; Ladbury, J.E.; Piper, P.W.; Pearl, L.H. Identification and Structural Characterization of the ATP/ADP-Binding Site in the Hsp90 Molecular Chaperone. *Cell* **1997**, *90*, 65–75. [CrossRef]
139. Plescia, J.; Salz, W.; Xia, F.; Pennati, M.; Zaffaroni, N.; Daidone, M.G.; Meli, M.; Dohi, T.; Fortugno, P.; Nefedova, Y.; et al. Rational Design of Shepherdin, a Novel Anticancer Agent. *Cancer Cell* **2005**, *7*, 457–468. [CrossRef]
140. Fortugno, P.; Beltrami, E.; Plescia, J.; Fontana‡, J.; Pradhan§, D.; Marchisio, P.C.; Sessa, W.C.; Altieri, D.C. Regulation of Survivin Function by Hsp90. *Proc. Natl. Acad. Sci. USA* **2003**, *100*, 13791–13796. [CrossRef]
141. Meli, M.; Pennati, M.; Curto, M.; Daidone, M.G.; Plescia, J.; Toba, S.; Altieri, D.C.; Zaffaroni, N.; Colombo, G. Small-Molecule Targeting of Heat Shock Protein 90 Chaperone Function: Rational Identification of a New Anticancer Lead. *J. Med. Chem.* **2006**, *49*, 7721–7730. [CrossRef] [PubMed]
142. Tomaselli, S.; Meli, M.; Plescia, J.; Zetta, L.; Altieri, D.C.; Colombo, G.; Ragona, L. Combined in Silico and Experimental Approach for Drug Design: The Binding Mode of Peptidic and Non-Peptidic Inhibitors to Hsp90 N-Terminal Domain: NMR and MD Studies of Hsp90 Inhibitors. *Chem. Biol. Drug Des.* **2010**, *76*, 382–391. [CrossRef] [PubMed]
143. Moroni, E.; Agard, D.A.; Colombo, G. The Structural Asymmetry of Mitochondrial Hsp90 (Trap1) Determines Fine Tuning of Functional Dynamics. *J. Chem. Theory Comput.* **2018**, *14*, 1033–1044. [CrossRef] [PubMed]
144. Hanahan, D.; Weinberg, R.A. Hallmarks of Cancer: The Next Generation. *Cell* **2011**, *144*, 646–674. [CrossRef] [PubMed]
145. Neckers, L.; Kern, A.; Tsutsumi, S. Hsp90 Inhibitors Disrupt Mitochondrial Homeostasis in Cancer Cells. *Chem. Biol.* **2007**, *14*, 1204–1206. [CrossRef] [PubMed]
146. Fu, Y.; Xu, X.; Huang, D.; Cui, D.; Liu, L.; Liu, J.; He, Z.; Liu, J.; Zheng, S.; Luo, Y. Plasma Heat Shock Protein 90alpha as a Biomarker for the Diagnosis of Liver Cancer: An Official, Large-Scale, and Multicenter Clinical Trial. *EBioMedicine* **2017**, *24*, 56–63. [CrossRef]
147. Ocaña, G.J.; Sims, E.K.; Watkins, R.A.; Ragg, S.; Mather, K.J.; Oram, R.A.; Mirmira, R.G.; DiMeglio, L.A.; Blum, J.S.; Evans-Molina, C. Analysis of Serum Hsp90 as a Potential Biomarker of β Cell Autoimmunity in Type 1 Diabetes. *PLoS ONE* **2019**, *14*, e0208456. [CrossRef]
148. Štorkánová, H.; Oreská, S.; Špiritović, M.; Heřmánková, B.; Bubová, K.; Komarc, M.; Pavelka, K.; Vencovský, J.; Distler, J.H.W.; Šenolt, L.; et al. Plasma Hsp90 Levels in Patients with Systemic Sclerosis and Relation to Lung and Skin Involvement: A Cross-Sectional and Longitudinal Study. *Sci. Rep.* **2021**, *11*, 1. [CrossRef]
149. Saisawat, P.; Kohl, S.; Hilger, A.C.; Hwang, D.-Y.; Yung Gee, H.; Dworschak, G.C.; Tasic, V.; Pennimpede, T.; Natarajan, S.; Sperry, E.; et al. Whole-Exome Resequencing Reveals Recessive Mutations in TRAP1 in Individuals with CAKUT and VACTERL Association. *Kidney Int.* **2014**, *85*, 1310–1317. [CrossRef]
150. Standing, A.S.; Hong, Y.; Paisan-Ruiz, C.; Omoyinmi, E.; Medlar, A.; Stanescu, H.; Kleta, R.; Rowcenzio, D.; Hawkins, P.; Lachmann, H.; et al. TRAP1 Chaperone Protein Mutations and Autoinflammation. *Life Sci. Alliance* **2020**, *3*, e201900376. [CrossRef]
151. Zhang, Y.; Jiang, D.-S.; Yan, L.; Cheng, K.-J.; Bian, Z.-Y.; Lin, G.-S. HSP75 Protects against Cardiac Hypertrophy and Fibrosis. *J. Cell. Biochem.* **2011**, *112*, 1787–1794. [CrossRef] [PubMed]
152. Takamura, H.; Koyama, Y.; Matsuzaki, S.; Yamada, K.; Hattori, T.; Miyata, S.; Takemoto, K.; Tohyama, M.; Katayama, T. TRAP1 Controls Mitochondrial Fusion/Fission Balance through Drp1 and Mff Expression. *PLoS ONE* **2012**, *7*, e51912. [CrossRef] [PubMed]
153. Ramos Rego, I.; Santos Cruz, B.; Ambrósio, A.F.; Alves, C.H. TRAP1 in Oxidative Stress and Neurodegeneration. *Antioxidants* **2021**, *10*, 1829. [CrossRef] [PubMed]
154. Hornbeck, P.V.; Zhang, B.; Murray, B.; Kornhauser, J.M.; Latham, V.; Skrzypek, E. PhosphoSitePlus, 2014: Mutations, PTMs and Recalibrations. *Nucleic Acids Res.* **2015**, *43*, D512–D520. [CrossRef]

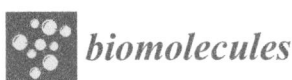

Review

The Mitochondrial HSP90 Paralog TRAP1: Structural Dynamics, Interactome, Role in Metabolic Regulation, and Inhibitors

Abhinav Joshi [1], Takeshi Ito [1], Didier Picard [2] and Len Neckers [1,*]

[1] Urologic Oncology Branch, Center for Cancer Research, National Cancer Institute (NCI), Bethesda, MD 20892, USA; aj.joshi@nih.gov (A.J.); takeshi.ito@nih.gov (T.I.)
[2] Department of Molecular and Cellular Biology, Université de Genève, Sciences III, 30 Quai Ernest-Ansermet, CH-1211 Geneva, Switzerland; didier.picard@unige.ch
* Correspondence: neckersl@mail.nih.gov; Tel.: +1-240-858-3918

Abstract: The HSP90 paralog TRAP1 was discovered more than 20 years ago; yet, a detailed understanding of the function of this mitochondrial molecular chaperone remains elusive. The dispensable nature of TRAP1 in vitro and in vivo further complicates an understanding of its role in mitochondrial biology. TRAP1 is more homologous to the bacterial HSP90, HtpG, than to eukaryotic HSP90. Lacking co-chaperones, the unique structural features of TRAP1 likely regulate its temperature-sensitive ATPase activity and shed light on the alternative mechanisms driving the chaperone's nucleotide-dependent cycle in a defined environment whose physiological temperature approaches 50 °C. TRAP1 appears to be an important bioregulator of mitochondrial respiration, mediating the balance between oxidative phosphorylation and glycolysis, while at the same time promoting mitochondrial homeostasis and displaying cytoprotective activity. Inactivation/loss of TRAP1 has been observed in several neurodegenerative diseases while TRAP1 expression is reported to be elevated in multiple cancers and, as with HSP90, evidence of addiction to TRAP1 has been observed. In this review, we summarize what is currently known about this unique HSP90 paralog and why a better understanding of TRAP1 structure, function, and regulation is likely to enhance our understanding of the mechanistic basis of mitochondrial homeostasis.

Keywords: HSP90; TRAP1; molecular chaperone; mitochondria; metabolism; OxPhos; tetramers

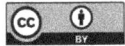

1. Introduction

Molecular chaperones form one of the central pillars of the cellular proteostasis network [1,2]. Depending upon their function, these molecules fall into three fundamental classes: foldases, holdases, and disaggregases [1–7]. Under certain circumstances, some molecular chaperones also deliver damaged and impossible to fold client proteins for degradation by proteosomes or autophagy [8–10]. Foldases are ATP-dependent chaperones that actively fold nascent proteins into their native functional conformations and refold unfolded proteins under cellular stress. Heat shock protein 90 (HSP90) is an ATP-dependent foldase that is remarkably conserved from bacteria to humans [11]. It regulates folding, maturation, and stability of proteins (in HSP90's case, termed "clients") that are involved in cell growth, survival, apoptosis, and adaptation to stress [12–14].

In mammalian cells there are four different HSP90 paralogs: HSP90α, HSP90β, GRP94, and TRAP1. HSP90α and HSP90β are primarily cytosolic with a small component in the nucleus. HSP90α is stress induced while HSP90β is constitutively expressed [15]. GRP94 is localized in the endoplasmic reticulum [16] and TRAP1 (or HSP75), the paralog on which we focused in this review, is primarily localized in mitochondria [17,18]. TRAP1 was initially identified in 2000 [17] and was widely presumed to facilitate late-stage folding of clients in the mitochondrial matrix. However, it increasingly became clear that this may not be the case. TRAP1 has since been implicated in metabolic regulation [19–25], mitochondrial dynamics [26], mitophagy [27,28], protection from oxidative stress [23,29–32], and protection from cell death [33].

2. TRAP1: Cytoprotective or Pro-Neoplastic?

Although TRAP1 may have regulatory roles in organellar processes, whether it is ultimately cytoprotective in the context of neurodegenerative diseases or pro-neoplastic in the context of many cancers may reflect two sides of the same coin. This molecule has been reported to play a crucial role in inhibiting oxidative stress-induced tissue damage in the ischemic brain [34], hypoxia-induced injury in cardiomyocytes [35], myocardial ischemia/reperfusion injury [36], motor neuron degeneration in oxidative stress-induced amyotrophic lateral sclerosis (ALS) [37], and acidosis-induced injury in cardiomyocytes [38]. Likewise, TRAP1 appears to be protective in genetic models of neurodegeneration such as Parkinson's disease [27,28,39] where protein quality control in mitochondria plays a critical role [40]. TRAP1 was also shown to be mitoprotective in models of kidney fibrosis and renal cell carcinoma [41,42]. Finally, loss-of-function TRAP1 mutations have been identified in the brain of a patient with Parkinson's disease [43], Leigh syndrome [44], and chronic functional symptomatology including pain, fatigue, and gastrointestinal dysmotility [45], and in congenital abnormalities associated with the kidney (CAKUT) [46].

While these studies identify TRAP1 as cytoprotective in mitochondrial-associated neuropathologies, other studies have highlighted a potential pro-neoplastic role of TRAP1 in cancer, where it can also display cytoprotective and other pro-tumorigenic activities. Thus, TRAP1 expression was found to be increased in hepatocellular carcinoma [47], breast cancer [48], glioma [49], small cell lung cancer [50], and kidney, prostrate, ovarian, colorectal, and esophageal cancer, and it is correlated with advanced-stage metastatic tumors with poor prognosis [51–57]. In colorectal cancer and its animal models, increased TRAP1 expression was found to be localized to pro-neoplastic lesions in the tumor [58,59]. While data supporting the importance of TRAP1 are numerous [24,47–57,59,60], these findings are challenged by other reports where TRAP1 expression inversely correlates with tumor stage [19] or is seemingly unimpactful in carcinogenesis models in TRAP1 knockout (KO) mice [61]. This has led to a general consensus that TRAP1's role may be more context dependent.

Nevertheless, TRAP1 does appear to play a role in the metabolic adaptation that may sustain neoplastic growth in a nutrient- and oxygen-poor environment; this hypothesis has driven research to mechanistically elucidate a role played by TRAP1 that is common to various cancers. Thus, TRAP1 was reported to play a critical role in the metabolic switch from oxidative phosphorylation (OxPhos) to aerobic glycolysis [19]. This relationship of TRAP1 to metabolic plasticity sparked an interest in exploring the details of TRAP1 structure, interactome, mode of action, and inhibitors. The data that has emerged since has definitively highlighted TRAP1 as a major player in mitochondrial bioenergetics. In this review, we hoped to provide a foundation for understanding the importance of TRAP1 in modulating mitochondrial homeostasis and the balance between oxidative phosphorylation and glycolysis.

3. Structure, ATPase Cycle, Dimers, and Tetramers

The TRAP1 gene is evolutionarily conserved [62] and is found in both metazoans and protozoans but not in the budding yeast. Unlike HSP90, TRAP1 is not an essential protein, and TRAP1 KO mice or cells derived therefrom are viable [19,63]. Likewise, loss of TRAP1 function in a patient with Parkinson's disease was unimpactful [43]. Similar to all members of the HSP90 family, TRAP1 has been primarily reported to form and function as a homodimer, with each protomer being comprised of an N-terminal ATPase domain (NTD), a middle domain (MD), and a C-terminal dimerization domain (CTD) [11,64,65]. The N-terminal domain contains a 59-amino acid mitochondrial-targeting sequence that is cleaved upon import [66]. Interestingly, TRAP1 more closely resembles bacterial HSP90 (HtpG) than human HSP90 [17,67]. As with HtpG, but unlike HSP90, TRAP1 lacks both a charged linker domain between the NTD and MD and a C-terminal EEVD motif that serves as a co-chaperone interaction domain in HSP90. TRAP1 also features an extended β-strand in the NTD, called "strap", that facilitates a cross protomer interaction in *trans* in the closed state of TRAP1. Removal of the "strap" domain dramatically upregulates ATPase activity; this extension is considered to be involved in the thermoregulation of the TRAP1 ATPase and to be potentially inhibitory for TRAP1 function under low temperatures [68].

TRAP1 is a nucleotide-dependent and nucleotide-activated chaperone that exists as a coiled-coil dimer in an autoinhibited state in the absence of ATP [69]. The presence of ATP activates the TRAP1 homodimer, which cycles between an open "apo" state and a closed state involving a series of ATP-dependent steps that promote large conformational changes within the molecule [70]. Unlike the rest of the HSP90 family, TRAP1 has a unique ATP-bound catalytically active state that adopts a strained asymmetric conformation [71]. This unique asymmetry is most pronounced in the highly conserved client binding region and results from the buckling of one of the protomers onto the other [71]. Interestingly, ATP hydrolysis is sequential between the two protomers, with the dimer undergoing a "flip" in the asymmetry while still remaining in the closed state [71]. The first ATP hydrolysis step facilitates client folding while the second leads to client unloading and return to an apo state [68]. The Mg^{2+} ion is the primary choice of cofactor for the TRAP1 ATPase, but it can be replaced by Ca^{2+} [72]. Surprisingly, Ca^{2+}-bound TRAP1 displays cooperative ATP hydrolysis and avoids asymmetric flipping of its protomers [72]. This may indicate that TRAP1 can function both as a foldase and a holdase, depending on its ionic environment.

Recently, TRAP1 was reported to form tetramers (dimer of dimers) [22], and it was proposed that the TRAP1 molecule exists in a dynamic equilibrium between a dimeric and a tetrameric state within mitochondria [22]. Analytical ultracentrifugation (AUC) with recombinant proteins further confirmed the existence of TRAP1 tetramers, which also seem to be stabilized in vitro by AMPPNP [73], a non-hydrolyzable structural homolog of ATP. Finally, cryo-EM analyses with purified proteins showed that the TRAP1 tetramer may adopt an orthogonal (butterfly), parallel, or antiparallel conformation (Figure 1) [73]. It should be noted that these observations are recent; any functional relevance of TRAP1 tetramers or for the potential transition between configurations remains unknown. Nevertheless, these observations are not entirely surprising when considering that crystallization of bacterial HtpG found the chaperone to exist as a dimer of dimers [74]. Similarly, HSP90 has also been reported to form such "oligomers" [75,76] under certain stimuli including elevated temperatures [77–79] and in the presence of non-ionic detergents or divalent cations [78,80].

Temperature-induced oligomerization of HSP90 is of particular interest in the context of TRAP1. This is because mitochondria operate close to 50 °C under physiological conditions, which is much higher than the 37 °C that is maintained in the adjacent cytosol [81]. To understand a physiological role of temperature-induced HSP90 oligomers, one study showed that self-oligomerized HSP90 under higher temperatures (>46 °C) readily binds to chemically unfolded dihydrofolate reductase (DHFR), a protein that could spontaneously refold by itself, to maintain it in a "folding-competent" state [79]. The binding of such a quaternary structure formed by HSP90 may actually provide an ideal environment for protein accommodation prior to folding and is consistent with a holdase function [82]. This hypothesis, while intriguing, definitely needs further experimental support. In the case of TRAP1, the existence of tetramers in "hot" mitochondria, the alterations in its asymmetry based on the availability of Mg^{2+} or Ca^{2+} ions, and a lack of significant proteome imbalance in TRAP1 KO cells [22] are consistent with the ability to adopt a holdase function in the mitochondrial environment. Additional experiments are needed to support or refute this hypothesis.

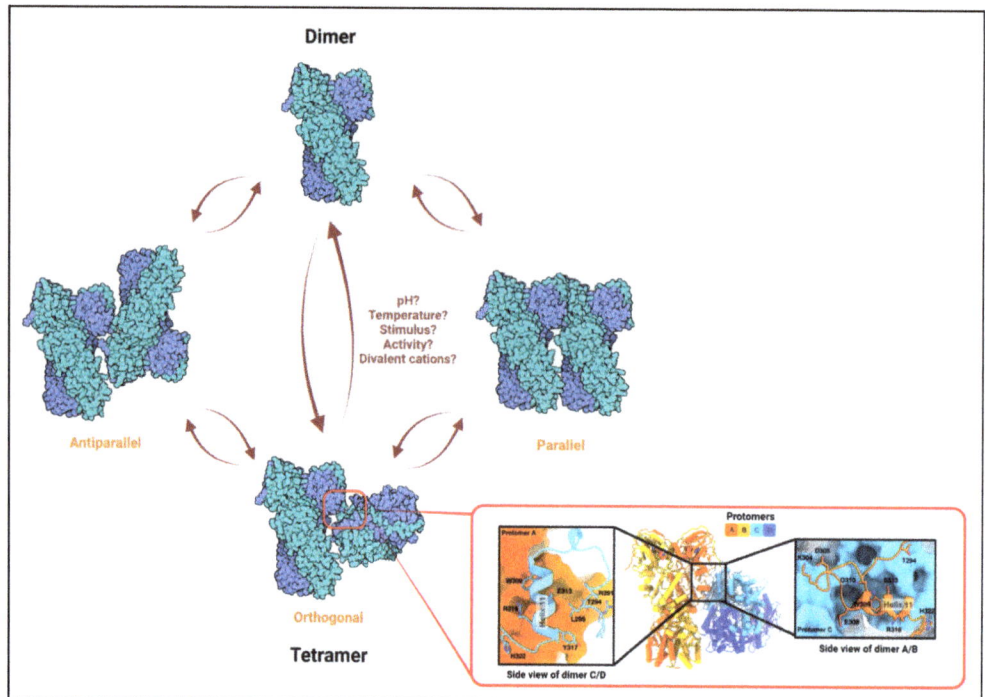

Figure 1. The TRAP1 tetramer. Based on in vitro studies on HSP90 oligomerization, rapid alterations in temperature, chaperone activity, or local concentration of divalent cations, which are common occurrences in the mitochondria, may influence dimer–tetramer transition. Three distinct conformations have been observed for the TRAP1 tetramer in vitro: orthogonal, parallel, and antiparallel [22,73]. The conditions required for the adoption of or transition to a particular configuration are only predicted and remain unclear. A high-resolution MD-MD dimer–dimer interface has only been shown for the orthogonal structure (shown in the inset; adapted from Liu et. al., Biorxiv, 2020 [73]). Left and right sub-insets show interacting residues from protomer C (blue) to A (orange) and from A to C at the dimer–dimer interface, respectively.

4. Cancer and Metabolic Rewiring

Cancers are generally characterized by a dramatic metabolic shift from OxPhos to aerobic glycolysis, a phenomenon that is commonly referred to as the Warburg phenotype [83–86]. The first indication that mitochondrial HSP90 is involved in cancer metabolism came from a study in 2012 reporting that this chaperone maintained metabolic homeostasis in neoplastic cells by inhibiting nutrient-sensing AMP kinase (AMPK), autophagy, and the unfolded protein response [87]. In the past 10 years, TRAP1 has been found to be highly expressed in a variety of neoplasms [24,47–57,59,60]. In 2013, an important observation provided a mechanistic basis for TRAP1 regulation of the balance between OxPhos and glycolysis in a variety of cell types [19]. More specifically, loss of TRAP1 led to an increase in mitochondrial respiration with a concomitant increase in oxygen-coupled ATP production, tricarboxylic acid (TCA) cycle activity, and fatty acid oxidation and the production of reactive oxygen species [19]. The re-introduction of TRAP1 restored this altered metabolic state to WT. Based on these observations and other supporting data, TRAP1 was proposed to act as a negative regulator of mitochondrial respiration, which exerted its effects via the inhibition of cytochrome C oxidase (Complex IV) and the mitochondrial pool of c-Src molecules [19]. Another independent study showed that TRAP1 directly binds to and inhibits the succinate dehydrogenase complex (SDH) [20], thereby downregulating mitochondrial respiration and the TCA cycle through a negative feedback generated by succinate accumulation [20,88–90]. Further, succinate accumulation inhibits hypoxia inducible factor (HIF) prolyl hydroxylation [91], stabilizing HIF1α [90] and creating a "pseudo-hypoxic" environment, which rewires cell metabolism towards glycolysis [90,92,93].

The early studies from Yoshida, Sciacovelli, and their colleagues [19,20] supported the hypothesis that TRAP1, by favoring a metabolic shift to glycolysis, is pro-tumorigenic. While this model is consistent with the reports highlighting the increased expression of TRAP1 in cancer, it is now clear that this molecule's role in mitochondrial metabolism and function is likely more complex than originally predicted (Figure 2). Thus, a separate report proposed that TRAP1 was actually required for the maintenance of mitochondrial metabolism under nutrient-limiting conditions [21]. Further, Chae and coworkers suggested that TRAP1 does not inhibit SDH activity but instead promotes it to stabilize mitochondrial OxPhos [21]. Similarly, a very recent study reported that TRAP1 may also compete with the peptidyl-prolyl cis-trans isomerase cyclophilin D (CypD) for binding to the oligomycin sensitivity-conferring protein (OSCP) subunit of the ATP–synthase complex to increase its catalytic activity and to suppress the inhibitory effects of CypD [94]. Further, Park et al. recently reported that a dynamic interplay between TRAP1 and the histone deacetylase sirtuin 3 (SIRT3) not only promoted mitochondrial respiration but also maintained metabolic plasticity, stemness, and increased adaptation to stress in glioblastoma cells [23]. In this study, the loss of TRAP1 ameliorated the tumor-forming ability of glioblastomas in vivo [23]. A similar, but not identical, in vivo consequence of TRAP1 loss was reported in a TRAP1-deficient mouse model of breast cancer [61]. While TRAP1 was not required for tumor initiation, growth, or metastases induced by polyoma middle T-antigen, its loss was associated with a delay of tumor initiation in vivo and in inhibition of proliferation, migration, and invasion in vitro when compared to WT [61].

A mechanistic insight that can explain the physiological consequences of metabolic rewiring by TRAP1, both from a cancer and non-cancer perspective, remains elusive. This gap in our understanding may be partially attributed to the cell type or context-dependent effects of TRAP1 on metabolism and/or other aspects of mitochondrial dynamics. While its presence is certainly inhibitory for OxPhos in some scenarios [19,20,22], it is actually required for OxPhos maintenance in other contexts [21,23]. In an attempt to dissect common alterations in the central carbon metabolism of cells lacking TRAP1 (compared to isogenic WT cells), multiple cancer-derived cell lines were grown in otherwise non-limiting conditions but were limited as to the carbon sources that feed glycolysis and OxPhos [22]. Cells having different metabolic phenotypes, with or without TRAP1, were forced to rely on either glucose, pyruvate, or glutamine as the sole carbon source. Surprisingly, consistent among all the cell types considered, TRAP1-deficient cells were unable to support OxPhos with either glucose or pyruvate, instead relying on glutamine, which served as an anaplerotic molecule [95] to support the TCA cycle and OxPhos upon conversion to α-ketoglutarate in mitochondria. Confusingly, all these metabolic behaviors are pro-neoplastic [85,96–98]. This apparent paradox remains to be reconciled but may provide a basis for understanding the conflicting reports that TRAP1 may be pro- or anti-tumorigenic depending on cellular and environmental contexts. In another recent report consistent with the model proposed by Joshi et al. [22], glucose uptake and lactate production were also shown to be impaired in TRAP1-silenced colorectal cancer (CRC) cells exposed to hypoxic conditions [99].

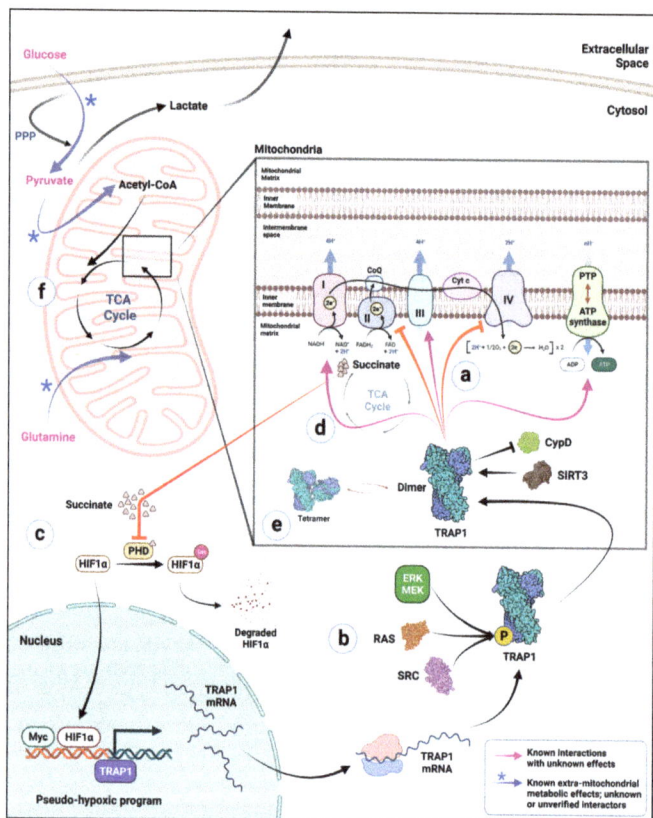

Figure 2. Potential mechanisms of TRAP1 participation in metabolic rewiring. (a) TRAP1 binds to and inhibits electron transport chain (ETC) complexes II and IV in the mitochondria. TRAP1 interacts with protein deacetylase SIRT3 in mitochondria and is reported to inhibit cyclophilin D (CypD), thereby preventing permeability transition pore (PTP) opening and inhibiting apoptosis due to cytochrome c release. (b) Further, TRAP1 activity is enhanced by phosphorylation via several pathways. Note that it remains unclear whether this happens before or after mitochondrial import of TRAP1. (c) ETC complex II inhibition by TRAP1 leads to succinate accumulation, which in turn inhibits prolyl hydroxylases in the cytosol to stabilize HIF1α. Stabilized HIF1α and Myc together activate a pseudo-hypoxic program, which further upregulates TRAP1 gene expression. (d) Inside mitochondria, TRAP1 also binds to ETC complexes I, III, and V (ATP synthase), but with unknown effects. (e) While TRAP1 tetramers exist alongside TRAP1 dimers in the mitochondrial matrix, determinants of the ratio of dimer to tetramer and any functional significance remain enigmatic. (f) TRAP1 presence and absence affect mitochondrial carbon preference. TRAP1 KO cells downregulate glucose- and pyruvate-derived carbon entry into the TCA cycle. A significant proportion of glucose is diverted to the pentose phosphate pathway (PPP) where it is used for the synthesis of NADPH reducing equivalents, perhaps to counter increased reactive oxygen species (ROS) that are characteristic of TRAP1 KO cells, and for the synthesis of ribose sugars. Pyruvate, upon decarboxylation, normally enters the TCA cycle and contributes to formation of acetyl-CoA, an important TCA cycle intermediate. In glycolysis, pyruvate is preferentially metabolized to lactate, generating NAD+ as a by-product of the reaction, at the expense of NADH. As with NADPH, increased levels of NADH provide more reducing equivalents to counter the increased ROS characteristic of TRAP1 KO. In contrast, TRAP1 KO cells utilize anaplerotic glutamine metabolism to maintain a functional TCA cycle by providing glutamine-derived carbon.

5. Defining a TRAP1 Interactome

How TRAP1 ATP hydrolysis is coupled to its mitochondrial protein interactome has remained unclear. In a first attempt to address this question, Joshi and colleagues examined the TRAP1 interactome as a function of the chaperone's ATPase activity [22]. Using a set of TRAP1 mutants displaying a 30-fold range of ATPase activity [69] and WT TRAP1 in a series of immunoprecipitation experiments followed by mass spectrometric analysis (IP-MS), the authors identified two distinct sets of interactors. The most abundant interactors were the mitochondrial chaperones mtHSP70/mortalin, HSP60, and prohibitin, whose binding to TRAP1 was not affected by TRAP1 ATPase activity. In contrast, a second, more diverse set of interactors, including the ATP synthase complex, translocases, proteins involved in mitochondrial membrane organization, and multiple subunits from mitochondrial electron transport chain complexes [22], displayed a strong negative correlation with the TRAP1 hydrolysis rate.

This second observation is in broad agreement with work done on HSP90 clients. In this case, HSP90 ATPase activity is inversely correlated with client binding and dwell time as part of the HSP90 complex [100]. Further, HSP90 mutants that bind ATP but cannot hydrolyze it demonstrate the strongest affinity for the HSP90 clients, HER2 and HSF1 [101,102]. These data suggest that TRAP1 interactors reflect the response of HSP90 clients to the chaperone's ATPase activity. However, the lack of correlation between TRAP1 ATPase activity and interaction with other mitochondrial chaperones does not share obvious similarities with HSP90; the significance of this differential response requires further experimental study.

6. TRAP1 Inhibitors

Most inhibitors of the HSP90 family competitively bind to the N-terminal ATP pocket. This mode of action was exploited to create the first set of inhibitors for TRAP1, whose ATPase domain has homology with other members of the HSP90 family. However, since the mitochondrial membrane is impervious to traditional HSP90 inhibitors, a mitochondrial-targeting moiety such as one to four tandem repeats of cyclic guanidium or triphenylphosphonium (TPP) had to be added in order for these inhibitors to reach the mitochondrial matrix [33,103,104]. The first TRAP1 inhibitor was based on the benzoquinone ansamycin geldanamycin (specifically, 17-AAG), which was linked to a TPP moiety to create a "Gamitrinib" or a geldanamycin-based mitochondrial matrix inhibitor. Gamitrinibs accumulate in mitochondria and were shown to be anti-neoplastic in tumor xenografts and in mouse models of prostate cancer [105]. A similar TPP tagged derivative, SMTIN-P01, was also designed from PU-H71, a purine-based HSP90 inhibitor [106]. SMTIN-P01 also concentrated in mitochondria and was found to be cytotoxic to cancer cells [106]. Further, PU-H71-based TRAP1 inhibitors were shown to induce strong mitochondrial depolarization and apoptosis in acute myeloid leukemia cells [107]. PU-H71-based SMTIN-P01 was further modified with carbon spacers to create multiple analogs [108]. Of these, a 10-carbon spacer analog, SMTIN-C10, displayed both orthosteric and allosteric interactions with TRAP1 and changed its conformation from apo to closed state. While SMTIN-C10 increased TRAP1 ATPase activity, it perturbed TRAP1 function, decreased client protein levels, and exhibited anticancer activity both in vitro and in vivo [108]. These results are consistent with the previously discussed negative correlation between non-chaperone TRAP1 interactors and TRAP1 ATPase activity [22]. Importantly, to move forward, it will be necessary to determine systematically whether TRAP1 inhibitors phenocopy any of the consequences resulting from a stable TRAP1 KO.

While many TRAP1 inhibitors that have been reported or continue to be tested are linked to mitochondrial-targeting motifs such as TPPs, it is important to note that TPP itself is toxic to mitochondria [109]. TPP downregulates mitochondrial OxPhos; its non-specific effects likely would be additive to the consequences of specific TRAP1 inhibition. Moreover, such inhibitors *en route* to the mitochondrial matrix are expected to interact to some extent with the much more abundant HSP90 in the cytosol before even reaching the mitochondria [110]. As such, the possibility of substantial HSP90 inhibition with these TRAP1 inhibitors can never be ruled out. These issues were partially circumvented with the introduction of DN401, a BIIB021 [111]-derived pyrazolopyrimidine [110]. This molecule displayed increased TRAP1 selectivity over HSP90, exhibited potent in vivo anticancer activity, and lacked any mitochondrial-targeting motifs [110].

Such a continued rational design approach is likely to identify additional allosteric inhibitors of TRAP1, which either do not or poorly bind to HSP90. To this end, molecular dynamics simulations have been performed to understand the dynamic coordination between any two residues within the TRAP1 molecule as a function of the fluctuations between their distance [112,113]. Residues with high coordination were associated with low pair-distance fluctuations. Based on such simulations, a putative allosteric site responsible for structural reorganization of TRAP1 after ATP hydrolysis was identified in the middle domain of the chaperone. A pharmacophore model of this site was used to screen drug databases, and several TRAP1 selective inhibitors were identified [114]. These molecules specifically inhibit TRAP1 ATPase activity with minimal effects on HSP90 and were found to inhibit in vitro growth of malignant peripheral nerve sheath tumor (MPNST) cells [114]. A similar approach was used to identify a honokiol derivative, HDCA (honokiol bis-dichloroacetate), which was observed to bind to the same TRAP1 allosteric binding pocket, inhibiting its ATPase activity and its neoplastic potential in MPNST cells [115].

Recently, studies have explored whether TRAP1 inhibitors may be synergistic with other anticancer drugs. Gamitrinibs have been found to amplify the efficacy of inhibitors of mitogen-activated protein kinases in models of BRAFV600E melanoma and on drug-resistant melanoma cells [116]. Bromodomain and extraterminal (BET) family protein inhibitors JQ1 and OTX015 were also found to synergize with Gamitrinibs and to induce apoptosis in malignant glioma cells [117]. Gamitrinibs also augment the effect of histone deacetylase inhibitors in inducing apoptosis in patient-derived glioblastoma xenografts [118].

7. Conclusions

TRAP1 provides a link between mitochondrial homeostasis and metabolism. Although it is a member of the HSP90 family, which is well known for its roles in cellular proteostasis, cumulative studies over the last 20 years suggest that TRAP1 functions diverge from those of other HSP90 paralogs. It appears to be more closely related to the prokaryotic HtpG. TRAP1 does not bind to any known eukaryotic HSP90 co-chaperone and, unlike HSP90, it is essential neither in vitro nor in vivo. Further distinguishing TRAP1 from HSP90, a loss of TRAP1 does not significantly destabilize the mitochondrial proteome, but it impacts the mitochondrial matrix structure and modulates mitochondrial metabolism to maintain metabolic plasticity. Unlike other members of the HSP90 family, TRAP1 molecules readily form tetramers in the "hot" mitochondrial matrix. Whether this is a direct consequence of elevated temperature and whether these tetramers may promote assembly and/or stabilization of large macromolecular structures common to mitochondria, their functional relevance, dynamics, and regulation remain unknown.

Even with all these questions and challenges, understanding the TRAP1 function and how it integrates dynamic alterations in the mitochondrial structure and cell metabolism, survival, and growth from neoplastic and non-neoplastic perspectives is a rapidly evolving field that retains great interest, especially in light of the emerging importance of mitochondria in many unexpected cellular processes. Continued deep analysis of TRAP1 dynamics, interactors, and functions is likely to prove rewarding in this context.

Author Contributions: Conceptualization and original draft preparation, A.J.; review and editing, L.N., D.P., A.J. and T.I. All authors have read and agreed to the published version of the manuscript.

Funding: L.N. was supported by funds from the intramural research program of the National Cancer Institute (project number ZIA SC 010074).

Institutional Review Board Statement: Not applicable.

Informed Consent Statement: Not applicable.

Acknowledgments: The figures for this review were created using Biorender.com (accessed on 22 June 2022) using an NCI institutional license.

Conflicts of Interest: The authors declare no conflict of interest.

References

1. Hartl, F.U.; Bracher, A.; Hayer-Hartl, M. Molecular chaperones in protein folding and proteostasis. *Nature* **2011**, *475*, 324–332. [CrossRef]
2. Kim, Y.E.; Hipp, M.S.; Bracher, A.; Hayer-Hartl, M.; Hartl, F.U. Molecular chaperone functions in protein folding and proteostasis. *Annu. Rev. Biochem.* **2013**, *82*, 323–355. [CrossRef]
3. Richter, K.; Haslbeck, M.; Buchner, J. The heat shock response: Life on the verge of death. *Mol. Cell* **2010**, *40*, 253–266. [CrossRef] [PubMed]
4. Gao, X.; Carroni, M.; Nussbaum-Krammer, C.; Mogk, A.; Nillegoda, N.B.; Szlachcic, A.; Guilbride, D.L.; Saibil, H.R.; Mayer, M.P.; Bukau, B. Human Hsp70 Disaggregase Reverses Parkinson's-Linked α-Synuclein Amyloid Fibrils. *Mol. Cell* **2015**, *59*, 781–793. [CrossRef] [PubMed]
5. Nillegoda, N.B.; Bukau, B. Metazoan Hsp70-based protein disaggregases: Emergence and mechanisms. *Front. Mol. Biosci.* **2015**, *2*, 57. [CrossRef] [PubMed]
6. Fernandez-Funez, P.; Sanchez-Garcia, J.; de Mena, L.; Zhang, Y.; Levites, Y.; Khare, S.; Golde, T.E.; Rincon-Limas, D.E. Holdase activity of secreted Hsp70 masks amyloid-β42 neurotoxicity in *Drosophila*. *Proc. Natl. Acad. Sci. USA* **2016**, *113*, E5212–E5221. [CrossRef]
7. Thoma, J.; Burmann, B.M.; Hiller, S.; Müller, D.J. Impact of holdase chaperones Skp and SurA on the folding of β-barrel outer-membrane proteins. *Nat. Struct. Mol. Biol.* **2015**, *22*, 795–802. [CrossRef]
8. Demand, J.; Alberti, S.; Patterson, C.; Höhfeld, J. Cooperation of a ubiquitin domain protein and an E3 ubiquitin ligase during chaperone/proteasome coupling. *Curr. Biol.* **2001**, *11*, 1569–1577. [CrossRef]
9. Gamerdinger, M.; Hajieva, P.; Kaya, A.M.; Wolfrum, U.; Hartl, F.U.; Behl, C. Protein quality control during aging involves recruitment of the macroautophagy pathway by BAG3. *EMBO J.* **2009**, *28*, 889–901. [CrossRef]
10. Hartmann-Petersen, R.; Seeger, M.; Gordon, C. Transferring substrates to the 26S proteasome. *Trends Biochem. Sci.* **2003**, *28*, 26–31. [CrossRef]
11. Csermely, P.; Schnaider, T.; Soti, C.; Prohászka, Z.; Nardai, G. The 90-kDa molecular chaperone family: Structure, function, and clinical applications. A comprehensive review. *Pharmacol. Ther.* **1998**, *79*, 129–168. [CrossRef]
12. Schopf, F.H.; Biebl, M.M.; Buchner, J. The HSP90 chaperone machinery. *Nat. Rev. Mol. Cell Biol.* **2017**, *18*, 345–360. [CrossRef] [PubMed]
13. Radli, M.; Rüdiger, S.G.D. Dancing with the Diva: Hsp90–Client Interactions. *J. Mol. Biol.* **2018**, *430*, 3029–3040. [CrossRef] [PubMed]
14. Taipale, M.; Jarosz, D.F.; Lindquist, S. HSP90 at the hub of protein homeostasis: Emerging mechanistic insights. *Nat. Rev. Mol. Cell Biol.* **2010**, *11*, 515–528. [CrossRef] [PubMed]
15. Zuehlke, A.D.; Beebe, K.; Neckers, L.; Prince, T. Regulation and function of the human HSP90AA1 gene. *Gene* **2015**, *570*, 8–16. [CrossRef]
16. Marzec, M.; Eletto, D.; Argon, Y. GRP94: An HSP90-like protein specialized for protein folding and quality control in the endoplasmic reticulum. *Biochim. Biophys. Acta* **2012**, *1823*, 774–787. [CrossRef]
17. Felts, S.J.; Owen, B.A.; Nguyen, P.; Trepel, J.; Donner, D.B.; Toft, D.O. The hsp90-related protein TRAP1 is a mitochondrial protein with distinct functional properties. *J. Biol. Chem.* **2000**, *275*, 3305–3312. [CrossRef]
18. Cechetto, J.D.; Gupta, R.S. Immunoelectron microscopy provides evidence that tumor necrosis factor receptor-associated protein 1 (TRAP-1) is a mitochondrial protein which also localizes at specific extramitochondrial sites. *Exp. Cell Res.* **2000**, *260*, 30–39. [CrossRef]
19. Yoshida, S.; Tsutsumi, S.; Muhlebach, G.; Sourbier, C.; Lee, M.-J.; Lee, S.; Vartholomaiou, E.; Tatokoro, M.; Beebe, K.; Miyajima, N.; et al. Molecular chaperone TRAP1 regulates a metabolic switch between mitochondrial respiration and aerobic glycolysis. *Proc. Natl. Acad. Sci. USA* **2013**, *110*, E1604–E1612. [CrossRef]
20. Sciacovelli, M.; Guzzo, G.; Morello, V.; Frezza, C.; Zheng, L.; Nannini, N.; Calabrese, F.; Laudiero, G.; Esposito, F.; Landriscina, M.; et al. The Mitochondrial Chaperone TRAP1 Promotes Neoplastic Growth by Inhibiting Succinate Dehydrogenase. *Cell Metab.* **2013**, *17*, 988–999. [CrossRef]
21. Chae, Y.C.; Angelin, A.; Lisanti, S.; Kossenkov, A.V.; Speicher, K.D.; Wang, H.; Powers, J.F.; Tischler, A.S.; Pacak, K.; Fliedner, S.; et al. Landscape of the mitochondrial Hsp90 metabolome in tumours. *Nat. Commun.* **2013**, *4*, 2139. [CrossRef]
22. Joshi, A.; Dai, L.; Liu, Y.; Lee, J.; Ghahhari, N.M.; Segala, G.; Beebe, K.; Jenkins, L.M.; Lyons, G.C.; Bernasconi, L.; et al. The mitochondrial HSP90 paralog TRAP1 forms an OXPHOS-regulated tetramer and is involved in mitochondrial metabolic homeostasis. *BMC Biol.* **2020**, *18*, 10. [CrossRef]

23. Park, H.K.; Hong, J.H.; Oh, Y.T.; Kim, S.S.; Yin, J.; Lee, A.J.; Chae, Y.C.; Kim, J.H.; Park, S.H.; Park, C.K.; et al. Interplay between TRAP1 and Sirtuin-3 Modulates Mitochondrial Respiration and Oxidative Stress to Maintain Stemness of Glioma Stem Cells. *Cancer Res.* **2019**, *79*, 1369–1382. [CrossRef]
24. Rasola, A.; Neckers, L.; Picard, D. Mitochondrial oxidative phosphorylation TRAP(1)ped in tumor cells. *Trends Cell Biol.* **2014**, *24*, 455–463. [CrossRef]
25. Masgras, I.; Laquatra, C.; Cannino, G.; Serapian, S.A.; Colombo, G.; Rasola, A. The molecular chaperone TRAP1 in cancer: From the basics of biology to pharmacological targeting. *Semin. Cancer Biol.* **2021**, *76*, 45–53. [CrossRef]
26. Takamura, H.; Koyama, Y.; Matsuzaki, S.; Yamada, K.; Hattori, T.; Miyata, S.; Takemoto, K.; Tohyama, M.; Katayama, T. TRAP1 controls mitochondrial fusion/fission balance through Drp1 and Mff expression. *PLoS ONE* **2012**, *7*, e51912. [CrossRef]
27. Costa, A.C.; Loh, S.H.Y.; Martins, L.M. Drosophila Trap1 protects against mitochondrial dysfunction in a PINK1/parkin model of Parkinson's disease. *Cell Death Dis.* **2013**, *4*, e467. [CrossRef]
28. Zhang, L.; Karsten, P.; Hamm, S.; Pogson, J.H.; Müller-Rischart, A.K.; Exner, N.; Haass, C.; Whitworth, A.J.; Winklhofer, K.F.; Schulz, J.B.; et al. TRAP1 rescues PINK1 loss-of-function phenotypes. *Hum. Mol. Genet.* **2013**, *22*, 2829–2841. [CrossRef]
29. Hua, G.; Zhang, Q.; Fan, Z. Heat Shock Protein 75 (TRAP1) Antagonizes Reactive Oxygen Species Generation and Protects Cells from Granzyme M-mediated Apoptosis. *J. Biol. Chem.* **2007**, *282*, 20553–20560. [CrossRef]
30. Montesano Gesualdi, N.; Chirico, G.; Pirozzi, G.; Costantino, E.; Landriscina, M.; Esposito, F. Tumor necrosis factor-associated protein 1 (TRAP-1) protects cells from oxidative stress and apoptosis. *Stress* **2007**, *10*, 342–350. [CrossRef]
31. Pridgeon, J.W.; Olzmann, J.A.; Chin, L.-S.; Li, L. PINK1 Protects against Oxidative Stress by Phosphorylating Mitochondrial Chaperone TRAP1. *PLoS Biol.* **2007**, *5*, e172. [CrossRef]
32. Ramos Rego, I.; Santos Cruz, B.; Ambrósio, A.F.; Alves, C.H. TRAP1 in Oxidative Stress and Neurodegeneration. *Antioxidants* **2021**, *10*, 1829. [CrossRef]
33. Kang, B.H.; Plescia, J.; Dohi, T.; Rosa, J.; Doxsey, S.J.; Altieri, D.C. Regulation of Tumor Cell Mitochondrial Homeostasis by an Organelle-Specific Hsp90 Chaperone Network. *Cell* **2007**, *131*, 257–270. [CrossRef]
34. Xu, L.; Voloboueva, L.A.; Ouyang, Y.; Emery, J.F.; Giffard, R.G. Overexpression of mitochondrial Hsp70/Hsp75 in rat brain protects mitochondria, reduces oxidative stress, and protects from focal ischemia. *J. Cereb. Blood Flow Metab.* **2009**, *29*, 365–374. [CrossRef]
35. Xiang, F.; Huang, Y.S.; Shi, X.H.; Zhang, Q. Mitochondrial chaperone tumour necrosis factor receptor-associated protein 1 protects cardiomyocytes from hypoxic injury by regulating mitochondrial permeability transition pore opening. *FEBS J.* **2010**, *277*, 1929–1938. [CrossRef]
36. Zhang, P.; Lu, Y.; Yu, D.; Zhang, D.; Hu, W. TRAP1 Provides Protection Against Myocardial Ischemia-Reperfusion Injury by Ameliorating Mitochondrial Dysfunction. *Cell. Physiol. Biochem. Int. J. Exp. Cell. Physiol. Biochem. Pharmacol.* **2015**, *36*, 2072–2082. [CrossRef]
37. Clarke, B.E.; Kalmar, B.; Greensmith, L. Enhanced Expression of TRAP1 Protects Mitochondrial Function in Motor Neurons under Conditions of Oxidative Stress. *Int. J. Mol. Sci.* **2022**, *23*, 1789. [CrossRef]
38. Zhang, L.; Su, N.; Luo, Y.; Chen, S.; Zhao, T. TRAP1 inhibits MIC60 ubiquitination to mitigate the injury of cardiomyocytes and protect mitochondria in extracellular acidosis. *Cell Death Discov.* **2021**, *7*, 389. [CrossRef]
39. Butler, E.K.; Voigt, A.; Lutz, A.K.; Toegel, J.P.; Gerhardt, E.; Karsten, P.; Falkenburger, B.; Reinartz, A.; Winklhofer, K.F.; Schulz, J.B. The mitochondrial chaperone protein TRAP1 mitigates α-Synuclein toxicity. *PLoS Genet.* **2012**, *8*, e1002488. [CrossRef]
40. Malpartida, A.B.; Williamson, M.; Narendra, D.P.; Wade-Martins, R.; Ryan, B.J. Mitochondrial Dysfunction and Mitophagy in Parkinson's Disease: From Mechanism to Therapy. *Trends Biochem. Sci.* **2021**, *46*, 329–343. [CrossRef]
41. Chen, J.F.; Wu, Q.S.; Xie, Y.X.; Si, B.L.; Yang, P.P.; Wang, W.Y.; Hua, Q.; He, Q. TRAP1 ameliorates renal tubulointerstitial fibrosis in mice with unilateral ureteral obstruction by protecting renal tubular epithelial cell mitochondria. *FASEB J.* **2017**, *31*, 4503–4514. [CrossRef]
42. Nicolas, E.; Demidova, E.V.; Iqbal, W.; Serebriiskii, I.G.; Vlasenkova, R.; Ghatalia, P.; Zhou, Y.; Rainey, K.; Forman, A.F.; Dunbrack, R.L., Jr.; et al. Interaction of germline variants in a family with a history of early-onset clear cell renal cell carcinoma. *Mol. Genet. Genom. Med.* **2019**, *7*, e556. [CrossRef]
43. Fitzgerald, J.C.; Zimprich, A.; Carvajal Berrio, D.A.; Schindler, K.M.; Maurer, B.; Schulte, C.; Bus, C.; Hauser, A.K.; Kübler, M.; Lewin, R.; et al. Metformin reverses TRAP1 mutation-associated alterations in mitochondrial function in Parkinson's disease. *Brain J. Neurol.* **2017**, *140*, 2444–2459. [CrossRef]
44. Skinner, S.J.; Doonanco, K.R.; Boles, R.G.; Chan, A.K.J. Homozygous TRAP1 sequence variant in a child with Leigh syndrome and normal kidneys. *Kidney Int.* **2014**, *86*, 860. [CrossRef]
45. Boles, R.G.; Hornung, H.A.; Moody, A.E.; Ortiz, T.B.; Wong, S.A.; Eggington, J.M.; Stanley, C.M.; Gao, M.; Zhou, H.; McLaughlin, S.; et al. Hurt, tired and queasy: Specific variants in the ATPase domain of the TRAP1 mitochondrial chaperone are associated with common, chronic "functional" symptomatology including pain, fatigue and gastrointestinal dysmotility. *Mitochondrion* **2015**, *23*, 64–70. [CrossRef]
46. Saisawat, P.; Kohl, S.; Hilger, A.C.; Hwang, D.Y.; Yung Gee, H.; Dworschak, G.C.; Tasic, V.; Pennimpede, T.; Natarajan, S.; Sperry, E.; et al. Whole-exome resequencing reveals recessive mutations in TRAP1 in individuals with CAKUT and VACTERL association. *Kidney Int.* **2014**, *85*, 1310–1317. [CrossRef]

47. Megger, D.A.; Bracht, T.; Kohl, M.; Ahrens, M.; Naboulsi, W.; Weber, F.; Hoffmann, A.-C.; Stephan, C.; Kuhlmann, K.; Eisenacher, M.; et al. Proteomic differences between hepatocellular carcinoma and nontumorous liver tissue investigated by a combined gel-based and label-free quantitative proteomics study. *Mol. Cell. Proteom.* **2013**, *12*, 2006–2020. [CrossRef]
48. Zhang, B.; Wang, J.; Huang, Z.; Wei, P.; Liu, Y.; Hao, J.; Zhao, L.; Zhang, F.; Tu, Y.; Wei, T. Aberrantly upregulated TRAP1 is required for tumorigenesis of breast cancer. *Oncotarget* **2015**, *6*, 44495. [CrossRef]
49. Li, S.; Lv, Q.; Sun, H.; Xue, Y.; Wang, P.; Liu, L.; Li, Z.; Li, Z.; Tian, X.; Liu, Y.H. Expression of TRAP1 predicts poor survival of malignant glioma patients. *J. Mol. Neurosci.* **2015**, *55*, 62–68. [CrossRef]
50. Lee, J.H.; Kang, K.W.; Kim, J.-E.; Hwang, S.W.; Park, J.H.; Kim, S.-H.; Ji, J.H.; Kim, T.G.; Nam, H.-Y.; Roh, M.S.; et al. Differential expression of heat shock protein 90 isoforms in small cell lung cancer. *Int. J. Clin. Exp. Pathol.* **2015**, *8*, 9487–9493.
51. Gao, C.; Li, M.; Jiang, A.-L.; Sun, R.; Jin, H.-L.; Gui, H.-W.; Xiao, F.; Ding, X.-W.; Fu, Z.-M.; Feng, J.-P. Overexpression of the mitochondrial chaperone tumor necrosis factor receptor-associated protein 1 is associated with the poor prognosis of patients with colorectal cancer. *Oncol. Lett.* **2018**, *15*, 5451–5458. [CrossRef] [PubMed]
52. Gao, J.-Y.; Song, B.-R.; Peng, J.-J.; Lu, Y.-M. Correlation between mitochondrial TRAP-1 expression and lymph node metastasis in colorectal cancer. *World J. Gastroenterol.* **2012**, *18*, 5965–5971. [CrossRef] [PubMed]
53. Leav, I.; Plescia, J.; Goel, H.L.; Li, J.; Jiang, Z.; Cohen, R.J.; Languino, L.R.; Altieri, D.C. Cytoprotective mitochondrial chaperone TRAP-1 as a novel molecular target in localized and metastatic prostate cancer. *Am. J. Pathol.* **2010**, *176*, 393–401. [CrossRef] [PubMed]
54. Lv, Q.; Sun, H.; Cao, C.; Gao, B.; Qi, Y. Overexpression of tumor necrosis factor receptor-associated protein 1 (TRAP1) are associated with poor prognosis of epithelial ovarian cancer. *Tumor Biol. J. Int. Soc. Oncodev. Biol. Med.* **2016**, *37*, 2721–2727. [CrossRef] [PubMed]
55. Ou, Y.; Liu, L.; Xue, L.; Zhou, W.; Zhao, Z.; Xu, B.; Song, Y.; Zhan, Q. TRAP1 shows clinical significance and promotes cellular migration and invasion through STAT3/MMP2 pathway in human esophageal squamous cell cancer. *J. Genet. Genom. Yi Chuan Xue Bao* **2014**, *41*, 529–537. [CrossRef]
56. Pak, M.G.; Koh, H.J.; Roh, M.S. Clinicopathologic significance of TRAP1 expression in colorectal cancer: A large scale study of human colorectal adenocarcinoma tissues. *Diagn. Pathol.* **2017**, *12*, 6. [CrossRef]
57. Si, T.; Yang, G.; Qiu, X.; Luo, Y.; Liu, B.; Wang, B. Expression of tumor necrosis factor receptor-associated protein 1 and its clinical significance in kidney cancer. *Int. J. Clin. Exp. Pathol.* **2015**, *8*, 13090–13095.
58. Chen, R.; Pan, S.; Lai, K.; Lai, L.A.; Crispin, D.A.; Bronner, M.P.; Brentnall, T.A. Up-regulation of mitochondrial chaperone TRAP1 in ulcerative colitis associated colorectal cancer. *World J. Gastroenterol.* **2014**, *20*, 17037–17048. [CrossRef]
59. Kowalik, M.A.; Guzzo, G.; Morandi, A.; Perra, A.; Menegon, S.; Masgras, I.; Trevisan, E.; Angioni, M.M.; Fornari, F.; Quagliata, L.; et al. Metabolic reprogramming identifies the most aggressive lesions at early phases of hepatic carcinogenesis. *Oncotarget* **2016**, *7*, 32375–32393. [CrossRef]
60. Wallace, D.C. Mitochondria and cancer. *Nat. Rev. Cancer* **2012**, *12*, 685–698. [CrossRef]
61. Vartholomaiou, E.; Madon-Simon, M.; Hagmann, S.; Mühlebach, G.; Wurst, W.; Floss, T.; Picard, D. Cytosolic Hsp90α and its mitochondrial isoform Trap1 are differentially required in a breast cancer model. *Oncotarget* **2017**, *8*, 17428. [CrossRef]
62. Chen, B.; Piel, W.H.; Gui, L.; Bruford, E.; Monteiro, A. The HSP90 family of genes in the human genome: Insights into their divergence and evolution. *Genomics* **2005**, *86*, 627–637. [CrossRef]
63. Lisanti, S.; Tavecchio, M.; Chae, Y.C.; Liu, Q.; Brice, A.K.; Thakur, M.L.; Languino, L.R.; Altieri, D.C. Deletion of the Mitochondrial Chaperone TRAP-1 Uncovers Global Reprogramming of Metabolic Networks. *Cell Rep.* **2014**, *8*, 671–677. [CrossRef]
64. Jackson, S.E. Hsp90: Structure and function. *Top. Curr. Chem.* **2013**, *328*, 155–240. [CrossRef]
65. Lavery, L.A.; Partridge, J.R.; Ramelot, T.A.; Elnatan, D.; Kennedy, M.A.; Agard, D.A. Structural asymmetry in the closed state of mitochondrial Hsp90 (TRAP1) supports a two-step ATP hydrolysis mechanism. *Mol. Cell* **2014**, *53*, 330–343. [CrossRef]
66. Kang, B.H. TRAP1 regulation of mitochondrial life or death decision in cancer cells and mitochondria-targeted TRAP1 inhibitors. *BMB Rep.* **2012**, *45*, 1–6. [CrossRef]
67. Tsutsumi, S.; Mollapour, M.; Prodromou, C.; Lee, C.T.; Panaretou, B.; Yoshida, S.; Mayer, M.P.; Neckers, L.M. Charged linker sequence modulates eukaryotic heat shock protein 90 (Hsp90) chaperone activity. *Proc. Natl. Acad. Sci. USA* **2012**, *109*, 2937–2942. [CrossRef]
68. Partridge, J.R.; Lavery, L.A.; Elnatan, D.; Naber, N.; Cooke, R.; Agard, D.A. A novel N-terminal extension in mitochondrial TRAP1 serves as a thermal regulator of chaperone activity. *eLife* **2014**, *3*, e03487. [CrossRef]
69. Sung, N.; Lee, J.; Kim, J.-H.; Chang, C.; Joachimiak, A.; Lee, S.; Tsai, F.T.F. Mitochondrial Hsp90 is a ligand-activated molecular chaperone coupling ATP binding to dimer closure through a coiled-coil intermediate. *Proc. Natl. Acad. Sci. USA* **2016**, *113*, 2952–2957. [CrossRef]
70. Leskovar, A.; Wegele, H.; Werbeck, N.D.; Buchner, J.; Reinstein, J. The ATPase cycle of the mitochondrial Hsp90 analog Trap1. *J. Biol. Chem.* **2008**, *283*, 11677–11688. [CrossRef]
71. Elnatan, D.; Betegon, M.; Liu, Y.; Ramelot, T.; Kennedy, M.A.; Agard, D.A. Symmetry broken and rebroken during the ATP hydrolysis cycle of the mitochondrial Hsp90 TRAP1. *eLife* **2017**, *6*, e25235. [CrossRef]
72. Elnatan, D.; Agard, D.A. Calcium binding to a remote site can replace magnesium as cofactor for mitochondrial Hsp90 (TRAP1) ATPase activity. *J. Biol. Chem.* **2018**, *293*, 13717–13724. [CrossRef]

73. Liu, Y.; Sun, M.; Elnatan, D.; Larson, A.G.; Agard, D.A. Cryo-EM analysis of human mitochondrial Hsp90 in multiple tetrameric states. *bioRxiv* **2020**. [CrossRef]
74. Shiau, A.K.; Harris, S.F.; Southworth, D.R.; Agard, D.A. Structural Analysis of E. coli hsp90 reveals dramatic nucleotide-dependent conformational rearrangements. *Cell* **2006**, *127*, 329–340. [CrossRef]
75. Nemoto, T.; Sato, N. Oligomeric forms of the 90-kDa heat shock protein. *Biochem. J.* **1998**, *330*, 989–995. [CrossRef]
76. Lee, C.-C.; Lin, T.-W.; Ko, T.-P.; Wang, A.H.J. The Hexameric Structures of Human Heat Shock Protein 90. *PLoS ONE* **2011**, *6*, e19961. [CrossRef]
77. Chadli, A.; Ladjimi, M.M.; Baulieu, E.-E.; Catelli, M.G. Heat-induced Oligomerization of the Molecular Chaperone Hsp90: Inhibition by atp and geldanamycin and activation by transition metal oxyanions. *J. Biol. Chem.* **1999**, *274*, 4133–4139. [CrossRef]
78. Moullintraffort, L.; Bruneaux, M.; Nazabal, A.; Allegro, D.; Giudice, E.; Zal, F.; Peyrot, V.; Barbier, P.; Thomas, D.; Garnier, C. Biochemical and Biophysical Characterization of the Mg^{2+}-induced 90-kDa Heat Shock Protein Oligomers. *J. Biol. Chem.* **2010**, *285*, 15100–15110. [CrossRef]
79. Yonehara, M.; Minami, Y.; Kawata, Y.; Nagai, J.; Yahara, I. Heat-induced Chaperone Activity of HSP90. *J. Biol. Chem.* **1996**, *271*, 2641–2645. [CrossRef]
80. Jakob, U.; Meyer, I.; Bügl, H.; André, S.; Bardwell, J.C.A.; Buchner, J. Structural Organization of Procaryotic and Eucaryotic Hsp90. Influence of divalent cations on structure and function. *J. Biol. Chem.* **1995**, *270*, 14412–14419. [CrossRef]
81. Chrétien, D.; Bénit, P.; Ha, H.-H.; Keipert, S.; El-Khoury, R.; Chang, Y.-T.; Jastroch, M.; Jacobs, H.T.; Rustin, P.; Rak, M. Mitochondria are physiologically maintained at close to 50 °C. *PLoS Biol.* **2018**, *16*, e2003992. [CrossRef]
82. Lepvrier, E.; Thomas, D.; Garnier, C. Hsp90 Quaternary Structures and the Chaperone Cycle: Highly Flexible Dimeric and Oligomeric Structures and Their Regulation by Co-Chaperones. *Curr. Proteom.* **2019**, *16*, 5–11. [CrossRef]
83. Hsu, P.P.; Sabatini, D.M. Cancer cell metabolism: Warburg and beyond. *Cell* **2008**, *134*, 703–707. [CrossRef]
84. Vander Heiden, M.G.; Cantley, L.C.; Thompson, C.B. Understanding the Warburg effect: The metabolic requirements of cell proliferation. *Science* **2009**, *324*, 1029–1033. [CrossRef]
85. Warburg, O. On the Origin of Cancer Cells. *Science* **1956**, *123*, 309–314. [CrossRef]
86. Warburg, O.; Wind, F.; Negelein, E. The metabolism of tumors in the body. *J. Gen. Physiol.* **1927**, *8*, 519–530. [CrossRef]
87. Chae, Y.C.; Caino, M.C.; Lisanti, S.; Ghosh, J.C.; Dohi, T.; Danial, N.N.; Villanueva, J.; Ferrero, S.; Vaira, V.; Santambrogio, L.; et al. Control of tumor bioenergetics and survival stress signaling by mitochondrial HSP90s. *Cancer Cell* **2012**, *22*, 331–344. [CrossRef]
88. King, A.; Selak, M.A.; Gottlieb, E. Succinate dehydrogenase and fumarate hydratase: Linking mitochondrial dysfunction and cancer. *Oncogene* **2006**, *25*, 4675–4682. [CrossRef]
89. Tretter, L.; Patocs, A.; Chinopoulos, C. Succinate, an intermediate in metabolism, signal transduction, ROS, hypoxia, and tumorigenesis. *Biochim. Biophys. Acta (BBA)-Bioenerg.* **2016**, *1857*, 1086–1101. [CrossRef]
90. Hayashi, Y.; Yokota, A.; Harada, H.; Huang, G. Hypoxia/pseudohypoxia-mediated activation of hypoxia-inducible factor-1α in cancer. *Cancer Sci.* **2019**, *110*, 1510–1517. [CrossRef]
91. Selak, M.A.; Armour, S.M.; MacKenzie, E.D.; Boulahbel, H.; Watson, D.G.; Mansfield, K.D.; Pan, Y.; Simon, M.C.; Thompson, C.B.; Gottlieb, E. Succinate links TCA cycle dysfunction to oncogenesis by inhibiting HIF-alpha prolyl hydroxylase. *Cancer Cell* **2005**, *7*, 77–85. [CrossRef]
92. Mao, H.; Yang, A.; Zhao, Y.; Lei, L.; Li, H. Succinate Supplement Elicited "Pseudohypoxia" Condition to Promote Proliferation, Migration, and Osteogenesis of Periodontal Ligament Cells. *Stem Cells Int.* **2020**, *2020*, 2016809. [CrossRef]
93. Al Tameemi, W.; Dale, T.P.; Al-Jumaily, R.M.K.; Forsyth, N.R. Hypoxia-Modified Cancer Cell Metabolism. *Front. Cell Dev. Biol.* **2019**, *7*, 4. [CrossRef]
94. Cannino, G.; Urbani, A.; Gaspari, M.; Varano, M.; Negro, A.; Filippi, A.; Ciscato, F.; Masgras, I.; Gerle, C.; Tibaldi, E.; et al. The mitochondrial chaperone TRAP1 regulates F-ATP synthase channel formation. *Cell Death Differ.* **2022**. [CrossRef]
95. Martins, F.; Gonçalves, L.G.; Pojo, M.; Serpa, J. Take Advantage of Glutamine Anaplerosis, the Kernel of the Metabolic Rewiring in Malignant Gliomas. *Biomolecules* **2020**, *10*, 1370. [CrossRef]
96. Wise, D.R.; Thompson, C.B. Glutamine addiction: A new therapeutic target in cancer. *Trends Biochem. Sci.* **2010**, *35*, 427–433. [CrossRef]
97. Altman, B.J.; Stine, Z.E.; Dang, C.V. From Krebs to clinic: Glutamine metabolism to cancer therapy. *Nat. Rev. Cancer* **2016**, *16*, 619–634. [CrossRef]
98. Cluntun, A.A.; Lukey, M.J.; Cerione, R.A.; Locasale, J.W. Glutamine Metabolism in Cancer: Understanding the Heterogeneity. *Trends Cancer* **2017**, *3*, 169–180. [CrossRef]
99. Bruno, G.; Li Bergolis, V.; Piscazzi, A.; Crispo, F.; Condelli, V.; Zoppoli, P.; Maddalena, F.; Pietrafesa, M.; Giordano, G.; Matassa, D.S.; et al. TRAP1 regulates the response of colorectal cancer cells to hypoxia and inhibits ribosome biogenesis under conditions of oxygen deprivation. *Int. J. Oncol.* **2022**, *60*, 79. [CrossRef]
100. Wang, X.; Venable, J.; LaPointe, P.; Hutt, D.M.; Koulov, A.V.; Coppinger, J.; Gurkan, C.; Kellner, W.; Matteson, J.; Plutner, H.; et al. Hsp90 cochaperone Aha1 downregulation rescues misfolding of CFTR in cystic fibrosis. *Cell* **2006**, *127*, 803–815. [CrossRef]
101. Prince, T.L.; Kijima, T.; Tatokoro, M.; Lee, S.; Tsutsumi, S.; Yim, K.; Rivas, C.; Alarcon, S.; Schwartz, H.; Khamit-Kush, K.; et al. Client Proteins and Small Molecule Inhibitors Display Distinct Binding Preferences for Constitutive and Stress-Induced HSP90 Isoforms and Their Conformationally Restricted Mutants. *PLoS ONE* **2015**, *10*, e0141786. [CrossRef] [PubMed]

102. Kijima, T.; Prince, T.L.; Tigue, M.L.; Yim, K.H.; Schwartz, H.; Beebe, K.; Lee, S.; Budzynski, M.A.; Williams, H.; Trepel, J.B.; et al. HSP90 inhibitors disrupt a transient HSP90-HSF1 interaction and identify a noncanonical model of HSP90-mediated HSF1 regulation. *Sci. Rep.* **2018**, *8*, 6976. [CrossRef] [PubMed]
103. Kang, B.H.; Plescia, J.; Song, H.Y.; Meli, M.; Colombo, G.; Beebe, K.; Scroggins, B.; Neckers, L.; Altieri, D.C. Combinatorial drug design targeting multiple cancer signaling networks controlled by mitochondrial Hsp90. *J. Clin. Investig.* **2009**, *119*, 454–464. [CrossRef] [PubMed]
104. Hoye, A.T.; Davoren, J.E.; Wipf, P.; Fink, M.P.; Kagan, V.E. Targeting mitochondria. *Acc. Chem. Res.* **2008**, *41*, 87–97. [CrossRef]
105. Kang, B.H.; Siegelin, M.D.; Plescia, J.; Raskett, C.M.; Garlick, D.S.; Dohi, T.; Lian, J.B.; Stein, G.S.; Languino, L.R.; Altieri, D.C. Preclinical characterization of mitochondria-targeted small molecule hsp90 inhibitors, gamitrinibs, in advanced prostate cancer. *Clin. Cancer Res. Off. J. Am. Assoc. Cancer Res.* **2010**, *16*, 4779–4788. [CrossRef]
106. Lee, C.; Park, H.K.; Jeong, H.; Lim, J.; Lee, A.J.; Cheon, K.Y.; Kim, C.S.; Thomas, A.P.; Bae, B.; Kim, N.D.; et al. Development of a mitochondria-targeted Hsp90 inhibitor based on the crystal structures of human TRAP1. *J. Am. Chem. Soc.* **2015**, *137*, 4358–4367. [CrossRef]
107. Bryant, K.G.; Chae, Y.C.; Martinez, R.L.; Gordon, J.C.; Elokely, K.M.; Kossenkov, A.V.; Grant, S.; Childers, W.E.; Abou-Gharbia, M.; Altieri, D.C. A Mitochondrial-targeted purine-based HSP90 antagonist for leukemia therapy. *Oncotarget* **2017**, *8*, 112184–112198. [CrossRef]
108. Hu, S.; Ferraro, M.; Thomas, A.P.; Chung, J.M.; Yoon, N.G.; Seol, J.-H.; Kim, S.; Kim, H.-u.; An, M.Y.; Ok, H.; et al. Dual Binding to Orthosteric and Allosteric Sites Enhances the Anticancer Activity of a TRAP1-Targeting Drug. *J. Med. Chem.* **2020**, *63*, 2930–2940. [CrossRef]
109. Trnka, J.; Elkalaf, M.; Anděl, M. Lipophilic triphenylphosphonium cations inhibit mitochondrial electron transport chain and induce mitochondrial proton leak. *PLoS ONE* **2015**, *10*, e0121837. [CrossRef]
110. Park, H.-K.; Jeong, H.; Ko, E.; Lee, G.; Lee, J.-E.; Lee, S.K.; Lee, A.-J.; Im, J.Y.; Hu, S.; Kim, S.H.; et al. Paralog Specificity Determines Subcellular Distribution, Action Mechanism, and Anticancer Activity of TRAP1 Inhibitors. *J. Med. Chem.* **2017**, *60*, 7569–7578. [CrossRef]
111. Lundgren, K.; Zhang, H.; Brekken, J.; Huser, N.; Powell, R.E.; Timple, N.; Busch, D.J.; Neely, L.; Sensintaffar, J.L.; Yang, Y.C.; et al. BIIB021, an orally available, fully synthetic small-molecule inhibitor of the heat shock protein Hsp90. *Mol. Cancer Ther.* **2009**, *8*, 921–929. [CrossRef] [PubMed]
112. Moroni, E.; Agard, D.A.; Colombo, G. The Structural Asymmetry of Mitochondrial Hsp90 (Trap1) Determines Fine Tuning of Functional Dynamics. *J. Chem. Theory Comput.* **2018**, *14*, 1033–1044. [CrossRef]
113. Montefiori, M.; Pilotto, S.; Marabelli, C.; Moroni, E.; Ferraro, M.; Serapian, S.A.; Mattevi, A.; Colombo, G. Impact of Mutations on NPAC Structural Dynamics: Mechanistic Insights from MD Simulations. *J. Chem. Inf. Modeling* **2019**, *59*, 3927–3937. [CrossRef] [PubMed]
114. Sanchez-Martin, C.; Moroni, E.; Ferraro, M.; Laquatra, C.; Cannino, G.; Masgras, I.; Negro, A.; Quadrelli, P.; Rasola, A.; Colombo, G. Rational Design of Allosteric and Selective Inhibitors of the Molecular Chaperone TRAP1. *Cell Rep.* **2020**, *31*, 107531. [CrossRef] [PubMed]
115. Sanchez-Martin, C.; Menon, D.; Moroni, E.; Ferraro, M.; Masgras, I.; Elsey, J.; Arbiser, J.L.; Colombo, G.; Rasola, A. Honokiol Bis-Dichloroacetate Is a Selective Allosteric Inhibitor of the Mitochondrial Chaperone TRAP1. *Antioxid. Redox Signal.* **2021**, *34*, 505–516. [CrossRef]
116. Zhang, G.; Frederick, D.T.; Wu, L.; Wei, Z.; Krepler, C.; Srinivasan, S.; Chae, Y.C.; Xu, X.; Choi, H.; Dimwamwa, E.; et al. Targeting mitochondrial biogenesis to overcome drug resistance to MAPK inhibitors. *J. Clin. Investig.* **2016**, *126*, 1834–1856. [CrossRef]
117. Ishida, C.T.; Shu, C.; Halatsch, M.-E.; Westhoff, M.-A.; Altieri, D.C.; Karpel-Massler, G.; Siegelin, M.D. Mitochondrial matrix chaperone and c-myc inhibition causes enhanced lethality in glioblastoma. *Oncotarget* **2017**, *8*, 37140–37153. [CrossRef]
118. Nguyen, T.T.T.; Zhang, Y.; Shang, E.; Shu, C.; Quinzii, C.M.; Westhoff, M.A.; Karpel-Massler, G.; Siegelin, M.D. Inhibition of HDAC1/2 Along with TRAP1 Causes Synthetic Lethality in Glioblastoma Model Systems. *Cells* **2020**, *9*, 1661. [CrossRef]

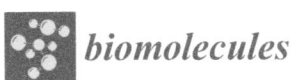

Review

Regulation of Protein Transport Pathways by the Cytosolic Hsp90s

Anna G. Mankovich and Brian C. Freeman *

School of Molecular and Cellular Biology, University of Illinois, Urbana-Champaign, Urbana, IL 61801, USA
* Correspondence: bfree@illinois.edu

Abstract: The highly conserved molecular chaperone heat shock protein 90 (Hsp90) is well-known for maintaining metastable proteins and mediating various aspects of intracellular protein dynamics. Intriguingly, high-throughput interactome studies suggest that Hsp90 is associated with a variety of other pathways. Here, we will highlight the potential impact of Hsp90 in protein transport. Currently, a limited number of studies have defined a few mechanistic contributions of Hsp90 to protein transport, yet the relevance of hundreds of additional connections between Hsp90 and factors known to aid this process remains unresolved. These interactors broadly support transport pathways including endocytic and exocytic vesicular transport, the transfer of polypeptides across membranes, or unconventional protein secretion. In resolving how Hsp90 contributes to the protein transport process, new therapeutic targets will likely be obtained for the treatment of numerous human health issues, including bacterial infection, cancer metastasis, and neurodegeneration.

Keywords: Hsp90; molecular chaperone; protein transport

Citation: Mankovich, A.G.; Freeman, B.C. Regulation of Protein Transport Pathways by the Cytosolic Hsp90s. *Biomolecules* 2022, 12, 1077. https://doi.org/10.3390/biom12081077

Academic Editor: Chrisostomos Prodromou

Received: 27 June 2022
Accepted: 27 July 2022
Published: 5 August 2022

Publisher's Note: MDPI stays neutral with regard to jurisdictional claims in published maps and institutional affiliations.

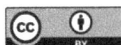

Copyright: © 2022 by the authors. Licensee MDPI, Basel, Switzerland. This article is an open access article distributed under the terms and conditions of the Creative Commons Attribution (CC BY) license (https://creativecommons.org/licenses/by/4.0/).

1. Introduction

For decades, molecular chaperones have been recognized as essential agents in the maintenance of protein homeostasis (proteostasis). One of the earliest-identified molecular chaperones is the highly conserved heat shock protein 90 (Hsp90) [1,2]. Apart from Archaea, Hsp90 is present in almost all bacterial and eukaryotic life [3,4]. In general, the number of Hsp90 homologues expands in parallel with increased cellular complexity [4,5]. For example, the majority of bacteria only contain one nonessential Hsp90 homologue often referred to as high-temperature protein G (HtpG) while eukaryotes can have multiple Hsp90 proteins including several cytoplasmic/nucleoplasmic Hsp90s, mitochondrial TRAP1 (tumor necrosis factor receptor-associated protein 1), endoplasmic reticulum (ER) GRP94 (94 kDa glucose-regulated protein), and chloroplast HSP90C (plastid heat shock protein 90) [5]. Each of the homologues, except for cytoplasmic/nucleoplasmic Hsp90s, is retained in its respective organelle to help maintain protein quality control within that compartment [6–8]. Here, we will focus on how the cytoplasmic/nucleoplasmic Hsp90 proteins contribute to the protein transport process.

Although compartmentalization has many benefits, it does require a multi-faceted delivery mechanism to transport biological molecules into, out of, within, and between organelles. Despite being historically implicated as a signaling pathway regulator of steroid hormone receptors and kinases [9,10], Hsp90 is increasingly associated with many other cellular processes, including protein transport [11–13]. Given the physiological relevance of protein transport to health and disease, including implications in neurotransmitter release, cell differentiation, bacterial infection, and autophagy [14–17], it is important to better understand how and when Hsp90 contributes to this process.

To gain insights into how one of the most abundant proteins in a cell cytoplasm/nucleoplasm contributes to life, multiple studies have attempted to identify the physical, genetic, and chemical–genetic interactors of Hsp90 using a variety of unbiased high-throughput screens including two-hybrid, synthetic genetic arrays and mass spectrometry-based tactics [11–13,18,19]. Significantly, within the conundrum of hits, there are numerous players with established roles in the transport and secretion pathways [11–13]. These connections include proteins involved in various aspects of exocytosis and endocytosis [13]. Focusing on the physical and genetic interactors of budding yeast's only two isomers, cytoplasmic/nucleoplasmic Hsc82 and Hsp82, Hsp90 is linked to 202 different proteins driving most aspects of intracellular transport and secretion (Figure 1). Hence, Hsp90 likely has a significant influence on the transport process that goes well beyond our current understanding. Perhaps of note, the human homologs of many of the yeast Hsp90-interactors are associated with various diseases, including bacterial infections (e.g., tetanus (SEC18/NSF), infant botulism (YKT6/YKT6), and diphtheria (RRT2/DPH7)), cancer (e.g., breast mucinous carcinoma (TRX2/TXN), primary bone cancer (SLT2/MAPK7), and endometrial cancer (PKH1/PDPK1)), and neurodegeneration (amyotrophic lateral sclerosis (VPS21/RAB5A, CDC48/VCP, VPS60/CHMP5), Parkinson's disease (BET4/RABGGTA, VPS35/VPS35, RIC1/RIC1), and dementia (CDC48/VCP, VPS60/CHMP5)) [20]. Unfortunately, for the majority of the connections, the molecular/physiological basis for the interaction has not been revealed. In this review, we will highlight the few established roles of Hsp90 in transport as well as underscore areas linked to Hsp90 through a variety of high-throughput screens [11–13,18,19].

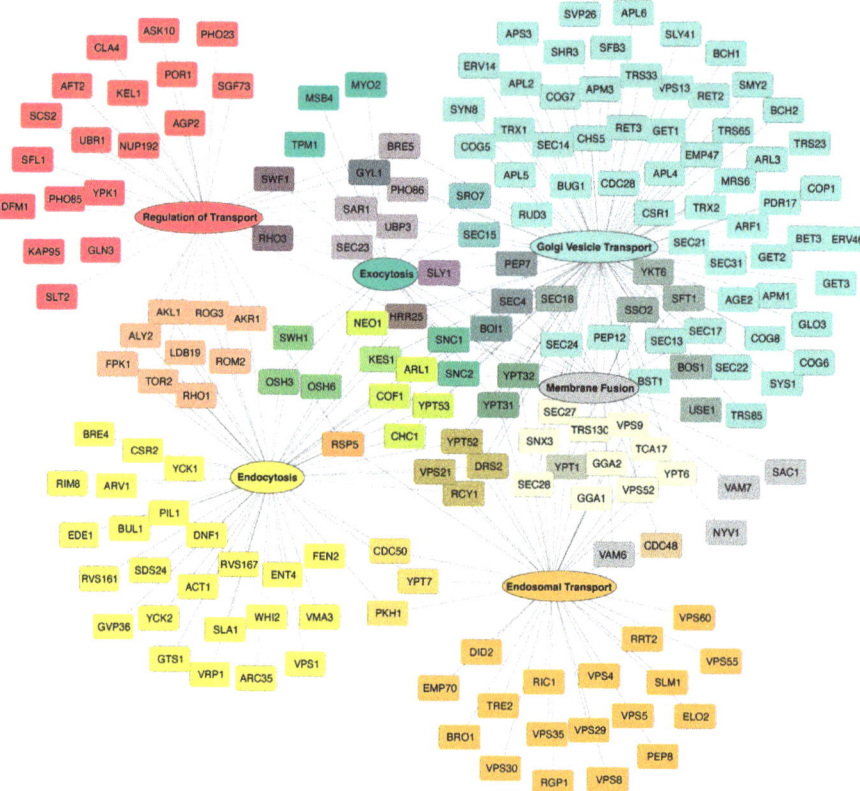

Figure 1. Protein transport factors linked to yeast Hsp90. The transport pathways mediated by the physical and genetic interactors of Hsc82 and Hsp82 were determined using the Gene Ontology

Slim Term Mapper from Saccharomyces Genome Database (http://genome-www.stanford.edu/Saccharomyces/ accessed on 6 June 2022). Six Gene Ontology terms relevant to protein transport were selected including Golgi Vesicle Transport, Endocytosis, Endosomal Transport, Regulation of Transport, Exocytosis, and Membrane Fusion. The interactors were organized into the shown interaction map using Cytoscape [21] by setting the Gene Ontology term as a source interactor and each gene as a target interactor.

2. Hsp90 and General Principles of Protein Transport

The physical flow of proteins among cellular compartments is a highly proteostasis-dependent process. Depending upon the precise transport step, the contribution from the proteostasis system will vary, including protein unfolding (even partial) to allow transfer, the maintenance of unfolded clients during transfer, polypeptide refolding after transfer, assembling large macromolecular complexes (e.g., vesicle formation), disassembling protein structures (e.g., vesicle fusion), monitoring the health of the transport machinery itself, and mediating the removal of damaged factors including clients or machinery components. If or how Hsp90 might contribute to these or other transport steps is an open investigation. To better understand where Hsp90 might contribute, we will briefly review the primary pathways used in the transport process, and then we will discuss established contributions of Hsp90 relative to protein transport.

Two major intracellular trafficking mechanisms are the endocytic and exocytic pathways [22]. Notably, both mechanisms rely heavily on vesicles, and Hsp90 has been linked to 106 different factors governing vesicle transport, including coat proteins, Rabs, soluble N-ethylmaleimide-sensitive factor attachment protein receptors (SNAREs), and Golgi complex proteins (Figure 1). The endocytic pathway allows for the internalization, recycling, and modification of membrane bound surface proteins such as signaling receptors as well as other cargo from the environment. Significantly, Hsp90 shares a total of 96 linkages to endocytosis and endosomal transport, including vacuolar protein sorting proteins, sorting nexin family proteins, and actin (Figure 1). Proteins are endocytosed through a variety of mechanisms whereby the plasma membrane invaginates to form a vesicle prior to being delivered to an early endosome [23]. At the early endosome, an initial decision is made to either recycle membrane proteins, such as receptors, back to the plasma membrane via recycling endosomes to direct proteins to the trans-Golgi network via the retromer, or to degrade proteins via the lysosome. To accomplish this sorting, cargo leaves the early endosome in intraluminal vesicles to become multivesicular bodies, endosomal carrier vesicles, or late endosomes, which can be sorted into lysosomes or fuse with autophagosomes [24–27] (Figure 2).

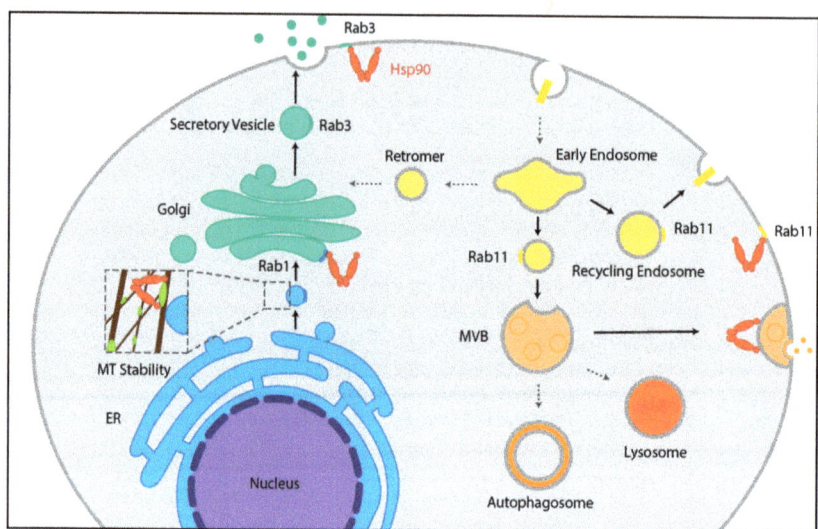

Figure 2. Hsp90 contributions to exocytic and endocytic trafficking. In the exocytic pathway (left), Hsp90 (red) aides in anterograde vesicle trafficking between the ER and Golgi by supporting microtubule stability through the binding of MAP4 (light green) [28–32], and the recycling of Rab1 and Rab3 to enable vesicle targeting and fusion with the Golgi and plasma membrane [28,29,33–35]. In the endocytic pathway (right), Hsp90 supports the transport of recycling endosomes as well as transport from early to late endosomes/multivesicular bodies (MVB) through the recycling of Rab11 [15,36,37]. Hsp90 also allows for the fusion of MVB with the plasma membrane by aiding in membrane deformations [38]. Transport events that Hsp90 is involved in are noted by solid black arrows.

The exocytic or secretory pathway is responsible for the synthesis, folding, modification, and trafficking of proteins that are members of the endomembrane system or destined for secretion. In exocytosis, newly synthesized proteins are inserted into the ER where they undergo maturation through folding and modifications, such as glycosylation and disulfide bond formation [39,40]. Across the exocytosis pathway, Hsp90 is connected to 23 different proteins comprising some myosins, Rabs, and exocyst complex components (Figure 1). From the ER, cargo is transported to the ER-Golgi Intermediate Compartments (ERGICs) via vesicles and then to the cis-Golgi where ER resident proteins are returned to the ER via retrograde transport [41]. In the Golgi, proteins undergo additional carbohydrate modifications and proteolytic processing as the cargo travels from the cis- to trans-Golgi either by vesicular transport or cisternal maturation [39,41]. From the trans-Golgi, cargo vesicles are trafficked to the plasma membrane where they fuse to release secretory proteins or deliver membrane proteins [41] (Figure 2). Hsp90 has been linked to 23 different proteins mediating these late secretory events including syntaxin and vesicle-associated membrane proteins (Figure 1). Furthermore, Hsp90 interacts with an additional 41 proteins that are known to regulate the overall protein transport process comprising Rho GTPase, mitogen-activated protein kinase (MAPK), cyclin-dependent kinase (CDK) and E3 ubiquitin–protein ligase (Figure 1). Although endocytic and exocytic transport mechanisms are well-studied pathways essential to the production, processing, and trafficking of proteins in cells, there is still much to be learned about the underlying mechanisms driving these events, including the contributions of the Hsp90 molecular chaperone.

3. Hsp90 Input with Mitochondria and Chloroplast Protein Import

The transport of proteins into mitochondria or chloroplasts requires the assistance of molecular chaperones. As ~95% of mitochondrial and chloroplast proteins are encoded by the nuclear genome and translated by cytoplasmic ribosomes, the post-translational import of proteins is considerable [42]. To successfully transport the various preproteins into these organelles, chaperones, including Hsp90, have been shown to deliver both mitochondrial and chloroplast preproteins to the respective outer membrane translocases [43,44]. In the case of mitochondrial import, Hsp90 works with Hsp70 to target and transport unfolded or hydrophobic preproteins to the translocase of the mitochondrial outer membrane (TOM) complex for import [43,45]. Specifically, Hsp90 docks onto a peripherally associated receptor subunit, Tom70, releasing the preprotein in an ATP-dependent manner either to be bound first by Tom70 or directly to the TOM pore complex [45,46]. To facilitate chloroplast import, Hsp90 binds precursor proteins and interacts with Toc64, a receptor subunit of the translocon of the outer envelope of chloroplasts (TOC) complex [44]. Similarly to mitochondrial transfer, the import of preproteins into the chloroplasts is Hsp90- and ATP-dependent [44] (Figure 3A,B).

Interestingly, Hsp90 fosters transfer across either the organelle's outer membrane by docking onto a receptor (Toc64 for chloroplasts or Tom70 for mitochondria) using a similar clamp-type tetratricopeptide repeat (TPR) domain present in the receptors [43,44,47]. At least within chloroplasts, client proteins can remain reliant on an Hsp90 homolog after crossing the outer membrane. Within the stroma, HSP90C and chloroplast Hsp90 (cpHsp70) and Hsp93 aid the translocation of proteins across the inner chloroplast membrane while Hsp90C also targets thylakoid lumen proteins to the thylakoid membrane translocase SecY1 [8,48–50] (Figure 3A,B). Hsp90's common role in preprotein targeting and transport to endosymbiotically derived organelles may indicate that in eukaryotic evolution, chaperones were used as an effective solution to import preproteins translated in the cytosol [42,47].

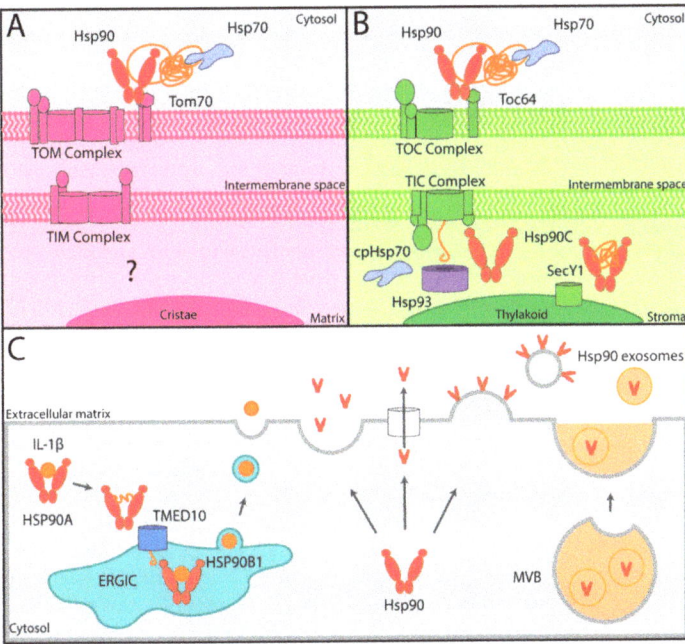

Figure 3. The role of Hsp90 in mitochondrial and chloroplast import as well as unconventional protein secretion (UPS). (**A**) Hsp90 with the aid of Hsp70 delivers preproteins to the TOM complex in

the outer membrane of mitochondria through interactions with the TPR domain (hexagon) of peripherally associated Tom70 [43,45]. (**B**) Hsp90 with the aid of Hsp70 delivers preproteins to the TOC complex in the outer membrane of chloroplasts through interactions with the TPR domain (hexagon) of peripherally associated Toc64 [44]. Chaperones in the chloroplast stroma including cpHsp70, Hsp93, and Hsp90C aid in protein transport through the TIC complex in the inner membrane and Hsp90C additionally targets proteins to the SecY1 translocase in the thylakoid membrane [8,48–50]. (**C**) HSP90A mediates UPS of IL-1β by unfolding the protein to allow for its transport into the ERGIC through the TMED10 translocase aided by HSP0B1, and then from ERGIC, IL-1β is secreted in vesicles (left) [51]. eHsp90 is thought to be secreted by UPS through vesicle fusion, across membrane transporters, on the surface of exosomes, and/or fusion of MVBs with the plasma membrane (right) [52,53].

4. Hsp90 and Unconventional Protein Secretion

Classically, secreted proteins have a signal peptide or leader sequence that targets the polypeptides for ER–Golgi trafficking via vesicles to eventually export the factors out of a cell [54,55]. Still, there are secreted proteins that lack such sequences and bypass the ER–Golgi route. These "leaderless" proteins are exported by unconventional protein secretion (UPS) that uses both non-vesicular and vesicular paths to export proteins [56]. One mechanism, which is dependent upon Hsp90, is the secretion of interleukin-1β (IL-1β) by mammalian cells during autophagy known as the TMED10-channeled UPS (THU) [17,51]. Following autophagy induction, IL-1β is produced and captured in its mature form by cytosolic HSP90A, potentially though the binding of KFERQ-like motifs in IL-1β [17,51]. It has been suggested that HSP90A then unfolds IL-1β to expose a signal motif allowing direct translocations into the ERGIC through transmembrane Emp24 domain-containing protein 10 (TMED10) [51] (Figure 3C). Of note, the import of IL-1β by TMED10 is also aided by HSP90B1, although HSP90B1 mechanistic contributions are less well understood [51]. The idea that Hsp90 recognizes Hsp90 through its KFERQ-like motifs is questionable, however, because so far only Hsc70, an Hsp70 family member, has been shown to bind KFERQ motifs, which are primarily used to target proteins to lysosomes for degradation in Chaperone-Mediated Autophagy (CMA) [57]. In CMA, Hsp90 plays a more indirect role through the stabilization and oligomerization of lysosome-associated membrane protein type 2A (LAMP2A) from inside the lysosome to allow for the Hsc70-delivered proteins to enter the lysosome through the LAMP2A translocation complex [58,59]. Thus, it is possible that Hsp90 may recognize IL-1β for UPS through another mechanism other than its KFERQ-like motifs.

Intriguingly, many heat shock proteins including Hsp60, Hsp27, Hsp20, Hsp70, and Hsp90 itself are likely exported out of cells via UPS [60]. Migratory cells during wound healing or cancerous growth continuously secrete Hsp90 [61–63] and normal cells exposed to a variety of stresses, including heat, hypoxia, serum starvation, reactive oxygen, or virus infection, transiently export Hsp90 [62,64–68]. Minimally, extracellular Hsp90 (eHsp90) increases cell motility. In the case of wound healing, Hsp90 is secreted in response to hypoxia at the wound site where Hypoxia-Inducible Factor-1alpha (HIF-1α) promotes the secretion of Hsp90α [62]. Notably, eHsp90 accelerates wound healing by inducing the migration of dermal fibroblasts, including facilitating wound healing in mice when applied topically [62,69].

In contrast to the beneficial role in wound healing, the secretion of Hsp90 on its own or on the outer surface of vesicles has been shown to increase cancer metastasis [70]. The eHsp90 enhances metastasis by dysregulating the extracellular matrix (ECM) through the activation of ECM-modifying proteases [52,71]. Thus, there is growing interest in utilizing eHsp90 as a biomarker and/or target for cancer treatment [52]. Despite the potential importance of eHsp90, the mechanism by which Hsp90 is secreted from cells is not fully understood. Minimally, Hsp90 can exit a cell via exosomes generated in the endocytic pathway rather than the canonical secretory pathway [72] (Figure 3C). How Hsp90 is loaded into these exosomes prior to export is not clear [52]. Nevertheless, Hsp90's influence with other types of vesicles has been shown.

5. Influence of Hsp90 in Endocytic Vesicle Transport

Hsp90 has been implicated in several endocytic mechanisms including endosome vesicle transport and recycling. A well-studied impact of Hsp90 is on the regulation of Rab recycling—Rabs are members of the Ras GTPase family [73]. Rab-GTPases generally regulate the assembly and disassembly of complexes that enable vesicle targeting and fusion [30]. Following the activation of Rab by GTPase-activating proteins (GAPs), GDP-bound Rab is retrieved from membranes by GDP-dissociation inhibitors (GDIs), thus enabling continuous vesicle transport [74,75]. Hsp90 modulates this recycling process by binding to GDI and Rab. Hsp90 recruits GDI to the membrane and configures GDI into an open confirmation to bind the geranylgeranyl (GG) lipids anchoring Rab-GDP to the membrane, triggering its release into the cytosol [73]. Hsp90 has been shown to interact with Rab11b in osteoclasts to mediate the transport of macrophage colony-stimulating factor receptor (c-fms) and receptor activator of nuclear factor kappa B (RANK) surface receptors in early to late endosomes and also to lysosomes for degradation [15] (Figure 2). This Hsp90-mediated endosomal transport of receptors to lysosomes allows for the proper regulation of osteoclastogenesis and the differentiation of hematopoietic precursors to osteoclasts that are critical for bone homeostasis [15,76].

The endocytic pathway mediated by Rab11 and Hsp90 can be hijacked by *Neisseria meningitidis* to aid in bacterial internalization [36]. In this study, endocytic vesicles containing both *Neisseria meningitidis* adhesin A (NadA) protein and Hsp90 recruited Rab11 in human epithelial cells, causing the NadA endosomes to be recycled to the cell's surface. Using the membrane-impermeable Hsp90 inhibitor FITC-GA to selectively inhibit the eHsp90 prevented the recruitment of Rab11 and subsequent endosomal recycling [36]. Hsp90 has been shown to bind NadA and interfere with bacterial attachment [16,36]. Hence, eHsp90 might serve as an interesting target to combat bacterial infection for agents entering through an endosomal transport mechanism. Significantly, disruption of membrane proteins recycling upon Hsp90 inhibition also has been observed with the cancer-associated ErbB2 tyrosine kinase receptor [37,77,78]. Normally ErbB2 is trafficked in early endosomes for recycling; however, upon treatment with an Hsp90 inhibitor, these receptors are instead routed to multivesicular endosomes and lysosomal compartments [37]. These compartments were found to have a modified ultrastructure, which is more tubular than under normal conditions [37]. It is speculated that this disruption of normal transport and structure is due to Hsp90's interactions with Rab12, which normally localizes to early/recycling endosomes and lysosomes or through Hsp90's regulation of cytoskeletal dynamics [37,78].

6. Modulation of Exocytic Intracellular Transport by Hsp90

In addition to endocytic events, Hsp90 aids exocytic pathways, including ER-Golgi vesicular transport and protein secretion. The influence of Hsp90 on these events has been primarily delineated by tracking the transport of vesicular stomatitis virus glycoprotein (VSV-G) in mammalian cells [31,32,73]. In these studies, the loss of Hsp90 blocks ER to Golgi and intra-Golgi transport, as evidenced by an impaired anterograde vesicle transport and Golgi fragmentation [31,32]. Of note, these observations have been attributed to multiple Hsp90 roles, including the following: (1) Hsp90's regulation of vesicular transport by associating with the membrane-bound protein VAPA in complex with the co-chaperone tetratricopeptide repeat protein TTC1 [31]; (2) Hsp90's modulation of microtubule stability by controlling microtubule-associated protein 4 (MAP4), which is essential for maintaining microtubule acetylation and stability [32]; and (3) Hsp90's control of Rab1 recycling. Rab1 is responsible for ER to Golgi trafficking with mammalian Rab1b also dictating the transport of proteins through the cis- and medial-Golgi compartments [28–30] (Figure 2). Hence, Hsp90 facilitates ER to Golgi vesicular transport by both promoting vesicle targeting and maintaining the structure of the Golgi.

In the secretory pathway Hsp90 has been shown to have diverse functions with exosome release. For instance, Hsp90 influences membrane conformation to promote the fusion of multivesicular bodies and the plasma membrane [38] (Figure 2). This membrane-remodeling activity is dependent upon an evolutionarily conserved amphipathic helix in Hsp90 both in vitro and in vivo at synapses and is further promoted by the Hsp90 cochaperone HOP [38]. Besides HOP, the AHA1 cochaperone fosters the release of secretory vesicles associated with Rab3, which supports the cell migration of cancer cells [33]. The involvement of Hsp90 with Rab3 is a common thread in many exocytosis events (Figure 2). For example, Hsp90 is key to Ca^{2+}-triggered neurotransmitter release through the αGDI-dependent recycling of Rab3A [34]. Similarly to other Rabs, Hsp90 forms a complex with αGDI to remove Rab3A from the lipid bilayer during neurotransmitter release [34]. Significantly, the Hsp90-αGDI regulation of Rab3A controls the association of α-Synuclein, a presynaptic protein linked to neurodegeneration, with the synaptic membrane [35]. At the pre-synaptic membrane, α-synuclein associates preferentially with Rab3A-GTP and is subsequently released from the membrane following the actions of GDI and Hsp90 [35]. Of note, the Hsp90-GDI regulation of Rab11A, which is typically involved in the recycling of endosomes, has been linked to the secretion of α-synuclein, and the Hsp90-dependent release of α-synuclein is associated with increased neurotoxicity [79]. Although not specifically connected to Rab recycling, Hsp90 has also been found to mediate the transport of Aldo-Keto Reductase 1B10 (AKR1B10), a tumor biomarker, by regulating its transport to lysosomes or secretion out of the cell [80]. Hence, an improved understanding of how Hsp90 governs secretion may lead to improved future therapies for treating cancer and neurodegeneration.

7. Conclusions

The cytoplasmic/nucleoplasmic Hsp90 interactome contains hundreds of connections to factors working in various aspects of the protein-transport process (Figure 1). Yet, the defined contributions of Hsp90 to the various transport pathways remains limited. Nevertheless, it is clear that Hsp90 facilitates central features of protein transport, including promoting endocytic and exocytic vesicular transport, docking clients onto membrane translocation machinery, and fostering unconventional protein secretion [32,43,44,73]. Perhaps significantly, the established roles of Hsp90 in transport have important health implications as the chaperone-dependent steps link to wound healing, bacterial infection, cancer metastasis, and neurodegenerative diseases [16,35,36,62,70,79]. Given the number of connections that have yet to be resolved both mechanistically and physiologically, it is probable that the relevance of the cytoplasmic/nucleoplasmic Hsp90s with protein transports will continue to grow. Beyond these Hsp90 homologues, it is important to consider how organelle Hsp90s (GRP94, TRAP1, and HSP90C) add to the influence of the Hsp90 system on protein transport. For instance, does the dependence of SARS-CoV-2 on Hsp90 [74–77] relate to its influence on the protein transport process? Minimally, it is apparent that Hsp90's role in proteostasis will extend well beyond the maintenance of metastable clients.

Author Contributions: Conceptualization, A.G.M. and B.C.F.; formal analysis, A.G.M.; writing—original draft preparation, A.G.M.; writing—review and editing, A.G.M. and B.C.F.; funding acquisition, B.C.F. All authors have read and agreed to the published version of the manuscript.

Funding: This research was funded by NIH Public Service grant, grant number GM136660.

Institutional Review Board Statement: Not applicable.

Informed Consent Statement: Not applicable.

Data Availability Statement: Not applicable.

Acknowledgments: We thank Janhavi A. Kolhe, Audrey Yi Tyan Peng, and Neethu Babu for their critical reading of this manuscript.

Conflicts of Interest: The authors declare no conflict of interest. The funders had no role in the design of the study; in the collection, analyses, or interpretation of data; in the writing of the manuscript; or in the decision to publish the results.

References

1. Lindquist, S.; Craig, E.A. The Heat-Shock Proteins. *Annu. Rev. Genet.* **1988**, *22*, 631–677. [CrossRef] [PubMed]
2. Tissiéres, A.; Mitchell, H.K.; Tracy, U.M. Protein Synthesis in Salivary Glands of Drosophila Melanogaster: Relation to Chromosome Puffs. *J. Mol. Biol.* **1974**, *84*, 389–398. [CrossRef]
3. Large, A.T.; Goldberg, M.D.; Lund, P.A. Chaperones and Protein Folding in the Archaea. *Biochem. Soc. Trans.* **2009**, *37*, 46–51. [CrossRef] [PubMed]
4. Johnson, J.L. Evolution and Function of Diverse Hsp90 Homologs and Cochaperone Proteins. *Biochim. Biophys. Acta BBA Mol. Cell Res.* **2012**, *1823*, 607–613. [CrossRef] [PubMed]
5. Chen, B.; Zhong, D.; Monteiro, A. Comparative Genomics and Evolution of the HSP90 Family of Genes across All Kingdoms of Organisms. *BMC Genom.* **2006**, *7*, 156. [CrossRef]
6. Eletto, D.; Dersh, D.; Argon, Y. GRP94 in ER Quality Control and Stress Responses. *Semin. Cell Dev. Biol.* **2010**, *21*, 479–485. [CrossRef]
7. Altieri, D.C.; Stein, G.S.; Lian, J.B.; Languino, L.R. TRAP-1, the Mitochondrial Hsp90. *Biochim. Biophys. Acta BBA Mol. Cell Res.* **2012**, *1823*, 767–773. [CrossRef]
8. Jiang, T.; Mu, B.; Zhao, R. Plastid Chaperone HSP90C Guides Precursor Proteins to the SEC Translocase for Thylakoid Transport. *J. Exp. Bot.* **2020**, *71*, 7073–7087. [CrossRef]
9. Dougherty, J.J.; Puri, R.K.; Toft, D.O. Polypeptide Components of Two 8 S Forms of Chicken Oviduct Progesterone Receptor. *J. Biol. Chem.* **1984**, *259*, 8004–8009. [CrossRef]
10. Brugge, J.S.; Erikson, E.; Erikson, R.L. The Specific Interaction of the Rous Sarcoma Virus Transforming Protein, Pp60src, with Two Cellular Proteins. *Cell* **1981**, *25*, 363–372. [CrossRef]
11. Franzosa, E.A.; Albanèse, V.; Frydman, J.; Xia, Y.; McClellan, A.J. Heterozygous Yeast Deletion Collection Screens Reveal Essential Targets of Hsp90. *PLoS ONE* **2011**, *6*, e28211. [CrossRef] [PubMed]
12. Millson, S.H.; Truman, A.W.; King, V.; Prodromou, C.; Pearl, L.H.; Piper, P.W. A Two-Hybrid Screen of the Yeast Proteome for Hsp90 Interactors Uncovers a Novel Hsp90 Chaperone Requirement in the Activity of a Stress-Activated Mitogen-Activated Protein Kinase, Slt2p (Mpk1p). *Eukaryot. Cell* **2005**, *4*, 849–860. [CrossRef] [PubMed]
13. McClellan, A.J.; Xia, Y.; Deutschbauer, A.M.; Davis, R.W.; Gerstein, M.; Frydman, J. Diverse Cellular Functions of the Hsp90 Molecular Chaperone Uncovered Using Systems Approaches. *Cell* **2007**, *131*, 121–135. [CrossRef]
14. Gerges, N.Z. Independent Functions of Hsp90 in Neurotransmitter Release and in the Continuous Synaptic Cycling of AMPA Receptors. *J. Neurosci.* **2004**, *24*, 4758–4766. [CrossRef] [PubMed]
15. Tran, M.T.; Okusha, Y.; Feng, Y.; Sogawa, C.; Eguchi, T.; Kadowaki, T.; Sakai, E.; Tsukuba, T.; Okamoto, K. A Novel Role of HSP90 in Regulating Osteoclastogenesis by Abrogating Rab11b-Driven Transport. *Biochim. Biophys. Acta BBA Mol. Cell Res.* **2021**, *1868*, 119096. [CrossRef]
16. Montanari, P.; Bozza, G.; Capecchi, B.; Caproni, E.; Barrile, R.; Norais, N.; Capitani, M.; Sallese, M.; Cecchini, P.; Ciucchi, L.; et al. Human Heat Shock Protein (Hsp) 90 Interferes with Neisseria Meningitidis Adhesin A (NadA)-mediated Adhesion and Invasion. *Cell. Microbiol.* **2012**, *14*, 368–385. [CrossRef]
17. Zhang, M.; Kenny, S.J.; Ge, L.; Xu, K.; Schekman, R. Translocation of Interleukin-1β into a Vesicle Intermediate in Autophagy-Mediated Secretion. *Elife* **2015**, *4*, e11205. [CrossRef]
18. Tsaytler, P.A.; Krijgsveld, J.; Goerdayal, S.S.; Rüdiger, S.; Egmond, M.R. Novel Hsp90 Partners Discovered Using Complementary Proteomic Approaches. *Cell Stress Chaperones* **2009**, *14*, 629. [CrossRef]
19. Zhao, R.; Davey, M.; Hsu, Y.-C.; Kaplanek, P.; Tong, A.; Parsons, A.B.; Krogan, N.; Cagney, G.; Mai, D.; Greenblatt, J.; et al. Navigating the Chaperone Network: An Integrative Map of Physical and Genetic Interactions Mediated by the Hsp90 Chaperone. *Cell* **2005**, *120*, 715–727. [CrossRef]
20. Safran, M.; Rosen, N.; Twik, M.; BarShir, R.; Stein, T.I.; Dahary, D.; Fishilevich, S.; Lancet, D. The GeneCards Suite. In *Practical Guide to Life Science Databases*; Springer: Singapore, 2022; pp. 27–56. [CrossRef]
21. Shannon, P.; Markiel, A.; Ozier, O.; Baliga, N.S.; Wang, J.T.; Ramage, D.; Amin, N.; Schwikowski, B.; Ideker, T. Cytoscape: A Software Environment for Integrated Models of Biomolecular Interaction Networks. *Genome Res.* **2003**, *13*, 2498–2504. [CrossRef]
22. Tokarev, A.A.; Alfonso, A.; Segev, N. Overview of Intracellular Compartments and Trafficking Pathways. In *Trafficking Inside Cells, Pathways, Mechanisms and Regulation*; Springer: New York, NY, USA, 2009; pp. 3–14. [CrossRef]
23. Kumari, S.; MG, S.; Mayor, S. Endocytosis Unplugged: Multiple Ways to Enter the Cell. *Cell Res.* **2010**, *20*, 256–275. [CrossRef] [PubMed]
24. Scott, C.C.; Vacca, F.; Gruenberg, J. Endosome Maturation, Transport and Functions. *Semin. Cell Dev. Biol.* **2014**, *31*, 2–10. [CrossRef] [PubMed]
25. Sorkin, A.; von Zastrow, M. Endocytosis and Signalling: Intertwining Molecular Networks. *Nat. Rev. Mol. Cell Biol.* **2009**, *10*, 609–622. [CrossRef] [PubMed]

26. Elkin, S.R.; Lakoduk, A.M.; Schmid, S.L. Endocytic Pathways and Endosomal Trafficking: A Primer. *Wien. Med. Wochenschr.* **2016**, *166*, 196–204. [CrossRef]
27. Naslavsky, N.; Caplan, S. The Enigmatic Endosome—Sorting the Ins and Outs of Endocytic Trafficking. *J. Cell Sci.* **2018**, *131*, jcs216499. [CrossRef] [PubMed]
28. Plutner, H.; Cox, A.D.; Pind, S.; Khosravi-Far, R.; Bourne, J.R.; Schwaninger, R.; Der, C.J.; Balch, W.E. Rab1b Regulates Vesicular Transport between the Endoplasmic Reticulum and Successive Golgi Compartments. *J. Cell Biol.* **1991**, *115*, 31–43. [CrossRef]
29. Allan, B.B.; Moyer, B.D.; Balch, W.E. Rab1 Recruitment of P115 into a Cis-SNARE Complex: Programming Budding COPII Vesicles for Fusion. *Science* **2000**, *289*, 444–448. [CrossRef]
30. Gurkan, C.; Lapp, H.; Alory, C.; Su, A.I.; Hogenesch, J.B.; Balch, W.E. Large-Scale Profiling of Rab GTPase Trafficking Networks: The Membrome. *Mol. Biol. Cell* **2005**, *16*, 3847–3864. [CrossRef]
31. Lotz, G.P.; Brychzy, A.; Heinz, S.; Obermann, W.M.J. A Novel HSP90 Chaperone Complex Regulates Intracellular Vesicle Transport. *J. Cell Sci.* **2008**, *121*, 717–723. [CrossRef]
32. Wu, Y.; Ding, Y.; Zheng, X.; Liao, K. The Molecular Chaperone Hsp90 Maintains Golgi Organization and Vesicular Trafficking by Regulating Microtubule Stability. *J. Mol. Cell Biol.* **2019**, *12*, 448–461. [CrossRef]
33. Ghosh, S.; Shinogle, H.E.; Garg, G.; Vielhauer, G.A.; Holzbeierlein, J.M.; Dobrowsky, R.T.; Blagg, B.S.J. Hsp90 C-Terminal Inhibitors Exhibit Antimigratory Activity by Disrupting the Hsp90α/Aha1 Complex in PC3-MM2 Cells. *ACS Chem. Biol.* **2015**, *10*, 577–590. [CrossRef] [PubMed]
34. Sakisaka, T.; Meerlo, T.; Matteson, J.; Plutner, H.; Balch, W.E. Rab-αGDI Activity Is Regulated by a Hsp90 Chaperone Complex. *EMBO J.* **2002**, *21*, 6125–6135. [CrossRef] [PubMed]
35. Chen, R.H.C.; Wislet-Gendebien, S.; Samuel, F.; Visanji, N.P.; Zhang, G.; Marsilio, D.; Langman, T.; Fraser, P.E.; Tandon, A. α-Synuclein Membrane Association Is Regulated by the Rab3a Recycling Machinery and Presynaptic Activity. *J. Biol. Chem.* **2013**, *288*, 7438–7449. [CrossRef] [PubMed]
36. Bozza, G.; Capitani, M.; Montanari, P.; Benucci, B.; Biancucci, M.; Nardi-Dei, V.; Caproni, E.; Barrile, R.; Picciani, B.; Savino, S.; et al. Role of ARF6, Rab11 and External Hsp90 in the Trafficking and Recycling of Recombinant-Soluble Neisseria Meningitidis Adhesin A (RNadA) in Human Epithelial Cells. *PLoS ONE* **2014**, *9*, e110047. [CrossRef] [PubMed]
37. Cortese, K.; Howes, M.T.; Lundmark, R.; Tagliatti, E.; Bagnato, P.; Petrelli, A.; Bono, M.; McMahon, H.T.; Parton, R.G.; Tacchetti, C. The HSP90 Inhibitor Geldanamycin Perturbs Endosomal Structure and Drives Recycling ErbB2 and Transferrin to Modified MVBs/Lysosomal Compartments. *Mol. Biol. Cell* **2013**, *24*, 129–144. [CrossRef]
38. Lauwers, E.; Wang, Y.-C.; Gallardo, R.; der Kant, R.V.; Michiels, E.; Swerts, J.; Baatsen, P.; Zaiter, S.S.; McAlpine, S.R.; Gounko, N.V.; et al. Hsp90 Mediates Membrane Deformation and Exosome Release. *Mol. Cell* **2018**, *71*, 689–702.e9. [CrossRef]
39. Barlowe, C.K.; Miller, E.A. Secretory Protein Biogenesis and Traffic in the Early Secretory Pathway. *Genetics* **2013**, *193*, 383–410. [CrossRef]
40. Schwarz, D.S.; Blower, M.D. The Endoplasmic Reticulum: Structure, Function and Response to Cellular Signaling. *Cell. Mol. Life Sci.* **2016**, *73*, 79–94. [CrossRef]
41. Mogre, S.S.; Brown, A.I.; Koslover, E.F. Getting around the Cell: Physical Transport in the Intracellular World. *Phys. Biol.* **2020**, *17*, 061003. [CrossRef]
42. Schleiff, E.; Becker, T. Common Ground for Protein Translocation: Access Control for Mitochondria and Chloroplasts. *Nat. Rev. Mol. Cell Biol.* **2011**, *12*, 48–59. [CrossRef]
43. Young, J.C.; Hoogenraad, N.J.; Hartl, F.U. Molecular Chaperones Hsp90 and Hsp70 Deliver Preproteins to the Mitochondrial Import Receptor Tom70. *Cell* **2003**, *112*, 41–50. [CrossRef]
44. Qbadou, S.; Becker, T.; Mirus, O.; Tews, I.; Soll, J.; Schleiff, E. The Molecular Chaperone Hsp90 Delivers Precursor Proteins to the Chloroplast Import Receptor Toc64. *EMBO J.* **2006**, *25*, 1836–1847. [CrossRef] [PubMed]
45. Fan, A.C.Y.; Bhangoo, M.K.; Young, J.C. Hsp90 Functions in the Targeting and Outer Membrane Translocation Steps of Tom70-Mediated Mitochondrial Import*. *J. Biol. Chem.* **2006**, *281*, 33313–33324. [CrossRef]
46. Wu, Y.; Sha, B. Crystal Structure of Yeast Mitochondrial Outer Membrane Translocon Member Tom70p. *Nat. Struct. Mol. Biol.* **2006**, *13*, 589–593. [CrossRef] [PubMed]
47. Schlegel, T.; Mirus, O.; von Haeseler, A.; Schleiff, E. The Tetratricopeptide Repeats of Receptors Involved in Protein Translocation across Membranes. *Mol. Biol. Evol.* **2007**, *24*, 2763–2774. [CrossRef]
48. Inoue, H.; Li, M.; Schnell, D.J. An Essential Role for Chloroplast Heat Shock Protein 90 (Hsp90C) in Protein Import into Chloroplasts. *Proc. Natl. Acad. Sci. USA* **2013**, *110*, 3173–3178. [CrossRef]
49. Jiang, T.; Oh, E.S.; Bonea, D.; Zhao, R. HSP90C Interacts with PsbO1 and Facilitates Its Thylakoid Distribution from Chloroplast Stroma in Arabidopsis. *PLoS ONE* **2017**, *12*, e0190168. [CrossRef]
50. Flores-Pérez, Ú.; Jarvis, P. Molecular Chaperone Involvement in Chloroplast Protein Import. *Biochim. Biophys. Acta BBA Mol. Cell Res.* **2013**, *1833*, 332–340. [CrossRef]
51. Zhang, M.; Liu, L.; Lin, X.; Wang, Y.; Li, Y.; Guo, Q.; Li, S.; Sun, Y.; Tao, X.; Zhang, D.; et al. A Translocation Pathway for Vesicle-Mediated Unconventional Protein Secretion. *Cell* **2020**, *181*, 637–652.e15. [CrossRef]
52. Wong, D.S.; Jay, D.G. Chapter Six Emerging Roles of Extracellular Hsp90 in Cancer. *Adv. Cancer Res.* **2016**, *129*, 141–163. [CrossRef]
53. Seclì, L.; Fusella, F.; Avalle, L.; Brancaccio, M. The Dark-Side of the Outside: How Extracellular Heat Shock Proteins Promote Cancer. *Cell. Mol. Life Sci.* **2021**, *78*, 4069–4083. [CrossRef] [PubMed]

54. Rothman, J.E. Mechanisms of Intracellular Protein Transport. *Nature* **1994**, *372*, 55–63. [CrossRef] [PubMed]
55. Palade, G. Intracellular Aspects of the Process of Protein Synthesis. *Science* **1975**, *189*, 347–358. [CrossRef] [PubMed]
56. Balmer, E.A.; Faso, C. The Road Less Traveled? Unconventional Protein Secretion at Parasite–Host Interfaces. *Front. Cell Dev. Biol.* **2021**, *9*, 662711. [CrossRef] [PubMed]
57. Kaushik, S.; Cuervo, A.M. The Coming of Age of Chaperone-Mediated Autophagy. *Nat. Rev. Mol. Cell Biol.* **2018**, *19*, 365–381. [CrossRef]
58. Agarraberes, F.A.; Dice, J.F. A Molecular Chaperone Complex at the Lysosomal Membrane Is Required for Protein Translocation. *J. Cell Sci.* **2001**, *114*, 2491–2499. [CrossRef]
59. Bandyopadhyay, U.; Kaushik, S.; Varticovski, L.; Cuervo, A.M. The Chaperone-Mediated Autophagy Receptor Organizes in Dynamic Protein Complexes at the Lysosomal Membrane. *Mol. Cell. Biol.* **2008**, *28*, 5747–5763. [CrossRef]
60. Santos, T.G.; Martins, V.R.; Hajj, G.N.M. Unconventional Secretion of Heat Shock Proteins in Cancer. *Int. J. Mol. Sci.* **2017**, *18*, 946. [CrossRef]
61. Eustace, B.K.; Sakurai, T.; Stewart, J.K.; Yimlamai, D.; Unger, C.; Zehetmeier, C.; Lain, B.; Torella, C.; Henning, S.W.; Beste, G.; et al. Functional Proteomic Screens Reveal an Essential Extracellular Role for Hsp90α in Cancer Cell Invasiveness. *Nat. Cell Biol.* **2004**, *6*, 507–514. [CrossRef]
62. Li, W.; Li, Y.; Guan, S.; Fan, J.; Cheng, C.; Bright, A.M.; Chinn, C.; Chen, M.; Woodley, D.T. Extracellular Heat Shock Protein-90α: Linking Hypoxia to Skin Cell Motility and Wound Healing. *EMBO J.* **2007**, *26*, 1221–1233. [CrossRef]
63. Tsutsumi, S.; Scroggins, B.; Koga, F.; Lee, M.-J.; Trepel, J.; Felts, S.; Carreras, C.; Neckers, L. A Small Molecule Cell-Impermeant Hsp90 Antagonist Inhibits Tumor Cell Motility and Invasion. *Oncogene* **2008**, *27*, 2478–2487. [CrossRef] [PubMed]
64. Hightower, L.E.; Guidon, P.T. Selective Release from Cultured Mammalian Cells of Heat-shock (Stress) Proteins That Resemble Glia-axon Transfer Proteins. *J. Cell. Physiol.* **1989**, *138*, 257–266. [CrossRef] [PubMed]
65. Liao, D.-F.; Jin, Z.-G.; Baas, A.S.; Daum, G.; Gygi, S.P.; Aebersold, R.; Berk, B.C. Purification and Identification of Secreted Oxidative Stress-Induced Factors from Vascular Smooth Muscle Cells. *J. Biol. Chem.* **2000**, *275*, 189–196. [CrossRef] [PubMed]
66. Clayton, A.; Turkes, A.; Navabi, H.; Mason, M.D.; Tabi, Z. Induction of Heat Shock Proteins in B-Cell Exosomes. *J. Cell Sci.* **2005**, *118*, 3631–3638. [CrossRef] [PubMed]
67. Woodley, D.T.; Fan, J.; Cheng, C.-F.; Li, Y.; Chen, M.; Bu, G.; Li, W. Participation of the Lipoprotein Receptor LRP1 in Hypoxia-HSP90α Autocrine Signaling to Promote Keratinocyte Migration. *J. Cell Sci.* **2009**, *122*, 1495–1498. [CrossRef]
68. Hung, C.-Y.; Tsai, M.-C.; Wu, Y.-P.; Wang, R.Y.L. Identification of Heat-Shock Protein 90 Beta in Japanese Encephalitis Virus-Induced Secretion Proteins. *J. Gen. Virol.* **2011**, *92*, 2803–2809. [CrossRef]
69. Cheng, C.-F.; Sahu, D.; Tsen, F.; Zhao, Z.; Fan, J.; Kim, R.; Wang, X.; O'Brien, K.; Li, Y.; Kuang, Y.; et al. A Fragment of Secreted Hsp90α Carries Properties That Enable It to Accelerate Effectively Both Acute and Diabetic Wound Healing in Mice. *J. Clin. Investig.* **2011**, *121*, 4348–4361. [CrossRef]
70. Tsutsumi, S.; Neckers, L. Extracellular Heat Shock Protein 90: A Role for a Molecular Chaperone in Cell Motility and Cancer Metastasis. *Cancer Sci.* **2007**, *98*, 1536–1539. [CrossRef]
71. Chakraborty, A.; Edkins, A.L. HSP90 as a Regulator of Extracellular Matrix Dynamics. *Biochem. Soc. Trans.* **2021**, *49*, 2611–2625. [CrossRef]
72. Sarkar, A.A.; Zohn, I.E. Hectd1 Regulates Intracellular Localization and Secretion of Hsp90 to Control Cellular Behavior of the Cranial Mesenchyme. *J. Cell Biol.* **2012**, *196*, 789–800. [CrossRef]
73. Chen, C.Y.; Balch, W.E. The Hsp90 Chaperone Complex Regulates GDI-Dependent Rab Recycling. *Mol. Biol. Cell* **2006**, *17*, 3494–3507. [CrossRef] [PubMed]
74. Sasaki, T.; Takai, Y. [9] Purification and Properties of Bovine Rab-GDP Dissociation Inhibitor. *Methods Enzymol.* **1995**, *257*, 70–79. [CrossRef]
75. Nishimura, N.; Goji, J.; Nakamura, H.; Orita, S.; Takai, Y.; Sano, K. Cloning of a Brain-Type Isoform of Human Rab GDI and Its Expression in Human Neuroblastoma Cell Lines and Tumor Specimens. *Cancer Res.* **1995**, *55*, 5445–5450. [PubMed]
76. Ono, T.; Nakashima, T. Recent Advances in Osteoclast Biology. *Histochem. Cell Biol.* **2018**, *149*, 325–341. [CrossRef] [PubMed]
77. Raja, S.M.; Desale, S.S.; Mohapatra, B.; Luan, H.; Soni, K.; Zhang, J.; Storck, M.A.; Feng, D.; Bielecki, T.A.; Band, V.; et al. Marked Enhancement of Lysosomal Targeting and Efficacy of ErbB2-Targeted Drug Delivery by HSP90 Inhibition. *Oncotarget* **2016**, *7*, 10522–10535. [CrossRef]
78. Matsui, T.; Itoh, T.; Fukuda, M. Small GTPase Rab12 Regulates Constitutive Degradation of Transferrin Receptor. *Traffic* **2011**, *12*, 1432–1443. [CrossRef]
79. Liu, J.; Zhang, J.-P.; Shi, M.; Quinn, T.; Bradner, J.; Beyer, R.; Chen, S.; Zhang, J. Rab11a and HSP90 Regulate Recycling of Extracellular α-Synuclein. *J. Neurosci.* **2009**, *29*, 1480–1485. [CrossRef]
80. Luo, D.; Bu, Y.; Ma, J.; Rajput, S.; He, Y.; Cai, G.; Liao, D.-F.; Cao, D. Heat Shock Protein 90-α Mediates Aldo-Keto Reductase 1B10 (AKR1B10) Protein Secretion through Secretory Lysosomes. *J. Biol. Chem.* **2013**, *288*, 36733–36740. [CrossRef]

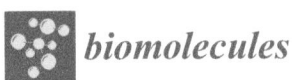

Review

The Role of Hsp90-R2TP in Macromolecular Complex Assembly and Stabilization

Jeffrey Lynham [1] and Walid A. Houry [1,2],*

[1] Department of Biochemistry, University of Toronto, Toronto, ON M5G 1M1, Canada; jeffrey.lynham@mail.utoronto.ca
[2] Department of Chemistry, University of Toronto, Toronto, ON M5S 3H6, Canada
* Correspondence: walid.houry@utoronto.ca; Tel.: +1-(416)-946-7141; Fax: +1-(416)-978-8548

Abstract: Hsp90 is a ubiquitous molecular chaperone involved in many cell signaling pathways, and its interactions with specific chaperones and cochaperones determines which client proteins to fold. Hsp90 has been shown to be involved in the promotion and maintenance of proper protein complex assembly either alone or in association with other chaperones such as the R2TP chaperone complex. Hsp90-R2TP acts through several mechanisms, such as by controlling the transcription of protein complex subunits, stabilizing protein subcomplexes before their incorporation into the entire complex, and by recruiting adaptors that facilitate complex assembly. Despite its many roles in protein complex assembly, detailed mechanisms of how Hsp90-R2TP assembles protein complexes have yet to be determined, with most findings restricted to proteomic analyses and in vitro interactions. This review will discuss our current understanding of the function of Hsp90-R2TP in the assembly, stabilization, and activity of the following seven classes of protein complexes: L7Ae snoRNPs, spliceosome snRNPs, RNA polymerases, PIKKs, MRN, TSC, and axonemal dynein arms.

Keywords: molecular chaperones; Hsp90; R2TP; PAQosome; TTT; snoRNP; snRNP; RNA polymerase; PIKK; TSC; dynein arm

Citation: Lynham, J.; Houry, W.A. The Role of Hsp90-R2TP in Macromolecular Complex Assembly and Stabilization. *Biomolecules* **2022**, *12*, 1045. https://doi.org/10.3390/biom12081045

Academic Editor: Chrisostomos Prodromou

Received: 20 June 2022
Accepted: 25 July 2022
Published: 28 July 2022

Publisher's Note: MDPI stays neutral with regard to jurisdictional claims in published maps and institutional affiliations.

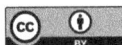

Copyright: © 2022 by the authors. Licensee MDPI, Basel, Switzerland. This article is an open access article distributed under the terms and conditions of the Creative Commons Attribution (CC BY) license (https://creativecommons.org/licenses/by/4.0/).

1. Overview of Hsp90 Structure and Its Function with R2TP

The Hsp90 molecular chaperone is a central regulator of protein homeostasis in eukaryotes under normal and stressed conditions. Hsp90 is involved in the final stages of client protein folding and maturation. In mammals, there are two cytoplasmic Hsp90 isoforms, Hsp90α and Hsp90β, while in yeast, Hsp82 and Hsc82 are the inducible and constitutively expressed Hsp90 isoforms, respectively [1]. Hsp90 isoforms (referred to here as Hsp90) exist as dynamic homodimers, with each protomer comprised of three domains: an N-terminal domain, the site of ATP binding and hydrolysis [2]; a middle domain, which interacts with Hsp90 substrates; and a C-terminal domain, which forms the Hsp90 dimerization interface (Figure 1A) [3]. The C-terminal domain also contains a MEEVD motif, which is important for interactions with Hsp90 cochaperones that contain TPR domains (see Table 1 for nomenclature). Hsp90 substrates are called clients, and the current set of Hsp90 clients includes steroid hormone receptors, kinases, transcription factors, E3 ubiquitin ligases, and many others that share no common features in terms of sequence, structure, or function [4]. Hsp90-mediated client folding and stabilization is a regulated process that requires the association and release of chaperones and cochaperones. Hsp90 client loading is largely dependent on Hsp70, which binds to nascent or partially folded polypeptides with exposed hydrophobic residues [5,6], and Hop, which functions as an adaptor between Hsp70 and Hsp90 [7].

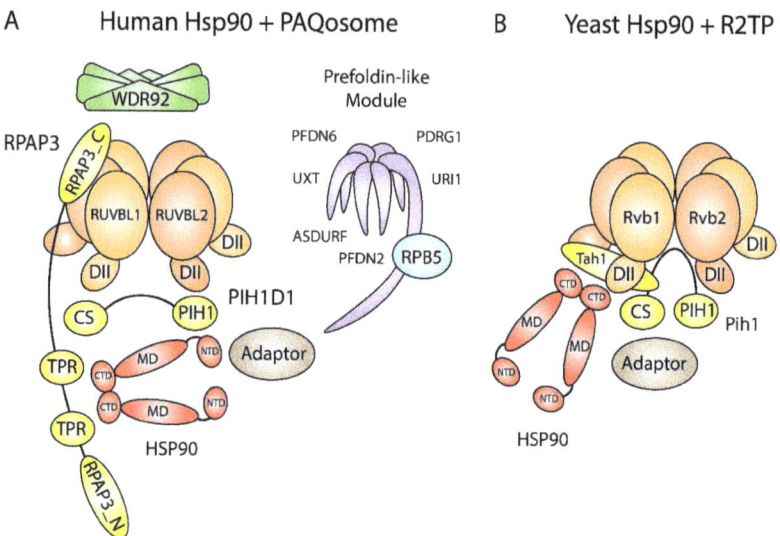

Figure 1. Schematic of Hsp90 and PAQosome subunits. (**A**) Human Hsp90 interacts with R2TP through the TPR domains on RPAP3. The RPAP3 C-terminal domain binds to the ATPase side of RUVBL2 and tethers Hsp90 and PIH1D1 to the rest of the R2TP complex. Some Hsp90 and RUVBL1/2 clients are recruited through adaptors. The PIH1 domain in PIH1D1 binds to proteins that contain a DpSDD/E motif. WDR92 and the prefoldin-like module (UPC) may also act as Hsp90 adaptors since they associate with human R2TP. CS, CHORD domain-containing protein Sgt1 domain; CTD, C-terminal domain; DII, Domain II; MD, middle domain; NTD, N-terminal domain; PIH1, Pih1 homology domain; RPAP3_C, RPAP3 C-terminal domain; RPAP3_N, RPAP3 N-terminal domain; TPR, tetratricopeptide domain. (**B**) Yeast Hsp90 interacts with R2TP through the RPAP3 yeast orthologue Tah1. Tah1 is much smaller than RPAP3, which gives yeast R2TP an open basket structure for client binding. An orthologous prefoldin-like module (UPC) and an orthologue for WDR92 are absent in yeast.

Table 1. Nomenclature.

17-AAG	17-(Allylamino)-17-demethoxygeldanamycin
AAA+	ATPases associated with diverse cellular activities
ASDURF	ASNSD1 upstream open reading frame protein
ATM	Ataxia-telangiectasia mutated
ATR	ATM- and RAD3-related
ATRIP	ATR-interacting protein
BRCA1	Breast cancer type 1 susceptibility protein
Cdc7	Cell division cycle 7-related protein kinase
CDK4	Cyclin-dependent kinase 4
CK2	Casein Kinase 2
COPS8	COP9 signalosome complex subunit 8
CS	CHORD domain-containing protein and Sgt1 domain
Cse4	Chromosome segregation protein 4

Table 1. Cont.

c-Src	Cellular proto-oncogene tyrosine-protein kinase Src
Dbf4	Protein DBF4 homolog A
DNAAF1	Dynein axonemal assembly factor 1
DNAAF2	Dynein axonemal assembly factor 2
DNAAF3	Dynein axonemal assembly factor 3
DNAAF4	Dynein axonemal assembly factor 4
DNAAF5	Dynein axonemal assembly factor 5
DNAAF6	Dynein axonemal assembly factor 6
DNAAF7	Dynein axonemal assembly factor 7
DNAAF8	Dynein axonemal assembly factor 8
DNAAF11	Dynein axonemal assembly factor 11
DNAI1	Dynein axonemal intermediate chain 1
DNAI2	Dynein axonemal intermediate chain 2
DNA-PKcs	DNA–protein kinase catalytic subunit
ECD	Ecdysoneless homolog
EFTUD2	Elongation factor Tu GTP binding domain containing 2
FKBP8	FK506-binding protein 8
GAR1	Glycine arginine rich protein 1
GPN2	GPN-Loop GTPase 2
GPN3	GPN-Loop GTPase 3
GrinL1A	Glutamate receptor-like protein 1A
Hop	Hsp organizing protein
Hsc82	Heat shock cognate protein 82
Hsp70	Heat shock protein 70
Hsp82	Heat shock protein 82
Hsp90	Heat shock protein 90
IFT1	Interferon-induced protein with tetratricopeptide repeats 1
Ku70	Lupus Ku autoantigen protein p70
Ku80	Lupus Ku autoantigen protein p80
LRRC6	Leucine rich repeat containing 6
MRE11	Meiotic recombination 11
MRN	MRE11-RAD50-NBS1
mRNP	Messenger ribonucleoprotein
mTOR	Mammalian target of rapamycin
mTORC1	Mammalian target of rapamycin complex 1
mTORC2	Mammalian target of rapamycin complex 2
NAF1	Nuclear assembly factor 1
NAP57	Nopp140-associated protein of 57 kDa

Table 1. *Cont.*

NBS1	Nibrin
NHP2	Non-Histone protein 2
NOP10	Nucleolar protein 10
NOP56	Nucleolar protein 56
NOP58	Nucleolar protein 58
NOPCHAP1	NOP protein chaperone 1
NUFIP1	Nuclear FMRP interacting protein 1
PAQosome	Particle for arrangement of quaternary structure
PDRG1	p53 and DNA damage regulated 1
PFDN2	Prefoldin subunit 2
PFDN6	Prefoldin subunit 6
Pih1	Protein interacting with Hsp90
PIH1D1	PIH1 domain-containing protein 1
PIH1D2	PIH1 domain-containing protein 2
PIKK	Phosphatidylinositol-3-kinase-related kinase
Prp19	Pre-mRNA-processing factor 19
PRPF31	Pre-mRNA-processing factor 31
PRPF8	Pre-mRNA-processing-splicing factor 8
R2SP	RUVBL1-RUVBL2-SPAG1-PIH1D2
R2TP	Rvb1–Rvb2–Tah1–Pih1
RAD50	Radiation sensitive 50
Rheb	Ras homolog enriched in brain
RNAP	RNA polymerase
RPA	Replication protein A 70 kDa DNA-binding subunit
RPA1	RNA polymerase I subunit A
RPA135	DNA-directed RNA polymerase I 135 kDa polypeptide
RPAP3	RNA polymerase II-associated protein 3
RPB1	RNA polymerase II subunit B1
RPB2	RNA polymerase II subunit B2
RPB3	RNA polymerase II subunit B3
RPB4	RNA polymerase II subunit B4
RPB5	RNA polymerase II subunit B5
RPB6	RNA polymerase II subunit B6
RPB7	RNA polymerase II subunit B7
RPB8	RNA polymerase II subunit B8
RPB9	RNA polymerase II subunit B9
RPB10	RNA polymerase II subunit B10
RPB11	RNA polymerase II subunit B11
RPB12	RNA polymerase II subunit B12
RPC1	RNA polymerase III subunit C160

Table 1. Cont.

RUVBL1	RuvB-like AAA ATPase 1
RUVBL2	RuvB-like AAA ATPase 2
Rvb1	RuvB-like protein 1
Rvb2	RuvB-like protein 2
SBP2	SECIS binding protein 2
SECIS	Selenocysteine insertion sequence
SHQ1	Small nucleolar RNAs of the box H/ACA family quantitative accumulation 1
Sgt1	Suppressor of G2 allele of SKP1 homolog
SMG1	Nonsense-mediated mRNA decay associated phosphatidylinositol-3-kinase-related kinase
snoRNA	Small nucleolar RNA
snoRNP	Small nucleolar ribonucleoprotein
snRNP	Small nuclear ribonucleoprotein
SNRNP200	Small nuclear ribonucleoprotein U5 subunit 200
SPAG1	Sperm-associated antigen 1
Tah1	TPR-containing protein associated with Hsp90
TBC1D7	Tre2-Bub2-Cdc16 domain family member 7
Tel2	Telomere maintenance 2
TELO2	Telomere length regulation protein TEL2 homolog
TERC	Telomerase RNA component
TERT	Telomerase reverse transcriptase
TPR	Tetratricopeptide repeat
Tra1	Transcription-associated protein 1
TRRAP	Transformation/transcription domain-associated protein
TSC	Tuberous sclerosis complex
TSC1	Tuberous sclerosis 1 protein
TSC2	Tuberous sclerosis 2 protein
TTC12	Tetratricopeptide repeat protein 12
TTI1	TEL2 interacting protein 1
TTI2	TEL2 interacting protein 2
TTT	TELO2-TTI1-TT2
UBR5	Ubiquitin protein ligase E3 component N-recognin 5
UPC	Unconventional prefoldin complex
URI1	Unconventional prefoldin RPB5 interactor 1
UXT	Ubiquitously expressed transcript
WAC	WW domain-containing adaptor protein with coiled-coil
WDR92	WD-40 repeat domain 92
ZNHIT2	Zinc finger HIT-type containing 2
ZNHIT3	Zinc finger HIT-type containing 3
ZNHIT6	Zinc finger HIT-type containing 6

In addition to stabilizing tertiary structure, Hsp90 and its cochaperones stabilize the quaternary structure of various macromolecular complexes. In 2005, our group identified Tah1 and Pih1 as Hsp90 interactors in yeast [8]. Tah1 and Pih1 form a heterodimer and interact with AAA+ proteins Rvb1 and Rvb2 to form the R2TP chaperone complex that is conserved in higher eukaryotes including humans. Most notably, the R2TP complex is involved in the assembly of L7Ae ribonucleoproteins [9–11], RNA polymerases [12], and PIKK complexes [13]. In humans, R2TP associates with RNA polymerase subunit RPB5, WD40 repeat protein WDR92, and the Unconventional Prefoldin Complex (UPC), comprising of URI1, UXT, PDRG1, PFDN2, PFDN6, and ASDURF [14–16]. Altogether, these 12 proteins constitute the PAQosome, Particle for Arrangement of Quaternary Structure (Figure 1A) [17]. The PAQosome is the largest and most intricate chaperone interacting with Hsp90. The R2TP complex is involved in all PAQosome-mediated pathways as the catalytic component, whereas the function of the other subunits is mostly unknown. WDR92 has a specialized role in dynein arm assembly [18], RPB5 likely bridges the interactions between the PAQosome and RNA polymerases, and the UPC may regulate R2TP in response to cell growth and proliferation [19]. Moreover, URI1 mediates nuclear and cytoplasmic shuttling of RNAP subunits, and it has been suggested to do so as part of the PAQosome [20,21]. Thus, PAQosome assembly may occur in the cytoplasm with URI1 facilitating its transport into the nucleus and vice-versa (Figure 2).

Within the PAQosome, RPAP3 and PIH1D1 are proposed to function as scaffolds for Hsp90 and its diverse client proteins. RPAP3 contains an RPAP3_N domain that mediates interactions with substrates enriched with helical-type domains [22]; two TPR domains, whereby TPR2 has high affinity for Hsp90 [23]; an intrinsically disordered region that makes contacts with RUVBL1 [22]; and an RPAP3_C domain that binds to the ATPase side of RUVBL2 [24]. PIH1D1 contains an N-terminal PIH1 domain that binds DpSDD/E motifs on clients [25,26] and a C-terminal CHORD and Sgt1 (CS) domain that binds RPAP3 [24,27]. Although it has been proposed that PIH1D1 binds to and regulates RUVBL2 ATPase activity as a nucleotide exchange factor, our group has shown that, within the R2TP complex, PIH1D1 binds exclusively to RPAP3 and that PIH1D1 has little effect on RUVBL1/2 ATPase activity and nucleotide binding affinity [22]. Interestingly, although our model suggests that PIH1D1 only interacts with RPAP3 within the R2TP complex, we have identified R2T and R2P complexes in vitro and *in cellulo* [22]. The significance of these findings in regard to Hsp90 function has yet to be determined.

In yeast, Tah1 is much smaller than RPAP3 and contains two TPR repeats followed by a C-helix and an unstructured region [28,29]. The TPR domain binds the Hsp90 C-terminal MEEVD motif, while the unstructured region binds Pih1. Yeast Pih1 is slightly larger than PIH1D1 and contains an N-terminal PIH1 domain, which also recruits clients with DpSDD/E motifs, and a C-terminal CS domain that binds Tah1 [26,28,30]. The Tah1-Pih1 dimer binds to the Rvb1/2 hexamer DII domains to form the R2TP complex [31,32]. Yeast R2TP forms an open basket that accommodates client proteins and Hsp90 (Figure 1B).

Although it has been established that human Hsp90 interacts with R2TP through RPAP3 [23,24], the details of Hsp90-mediated protein complex assembly are limited, with most of our knowledge restricted to proteomics and in vitro interaction analyses. This review will discuss our current understanding of Hsp90-R2TP in higher metazoans and its roles in protein complex assembly, stabilization, function, or localization for seven classes of protein complexes: L7Ae snoRNPs, spliceosome snRNPs, RNA polymerases, PIKKs, MRN, TSC, and axonemal dynein arms (Figure 2). Of note, human Hsp90 in these studies may refer to either isoform, Hsp90α or Hsp90β, since they have nearly identical structural and functional similarities that cannot be easily distinguished from one another.

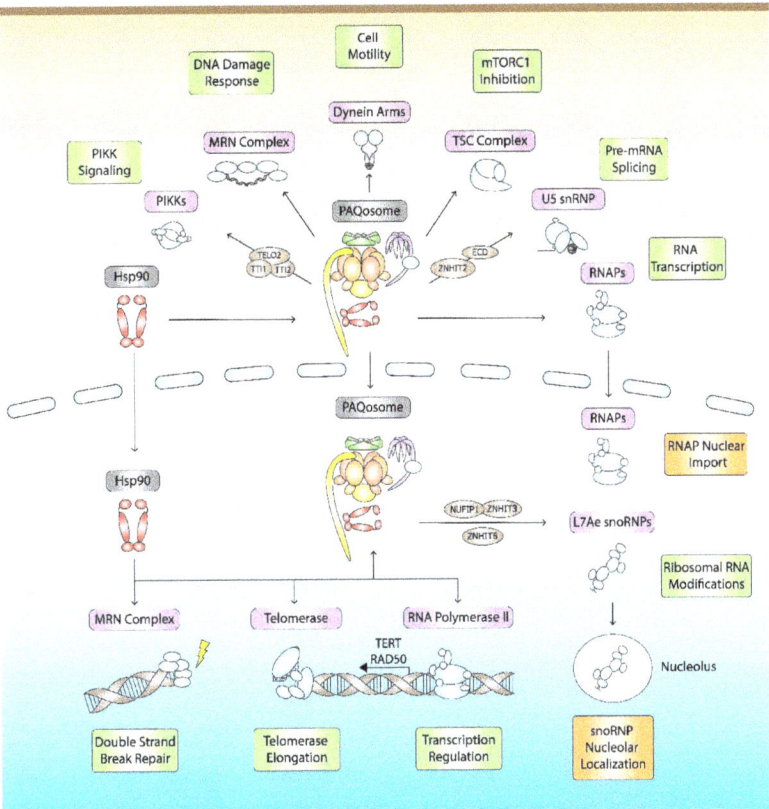

Figure 2. Hsp90- and PAQosome-mediated quaternary assembly and stabilization pathways. Hsp90 together with the PAQosome are involved in the assembly, stabilization, function (green), or localization (orange) of at least seven classes of protein complexes (purple), which include L7Ae snoRNPs, spliceosome snRNPs, RNA Polymerases, PIKKs, MRN, TSC, and dynein arms. RNAs within each RNP complex that are mentioned in the text are listed. R2TP/PAQosome assembly factors (brown) are shown.

2. snoRNP Biogenesis

Eukaryotic ribosomal RNA (rRNA) processing occurs in the nucleolus, which contains numerous small nucleolar RNAs (snoRNA). Most snoRNAs function as sequence-specific guides during rRNA modification [33], while others are involved in folding and cleavage events [34,35]. There are two major families of snoRNAs: box C/D and box H/ACA. Box C/D snoRNAs direct ribose 2′-O-methylation within rRNA and certain spliceosome small nuclear RNA (snRNA) [36,37], and box H/ACA snoRNAs direct the isomerization of uridine to pseudouridine [38]. They are classified based on conserved sequence motifs and their association with common core proteins. Mature snoRNP complexes are comprised of snoRNA and four common core proteins, namely, fibrillarin, NOP56, NOP58, and 15.5K for box C/D snoRNPs, and NHP2, NOP10, GAR1, and NAP57 for box H/ACA snoRNPs (Figure 3). During snoRNP biogenesis, Hsp90 stabilizes NOP58, 15.5K, and NHP2 [9].

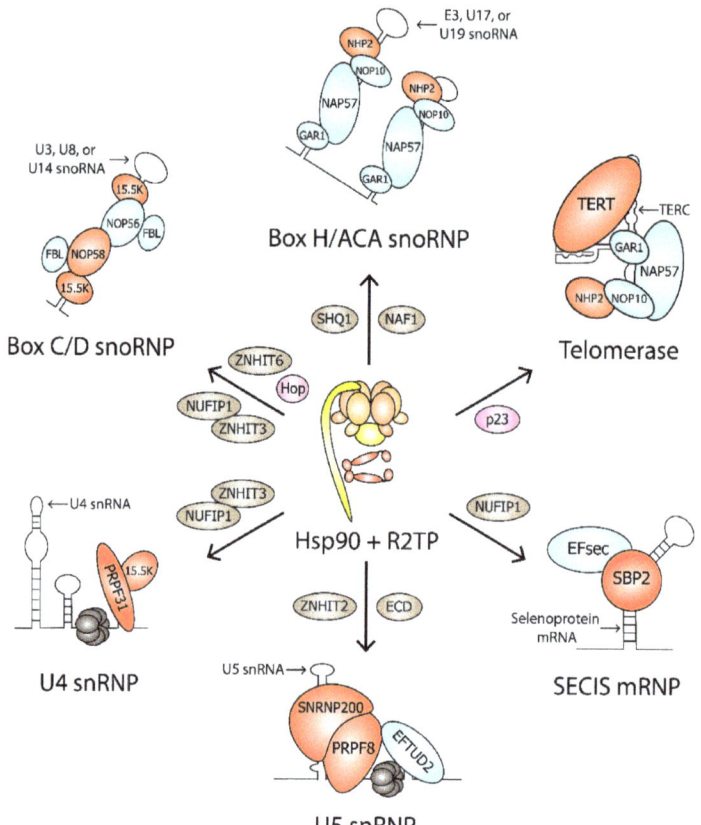

Figure 3. Hsp90 clients in RNP complexes. Hsp90, Hsp90 cochaperones (pink), R2TP, and assembly factors (brown) are involved in the biogenesis of Box C/D snoRNP, Box H/ACA snoRNP, Telomerase, U4 snRNP, U5 snRNP, and SECIS mRNP. Hsp90 clients are shown in red. Protein complex components that are not Hsp90 clients are shown in blue.

2.1. Box C/D snoRNP Assembly

2.1.1. Role of Hsp90 in Box C/D snoRNP Assembly

Regardless of their snoRNA component, box C/D snoRNPs have a highly conserved asymmetric arrangement of core proteins [39–42]. The 15.5K protein is part of the L7Ae family of ribosomal proteins and was first identified as a component of the U4/U6.U5 tri-snRNP that binds directly to the 5′ stem loop of U4 snRNA [43], which has a similar primary and secondary structure to box C/D and C′/D′ motifs [44]. 15.5K binding to the box C/D motif is essential for the recruitment of assembly factors RUVBL1 and RUVBL2 and other core proteins including NOP56, NOP58, and fibrillarin [45]. NOP56 and NOP58 are two paralogous proteins that contain NOP and coiled-coil (CC) domains [46]. The NOP domain exhibits RNA and protein binding, which allows NOP56 and NOP58 binding to 15.5K-box C/D snoRNA complexes [47], while the CC domain enables NOP56-NOP58 heterodimerization across the C/D and C′/D′ motifs [39,42]. The NOP56 and NOP58 N-terminal domains together recruit one copy of fibrillarin to the snoRNP complex [39].

Box C/D snoRNP formation requires Hsp90. In HeLa cell extracts, Hsp90, RPAP3, and PIH1D1 coprecipitated with precursor and mature forms of ectopically expressed rat U3 snoRNA [9]. HEK293 cells expressing rat U3 snoRNA and treated with geldanamycin, an Hsp90 inhibitor that blocks the ATP binding site [2,48], had less U3 snoRNA accumulation [9]. These findings were the first to indicate a role for Hsp90 in box C/D snoRNP biogenesis.

Subsequent experiments have suggested that the role of Hsp90 in box C/D snoRNP biogenesis is to stabilize core protein NOP58. When HEK293 cell lines expressing GFP-tagged proteins were treated with geldanamycin, NOP58 and 15.5K failed to accumulate, while a mild effect was seen for NOP56 [9]. NOP58 mutants, NOP58-K310A-A313R, and NOP58-A283P, which cannot assemble into mature snoRNPs, showed stronger interactions with Hsp90 than NOP58-WT [49]. NOP58-A283P also associated with the Hsp70-Hsp90 adaptor Hop [49]. Therefore, NOP58 is likely stabilized through the Hsp70-Hop-Hsp90 pathway during its maturation and assembly into snoRNPs. Interestingly, Hsp90 also stabilized the L7Ae protein SBP2, suggesting that Hsp90 is also involved in SECIS mRNP biogenesis (Figure 3) [9]. SECIS mRNPs associate with selenoprotein mRNAs for translational recoding of a UGA codon that enables the insertion of selenocysteine [50].

2.1.2. Role of R2TP in Box C/D snoRNP Assembly

NOP58 can be stabilized by other chaperones, namely the RUVBL1/2 complex and NOPCHAP1 [49]. RUVBL1 and RUVBL2 were identified as box C/D snoRNP biogenesis factors from an early study identifying mouse U14 snoRNA interactors [51]. Subsequent studies have shown that RUVBL1/2 interact with precursor and mature forms of rat U3 and human U8 snoRNA [9,52,53]. NOPCHAP1 was identified as a snoRNP assembly factor through Stable Isotope Labeling with Amino Acids in Cell Culture (SILAC) experiments, which showed that NOPCHAP1 and RUVBL1/2 associated with nascent NOP58 [54]. NOPCHAP1 binds to NOP58 through the CC-NOP fragment, while it binds to RUVBL1 through the DII domain [49]. The interaction between NOP58 and RUVBL1 is weak, but in the presence of NOPCHAP1, it is enhanced 20-fold [49]. RUVBL1 binds to NOPCHAP1 in the absence of ATP since ATPγS, a non-hydrolyzable ATP analogue, abolished NOPCHAP1 binding [49]. The interaction between NOPCHAP1 and RUVBL1/2 is likely transient and may serve only to direct NOP58 to RUVBL1/2. Interestingly, WT HEK293T cells treated with geldanamycin and NOPCHAP1 KO cells displayed similar levels of reduced NOP58, indicating that Hsp90 and NOPCHAP1 may act on the same pathway [49]. A caveat to consider is that geldanamycin may have additional binding targets that affect the viability of Hsp90 clients.

RUVBL1/2 may also act as a NOP58 chaperone as part of the R2TP complex. HeLa cell extracts separated on linear glycerol gradients showed the assembly factor NUFIP1 and core proteins NOP58 and fibrillarin to be in the same fractions as RUVBL1, RUVBL2, and RPAP3 [9]. Also, pulldown assays in rabbit reticulocyte lysates showed that PIH1D1 directly interacts with NOP56 and NOP58 [9], and that RUVBL1 and RUVBL2 interact with all four box C/D snoRNP proteins [55]. Moreover, the R2TP complex is involved in Cajal body and nucleolar localization of pre-snoRNPs and mature snoRNPs, respectively. In HeLa cells transfected with siRNA, depletion of RUVBL1 and RUVBL2 caused reductions of Cajal body and nucleolar U3 snoRNA [55].

Hsp90 inhibition in HEK293 cells resulted in the disappearance of both NOP58 and 15.5K [9], but the link between Hsp90 ATPase activity and 15.5K stabilization remains unclear. Hsp90 may indirectly stabilize 15.5K by stabilizing NOP58 first. Rather than interacting with Hsp90, 15.5K can bind RUVBL1, RUVBL2, and RUVBL1/2 in the presence of ATP [55,56]. Additionally, RUVBL1/2 was shown to bridge the interaction between 15.5K and core proteins NOP56 and NOP58 [55], which may be important for 15.5K stability. Taken together, Hsp70, Hop, Hsp90, R2TP, and NOPCHAP1 stabilize NOP58, and RUVBL1/2 subsequently recruits 15.5K to NOP56-NOP58, thereby stabilizing 15.5K.

2.1.3. R2TP-Associated Box C/D snoRNP Assembly Factors

The R2TP complex is a highly interactive chaperone complex that works together with other box C/D snoRNP assembly factors, namely, NUFIP1, ZNHIT3, and ZNHIT6 [54]. NUFIP1 acts mainly as a tethering protein, joining 15.5K with NOP56, NOP58, and fibrillarin [9,56]. However, NUFIP1 may also regulate R2TP function during snoRNP assembly since it interacts directly with RUVBL1, RUVBL2, and PIH1D1 [9,56]. For example, the coprecipitation of 15.5K with either NOP56 or NOP58 was enhanced with RUVBL1/2, but was repressed with both RUVBL1/2 and NUFIP1 [55].

NUFIP1 forms a heterodimer with ZNHIT3, an assembly factor belonging to the zf-HIT family, which are often observed in complexes containing RUVBL1 and RUVBL2 [54,57–60]. ZNHIT3 is required for NUFIP1 stability since siRNA-mediated depletion of ZNHIT3 in HeLa cells resulted in similar decreases in NUFIP1 levels [60]. ZNHIT3 was unable to bind precursor or mature forms of rat U3 snoRNA, but it was able to bind U3 snoRNA mutants that had decreased affinity for NOP56, NOP58, and fibrillarin [54].

Finally, in the presence of ATP, ZNHIT6 interacts with the RUVBL1/2 complex, but not with individual RUVBL1 and RUVBL2 proteins [55]. In addition, ZNHIT6 binds 15.5K, but not NOP56, NOP58, or fibrillarin [56].

2.2. Box H/ACA snoRNP Assembly

The assembly of box H/ACA snoRNPs has been well-established. The pseudouridine synthase NAP57 (also named dyskerin) and core proteins NOP10 and NHP2 form a trimer that binds directly to H/ACA RNA in the absence of GAR1 [61]. Early yeast genetic depletion studies have demonstrated that the core trimer is required for H/ACA RNA stability and that all four core proteins are essential for cell viability [62–66]. The assembly of mammalian H/ACA snoRNPs requires two assembly factors, NAF1 and SHQ1, which are needed for H/ACA RNA accumulation without being part of the mature particles [67,68]. NAF1 is structurally similar to GAR1 [69]. During snoRNP biogenesis, NAF1 and the core trimer associate with H/ACA RNA at the site of transcription [70]. Upon snoRNP maturation, snoRNP particles localize to Cajal bodies or nucleoli where GAR1 replaces NAF1 [68,70]. SHQ1 functions as a NAP57 chaperone by acting as an RNA placeholder, thereby protecting NAP57 from nonspecific RNA binding before its association with H/ACA RNA and other core RNP proteins [71].

2.2.1. Role of Hsp90 in Box H/ACA snoRNP Assembly

Hsp90 is involved in H/ACA snoRNP biogenesis since Hsp90 inhibition led to defects in H/ACA RNA production and core protein stability [9]. HEK293 cells treated with geldanamycin showed decreased levels of telomerase H/ACA RNA [9], which is consistent with TERT, the reverse transcriptase in the telomerase complex, being an Hsp90 client [72]. In addition, geldanamycin-treated cells showed a complete loss of core protein NHP2, indicating NHP2 as a potential Hsp90 client [9]. NAP57 levels were unaffected by geldanamycin [9], presumably because it was stabilized by SHQ1 [73].

Telomerase is a box H/ACA snoRNP complex that synthesizes the G-rich DNA at the 3′-ends of linear chromosomes [74]. In addition to the four box H/ACA core proteins, human telomerase contains reverse transcriptase TERT and telomerase RNA component TERC (Figure 3). Hsp90 and its cochaperone p23 bind TERT, and blocking this interaction inhibits the proper assembly of active telomerase in vitro [72]. TERT and TERC could bind to each other without Hsp90-p23, although this complex was inactive [75]. In addition, Hsp90 inhibitors geldanamycin and novobiocin inhibited telomerase even after telomerase was assembled [75]. Unlike most of their clients, Hsp90 and p23 remain associated with active telomerase [76]. In mammalian cells, Hsp90 regulates TERT expression. In SCC4 cells, a telomerase-positive oral cancer cell line, coprecipitation experiments showed an in vivo interaction between Hsp90 and the TERT promoter. Geldanamycin exposure decreased telomerase activity, TERT promoter activity, and TERT mRNA expression [77]. Additionally, in cerebral endothelial cells, siRNA-mediated Hsp90 depletion inhibited telomerase activity and decreased telomerase protein expression [78].

2.2.2. Role of R2TP in Box H/ACA snoRNP Assembly

Hsp90 chaperone function on telomerase may depend on R2TP, since RUVBL1 and RUVBL2 were reported to interact with TERT and NAP57 [79]. During telomerase assembly, RUVBL1 and RUVBL2 may stabilize NAP57 since depletion of RUVBL1 and RUVBL2 led to a significant reduction of NAP57 steady-state levels [79]. Moreover, RUVBL1 and RUVBL2 associated with TERC in HeLa cell extracts, and RUVBL1 ATPase activity was essential for TERC maintenance [79]. In addition, RUVBL1 and RUVBL2 are involved in the production of other H/ACA RNAs. RUVBL1- or RUVBL2-siRNA knockdown in HeLa cells caused a reduction in the H/ACA RNAs E3 and U17/E1 [10].

Regarding H/ACA snoRNP complex assembly, knockdown of RUVBL1 and RUVBL2 in HeLa cells resulted in a loss of NHP2 and NAP57 [10]. NHP2 makes a direct interaction with NUFIP1 [9], suggesting that NUFIP1 could bridge the interaction between NHP2 and RUVBL1/2 to mediate NHP2 assembly or stability. Similar to its role in box C/D snoRNPs, NUFIP1 may also be involved in bridging interactions between H/ACA snoRNA and core proteins. NUFIP1 coprecipitated with U19 H/ACA snoRNA, and its depletion reduced the levels of U19 and telomerase RNA [9].

During snoRNP assembly, NAP57 is stabilized by the RUVBL1/2 complex and SHQ1 [73,79], and NAP57 requires the R2TP complex to dissociate from SHQ1 [10]. SHQ1 exerts a clamp-like grip on NAP57 through binding to NAP57 *in trans*: the N-terminal CS domain of SHQ1 binds to the surface that is opposite from the RNA binding surface where the C-terminal SHQ1-specific domain binds [10]. NAP57 recruits the R2TP complex through its unstructured C-terminus [10]. RUVBL1, RUVBL2, and PIH1D1 bind to the same domain on NAP57 as SHQ1. RUVBL1 and RUVBL2 also bind to the CS domain of SHQ1 and remove it from NAP57 through an ATP-independent mechanism [10]. ATP binding and hydrolysis may only be required for the release of RUVBL1/2 from NAP57 after SHQ1 has been removed.

3. Spliceosome snRNP Assembly

The spliceosome is a molecular machine that catalyzes splicing, an essential post-transcriptional modification that removes introns from pre-mRNA. Spliceosomes are comprised of the Prp19 complex, U1 snRNP, U2 snRNP, and the U4/U6.U5 tri-RNP, with each snRNP having their own snRNA component and associated proteins. The spliceosome associates with more than 300 different proteins [80]. Proteomic analyses of purified spliceosomes have shown that the complex is highly conserved, with more than 85% of yeast proteins having a direct human orthologue [81]. Proteomic analyses in yeast and human cells have revealed a role for Hsp90 and R2TP in U4 and U5 snRNP assembly [54,58,59,82].

3.1. U4 snRNP Assembly

3.1.1. Similarities between U4 snRNP and Box C/D snoRNP Complexes

The U4 snRNP is comprised of U4 snRNA, L7Ae protein 15.5K, and splicing component PRPF31 (Figure 3). In addition, 15.5K binds to the 5' stem-loop of U4 snRNA in a manner similar to the box C/D motif [43,45], enabling PRPF31 recruitment [83]. Without 15.5K, PRPF31 weakly associates with U4 RNA [82]. The association between PRPF31 and 15.5K is essential because an A216P mutation in PRPF31, which abolished the PRPF31-15.5K interaction, resulted in PRPF31 cytoplasmic accumulation, indicating the prevention of PRPF31 incorporation into mature spliceosomes within the nucleus [82].

U4 snRNP shares a few similarities with box C/D snoRNP. In addition to both containing the RNA binding component 15.5K, the U4 snRNP splicing component PRPF31 is homologous to box C/D core proteins NOP56 and NOP58. These three proteins each have a NOP domain, which binds to preformed 15.5K-RNA complexes, and a CC domain, which mediate protein–protein interactions within RNP complexes [47]. Furthermore, U4 snRNA and box C/D snoRNA both associate with the assembly factor NUFIP1, but unlike box C/D snoRNA, U4 snRNA is not dependent on NUFIP1 for its assembly and maturation [9].

3.1.2. Role of Hsp90 and R2TP in U4 snRNP Assembly

Similar to box C/D snoRNP assembly, U4 snRNP assembly and stabilization is mediated by chaperones R2TP, Hsp90, and Hsp70. Co-IP experiments using antibodies against Hsp90, RUVBL1, RUVBL2, RPAP3, and PIH1D1 showed that each associated with U4 snRNA [9]. HEK293 cells treated with geldanamycin showed an almost complete loss of U4 snRNA, a moderate decrease of 15.5K, and a mild effect on PRPF31 [9]. In PRPF31, an A216P mutation prevents its nuclear localization [84], and a K243A/A246R double mutation prevents its interaction with 15.5K [82]. SILAC-IP experiments using HeLa cells expressing PRPF31-A216P or PRPF31-K243A/A246R showed that both PRPF31 mutants were enriched with Hop and Hsp70 [49]. Hsp90 was also present at low levels [49]. These findings show that PRPF31 binds to Hsp70 in the cytoplasm and suggest that the Hsp70-Hop-Hsp90 pathway mediates the PRPF31-15.5K interaction.

The assembly factors NUFIP1 and ZNHIT3 together with the R2TP complex are also involved in U4 snRNP biogenesis. In mammalian cells, NUFIP1 can mediate the interaction between 15.5K and PRPF31, and it may do so with help from the R2TP complex since NUFIP1 also binds to RUVBL1, RUVBL2, and PIH1D1 [9,56]. Moreover, coprecipitation experiments in HEK293T cells showed that NUFIP1, ZNHIT3, and RUVBL1 each associate with U4 snRNA and PRPF31, suggesting that they can mediate the interaction between U4 snRNA and PRPF31 [82]. Indeed, NUFIP1 knockout cells had a two-fold reduction in binding between PRPF31 and U4 snRNA [82].

3.2. U5 snRNP Assembly

3.2.1. Role of Hsp90 and R2TP in U5 snRNP Assembly

U5 snRNP is recruited to the spliceosome as part of the U4/U6.U5 tri-snRNP and is comprised of U5 snRNA, GTPase EFTUD2, helicase SNRNP200, and mRNA processing factor PRPF8 (Figure 3). The Hsp90/R2TP complex is mostly involved in the stabilization and assembly of PRPF8 into mature U5 snRNP particles. SILAC experiments showed that Hsp90 associates with PRPF8 and EFTUD2, as well as with assembly factors AAR2 and ECD [59]. In HeLa cells, Hsp90 ATPase activity was shown to stabilize PRPF8 and SNRNP200, but not EFTUD2 [59]. Hsp90 was also shown to mediate the interaction between PRPF8 and cytoplasmic RPAP3 [59].

PRPF8 is stabilized by the R2TP complex and U5 snRNP assembly factors. In vitro pull-down experiments have shown FLAG-tagged PRPF8 to simultaneously co-elute with purified RUVBL1-RUVBL2, RPAP3-PIH1D1, AAR2, ECD, and ZNHIT2 [85]. PRPF8 can make direct interactions with RUVBL1-RUVBL2 and RPAP3-PIH1D1. The PRPF8-RUVBL1/2 interaction is stronger than the PRPF8-RPAP3-PIH1D1 interaction [85]. PRPF8 mutants that cannot be integrated into mature U5 snRNPs associate more strongly with R2TP than WT PRPF8 [59]. PRPF8 binding to R2TP and AAR2 chaperones was increased in the absence of PIH1D1, suggesting that the formation of the R2TP complex through PIH1D1 binding is important for the release of PRPF8 from R2TP and AAR2 [59].

EFTUD2 may also be stabilized by the R2TP complex and AAR2. EFTUD2 has a DSDED motif, suggesting that it binds to PIH1D1; however, the PIH1D1 N-terminal domain was not sufficient to bind EFTUD2 [59]. Although, mutations in the EFTUD2 DSDED motif did affect EFTUD2 binding with AAR2, RUVBL1/2, and ZNHIT2 [59]. In addition, when PIH1D1, RUVBL2, and ZNHIT2 were depleted, there was less EFTUD2 [59]. EFTUD2 may be recruited to the R2TP complex through RPAP3 since EFTUD2 was shown to interact with ectopically expressed FLAG-RPAP3 in HEK293 lysates [58].

3.2.2. R2TP-Associated U5 snRNP Assembly Factors

ZNHIT2 and the R2TP complex mediate U5 snRNP subunit interactions during U5 snRNP assembly. SILAC experiments showed that ZNHIT2 interacts with R2TP, EFTUD2, PRPF8, SNRNP200, and yeast two-hybrid experiments confirmed direct interactions between ZNHIT2-EFTUD2 and ZNHIT2-RUVBL1 [59]. When ZNHIT2 is knocked out, the interactions between RPAP3-EFTUD2 and RPAP3-PRPF8 were absent [58]. ZNHIT2 is also needed to bridge the binding of RUVBL1/2 with EFTUD2 and PRPF8 [58]. The RUVBL1/2-ZNHIT2 cryo-EM structure shows that the RUVBL1/2 DII domains interact with the ZNHIT2 C-terminal end [85], which is in contrast to another study that showed that the ZNHIT2 HIT domain was essential for binding [58]. Rather than mediating the RUVBL1/2-ZNHIT2 interaction, the HIT domain may regulate the conformation and nucleotide state of RUVBL1/2 [85]. Through binding to the DII domains, ZNHIT2 disrupts the RUVBL1/2 dodecamer [85]. When ZNHIT2 was bound to the hexamer, RUVBL1 still had ADP bound while RUVBL2 was in the apo state [85]. Interestingly, the intrinsically low ATPase activity of RUVBL1/2 hexamers with one Walker B mutant, in either RUVBL1 or RUVBL2, was significantly increased with ZNHIT2 present, suggesting that ZNHIT2 affects the activity of both RUVBL1 and RUVBL2 subunits [85].

ECD is another adaptor protein involved in U5 snRNP biogenesis. In vitro pulldowns showed that ECD co-eluted with GST-ZNHIT2 and RUVBL1/2, and its association with this complex was enhanced when RPAP3 and PIH1D1 were added [85]. ECD can bind RUVBL1 and PIH1D1, either through its DpSDD motif or another uncharacterized binding site [25,86].

4. Hsp90- and R2TP-Mediated RNA Polymerase Assembly and Localization

The eukaryotic RNA polymerases, RNAP I, RNAP II, and RNAP III, are multiprotein complexes that synthesize ribosomal, messenger, and transfer RNA, respectively. The three RNA polymerases are structurally related. Within each complex, the two largest subunits form the catalytic core, while the smaller subunits are located on the periphery. They are also related through having five common subunits: RPB5, RPB6, RPB8, RPB10, and RPB12. Large-scale proteomic screens identified Hsp90, R2TP, and prefoldins as RNAP II interactors (Figure 1) [14,16,87,88]. RNAP II is assembled in the cytoplasm by Hsp90 and R2TP and then imported into the nucleus through URI1 [12,20]. To further analyze the interactions of RNAP II subunits during assembly, Boulon and colleagues performed triple-SILAC purifications on U2OS cells treated with α-amanitin, a small molecule that binds RPB1 and induces its degradation [12,89]. Their findings revealed the presence of two subcomplexes: RPB1-RPB8 and RPB2-RPB3-RPB10-RPB11-RPB12. In addition, each subcomplex associated with a specific set of assembly factors, such as RPAP2, GPN2, GPN3, and GrinL1A. RPB1-RPB8 also associated with R2TP/Prefoldin components RPAP3, PFDN2, and UXT [12].

RPB1 is the largest subunit in RNAP II and interacts with many RNAP II subunits and assembly factors. Coprecipitation and yeast two-hybrid experiments showed that Hsp90 interacts with RPB1 and with the TPR2 domain on RPAP3 [12]. RPB1 interacts with RPAP3 outside of the TPR2 domain [12], implying that RPAP3 stabilizes RPB1 by tethering the interaction between Hsp90 and RPB1. Indeed, long-term RPAP3 depletion in U2OS cells resulted in RPB1 loss [12]. Also, RPAP3 depletion resulted in RPB1 cytoplasmic accumulation in mouse intestinal epithelium cells and crypt base columnar stem cells [90]. Another study showed that RNAP II assembly in melanoma cells was dependent on RPB1 interacting with URI1 [91], but the role of the prefoldin-like module during RNAP II assembly is uncharacterized.

The depletion of RNAP subunits leads to the accumulation of unstable cytoplasmic RPB1. Boulon and colleagues showed that siRNA-mediated depletion of any RNAP II subunit in U2OS cells resulted in RPB1 cytoplasmic accumulation [12]. When cells were treated with geldanamycin, there was a significant decrease of RPB1 in RPB2-, RPB3-, RPB5-, RPB8-, RPB10-, RPB11-, and RPB12-depleted cells, but no significant changes of RPB1 in RPB4-, RPB6-, RPB7-, and RPB9-depleted cells [12]. Hsp90 is essential for stabilizing RPB1, however, Hsp90 binding to RPB1 occurred independent of its ATPase activity [12]. To stabilize RPB1, Hsp90 ATPase activity may mediate interactions between RPB1 and RNAP II subunits RPB5, RPB8, and the subcomplex RPB2-RPB3-RPB10-RPB11-RPB12. The remaining RNAP II subunits, RPB4, RPB6, RPB7, and RPB9, are likely nonessential for RPB1 stability and may be integrated at a later stage. Taken together, these findings show that Hsp90 and R2TP stabilize RPB1 by mediating its interactions with other RNAP II subunits.

R2TP may also be involved in RNAP I and RNAP III assembly since RPAP3-based purifications showed interactions with RPA1 and RPC1, the two largest subunits of RNAP I and RNAP III, respectively [12,16]. Depletion of RPA135, the second largest subunit in RNAP I, increased the interaction between RPA1 and RPAP3, demonstrating that RPAP3 preferentially binds to RPA1 when it is unassembled [12].

5. PIKK Complex Assembly and Stabilization

Phosphatidylinositol 3-kinase-related kinases (PIKKs) belong to the Ser/Thr kinase family and are required for cell proliferation, metabolism, and differentiation. The PIKK family is comprised of ATM, ATR, and DNA-PKcs, which are involved in DNA damage sensing, signaling, and repair (Figure 4); mTOR, a central regulator of cell metabolism, growth, and survival (Figure 4); SMG1, involved in nonsense-mediated mRNA decay; and TRRAP, a pseudokinase that lacks catalytic activity but functions as a large protein interaction hub. Although they have diverse functions, PIKKs share a common domain architecture where their N-termini carry long arrays of HEAT repeats [92], and their C-termini phosphorylate target proteins using a region related to the domain of PI3 kinase [93]. The PIKKs oligomerize with other proteins to form complexes, yet none of their binding partners or target proteins are common to all family members. During PIKK complex assembly and function, they each depend on Hsp90, the TTT complex, and the R2TP complex [13,94,95].

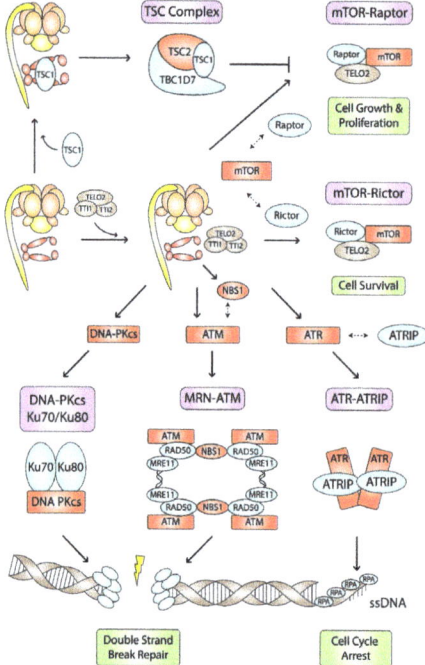

Figure 4. Hsp90- and R2TP-mediated PIKK, MRN, and TSC complex assembly pathways. Hsp90, R2TP, and the TTT (brown) are involved in the assembly, stabilization, or function (green) of several complexes (purple) involved in cell metabolism and DNA damage responses. Hsp90-R2TP stabilizes its clients (red) and mediates interactions (dashed double-sided arrows) between its clients and other complex subunits (blue).

5.1. Role of Hsp90-TTT in PIKK Complex Assembly

The TTT complex, comprising of TELO2, TTI1, and TTI2, was discovered through a large-scale proteomic analysis identifying Tel2 interactors in fission yeast [96,97]. Each component of the TTT complex is mutually dependent on each other for their stability [98]. TTI1 provides a platform for TELO2 and TTI2 to bind to its central and C-terminal regions, respectively [99]. Functional studies in yeast, *C. elegans*, and mammalian cells show that components of the TTT complex are essential for proper PIKK signaling pathways, namely, the DNA damage response [94,98,100–106], metabolic stress [107–113], nonsense-mediated mRNA decay [114,115], and transcriptional regulation [116,117]. The TTT complex recognizes and stabilizes PIKKs cotranslationally before mediating their assembly into larger complexes [95,111,118].

The TTT complex functions as an Hsp90 cochaperone. Co-IP experiments coupled with MALDI-TOF using HeLa S3 cell extracts revealed that FLAG-tagged TTT subunits associate with PIKKs, R2TP subunits, and Hsps [118]. TTI2 was shown to associate with Hsp90 [118]. Co-IPs in HEK293 cells showed that TELO2 and TTI1 could also associate with Hsp90, and Hsp90 ATPase activity was needed to stabilize TELO2 and TTI1 [94]. Thus, Hsp90 ATPase activity is essential for PIKK stabilization and proper PIKK signaling [94,119]. Hsp90 inhibition in HeLa cells interfered with TELO2-ATR and TELO2-mTOR interactions, which decreased the association of ATR with ATRIP, and mTOR with Raptor and Rictor [118]. These findings have important implications on overall cell metabolism. ATR-ATRIP interact with RPA on ssDNA to initiate cell cycle arrest [120]. mTOR and Raptor are part of the mTORC1 complex, which is involved in cell growth and proliferation, and mTOR and Rictor are part of the mTORC2 complex, which is involved in cell survival (Figure 4) [121]. Hsp90 inhibition coupled with glutaminase inhibition has been shown to be an effective therapeutic strategy against mTORC1-driven tumors [122]. Furthermore, Hsp90 inhibition also interfered with TELO2-ATM and TELO2-DNA-PKcs interactions [118]. Similar to ATR and mTOR, ATM and DNA-PKcs interactions with TELO2 may mediate ATM-MRN and DNA-PKcs-Ku70/Ku80 interactions. The ATM-MRN and DNA-PKcs-Ku70/Ku80 complexes are both involved in DNA double-strand break repair (Figure 4) [123–126].

5.2. Role of R2TP-TTT in PIKK Complex Assembly

In addition to Hsp90, the RUVBL1/2 complex also functions as a TTT cochaperone. The mechanism of RUVBL1/2-mediated mTORC1 complex assembly and activation has recently been elucidated. The cryo-EM structure of the human R2TP-TTT complex shows that TTT binds simultaneously with DII domains from consecutive RUVBL1 and RUVBL2 subunits of the RUVBL1/2 hexameric ring [127]. RUVBL1/2 and TTT cooperate to recruit mTOR to the complex. In vitro binding experiments showed that the human TTT complex coprecipitates with a mTOR C-terminal fragment, and the RUVBL1/2 complex coprecipitates with an mTOR N-terminal fragment [127]. Although TTT complex binding to RUVBL1/2 inhibited RUVBL1/2 ATPase activity in vitro [127], RUVBL1 ATPase activity is essential for TTT complex formation and mTOR complex activation *in cellulo* [112]. When endogenous RUVBL1 was knocked out in $TSC2^{-/-}$ MEFs, which have high mTORC1-driven translation, and rescued with a RUVBL1 ATPase-activity deficient mutant, mTORC1 complex dimerization was inhibited [112]. RUVBL1 ATPase inhibition prevented mTOR-TELO2, TTI1-TELO2, and RUVBL1-TELO2 interactions, indicating disassembly of the RUVBL1/2-mTOR-TTT complex [112]. Interestingly, piperlongumine, a cancer therapeutic for mTORC1-addicted cells, targets RUVBL1/2 to prevent the formation of the RUVBL1/2-TTT complex [128].

Several scaffold and adaptor proteins mediate RUVBL1/2-TTT-PIKK complex assembly. WAC was identified as an adaptor between RUVBL1/2 and TTT during energy-dependent mTORC1 dimerization [108]. Co-IPs in HeLa cell lysates showed that URI1 associates with TELO2, TTI1, TTI2, Hsp90, RUVBL1, RUVBL2, RPAP3, and PIH1D1 [94], suggesting that it may bridge interactions between TTT, Hsp90, and R2TP. Moreover, PIH1D1 within the R2TP complex acts as an adaptor between RUVBL1/2 and TTT. PIH1D1 binds to two constitutively phosphorylated serine residues (S487 and S491) on TELO2 [13]. Co-IPs using TELO2 knockout MEFs rescued with TELO2 S487A and S491A mutants showed compromised association between TELO2 with PIH1D1 and RUVBL1 [13]. In addition, compared to MEF knockout cells rescued with WT TELO2, cells rescued with the TELO2 substitution mutants had a complete reduction of SMG1, a significant reduction of mTOR, and a minor reduction of ATM, ATR, and DNA-PKcs [13]. Inhibition of CK2, the kinase that phosphorylates TELO2 [13], also reduced levels of endogenous SMG1 [114]. Further analysis of the PIH1D1 binding motif, DpSDD, on TELO2 showed that it was highly conserved from yeast to humans, suggesting a mechanism by which PIH1D1 recognizes its substrates [25]. As mentioned above, the DpSDD motif is present in other proteins involved in PAQosome-mediated assembly pathways [25], including the E3 ligase UBR5, which interacts with the H/ACA ribonucleoprotein complex and regulates ribosomal RNA biogenesis [129]; RNAP II subunit RPB1, the largest subunit in the RNAP II complex; EFTUD2, the splicing component of U5 snRNP; and ECD, an adaptor protein for U5 snRNP complex assembly [130].

6. Hsp90- and R2TP-Mediated MRN Complex Stabilization

The MRN complex is involved in sensing, processing, and repairing DNA strand breaks (DSBs). The complex is comprised of the nuclease MRE11, ATPase RAD50, and PIKK scaffold NBS1 (Figure 4). During the DNA damage response, the MRN complex binds to DSBs, recruits and activates the PIKKs ATM and ATR, and facilitates DNA repair by homologous recombination and non-homologous end-joining [131–135]. Hypomorphic mutations in MRE11, NBS1, and RAD50 cause ataxia-telangiectasia-like disease [136], Nijmegen breakage syndrome [137], and Nijmegen breakage syndrome-like disorder [138], respectively. Both ataxia-telangiectasia-like disease and Nijmegen breakage syndrome are characterized by genomic instability, hypersensitivity to radiation, and increased susceptibility to cancer.

MRE11 is a conserved 70–90 kDa dimeric protein that has endo- and exonuclease activity against single- and double-stranded DNA [139–141]. MRE11 stability was shown to be dependent on its interaction with PIH1D1 [142]. PIH1D1 interacts with MRE11 at S558/S561 or S688/S689 when both serines of each site are phosphorylated, with the latter being the major binding site [142]. Cells expressing MRE11 mutated at S688/S689 had reduced levels of stable MRE11 compared to WT cells [142]. In addition, RPE1, U2OS, and HCT116 cells treated with siRNA against *PIH1D1* had reduced levels of MRE11 and slightly reduced levels of RAD50 and NBS1 [142].

RAD50 is a 150 kDa protein that contains an ABC-type ATPase domain that binds and unwinds dsDNA termini [143,144]. Hsp90 ATPase activity is essential for RAD50 expression [145]. HO-8910 ovarian cancer cells treated with 17-AAG had significantly reduced levels of RAD50 [145]. Hsp90 is also important for RAD50-mediated BRCA1 recruitment to DSBs. BRCA1, a tumor suppressor protein linked to breast and ovarian cancer, interacts with RAD50 in vitro and in vivo and co-localizes with RAD50, MRE11, and NBS1 in irradiation-induced foci [146]. In MCF7 breast cancer cells, 17-AAG decreased BRCA1 protein levels in a dose- and time-dependent manner and impaired irradiation-induced homologous recombination and non-homologous end joining [147].

NBS1 is an 85 kDa protein containing two BRCT domains that bind pSDpTD motifs on interacting proteins, including repair and checkpoint proteins at DSBs [148,149]. Hsp90α stabilizes NBS1 and ATM, but not MRE11 and RAD50 [150]. Hsp90 also stabilizes the interaction between NBS1 and ATM and is needed for MRN translocation to nuclear foci after irradiation [151]. Upon irradiation-induced ATM activation, ATM phosphorylates both NBS1 and Hsp90α, and pNBS1 dissociates from pHsp90 and translocates to DSBs [150,152]. When PIKKs phosphorylate Hsp90 at Thr 7, Hsp90α also translocates to DSBs [153]. By contrast, another study showed that when ATM phosphorylates Hsp90 at Thr 5 and Thr 7, Hsp90α is not significantly recruited to DSBs [150]. In addition to regulating Hsp90 localization, Hsp90 phosphorylation is essential for MRN stabilization since Cdc7-Dbf4-mediated phosphorylation of S164 on Hsp90 was required for stabilizing the Hsp90-TELO2-MRN complex and resulted in enhanced ATM/ATR signaling [154].

7. Hsp90- and R2TP-Mediated TSC Complex Stabilization

The TSC complex, comprising of tumor-suppressor proteins TSC1, TSC2, and TBC1D7, inhibits the mTORC1 complex, which controls cell growth and proliferation (Figure 4) [155]. Loss-of-function mutations in TSC1 or TSC2 have been linked to tuberous sclerosis, a rare genetic disorder that causes tumor growth in multiple organs and neurological symptoms [156]. Within the TSC complex, TSC1 binds and stabilizes both TSC2 and TBC1D7 [157–159]. To inactivate mTORC1, TSC2, which contains a GAP domain, catalyzes the conversion of Rheb-GTP to Rheb-GDP [160,161].

TSC1 was reported to be an Hsp90 cochaperone that inhibits Hsp90 ATPase activity (Figure 4) [162]. TSC1 enables TSC2 binding to Hsp90, which prevents TSC2 ubiquitin-mediated proteasomal degradation [162]. TSC1 binding to Hsp90 was also important for stability and activity of kinase client proteins such as c-Src, CDK4, and Ulk1, as well as non-kinase client proteins such as glucocorticoid receptor and folliculin [162]. In bladder cancer cells, TSC1 facilitated Hsp90 acetylation at K407/K419, which increased its binding affinity for Hsp90 inhibitor ganetespib [163]. In contrast to bladder cancer cells, however, CAL-72 and PEER cells, which have a complete loss of TSC1 and reduced TSC2 expression, were also sensitized to ganetespib with IC_{50} values of 22 and 3 nM, respectively [164]. In addition, hepatocellular cancer cell lines SNU-398, SNU-878, and SNU-886, which have a complete loss of TSC2 and normal TSC1 expression, had IC_{50} values of 9, 14, and 35 nM, respectively [164]. Nevertheless, these findings show that TSC1 and TSC2 influence Hsp90 activity.

The TSC complex may be stabilized through the PAQosome. Co-IP experiments in HeLa cells showed that FLAG-tagged URI1 and RPAP3 interacted with endogenous TSC1 and TSC2 [58]. TAP-MS of each TSC complex subunit demonstrated high confidence interactions with RUVBL1, RUVBL2, RPAP3, PIH1D1, WDR92, and URI1 [58]. A SILAC proteomic analysis using the N-terminal domain of PIH1D1 showed that it associated with all three subunits of the TSC complex [59]. The significance of these interactions is unknown. The PAQosome may act as a loading dock that stabilizes each TSC subunit before combining them into a single complex. Moreover, the PAQosome may scaffold TSC1, to regulate Hsp90 ATPase activity, or it may scaffold TSC2, to facilitate loading onto Hsp90 [162].

8. Axonemal Dynein Arm Assembly

Motile cilia are small microtubule-based organelles required for fluid transport and cell motility in many organisms. In humans, motile cilia are essential for the generation of left-right asymmetry during embryonic development, sperm motility, and the movement of fluid in the respiratory tract, brain ventricular system, and oviducts [165]. Motile cilia contain a 9 + 2 axoneme comprised of nine outer doublet microtubules and a pair of central microtubules. Between each outer doublet, there are several multiprotein complexes, which include the inner dynein arms (IDA) and outer dynein arms (ODA). Dynein is a AAA+ ATPase that mediates microtubule sliding and subsequent ciliary movement [166]. Before being incorporated into the axoneme, dynein arms are preassembled in the cytoplasm [167,168].

8.1. DNAAFs Form Complexes with Hsp90

DNAAFs were discovered through genetic analyses of families with primary ciliary dyskinesia and mutation studies in animals [168–179]. Although most of their functions are still being investigated, it is clear that DNAAFs work together with Hsp90 to mediate IDA and ODA assembly [180]. DNAAF2, DNAAF4, DNAAF6, and DNAAF11 have domains that associate with Hsp90, including PIH1, CS, and TPR domains, while DNAAF1, DNAAF3, DNAAF5, and DNAAF7 lack Hsp90 association domains.

In vertebrates, the PIH1 domain is present in at least four proteins: DNAAF2, DNAAF6, PIH1D1, and PIH1D2 [181–183]. Each protein has been shown to be involved in ciliary dynein arm assembly [182]. DNAAF2 and DNAAF6 each contain an N-terminal PIH1 domain followed by a CS domain. In mouse testis extracts, DNAAF2 coprecipitated with Hsp70 but not Hsp90 [175], whereas DNAAF6 coprecipitated with both Hsp70 and Hsp90 [181]. In addition, a yeast two-hybrid analysis showed that DNAAF6 interacts with Hsp90, DNAAF2, and DNAAF4 [176].

DNAAF4 contains a C-terminal TPR domain, and a yeast two-hybrid screen showed that it interacts with Hsp70 and Hsp90 C-termini via the EEVD motif that binds TPR domains [184]. These interactions were confirmed through coprecipitation experiments in mouse trachea tissues [177]. In addition, DNAAF4 coprecipitated with DNAAF2 in HEK293 cells [177]. Based on their domains, DNAAF2 and DNAAF4 may form R2TP-like complexes that mediate Hsp90 involvement in dynein arm assembly (Figure 5) [26]. Moreover, TTC12 has recently emerged as another dynein arm assembly factor, and it contains a stretch of three TPR domains [185], suggesting that it may also be involved in forming R2TP-like complexes.

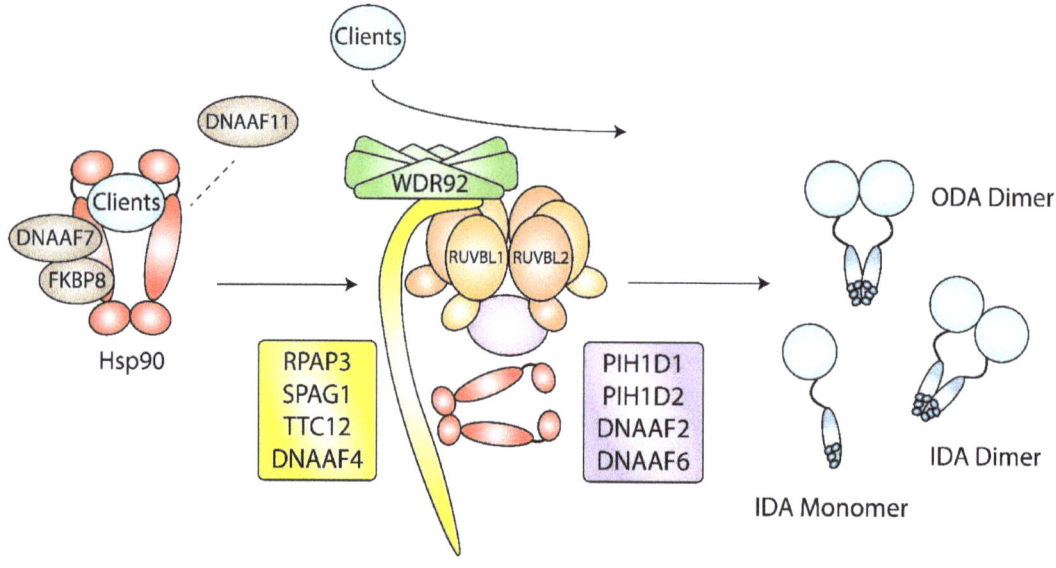

Figure 5. Hsp90- and R2TP/R2TP-like complex-mediated dynein arm assembly. During dynein arm assembly, DNAAF7 and FKBP8 act as Hsp90 cochaperones that are required for the folding of dynein arm clients. DNAAF11 may be needed for client release from Hsp90 to WDR92, R2TP, and R2TP-like complexes. Other clients may not require Hsp90 for folding and may interact with WDR92, R2TP, and R2TP-like complexes directly. R2TP-like complexes contain the RUVBL1/2 hexamer and may have a combination of RPAP3-like (yellow) and PIH1D1-like (purple) proteins. IDA, inner dynein arm; ODA; outer dynein arm.

DNAAF1 and DNAAF7, which lack Hsp90 binding domains, have been linked to Hsp90. Streptavidin-II/FLAG tandem affinity purification coupled with mass spectrometry (SF-TAP/MS) experiments using HEK293 lysates showed that DNAAF1 associates with several Hsps, including Hsp70 and Hsp90 [186]. Although DNAAF7 lacks an Hsp90 binding domain, endogenous DNAAF7 coprecipitations from P30 mouse testes, P7 mouse oviducts, and primary ciliated HEK293 cells revealed the presence of Hsp90 [187]. Hsp90 may have an indirect interaction with DNAAF7 through FKBP8, an immunophilin belonging to the FK506-binding protein family, thereby forming a DNAAF7-FKBP8-Hsp90 complex. FKBP8 contains a TPR domain that interacts with Hsp90 [188], and it was present in endogenous DNAAF7 coprecipitations from P30 mouse testes and differentiating human tracheal epithelial cultures [187]. There have been no reports linking DNAAF3 and DNAAF5 to Hsp90. Aside from it being essential for dynein arm assembly, little is known about DNAAF3 function, but it may have a role similar to DNAAF1 and DNAAF2 [168]. Coprecipitation experiments using human bronchial epithelial tissues showed that DNAAF5 does not interact with Hsp70 or Hsp90 [169].

DNAAF11 (formerly named LRRC6) is another essential protein for dynein arm assembly [189,190]. HEK293T cells co-expressing DNAAF7 and DNAAF11 and treated with protein synthesis inhibitor cycloheximide for 48 h had 44.4% of its DNAAF11 remaining, while DNAAF11 expressed alone had 7.8% remaining [191], indicating that DNAAF7 is needed to stabilize DNAAF11. DNAAF11 may interact with Hsp90 directly through its CS domain, or indirectly through its interactors DNAAF7 and RUVBL2 [173,178,187,192]. To release client proteins from Hsp90, p23 binding and ATP hydrolysis is required [193]. Thus, DNAAF11 binding to Hsp90 may promote the release of dynein arms from DNAAF7-FKBP8-Hsp90 to other chaperone complexes, including R2TP and R2TP-like complexes (Figure 5) [187].

8.2. R2TP and R2TP-like Complexes Are Dynein Arm Assembly Factors

The R2TP complex may be involved in late-stage dynein arm assembly. Similar to DNAAFs, the catalytic components of R2TP, RUVBL1 and RUVBL2, were demonstrated to be involved in dynein arm assembly through mutational analyses in animal models. Inducible deletion of RUVBL1 in mouse oviducts resulted in the absence of outer dynein arms and the appearance of undefined protein clusters [194]. Streptavidin-II/FLAG tandem affinity purification (SF-TAP) using HEK293 cell lysates showed that DNAAF1 interacts with RUVBL1 and RUVBL2, and that the RUVBL1 interaction was reduced with mutant DNAAF1 [186]. RUVBL1 knockdown in hTERT-RPE1 cells showed increased co-localization between intraflagellar transport protein IFT1 and DNAAF1, suggesting that RUVBL1 mediates DNAAF1 transport or localization [186]. In zebrafish, RUVBL1 and RUVBL2 are enriched in cytoplasmic puncta in zebrafish ciliated tissues, and cilia motility is lost in zebrafish with either RUVBL1 or RUVBL2 mutants [192,195]. RUVBL2 interacts with DNAAF11, which has a similar domain composition to DNAAF1 [192]. The RUVBL2-DNAAF11 complex was essential for dynein arm assembly in zebrafish [192]. Altogether, these findings suggest the presence of cytoplasmic R2TP-like complexes that mediate dynein arm assembly.

In a conditional mouse model, loss of RUVBL1 resulted in immotile spermatozoa due to reduced ODA components, DNAI1 and DNAI2 [195]. In mouse testes, RUVBL2 interacted with Hsp90, suggesting that RUVBL2 scaffolds DNAI1 and DNAI2 to Hsp90 [195]. RUVBL1 may also scaffold IDA and ODA components to Hsp90 through the R2TP-like complex R2SP, comprising of RUVBL1, RUVBL2, SPAG1, and PIH1D2 [196]. Both SPAG1 and RPAP3 contain RPAP3_C and TPR domains, while PIH1D1 and PIH1D2 both contain N-terminal PIH1 and C-terminal CS domains. In zebrafish, SPAG1 null mutations resulted in dorsal body curvature and hydrocephalus, indications of primary ciliary dyskinesia [197], while double-null mutations in PIH1D2 and DNAAF2 resulted in abnormal sperm motility [182]. RUVBL2, SPAG1, and PIH1D2 were found to be ubiquitously expressed in all human tissues and had moderate to high enrichment in the testes [196]. The R2SP complex was shown to facilitate the formation of liprin-α2 complexes [196], which are involved in synaptic vesicle release [198]. Interestingly, PIH1 domain-containing proteins DNAAF2 and DNAAF6 were also enriched in the testes, suggesting the presence of multiple R2TP-like complexes [196].

In addition to R2TP and R2TP-like complexes, proper dynein arm assembly requires WDR92 (recently renamed DNAAF10), which is also highly expressed in human testes [199].

In *Chlamydomonas*, experiments using insertion and truncation mutants showed that WDR92 is needed to stabilize ODA and IDA heavy chains during preassembly [200,201]. Co-IPs using HEK293 cells and in vitro pulldowns showed that WDR92 interacts directly with RPAP3 [200,202], suggesting that a WDR92-R2TP complex is needed for proper dynein arm assembly (Figure 5). In addition, *Drosophila* WDR92 was shown to interact with CG18472, the closest *Drosophila* orthologue of human SPAG1 [197,203]. A proteomic analysis also supports a possible interaction between human WDR92 and SPAG1 [58]. These findings suggest the possibility of a WDR92-R2SP complex.

RUVBL1 and RUVBL2 were recently demonstrated to be involved in the synthesis of cytoplasmic cilia, in which the axoneme is exposed to the cytoplasm [204,205]. Cytoplasmic cilia are found in male gametes, including human and *Drosophila* sperm. While investigating *Drosophila* spermiogenesis, Fingerhut and colleagues identified a novel RNP granule located at the axoneme distal end, the site of ciliogenesis [205]. The RNP granule contained RUVBL1 and RUVBL2, as well as mRNA that encodes axonemal dynein arms. By localizing translation, dynein arms can be integrated into the axoneme directly from the cytoplasm. RUVBL1 and RUVBL2 were essential for dynein arm integration and subsequent spermatozoa motility. Similar to their involvement with other RNPs, RUVBL1 and RUVBL2 were also essential for RNP granule formation [205].

9. Concluding Remarks

These studies demonstrate that Hsp90 and R2TP have many diverse and essential roles in macromolecular complex assembly that often complement each other. Before complex assembly, Hsp90 initiates subunit expression (e.g., RAD50, TERT transcription) and regulates RNA levels (e.g., U3 snoRNA, U4 snRNA). During complex assembly, Hsp90 stabilizes clients that compose multisubunit complexes (e.g., L7Ae proteins 15.5K, NHP2, SBP2; RNAP subunits RPA1, RPB1, RPC1; PIKK proteins ATM, ATR, DNA-PKcs, mTOR, SMG-1, TRRAP), while R2TP mediates important interactions between Hsp90 and clients (e.g., Hsp90-RPB1), adaptors and clients (e.g., TELO2-mTOR, TELO2-ATR), and complex subunits (e.g., 15.5K-NOP56, 15.5K-NOP58). After complex assembly, Hsp90 is critical for the function of some complexes (e.g., telomerase elongation, MRN-mediated recruitment of BRCA1 to DSBs), and R2TP together with its associated prefoldin-like module are involved in the localization of assembled protein complexes (i.e., R2TP-mediated Cajal body and nucleolar localization of snoRNPs, URI1-mediated nuclear localization of RNAP II). Thus, in addition to the canonical role of Hsp90 in client stabilization, these findings highlight the additional roles of Hsp90, together with R2TP, in quaternary complex assembly. Determining how Hsp90 integrates its clients into multiprotein complexes may facilitate the discovery of novel therapeutic drug targets. For example, inhibiting Hsp90-mediated TELO2-mTOR interactions may be an effective adjuvant against mTORC1-driven tumors. Thus, the role of Hsp90 during complex assembly and how it functions with its chaperones and cochaperones, especially TTT and R2TP, should be further investigated.

Author Contributions: Conceptualization, J.L. and W.A.H.; writing—original draft preparation, J.L.; writing—review and editing, W.A.H.; visualization, J.L.; supervision, W.A.H.; funding acquisition, W.A.H. All authors have read and agreed to the published version of the manuscript.

Funding: Research in the PI's lab on this project is funded by the Canadian Institutes of Health Research project grant (PJT-173491). The APC was funded by Canadian Institutes of Health Research project grant (PJT-173491).

Institutional Review Board Statement: Not applicable.

Informed Consent Statement: Not applicable.

Data Availability Statement: Not applicable.

Acknowledgments: J.L. held an Ontario Graduate Scholarship (2019–2020) and currently holds a fellowship from the Centre for Pharmaceutical Oncology at the University of Toronto (2021–2022).

The work in WAH's group on this subject is supported by the Canadian Institutes of Health Research project grant (PJT-173491).

Conflicts of Interest: The authors declare no conflict of interest.

References

1. Gupta, R.S. Phylogenetic analysis of the 90 kD heat shock family of protein sequences and an examination of the relationship among animals, plants, and fungi species. *Mol. Biol. Evol.* **1995**, *12*, 1063–1073. [CrossRef]
2. Prodromou, C.; Roe, S.M.; O'Brien, R.; Ladbury, J.E.; Piper, P.W.; Pearl, L.H. Identification and structural characterization of the ATP/ADP-binding site in the Hsp90 molecular chaperone. *Cell* **1997**, *90*, 65–75. [CrossRef]
3. Harris, S.F.; Shiau, A.K.; Agard, D.A. The crystal structure of the carboxy-terminal dimerization domain of htpG, the Escherichia coli Hsp90, reveals a potential substrate binding site. *Structure* **2004**, *12*, 1087–1097. [CrossRef] [PubMed]
4. Schopf, F.H.; Biebl, M.M.; Buchner, J. The HSP90 chaperone machinery. *Nat. Rev. Mol. Cell Biol.* **2017**, *18*, 345–360. [CrossRef] [PubMed]
5. Gragerov, A.; Zeng, L.; Zhao, X.; Burkholder, W.; Gottesman, M.E. Specificity of DnaK-peptide binding. *J. Mol. Biol.* **1994**, *235*, 848–854. [CrossRef]
6. Rudiger, S.; Germeroth, L.; Schneider-Mergener, J.; Bukau, B. Substrate specificity of the DnaK chaperone determined by screening cellulose-bound peptide libraries. *EMBO J.* **1997**, *16*, 1501–1507. [CrossRef] [PubMed]
7. Chen, S.; Smith, D.F. Hop as an adaptor in the heat shock protein 70 (Hsp70) and hsp90 chaperone machinery. *J. Biol. Chem.* **1998**, *273*, 35194–35200. [CrossRef] [PubMed]
8. Zhao, R.; Davey, M.; Hsu, Y.C.; Kaplanek, P.; Tong, A.; Parsons, A.B.; Krogan, N.; Cagney, G.; Mai, D.; Greenblatt, J.; et al. Navigating the chaperone network: An integrative map of physical and genetic interactions mediated by the hsp90 chaperone. *Cell* **2005**, *120*, 715–727. [CrossRef] [PubMed]
9. Boulon, S.; Marmier-Gourrier, N.; Pradet-Balade, B.; Wurth, L.; Verheggen, C.; Jady, B.E.; Rothe, B.; Pescia, C.; Robert, M.C.; Kiss, T.; et al. The Hsp90 chaperone controls the biogenesis of L7Ae RNPs through conserved machinery. *J. Cell Biol.* **2008**, *180*, 579–595. [CrossRef] [PubMed]
10. Machado-Pinilla, R.; Liger, D.; Leulliot, N.; Meier, U.T. Mechanism of the AAA+ ATPases pontin and reptin in the biogenesis of H/ACA RNPs. *RNA* **2012**, *18*, 1833–1845. [CrossRef] [PubMed]
11. Zhao, R.; Kakihara, Y.; Gribun, A.; Huen, J.; Yang, G.; Khanna, M.; Costanzo, M.; Brost, R.L.; Boone, C.; Hughes, T.R.; et al. Molecular chaperone Hsp90 stabilizes Pih1/Nop17 to maintain R2TP complex activity that regulates snoRNA accumulation. *J. Cell Biol.* **2008**, *180*, 563–578. [CrossRef] [PubMed]
12. Boulon, S.; Pradet-Balade, B.; Verheggen, C.; Molle, D.; Boireau, S.; Georgieva, M.; Azzag, K.; Robert, M.C.; Ahmad, Y.; Neel, H.; et al. HSP90 and its R2TP/Prefoldin-like cochaperone are involved in the cytoplasmic assembly of RNA polymerase II. *Mol. Cell* **2010**, *39*, 912–924. [CrossRef] [PubMed]
13. Horejsi, Z.; Takai, H.; Adelman, C.A.; Collis, S.J.; Flynn, H.; Maslen, S.; Skehel, J.M.; de Lange, T.; Boulton, S.J. CK2 phospho-dependent binding of R2TP complex to TEL2 is essential for mTOR and SMG1 stability. *Mol. Cell* **2010**, *39*, 839–850. [CrossRef]
14. Cloutier, P.; Al-Khoury, R.; Lavallee-Adam, M.; Faubert, D.; Jiang, H.; Poitras, C.; Bouchard, A.; Forget, D.; Blanchette, M.; Coulombe, B. High-resolution mapping of the protein interaction network for the human transcription machinery and affinity purification of RNA polymerase II-associated complexes. *Methods* **2009**, *48*, 381–386. [CrossRef] [PubMed]
15. Cloutier, P.; Poitras, C.; Faubert, D.; Bouchard, A.; Blanchette, M.; Gauthier, M.S.; Coulombe, B. Upstream ORF-Encoded ASDURF Is a Novel Prefoldin-like Subunit of the PAQosome. *J. Proteome Res.* **2020**, *19*, 18–27. [CrossRef] [PubMed]
16. Jeronimo, C.; Forget, D.; Bouchard, A.; Li, Q.; Chua, G.; Therien, C.; Bergeron, D.; Bourassa, S.; Greenblatt, J.; et al. Systematic analysis of the protein interaction network for the human transcription machinery reveals the identity of the 7SK capping enzyme. *Mol. Cell* **2007**, *27*, 262–274. [CrossRef]
17. Houry, W.A.; Bertrand, E.; Coulombe, B. The PAQosome, an R2TP-Based Chaperone for Quaternary Structure Formation. *Trends Biochem. Sci.* **2018**, *43*, 4–9. [CrossRef] [PubMed]
18. Patel-King, R.S.; King, S.M. A prefoldin-associated WD-repeat protein (WDR92) is required for the correct architectural assembly of motile cilia. *Mol. Biol. Cell* **2016**, *27*, 1204–1209. [CrossRef] [PubMed]
19. Lynham, J.; Houry, W.A. The Multiple Functions of the PAQosome: An R2TP- and URI1 Prefoldin-Based Chaperone Complex. *Adv. Exp. Med. Biol.* **2018**, *1106*, 37–72. [CrossRef] [PubMed]
20. Miron-Garcia, M.C.; Garrido-Godino, A.I.; Garcia-Molinero, V.; Hernandez-Torres, F.; Rodriguez-Navarro, S.; Navarro, F. The prefoldin bud27 mediates the assembly of the eukaryotic RNA polymerases in an rpb5-dependent manner. *PLoS Genet.* **2013**, *9*, e1003297. [CrossRef] [PubMed]
21. Mita, P.; Savas, J.N.; Ha, S.; Djouder, N.; Yates, J.R., 3rd; Logan, S.K. Analysis of URI nuclear interaction with RPB5 and components of the R2TP/prefoldin-like complex. *PLoS ONE* **2013**, *8*, e63879. [CrossRef] [PubMed]
22. Seraphim, T.V.; Nano, N.; Cheung, Y.W.S.; Aluksanasuwan, S.; Colleti, C.; Mao, Y.Q.; Bhandari, V.; Young, G.; Holl, L.; Phanse, S.; et al. Assembly principles of the human R2TP chaperone complex reveal the presence of R2T and R2P complexes. *Structure* **2022**, *30*, 156–171.e112. [CrossRef] [PubMed]

23. Henri, J.; Chagot, M.E.; Bourguet, M.; Abel, Y.; Terral, G.; Maurizy, C.; Aigueperse, C.; Georgescauld, F.; Vandermoere, F.; Saint-Fort, R.; et al. Deep Structural Analysis of RPAP3 and PIH1D1, Two Components of the HSP90 Co-chaperone R2TP Complex. *Structure* **2018**, *26*, 1196–1209.e1198. [CrossRef] [PubMed]
24. Martino, F.; Pal, M.; Munoz-Hernandez, H.; Rodriguez, C.F.; Nunez-Ramirez, R.; Gil-Carton, D.; Degliesposti, G.; Skehel, J.M.; Roe, S.M.; Prodromou, C.; et al. RPAP3 provides a flexible scaffold for coupling HSP90 to the human R2TP co-chaperone complex. *Nat. Commun.* **2018**, *9*, 1501. [CrossRef]
25. Horejsi, Z.; Stach, L.; Flower, T.G.; Joshi, D.; Flynn, H.; Skehel, J.M.; O'Reilly, N.J.; Ogrodowicz, R.W.; Smerdon, S.J.; Boulton, S.J. Phosphorylation-dependent PIH1D1 interactions define substrate specificity of the R2TP cochaperone complex. *Cell Rep.* **2014**, *7*, 19–26. [CrossRef] [PubMed]
26. Pal, M.; Morgan, M.; Phelps, S.E.; Roe, S.M.; Parry-Morris, S.; Downs, J.A.; Polier, S.; Pearl, L.H.; Prodromou, C. Structural basis for phosphorylation-dependent recruitment of Tel2 to Hsp90 by Pih1. *Structure* **2014**, *22*, 805–818. [CrossRef]
27. Munoz-Hernandez, H.; Pal, M.; Rodriguez, C.F.; Fernandez-Leiro, R.; Prodromou, C.; Pearl, L.H.; Llorca, O. Structural mechanism for regulation of the AAA-ATPases RUVBL1-RUVBL2 in the R2TP co-chaperone revealed by cryo-EM. *Sci. Adv.* **2019**, *5*, eaaw1616. [CrossRef] [PubMed]
28. Jimenez, B.; Ugwu, F.; Zhao, R.; Orti, L.; Makhnevych, T.; Pineda-Lucena, A.; Houry, W.A. Structure of minimal tetratricopeptide repeat domain protein Tah1 reveals mechanism of its interaction with Pih1 and Hsp90. *J. Biol. Chem.* **2012**, *287*, 5698–5709. [CrossRef]
29. Millson, S.H.; Vaughan, C.K.; Zhai, C.; Ali, M.M.; Panaretou, B.; Piper, P.W.; Pearl, L.H.; Prodromou, C. Chaperone ligand-discrimination by the TPR-domain protein Tah1. *Biochem. J.* **2008**, *413*, 261–268. [CrossRef] [PubMed]
30. Back, R.; Dominguez, C.; Rothe, B.; Bobo, C.; Beaufils, C.; Morera, S.; Meyer, P.; Charpentier, B.; Branlant, C.; Allain, F.H.; et al. High-resolution structural analysis shows how Tah1 tethers Hsp90 to the R2TP complex. *Structure* **2013**, *21*, 1834–1847. [CrossRef]
31. Rivera-Calzada, A.; Pal, M.; Munoz-Hernandez, H.; Luque-Ortega, J.R.; Gil-Carton, D.; Degliesposti, G.; Skehel, J.M.; Prodromou, C.; Pearl, L.H.; Llorca, O. The Structure of the R2TP Complex Defines a Platform for Recruiting Diverse Client Proteins to the HSP90 Molecular Chaperone System. *Structure* **2017**, *25*, 1145–1152.e1144. [CrossRef] [PubMed]
32. Tian, S.; Yu, G.; He, H.; Zhao, Y.; Liu, P.; Marshall, A.G.; Demeler, B.; Stagg, S.M.; Li, H. Pih1p-Tah1p Puts a Lid on Hexameric AAA+ ATPases Rvb1/2p. *Structure* **2017**, *25*, 1519–1529.e1514. [CrossRef]
33. Filipowicz, W.; Pelczar, P.; Pogacic, V.; Dragon, F. Structure and biogenesis of small nucleolar RNAs acting as guides for ribosomal RNA modification. *Acta Biochim. Pol.* **1999**, *46*, 377–389. [CrossRef]
34. Borovjagin, A.V.; Gerbi, S.A. U3 small nucleolar RNA is essential for cleavage at sites 1, 2 and 3 in pre-rRNA and determines which rRNA processing pathway is taken in Xenopus oocytes. *J. Mol. Biol.* **1999**, *286*, 1347–1363. [CrossRef] [PubMed]
35. Dutca, L.M.; Gallagher, J.E.; Baserga, S.J. The initial U3 snoRNA: Pre-rRNA base pairing interaction required for pre-18S rRNA folding revealed by in vivo chemical probing. *Nucleic Acids Res.* **2011**, *39*, 5164–5180. [CrossRef]
36. Jady, B.E.; Kiss, T. A small nucleolar guide RNA functions both in 2'-O-ribose methylation and pseudouridylation of the U5 spliceosomal RNA. *EMBO J.* **2001**, *20*, 541–551. [CrossRef] [PubMed]
37. Tycowski, K.T.; You, Z.H.; Graham, P.J.; Steitz, J.A. Modification of U6 spliceosomal RNA is guided by other small RNAs. *Mol. Cell* **1998**, *2*, 629–638. [CrossRef]
38. Ganot, P.; Bortolin, M.-L.; Kiss, T. Site-Specific Pseudouridine Formation in Preribosomal RNA Is Guided by Small Nucleolar RNAs. *Cell* **1997**, *89*, 799–809. [CrossRef]
39. Aittaleb, M.; Rashid, R.; Chen, Q.; Palmer, J.R.; Daniels, C.J.; Li, H. Structure and function of archaeal box C/D sRNP core proteins. *Nat. Struct. Biol.* **2003**, *10*, 256–263. [CrossRef] [PubMed]
40. Cahill, N.M.; Friend, K.; Speckmann, W.; Li, Z.H.; Terns, R.M.; Terns, M.P.; Steitz, J.A. Site-specific cross-linking analyses reveal an asymmetric protein distribution for a box C/D snoRNP. *EMBO J.* **2002**, *21*, 3816–3828. [CrossRef]
41. Lin, J.; Lai, S.; Jia, R.; Xu, A.; Zhang, L.; Lu, J.; Ye, K. Structural basis for site-specific ribose methylation by box C/D RNA protein complexes. *Nature* **2011**, *469*, 559–563. [CrossRef]
42. Qu, G.; van Nues, R.W.; Watkins, N.J.; Maxwell, E.S. The spatial-functional coupling of box C/D and C'/D' RNPs is an evolutionarily conserved feature of the eukaryotic box C/D snoRNP nucleotide modification complex. *Mol. Cell Biol.* **2011**, *31*, 365–374. [CrossRef]
43. Nottrott, S.; Hartmuth, K.; Fabrizio, P.; Urlaub, H.; Vidovic, I.; Ficner, R.; Luhrmann, R. Functional interaction of a novel 15.5kD [U4/U6.U5] tri-snRNP protein with the 5' stem-loop of U4 snRNA. *EMBO J.* **1999**, *18*, 6119–6133. [CrossRef]
44. Watkins, N.J.; Segault, V.; Charpentier, B.; Nottrott, S.; Fabrizio, P.; Bachi, A.; Wilm, M.; Rosbash, M.; Branlant, C.; Luhrmann, R. A common core RNP structure shared between the small nucleoar box C/D RNPs and the spliceosomal U4 snRNP. *Cell* **2000**, *103*, 457–466. [CrossRef]
45. Watkins, N.J.; Dickmanns, A.; Luhrmann, R. Conserved stem II of the box C/D motif is essential for nucleolar localization and is required, along with the 15.5K protein, for the hierarchical assembly of the box C/D snoRNP. *Mol. Cell Biol.* **2002**, *22*, 8342–8352. [CrossRef]
46. Gautier, T.; Berges, T.; Tollervey, D.; Hurt, E. Nucleolar KKE/D repeat proteins Nop56p and Nop58p interact with Nop1p and are required for ribosome biogenesis. *Mol. Cell Biol.* **1997**, *17*, 7088–7098. [CrossRef] [PubMed]
47. Liu, S.; Li, P.; Dybkov, O.; Nottrott, S.; Hartmuth, K.; Luhrmann, R.; Carlomagno, T.; Wahl, M.C. Binding of the human Prp31 Nop domain to a composite RNA-protein platform in U4 snRNP. *Science* **2007**, *316*, 115–120. [CrossRef]

48. Stebbins, C.E.; Russo, A.A.; Schneider, C.; Rosen, N.; Hartl, F.U.; Pavletich, N.P. Crystal structure of an Hsp90-geldanamycin complex: Targeting of a protein chaperone by an antitumor agent. *Cell* **1997**, *89*, 239–250. [CrossRef]
49. Abel, Y.; Paiva, A.C.F.; Bizarro, J.; Chagot, M.E.; Santo, P.E.; Robert, M.C.; Quinternet, M.; Vandermoere, F.; Sousa, P.M.F.; Fort, P.; et al. NOPCHAP1 is a PAQosome cofactor that helps loading NOP58 on RUVBL1/2 during box C/D snoRNP biogenesis. *Nucleic Acids Res.* **2021**, *49*, 1094–1113. [CrossRef]
50. Berry, M.J.; Banu, L.; Chen, Y.Y.; Mandel, S.J.; Kieffer, J.D.; Harney, J.W.; Larsen, P.R. Recognition of UGA as a selenocysteine codon in type I deiodinase requires sequences in the 3′ untranslated region. *Nature* **1991**, *353*, 273–276. [CrossRef] [PubMed]
51. Newman, D.R.; Kuhn, J.F.; Shanab, G.M.; Maxwell, E.S. Box C/D snoRNA-associated proteins: Two pairs of evolutionarily ancient proteins and possible links to replication and transcription. *RNA* **2000**, *6*, 861–879. [CrossRef]
52. Watkins, N.J.; Lemm, I.; Ingelfinger, D.; Schneider, C.; Hossbach, M.; Urlaub, H.; Luhrmann, R. Assembly and maturation of the U3 snoRNP in the nucleoplasm in a large dynamic multiprotein complex. *Mol. Cell* **2004**, *16*, 789–798. [CrossRef] [PubMed]
53. Watkins, N.J.; Lemm, I.; Luhrmann, R. Involvement of nuclear import and export factors in U8 box C/D snoRNP biogenesis. *Mol. Cell Biol.* **2007**, *27*, 7018–7027. [CrossRef]
54. Bizarro, J.; Charron, C.; Boulon, S.; Westman, B.; Pradet-Balade, B.; Vandermoere, F.; Chagot, M.E.; Hallais, M.; Ahmad, Y.; Leonhardt, H.; et al. Proteomic and 3D structure analyses highlight the C/D box snoRNP assembly mechanism and its control. *J. Cell Biol.* **2014**, *207*, 463–480. [CrossRef] [PubMed]
55. McKeegan, K.S.; Debieux, C.M.; Watkins, N.J. Evidence that the AAA+ proteins TIP48 and TIP49 bridge interactions between 15.5K and the related NOP56 and NOP58 proteins during box C/D snoRNP biogenesis. *Mol. Cell Biol.* **2009**, *29*, 4971–4981. [CrossRef]
56. McKeegan, K.S.; Debieux, C.M.; Boulon, S.; Bertrand, E.; Watkins, N.J. A dynamic scaffold of pre-snoRNP factors facilitates human box C/D snoRNP assembly. *Mol. Cell Biol.* **2007**, *27*, 6782–6793. [CrossRef]
57. Sardiu, M.E.; Cai, Y.; Jin, J.; Swanson, S.K.; Conaway, R.C.; Conaway, J.W.; Florens, L.; Washburn, M.P. Probabilistic assembly of human protein interaction networks from label-free quantitative proteomics. *Proc. Natl. Acad. Sci. USA* **2008**, *105*, 1454–1459. [CrossRef] [PubMed]
58. Cloutier, P.; Poitras, C.; Durand, M.; Hekmat, O.; Fiola-Masson, E.; Bouchard, A.; Faubert, D.; Chabot, B.; Coulombe, B. R2TP/Prefoldin-like component RUVBL1/RUVBL2 directly interacts with ZNHIT2 to regulate assembly of U5 small nuclear ribonucleoprotein. *Nat. Commun.* **2017**, *8*, 15615. [CrossRef] [PubMed]
59. Malinová, A.; Cvačková, Z.; Matějů, D.; Hořejší, Z.; Abéza, C.; Vandermoere, F.; Bertrand, E.; Staněk, D.; Verheggen, C. Assembly of the U5 snRNP component PRPF8 is controlled by the HSP90/R2TP chaperones. *J. Cell Biol.* **2017**, *216*, 1579–1596. [CrossRef] [PubMed]
60. Rothe, B.; Saliou, J.M.; Quinternet, M.; Back, R.; Tiotiu, D.; Jacquemin, C.; Loegler, C.; Schlotter, F.; Pena, V.; Eckert, K.; et al. Protein Hit1, a novel box C/D snoRNP assembly factor, controls cellular concentration of the scaffolding protein Rsa1 by direct interaction. *Nucleic Acids Res.* **2014**, *42*, 10731–10747. [CrossRef] [PubMed]
61. Wang, C.; Meier, U.T. Architecture and assembly of mammalian H/ACA small nucleolar and telomerase ribonucleoproteins. *EMBO J.* **2004**, *23*, 1857–1867. [CrossRef]
62. Dez, C.; Henras, A.; Faucon, B.; Lafontaine, D.; Caizergues-Ferrer, M.; Henry, Y. Stable expression in yeast of the mature form of human telomerase RNA depends on its association with the box H/ACA small nucleolar RNP proteins Cbf5p, Nhp2p and Nop10p. *Nucleic Acids Res.* **2001**, *29*, 598–603. [CrossRef]
63. Girard, J.P.; Lehtonen, H.; Caizergues-Ferrer, M.; Amalric, F.; Tollervey, D.; Lapeyre, B. GAR1 is an essential small nucleolar RNP protein required for pre-rRNA processing in yeast. *EMBO J.* **1992**, *11*, 673–682. [CrossRef] [PubMed]
64. Henras, A.; Henry, Y.; Bousquet-Antonelli, C.; Noaillac-Depeyre, J.; Gelugne, J.P.; Caizergues-Ferrer, M. Nhp2p and Nop10p are essential for the function of H/ACA snoRNPs. *EMBO J.* **1998**, *17*, 7078–7090. [CrossRef] [PubMed]
65. Jiang, W.; Middleton, K.; Yoon, H.J.; Fouquet, C.; Carbon, J. An essential yeast protein, CBF5p, binds in vitro to centromeres and microtubules. *Mol. Cell Biol.* **1993**, *13*, 4884–4893. [CrossRef] [PubMed]
66. Kolodrubetz, D.; Burgum, A. Sequence and genetic analysis of NHP2: A moderately abundant high mobility group-like nuclear protein with an essential function in Saccharomyces cerevisiae. *Yeast* **1991**, *7*, 79–90. [CrossRef]
67. Grozdanov, P.N.; Roy, S.; Kittur, N.; Meier, U.T. SHQ1 is required prior to NAF1 for assembly of H/ACA small nucleolar and telomerase RNPs. *RNA* **2009**, *15*, 1188–1197. [CrossRef] [PubMed]
68. Hoareau-Aveilla, C.; Bonoli, M.; Caizergues-Ferrer, M.; Henry, Y. hNaf1 is required for accumulation of human box H/ACA snoRNPs, scaRNAs, and telomerase. *RNA* **2006**, *12*, 832–840. [CrossRef] [PubMed]
69. Leulliot, N.; Godin, K.S.; Hoareau-Aveilla, C.; Quevillon-Cheruel, S.; Varani, G.; Henry, Y.; Van Tilbeurgh, H. The box H/ACA RNP assembly factor Naf1p contains a domain homologous to Gar1p mediating its interaction with Cbf5p. *J. Mol. Biol.* **2007**, *371*, 1338–1353. [CrossRef]
70. Darzacq, X.; Kittur, N.; Roy, S.; Shav-Tal, Y.; Singer, R.H.; Meier, U.T. Stepwise RNP assembly at the site of H/ACA RNA transcription in human cells. *J. Cell Biol.* **2006**, *173*, 207–218. [CrossRef]
71. Walbott, H.; Machado-Pinilla, R.; Liger, D.; Blaud, M.; Rety, S.; Grozdanov, P.N.; Godin, K.; van Tilbeurgh, H.; Varani, G.; Meier, U.T.; et al. The H/ACA RNP assembly factor SHQ1 functions as an RNA mimic. *Genes Dev.* **2011**, *25*, 2398–2408. [CrossRef] [PubMed]

72. Holt, S.E.; Aisner, D.L.; Baur, J.; Tesmer, V.M.; Dy, M.; Ouellette, M.; Trager, J.B.; Morin, G.B.; Toft, D.O.; Shay, J.W.; et al. Functional requirement of p23 and Hsp90 in telomerase complexes. *Genes Dev.* **1999**, *13*, 817–826. [CrossRef] [PubMed]
73. Godin, K.S.; Walbott, H.; Leulliot, N.; van Tilbeurgh, H.; Varani, G. The box H/ACA snoRNP assembly factor Shq1p is a chaperone protein homologous to Hsp90 cochaperones that binds to the Cbf5p enzyme. *J. Mol. Biol.* **2009**, *390*, 231–244. [CrossRef] [PubMed]
74. Morin, G.B. The human telomere terminal transferase enzyme is a ribonucleoprotein that synthesizes TTAGGG repeats. *Cell* **1989**, *59*, 521–529. [CrossRef]
75. Keppler, B.R.; Grady, A.T.; Jarstfer, M.B. The biochemical role of the heat shock protein 90 chaperone complex in establishing human telomerase activity. *J. Biol. Chem.* **2006**, *281*, 19840–19848. [CrossRef] [PubMed]
76. Forsythe, H.L.; Jarvis, J.L.; Turner, J.W.; Elmore, L.W.; Holt, S.E. Stable association of hsp90 and p23, but Not hsp70, with active human telomerase. *J. Biol. Chem.* **2001**, *276*, 15571–15574. [CrossRef] [PubMed]
77. Kim, R.H.; Kim, R.; Chen, W.; Hu, S.; Shin, K.H.; Park, N.H.; Kang, M.K. Association of hsp90 to the hTERT promoter is necessary for hTERT expression in human oral cancer cells. *Carcinogenesis* **2008**, *29*, 2425–2431. [CrossRef] [PubMed]
78. Chiu, W.T.; Shen, S.C.; Yang, L.Y.; Chow, J.M.; Wu, C.Y.; Chen, Y.C. Inhibition of HSP90-dependent telomerase activity in amyloid beta-induced apoptosis of cerebral endothelial cells. *J. Cell Physiol.* **2011**, *226*, 2041–2051. [CrossRef] [PubMed]
79. Venteicher, A.S.; Meng, Z.; Mason, P.J.; Veenstra, T.D.; Artandi, S.E. Identification of ATPases pontin and reptin as telomerase components essential for holoenzyme assembly. *Cell* **2008**, *132*, 945–957. [CrossRef] [PubMed]
80. Rappsilber, J.; Ryder, U.; Lamond, A.I.; Mann, M. Large-scale proteomic analysis of the human spliceosome. *Genome Res.* **2002**, *12*, 1231–1245. [CrossRef] [PubMed]
81. Fabrizio, P.; Dannenberg, J.; Dube, P.; Kastner, B.; Stark, H.; Urlaub, H.; Luhrmann, R. The evolutionarily conserved core design of the catalytic activation step of the yeast spliceosome. *Mol. Cell* **2009**, *36*, 593–608. [CrossRef] [PubMed]
82. Bizarro, J.; Dodre, M.; Huttin, A.; Charpentier, B.; Schlotter, F.; Branlant, C.; Verheggen, C.; Massenet, S.; Bertrand, E. NUFIP and the HSP90/R2TP chaperone bind the SMN complex and facilitate assembly of U4-specific proteins. *Nucleic Acids Res.* **2015**, *43*, 8973–8989. [CrossRef]
83. Nottrott, S.; Urlaub, H.; Luhrmann, R. Hierarchical, clustered protein interactions with U4/U6 snRNA: A biochemical role for U4/U6 proteins. *EMBO J.* **2002**, *21*, 5527–5538. [CrossRef] [PubMed]
84. Deery, E.C.; Vithana, E.N.; Newbold, R.J.; Gallon, V.A.; Bhattacharya, S.S.; Warren, M.J.; Hunt, D.M.; Wilkie, S.E. Disease mechanism for retinitis pigmentosa (RP11) caused by mutations in the splicing factor gene PRPF31. *Hum. Mol. Genet.* **2002**, *11*, 3209–3219. [CrossRef] [PubMed]
85. Serna, M.; Gonzalez-Corpas, A.; Cabezudo, S.; Lopez-Perrote, A.; Degliesposti, G.; Zarzuela, E.; Skehel, J.M.; Munoz, J.; Llorca, O. CryoEM of RUVBL1-RUVBL2-ZNHIT2, a complex that interacts with pre-mRNA-processing-splicing factor 8. *Nucleic Acids Res.* **2022**, *50*, 1128–1146. [CrossRef] [PubMed]
86. Mir, R.A.; Lovelace, J.; Schafer, N.P.; Simone, P.D.; Kellezi, A.; Kolar, C.; Spagnol, G.; Sorgen, P.L.; Band, H.; Band, V.; et al. Biophysical characterization and modeling of human Ecdysoneless (ECD) protein supports a scaffolding function. *AIMS Biophys* **2016**, *3*, 195–208. [CrossRef] [PubMed]
87. Cloutier, P.; Coulombe, B. New insights into the biogenesis of nuclear RNA polymerases? *Biochem. Cell Biol.* **2010**, *88*, 211–221. [CrossRef]
88. Forget, D.; Lacombe, A.A.; Cloutier, P.; Al-Khoury, R.; Bouchard, A.; Lavallee-Adam, M.; Faubert, D.; Jeronimo, C.; Blanchette, M.; Coulombe, B. The protein interaction network of the human transcription machinery reveals a role for the conserved GTPase RPAP4/GPN1 and microtubule assembly in nuclear import and biogenesis of RNA polymerase II. *Mol. Cell Proteom.* **2010**, *9*, 2827–2839. [CrossRef] [PubMed]
89. Nguyen, V.T.; Giannoni, F.; Dubois, M.F.; Seo, S.J.; Vigneron, M.; Kedinger, C.; Bensaude, O. In vivo degradation of RNA polymerase II largest subunit triggered by alpha-amanitin. *Nucleic Acids Res.* **1996**, *24*, 2924–2929. [CrossRef] [PubMed]
90. Maurizy, C.; Abeza, C.; Lemmers, B.; Gabola, M.; Longobardi, C.; Pinet, V.; Ferrand, M.; Paul, C.; Bremond, J.; Langa, F.; et al. The HSP90/R2TP assembly chaperone promotes cell proliferation in the intestinal epithelium. *Nat. Commun.* **2021**, *12*, 4810. [CrossRef]
91. Frischknecht, L.; Britschgi, C.; Galliker, P.; Christinat, Y.; Vichalkovski, A.; Gstaiger, M.; Kovacs, W.J.; Krek, W. BRAF inhibition sensitizes melanoma cells to alpha-amanitin via decreased RNA polymerase II assembly. *Sci. Rep.* **2019**, *9*, 7779. [CrossRef]
92. Perry, J.; Kleckner, N. The ATRs, ATMs, and TORs are giant HEAT repeat proteins. *Cell* **2003**, *112*, 151–155. [CrossRef]
93. Lavin, M.F.; Khanna, K.K.; Beamish, H.; Spring, K.; Watters, D.; Shiloh, Y. Relationship of the ataxia-telangiectasia protein ATM to phosphoinositide 3-kinase. *Trends Biochem. Sci.* **1995**, *20*, 382–383. [CrossRef]
94. Izumi, N.; Yamashita, A.; Hirano, H.; Ohno, S. Heat shock protein 90 regulates phosphatidylinositol 3-kinase-related protein kinase family proteins together with the RUVBL1/2 and Tel2-containing co-factor complex. *Cancer Sci.* **2012**, *103*, 50–57. [CrossRef] [PubMed]
95. Toullec, D.; Elias-Villalobos, A.; Faux, C.; Noly, A.; Lledo, G.; Seveno, M.; Helmlinger, D. The Hsp90 cochaperone TTT promotes cotranslational maturation of PIKKs prior to complex assembly. *Cell Rep.* **2021**, *37*, 109867. [CrossRef]
96. Hayashi, T.; Hatanaka, M.; Nagao, K.; Nakaseko, Y.; Kanoh, J.; Kokubu, A.; Ebe, M.; Yanagida, M. Rapamycin sensitivity of the *Schizosaccharomyces pombe* tor2 mutant and organization of two highly phosphorylated TOR complexes by specific and common subunits. *Genes Cells* **2007**, *12*, 1357–1370. [CrossRef] [PubMed]

97. Shevchenko, A.; Roguev, A.; Schaft, D.; Buchanan, L.; Habermann, B.; Sakalar, C.; Thomas, H.; Krogan, N.J.; Shevchenko, A.; Stewart, A.F. Chromatin Central: Towards the comparative proteome by accurate mapping of the yeast proteomic environment. *Genome Biol.* **2008**, *9*, R167. [CrossRef] [PubMed]
98. Hurov, K.E.; Cotta-Ramusino, C.; Elledge, S.J. A genetic screen identifies the Triple T complex required for DNA damage signaling and ATM and ATR stability. *Genes Dev.* **2010**, *24*, 1939–1950. [CrossRef]
99. Kim, Y.; Park, J.; Joo, S.Y.; Kim, B.G.; Jo, A.; Lee, H.; Cho, Y. Structure of the Human TELO2-TTI1-TTI2 Complex. *J. Mol. Biol.* **2022**, *434*, 167370. [CrossRef] [PubMed]
100. Ahmed, S.; Alpi, A.; Hengartner, M.O.; Gartner, A.C. Elegans RAD-5/CLK-2 defines a new DNA damage checkpoint protein. *Curr. Biol.* **2001**, *11*, 1934–1944. [CrossRef]
101. Anderson, C.M.; Korkin, D.; Smith, D.L.; Makovets, S.; Seidel, J.J.; Sali, A.; Blackburn, E.H. Tel2 mediates activation and localization of ATM/Tel1 kinase to a double-strand break. *Genes Dev.* **2008**, *22*, 854–859. [CrossRef]
102. Goto, G.H.; Ogi, H.; Biswas, H.; Ghosh, A.; Tanaka, S.; Sugimoto, K. Two separate pathways regulate protein stability of ATM/ATR-related protein kinases Mec1 and Tel1 in budding yeast. *PLoS Genet.* **2017**, *13*, e1006873. [CrossRef] [PubMed]
103. Rao, F.; Cha, J.; Xu, J.; Xu, R.; Vandiver, M.S.; Tyagi, R.; Tokhunts, R.; Koldobskiy, M.A.; Fu, C.; Barrow, R.; et al. Inositol pyrophosphates mediate the DNA-PK/ATM-p53 cell death pathway by regulating CK2 phosphorylation of Tti1/Tel2. *Mol. Cell* **2014**, *54*, 119–132. [CrossRef] [PubMed]
104. Shikata, M.; Ishikawa, F.; Kanoh, J. Tel2 is required for activation of the Mrc1-mediated replication checkpoint. *J. Biol. Chem.* **2007**, *282*, 5346–5355. [CrossRef] [PubMed]
105. Takai, H.; Wang, R.C.; Takai, K.K.; Yang, H.; de Lange, T. Tel2 regulates the stability of PI3K-related protein kinases. *Cell* **2007**, *131*, 1248–1259. [CrossRef] [PubMed]
106. Xu, Y.J.; Khan, S.; Didier, A.C.; Wozniak, M.; Liu, Y.; Singh, A.; Nakamura, T.M. A tel2 Mutation That Destabilizes the Tel2-Tti1-Tti2 Complex Eliminates Rad3(ATR) Kinase Signaling in the DNA Replication Checkpoint and Leads to Telomere Shortening in Fission Yeast. *Mol. Cell Biol.* **2019**, *39*, e00175-19. [CrossRef] [PubMed]
107. Brown, M.C.; Gromeier, M. MNK controls mTORC1: Substrate association through regulation of TELO2 binding with mTORC1. *Cell Rep.* **2017**, *18*, 1444–1457. [CrossRef] [PubMed]
108. David-Morrison, G.; Xu, Z.; Rui, Y.N.; Charng, W.L.; Jaiswal, M.; Yamamoto, S.; Xiong, B.; Zhang, K.; Sandoval, H.; Duraine, L.; et al. WAC Regulates mTOR Activity by Acting as an Adaptor for the TTT and Pontin/Reptin Complexes. *Dev. Cell* **2016**, *36*, 139–151. [CrossRef]
109. Fernández-Sáiz, V.; Targosz, B.-S.; Lemeer, S.; Eichner, R.; Langer, C.; Bullinger, L.; Reiter, C.; Slotta-Huspenina, J.; Schroeder, S.; Knorn, A.-M.; et al. SCFFbxo9 and CK2 direct the cellular response to growth factor withdrawal via Tel2/Tti1 degradation and promote survival in multiple myeloma. *Nat. Cell Biol.* **2012**, *15*, 72. [CrossRef]
110. Hoffman, K.S.; Duennwald, M.L.; Karagiannis, J.; Genereaux, J.; McCarton, A.S.; Brandl, C.J. *Saccharomyces cerevisiae* Tti2 Regulates PIKK Proteins and Stress Response. *G3* **2016**, *6*, 1649–1659. [CrossRef]
111. Kaizuka, T.; Hara, T.; Oshiro, N.; Kikkawa, U.; Yonezawa, K.; Takehana, K.; Iemura, S.; Natsume, T.; Mizushima, N. Tti1 and Tel2 are critical factors in mammalian target of rapamycin complex assembly. *J. Biol. Chem.* **2010**, *285*, 20109–20116. [CrossRef]
112. Kim, S.G.; Hoffman, G.R.; Poulogiannis, G.; Buel, G.R.; Jang, Y.J.; Lee, K.W.; Kim, B.Y.; Erikson, R.L.; Cantley, L.C.; Choo, A.Y.; et al. Metabolic stress controls mTORC1 lysosomal localization and dimerization by regulating the TTT-RUVBL1/2 complex. *Mol. Cell* **2013**, *49*, 172–185. [CrossRef]
113. Rozario, D.; Siede, W. *Saccharomyces cerevisiae* Tel2 plays roles in TORC signaling and telomere maintenance that can be mutationally separated. *Biochem. Biophys. Res. Commun.* **2012**, *417*, 1182–1187. [CrossRef]
114. Ahn, S.; Kim, J.; Hwang, J. CK2-mediated TEL2 phosphorylation augments nonsense-mediated mRNA decay (NMD) by increase of SMG1 stability. *Biochim. Biophys. Acta* **2013**, *1829*, 1047–1055. [CrossRef]
115. Guo, Y.; Tocchini, C.; Ciosk, R. CLK-2/TEL2 is a conserved component of the nonsense-mediated mRNA decay pathway. *PLoS ONE* **2021**, *16*, e0244505. [CrossRef] [PubMed]
116. Detilleux, D.; Raynaud, P.; Pradet-Balade, B.; Helmlinger, D. The TRRAP transcription cofactor represses interferon-stimulated genes in colorectal cancer cells. *Elife* **2022**, *11*, e69705. [CrossRef] [PubMed]
117. Elias-Villalobos, A.; Toullec, D.; Faux, C.; Seveno, M.; Helmlinger, D. Chaperone-mediated ordered assembly of the SAGA and NuA4 transcription co-activator complexes in yeast. *Nat. Commun.* **2019**, *10*, 5237. [CrossRef]
118. Takai, H.; Xie, Y.; de Lange, T.; Pavletich, N.P. Tel2 structure and function in the Hsp90-dependent maturation of mTOR and ATR complexes. *Genes Dev.* **2010**, *24*, 2019–2030. [CrossRef] [PubMed]
119. Izumi, N.; Yamashita, A.; Iwamatsu, A.; Kurata, R.; Nakamura, H.; Saari, B.; Hirano, H.; Anderson, P.; Ohno, S. AAA+ proteins RUVBL1 and RUVBL2 coordinate PIKK activity and function in nonsense-mediated mRNA decay. *Sci. Signal.* **2010**, *3*, ra27. [CrossRef] [PubMed]
120. Zou, L.; Elledge, S.J. Sensing DNA damage through ATRIP recognition of RPA-ssDNA complexes. *Science* **2003**, *300*, 1542–1548. [CrossRef]
121. Foster, K.G.; Fingar, D.C. Mammalian target of rapamycin (mTOR): Conducting the cellular signaling symphony. *J. Biol. Chem.* **2010**, *285*, 14071–14077. [CrossRef]
122. Li, J.; Csibi, A.; Yang, S.; Hoffman, G.R.; Li, C.; Zhang, E.; Yu, J.J.; Blenis, J. Synthetic lethality of combined glutaminase and Hsp90 inhibition in mTORC1-driven tumor cells. *Proc. Natl. Acad. Sci. USA* **2015**, *112*, E21–E29. [CrossRef] [PubMed]

123. Uziel, T.; Lerenthal, Y.; Moyal, L.; Andegeko, Y.; Mittelman, L.; Shiloh, Y. Requirement of the MRN complex for ATM activation by DNA damage. *EMBO J.* **2003**, *22*, 5612–5621. [CrossRef] [PubMed]
124. Lee, J.H.; Paull, T.T. ATM activation by DNA double-strand breaks through the Mre11-Rad50-Nbs1 complex. *Science* **2005**, *308*, 551–554. [CrossRef] [PubMed]
125. Singleton, B.K.; Torres-Arzayus, M.I.; Rottinghaus, S.T.; Taccioli, G.E.; Jeggo, P.A. The C terminus of Ku80 activates the DNA-dependent protein kinase catalytic subunit. *Mol. Cell Biol.* **1999**, *19*, 3267–3277. [CrossRef]
126. Sibanda, B.L.; Chirgadze, D.Y.; Ascher, D.B.; Blundell, T.L. DNA-PKcs structure suggests an allosteric mechanism modulating DNA double-strand break repair. *Science* **2017**, *355*, 520–524. [CrossRef]
127. Pal, M.; Munoz-Hernandez, H.; Bjorklund, D.; Zhou, L.; Degliesposti, G.; Skehel, J.M.; Hesketh, E.L.; Thompson, R.F.; Pearl, L.H.; Llorca, O.; et al. Structure of the TELO2-TTI1-TTI2 complex and its function in TOR recruitment to the R2TP chaperone. *Cell Rep.* **2021**, *36*, 109317. [CrossRef]
128. Shin, S.H.; Lee, J.S.; Zhang, J.M.; Choi, S.; Boskovic, Z.V.; Zhao, R.; Song, M.; Wang, R.; Tian, J.; Lee, M.H.; et al. Synthetic lethality by targeting the RUVBL1/2-TTT complex in mTORC1-hyperactive cancer cells. *Sci. Adv.* **2020**, *6*, eaay9131. [CrossRef]
129. Saez, I.; Gerbracht, J.V.; Koyuncu, S.; Lee, H.J.; Horn, M.; Kroef, V.; Denzel, M.S.; Dieterich, C.; Gehring, N.H.; Vilchez, D. The E3 ubiquitin ligase UBR5 interacts with the H/ACA ribonucleoprotein complex and regulates ribosomal RNA biogenesis in embryonic stem cells. *FEBS Lett.* **2020**, *594*, 175–188. [CrossRef]
130. Erkelenz, S.; Stankovic, D.; Mundorf, J.; Bresser, T.; Claudius, A.K.; Boehm, V.; Gehring, N.H.; Uhlirova, M. Ecd promotes U5 snRNP maturation and Prp8 stability. *Nucleic Acids Res.* **2021**, *49*, 1688–1707. [CrossRef]
131. Buis, J.; Wu, Y.; Deng, Y.; Leddon, J.; Westfield, G.; Eckersdorff, M.; Sekiguchi, J.M.; Chang, S.; Ferguson, D.O. Mre11 nuclease activity has essential roles in DNA repair and genomic stability distinct from ATM activation. *Cell* **2008**, *135*, 85–96. [CrossRef]
132. Milman, N.; Higuchi, E.; Smith, G.R. Meiotic DNA double-strand break repair requires two nucleases, MRN and Ctp1, to produce a single size class of Rec12 (Spo11)-oligonucleotide complexes. *Mol. Cell Biol.* **2009**, *29*, 5998–6005. [CrossRef]
133. You, Z.; Chahwan, C.; Bailis, J.; Hunter, T.; Russell, P. ATM activation and its recruitment to damaged DNA require binding to the C terminus of Nbs1. *Mol. Cell Biol.* **2005**, *25*, 5363–5379. [CrossRef] [PubMed]
134. Zhong, H.; Bryson, A.; Eckersdorff, M.; Ferguson, D.O. Rad50 depletion impacts upon ATR-dependent DNA damage responses. *Hum. Mol. Genet.* **2005**, *14*, 2685–2693. [CrossRef]
135. Zhuang, J.; Jiang, G.; Willers, H.; Xia, F. Exonuclease function of human Mre11 promotes deletional nonhomologous end joining. *J. Biol. Chem.* **2009**, *284*, 30565–30573. [CrossRef] [PubMed]
136. Stewart, G.S.; Maser, R.S.; Stankovic, T.; Bressan, D.A.; Kaplan, M.I.; Jaspers, N.G.; Raams, A.; Byrd, P.J.; Petrini, J.H.; Taylor, A.M. The DNA double-strand break repair gene hMRE11 is mutated in individuals with an ataxia-telangiectasia-like disorder. *Cell* **1999**, *99*, 577–587. [CrossRef]
137. Varon, R.; Vissinga, C.; Platzer, M.; Cerosaletti, K.M.; Chrzanowska, K.H.; Saar, K.; Beckmann, G.; Seemanova, E.; Cooper, P.R.; Nowak, N.J.; et al. Nibrin, a novel DNA double-strand break repair protein, is mutated in Nijmegen breakage syndrome. *Cell* **1998**, *93*, 467–476. [CrossRef]
138. Waltes, R.; Kalb, R.; Gatei, M.; Kijas, A.W.; Stumm, M.; Sobeck, A.; Wieland, B.; Varon, R.; Lerenthal, Y.; Lavin, M.F.; et al. Human RAD50 deficiency in a Nijmegen breakage syndrome-like disorder. *Am. J. Hum. Genet.* **2009**, *84*, 605–616. [CrossRef]
139. Paull, T.T.; Gellert, M. The 3′ to 5′ exonuclease activity of Mre 11 facilitates repair of DNA double-strand breaks. *Mol. Cell* **1998**, *1*, 969–979. [CrossRef]
140. Paull, T.T.; Gellert, M. Nbs1 potentiates ATP-driven DNA unwinding and endonuclease cleavage by the Mre11/Rad50 complex. *Genes Dev.* **1999**, *13*, 1276–1288. [CrossRef]
141. Williams, R.S.; Moncalian, G.; Williams, J.S.; Yamada, Y.; Limbo, O.; Shin, D.S.; Groocock, L.M.; Cahill, D.; Hitomi, C.; Guenther, G.; et al. Mre11 dimers coordinate DNA end bridging and nuclease processing in double-strand-break repair. *Cell* **2008**, *135*, 97–109. [CrossRef] [PubMed]
142. von Morgen, P.; Burdova, K.; Flower, T.G.; O'Reilly, N.J.; Boulton, S.J.; Smerdon, S.J.; Macurek, L.; Horejsi, Z. MRE11 stability is regulated by CK2-dependent interaction with R2TP complex. *Oncogene* **2017**, *36*, 4943–4950. [CrossRef] [PubMed]
143. de Jager, M.; van Noort, J.; van Gent, D.C.; Dekker, C.; Kanaar, R.; Wyman, C. Human Rad50/Mre11 is a flexible complex that can tether DNA ends. *Mol. Cell* **2001**, *8*, 1129–1135. [CrossRef]
144. Hopfner, K.P.; Karcher, A.; Shin, D.S.; Craig, L.; Arthur, L.M.; Carney, J.P.; Tainer, J.A. Structural biology of Rad50 ATPase: ATP-driven conformational control in DNA double-strand break repair and the ABC-ATPase superfamily. *Cell* **2000**, *101*, 789–800. [CrossRef]
145. Wang, Y.; Chen, Q.; Wu, D.; Chen, Q.; Gong, G.; He, L.; Wu, X. Lamin-A interacting protein Hsp90 is required for DNA damage repair and chemoresistance of ovarian cancer cells. *Cell Death Dis.* **2021**, *12*, 786. [CrossRef] [PubMed]
146. Zhong, Q.; Chen, C.F.; Li, S.; Chen, Y.; Wang, C.C.; Xiao, J.; Chen, P.L.; Sharp, Z.D.; Lee, W.H. Association of BRCA1 with the hRad50-hMre11-p95 complex and the DNA damage response. *Science* **1999**, *285*, 747–750. [CrossRef]
147. Stecklein, S.R.; Kumaraswamy, E.; Behbod, F.; Wang, W.; Chaguturu, V.; Harlan-Williams, L.M.; Jensen, R.A. BRCA1 and HSP90 cooperate in homologous and non-homologous DNA double-strand-break repair and G2/M checkpoint activation. *Proc. Natl. Acad. Sci. USA* **2012**, *109*, 13650–13655. [CrossRef]

148. Lloyd, J.; Chapman, J.R.; Clapperton, J.A.; Haire, L.F.; Hartsuiker, E.; Li, J.; Carr, A.M.; Jackson, S.P.; Smerdon, S.J. A supramodular FHA/BRCT-repeat architecture mediates Nbs1 adaptor function in response to DNA damage. *Cell* **2009**, *139*, 100–111. [CrossRef] [PubMed]
149. Williams, R.S.; Dodson, G.E.; Limbo, O.; Yamada, Y.; Williams, J.S.; Guenther, G.; Classen, S.; Glover, J.N.; Iwasaki, H.; Russell, P.; et al. Nbs1 flexibly tethers Ctp1 and Mre11-Rad50 to coordinate DNA double-strand break processing and repair. *Cell* **2009**, *139*, 87–99. [CrossRef]
150. Pennisi, R.; Antoccia, A.; Leone, S.; Ascenzi, P.; di Masi, A. Hsp90alpha regulates ATM and NBN functions in sensing and repair of DNA double-strand breaks. *FEBS J.* **2017**, *284*, 2378–2395. [CrossRef] [PubMed]
151. Dote, H.; Burgan, W.E.; Camphausen, K.; Tofilon, P.J. Inhibition of hsp90 compromises the DNA damage response to radiation. *Cancer Res.* **2006**, *66*, 9211–9220. [CrossRef]
152. Elaimy, A.L.; Ahsan, A.; Marsh, K.; Pratt, W.B.; Ray, D.; Lawrence, T.S.; Nyati, M.K. ATM is the primary kinase responsible for phosphorylation of Hsp90alpha after ionizing radiation. *Oncotarget* **2016**, *7*, 82450–82457. [CrossRef]
153. Quanz, M.; Herbette, A.; Sayarath, M.; de Koning, L.; Dubois, T.; Sun, J.S.; Dutreix, M. Heat shock protein 90alpha (Hsp90alpha) is phosphorylated in response to DNA damage and accumulates in repair foci. *J. Biol. Chem.* **2012**, *287*, 8803–8815. [CrossRef]
154. Cheng, A.N.; Fan, C.C.; Lo, Y.K.; Kuo, C.L.; Wang, H.C.; Lien, I.H.; Lin, S.Y.; Chen, C.H.; Jiang, S.S.; Chang, I.S.; et al. Cdc7-Dbf4-mediated phosphorylation of HSP90-S164 stabilizes HSP90-HCLK2-MRN complex to enhance ATR/ATM signaling that overcomes replication stress in cancer. *Sci. Rep.* **2017**, *7*, 17024. [CrossRef]
155. Huang, J.; Manning, B.D. The TSC1-TSC2 complex: A molecular switchboard controlling cell growth. *Biochem. J.* **2008**, *412*, 179–190. [CrossRef]
156. Henske, E.P.; Jozwiak, S.; Kingswood, J.C.; Sampson, J.R.; Thiele, E.A. Tuberous sclerosis complex. *Nat. Rev. Dis. Primers* **2016**, *2*, 16035. [CrossRef]
157. Benvenuto, G.; Li, S.; Brown, S.J.; Braverman, R.; Vass, W.C.; Cheadle, J.P.; Halley, D.J.; Sampson, J.R.; Wienecke, R.; DeClue, J.E. The tuberous sclerosis-1 (TSC1) gene product hamartin suppresses cell growth and augments the expression of the TSC2 product tuberin by inhibiting its ubiquitination. *Oncogene* **2000**, *19*, 6306–6316. [CrossRef]
158. Nakashima, A.; Yoshino, K.; Miyamoto, T.; Eguchi, S.; Oshiro, N.; Kikkawa, U.; Yonezawa, K. Identification of TBC7 having TBC domain as a novel binding protein to TSC1-TSC2 complex. *Biochem. Biophys. Res. Commun.* **2007**, *361*, 218–223. [CrossRef]
159. Sato, N.; Koinuma, J.; Ito, T.; Tsuchiya, E.; Kondo, S.; Nakamura, Y.; Daigo, Y. Activation of an oncogenic TBC1D7 (TBC1 domain family, member 7) protein in pulmonary carcinogenesis. *Genes Chromosomes Cancer* **2010**, *49*, 353–367. [CrossRef]
160. Inoki, K.; Li, Y.; Xu, T.; Guan, K.L. Rheb GTPase is a direct target of TSC2 GAP activity and regulates mTOR signaling. *Genes Dev.* **2003**, *17*, 1829–1834. [CrossRef]
161. Zhang, Y.; Gao, X.; Saucedo, L.J.; Ru, B.; Edgar, B.A.; Pan, D. Rheb is a direct target of the tuberous sclerosis tumour suppressor proteins. *Nat. Cell Biol.* **2003**, *5*, 578–581. [CrossRef]
162. Woodford, M.R.; Sager, R.A.; Marris, E.; Dunn, D.M.; Blanden, A.R.; Murphy, R.L.; Rensing, N.; Shapiro, O.; Panaretou, B.; Prodromou, C.; et al. Tumor suppressor Tsc1 is a new Hsp90 co-chaperone that facilitates folding of kinase and non-kinase clients. *EMBO J.* **2017**, *36*, 3650–3665. [CrossRef]
163. Woodford, M.R.; Hughes, M.; Sager, R.A.; Backe, S.J.; Baker-Williams, A.J.; Bratslavsky, M.S.; Jacob, J.M.; Shapiro, O.; Wong, M.; Bratslavsky, G.; et al. Mutation of the co-chaperone Tsc1 in bladder cancer diminishes Hsp90 acetylation and reduces drug sensitivity and selectivity. *Oncotarget* **2019**, *10*, 5824–5834. [CrossRef] [PubMed]
164. Mrozek, E.M.; Bajaj, V.; Guo, Y.; Malinowska, I.A.; Zhang, J.; Kwiatkowski, D.J. Evaluation of Hsp90 and mTOR inhibitors as potential drugs for the treatment of TSC1/TSC2 deficient cancer. *PLoS ONE* **2021**, *16*, e0248380. [CrossRef] [PubMed]
165. Fliegauf, M.; Benzing, T.; Omran, H. When cilia go bad: Cilia defects and ciliopathies. *Nat. Rev. Mol. Cell Biol.* **2007**, *8*, 880–893. [CrossRef]
166. Gibbons, I.R.; Rowe, A.J. Dynein: A Protein with Adenosine Triphosphatase Activity from Cilia. *Science* **1965**, *149*, 424–426. [CrossRef]
167. Fok, A.K.; Wang, H.; Katayama, A.; Aihara, M.S.; Allen, R.D. 22S axonemal dynein is preassembled and functional prior to being transported to and attached on the axonemes. *Cell Motil. Cytoskelet.* **1994**, *29*, 215–224. [CrossRef] [PubMed]
168. Mitchison, H.M.; Schmidts, M.; Loges, N.T.; Freshour, J.; Dritsoula, A.; Hirst, R.A.; O'Callaghan, C.; Blau, H.; Al Dabbagh, M.; Olbrich, H.; et al. Mutations in axonemal dynein assembly factor DNAAF3 cause primary ciliary dyskinesia. *Nat. Genet.* **2012**, *44*, 381–389. [CrossRef]
169. Diggle, C.P.; Moore, D.J.; Mali, G.; zur Lage, P.; Ait-Lounis, A.; Schmidts, M.; Shoemark, A.; Garcia Munoz, A.; Halachev, M.R.; Gautier, P.; et al. HEATR2 plays a conserved role in assembly of the ciliary motile apparatus. *PLoS Genet.* **2014**, *10*, e1004577. [CrossRef] [PubMed]
170. Duquesnoy, P.; Escudier, E.; Vincensini, L.; Freshour, J.; Bridoux, A.M.; Coste, A.; Deschildre, A.; de Blic, J.; Legendre, M.; Montantin, G.; et al. Loss-of-function mutations in the human ortholog of *Chlamydomonas reinhardtii* ODA7 disrupt dynein arm assembly and cause primary ciliary dyskinesia. *Am. J. Hum. Genet.* **2009**, *85*, 890–896. [CrossRef]
171. Guo, Z.; Chen, W.; Huang, J.; Wang, L.; Qian, L. Clinical and genetic analysis of patients with primary ciliary dyskinesia caused by novel DNAAF3 mutations. *J. Hum. Genet.* **2019**, *64*, 711–719. [CrossRef] [PubMed]

172. Horani, A.; Druley, T.E.; Zariwala, M.A.; Patel, A.C.; Levinson, B.T.; Van Arendonk, L.G.; Thornton, K.C.; Giacalone, J.C.; Albee, A.J.; Wilson, K.S.; et al. Whole-exome capture and sequencing identifies HEATR2 mutation as a cause of primary ciliary dyskinesia. *Am. J. Hum. Genet.* **2012**, *91*, 685–693. [CrossRef]
173. Moore, D.J.; Onoufriadis, A.; Shoemark, A.; Simpson, M.A.; zur Lage, P.I.; de Castro, S.C.; Bartoloni, L.; Gallone, G.; Petridi, S.; Woollard, W.J.; et al. Mutations in ZMYND10, a gene essential for proper axonemal assembly of inner and outer dynein arms in humans and flies, cause primary ciliary dyskinesia. *Am. J. Hum. Genet.* **2013**, *93*, 346–356. [CrossRef]
174. Olcese, C.; Patel, M.P.; Shoemark, A.; Kiviluoto, S.; Legendre, M.; Williams, H.J.; Vaughan, C.K.; Hayward, J.; Goldenberg, A.; Emes, R.D.; et al. X-linked primary ciliary dyskinesia due to mutations in the cytoplasmic axonemal dynein assembly factor PIH1D3. *Nat. Commun.* **2017**, *8*, 14279. [CrossRef] [PubMed]
175. Omran, H.; Kobayashi, D.; Olbrich, H.; Tsukahara, T.; Loges, N.T.; Hagiwara, H.; Zhang, Q.; Leblond, G.; O'Toole, E.; Hara, C.; et al. Ktu/PF13 is required for cytoplasmic pre-assembly of axonemal dyneins. *Nature* **2008**, *456*, 611. [CrossRef] [PubMed]
176. Paff, T.; Loges, N.T.; Aprea, I.; Wu, K.; Bakey, Z.; Haarman, E.G.; Daniels, J.M.A.; Sistermans, E.A.; Bogunovic, N.; Dougherty, G.W.; et al. Mutations in PIH1D3 Cause X-Linked Primary Ciliary Dyskinesia with Outer and Inner Dynein Arm Defects. *Am. J. Hum. Genet.* **2017**, *100*, 160–168. [CrossRef] [PubMed]
177. Tarkar, A.; Loges, N.T.; Slagle, C.E.; Francis, R.; Dougherty, G.W.; Tamayo, J.V.; Shook, B.; Cantino, M.; Schwartz, D.; Jahnke, C.; et al. DYX1C1 is required for axonemal dynein assembly and ciliary motility. *Nat. Genet.* **2013**, *45*, 995–1003. [CrossRef]
178. Zariwala, M.A.; Gee, H.Y.; Kurkowiak, M.; Al-Mutairi, D.A.; Leigh, M.W.; Hurd, T.W.; Hjeij, R.; Dell, S.D.; Chaki, M.; Dougherty, G.W.; et al. ZMYND10 is mutated in primary ciliary dyskinesia and interacts with LRRC6. *Am. J. Hum. Genet.* **2013**, *93*, 336–345. [CrossRef] [PubMed]
179. Zur Lage, P.; Xi, Z.; Lennon, J.; Hunter, I.; Chan, W.K.; Bolado Carrancio, A.; von Kriegsheim, A.; Jarman, A.P. The Drosophila orthologue of the primary ciliary dyskinesia-associated gene, DNAAF3, is required for axonemal dynein assembly. *Biol. Open* **2021**, *10*, bio058812. [CrossRef]
180. Fabczak, H.; Osinka, A. Role of the Novel Hsp90 Co-Chaperones in Dynein Arms' Preassembly. *Int. J. Mol. Sci.* **2019**, *20*, 6174. [CrossRef]
181. Dong, F.; Shinohara, K.; Botilde, Y.; Nabeshima, R.; Asai, Y.; Fukumoto, A.; Hasegawa, T.; Matsuo, M.; Takeda, H.; Shiratori, H.; et al. Pih1d3 is required for cytoplasmic preassembly of axonemal dynein in mouse sperm. *J. Cell Biol.* **2014**, *204*, 203–213. [CrossRef]
182. Yamaguchi, H.; Oda, T.; Kikkawa, M.; Takeda, H. Systematic studies of all PIH proteins in zebrafish reveal their distinct roles in axonemal dynein assembly. *Elife* **2018**, *7*, e36979. [CrossRef] [PubMed]
183. Yamamoto, R.; Hirono, M.; Kamiya, R. Discrete PIH proteins function in the cytoplasmic preassembly of different subsets of axonemal dyneins. *J. Cell Biol.* **2010**, *190*, 65–71. [CrossRef]
184. Chen, Y.; Zhao, M.; Wang, S.; Chen, J.; Wang, Y.; Cao, Q.; Zhou, W.; Liu, J.; Xu, Z.; Tong, G.; et al. A novel role for DYX1C1, a chaperone protein for both Hsp70 and Hsp90, in breast cancer. *J. Cancer Res. Clin. Oncol.* **2009**, *135*, 1265–1276. [CrossRef] [PubMed]
185. Thomas, L.; Bouhouche, K.; Whitfield, M.; Thouvenin, G.; Coste, A.; Louis, B.; Szymanski, C.; Bequignon, E.; Papon, J.F.; Castelli, M.; et al. TTC12 Loss-of-Function Mutations Cause Primary Ciliary Dyskinesia and Unveil Distinct Dynein Assembly Mechanisms in Motile Cilia Versus Flagella. *Am. J. Hum. Genet.* **2020**, *106*, 153–169. [CrossRef]
186. Hartill, V.L.; van de Hoek, G.; Patel, M.P.; Little, R.; Watson, C.M.; Berry, I.R.; Shoemark, A.; Abdelmottaleb, D.; Parkes, E.; Bacchelli, C.; et al. DNAAF1 links heart laterality with the AAA+ ATPase RUVBL1 and ciliary intraflagellar transport. *Hum. Mol. Genet.* **2018**, *27*, 529–545. [CrossRef]
187. Mali, G.R.; Yeyati, P.L.; Mizuno, S.; Dodd, D.O.; Tennant, P.A.; Keighren, M.A.; Zur Lage, P.; Shoemark, A.; Garcia-Munoz, A.; Shimada, A.; et al. ZMYND10 functions in a chaperone relay during axonemal dynein assembly. *Elife* **2018**, *7*, e34389. [CrossRef]
188. Okamoto, T.; Nishimura, Y.; Ichimura, T.; Suzuki, K.; Miyamura, T.; Suzuki, T.; Moriishi, K.; Matsuura, Y. Hepatitis C virus RNA replication is regulated by FKBP8 and Hsp90. *EMBO J.* **2006**, *25*, 5015–5025. [CrossRef] [PubMed]
189. Horani, A.; Ferkol, T.W.; Shoseyov, D.; Wasserman, M.G.; Oren, Y.S.; Kerem, B.; Amirav, I.; Cohen-Cymberknoh, M.; Dutcher, S.K.; Brody, S.L.; et al. LRRC6 mutation causes primary ciliary dyskinesia with dynein arm defects. *PLoS ONE* **2013**, *8*, e59436. [CrossRef] [PubMed]
190. Kott, E.; Duquesnoy, P.; Copin, B.; Legendre, M.; Dastot-Le Moal, F.; Montantin, G.; Jeanson, L.; Tamalet, A.; Papon, J.F.; Siffroi, J.P.; et al. Loss-of-function mutations in LRRC6, a gene essential for proper axonemal assembly of inner and outer dynein arms, cause primary ciliary dyskinesia. *Am. J. Hum. Genet.* **2012**, *91*, 958–964. [CrossRef] [PubMed]
191. Cho, K.J.; Noh, S.H.; Han, S.M.; Choi, W.I.; Kim, H.Y.; Yu, S.; Lee, J.S.; Rim, J.H.; Lee, M.G.; Hildebrandt, F.; et al. ZMYND10 stabilizes intermediate chain proteins in the cytoplasmic pre-assembly of dynein arms. *PLoS Genet.* **2018**, *14*, e1007316. [CrossRef]
192. Zhao, L.; Yuan, S.; Cao, Y.; Kallakuri, S.; Li, Y.; Kishimoto, N.; DiBella, L.; Sun, Z. Reptin/Ruvbl2 is a Lrrc6/Seahorse interactor essential for cilia motility. *Proc. Natl. Acad. Sci. USA* **2013**, *110*, 12697–12702. [CrossRef]
193. Li, J.; Richter, K.; Buchner, J. Mixed Hsp90-cochaperone complexes are important for the progression of the reaction cycle. *Nat. Struct. Mol. Biol.* **2011**, *18*, 61–66. [CrossRef] [PubMed]
194. Dafinger, C.; Rinschen, M.M.; Borgal, L.; Ehrenberg, C.; Basten, S.G.; Franke, M.; Hohne, M.; Rauh, M.; Gobel, H.; Bloch, W.; et al. Targeted deletion of the AAA-ATPase Ruvbl1 in mice disrupts ciliary integrity and causes renal disease and hydrocephalus. *Exp. Mol. Med.* **2018**, *50*, 1–17. [CrossRef] [PubMed]

195. Li, Y.; Zhao, L.; Yuan, S.; Zhang, J.; Sun, Z. Axonemal dynein assembly requires the R2TP complex component Pontin. *Dev.* **2017**, *144*, 4684–4693. [CrossRef]
196. Maurizy, C.; Quinternet, M.; Abel, Y.; Verheggen, C.; Santo, P.E.; Bourguet, M.; Paiva, A.C.F.; Bragantini, B.; Chagot, M.E.; Robert, M.C.; et al. The RPAP3-Cterminal domain identifies R2TP-like quaternary chaperones. *Nat. Commun.* **2018**, *9*, 2093. [CrossRef] [PubMed]
197. Knowles, M.R.; Ostrowski, L.E.; Loges, N.T.; Hurd, T.; Leigh, M.W.; Huang, L.; Wolf, W.E.; Carson, J.L.; Hazucha, M.J.; Yin, W.; et al. Mutations in SPAG1 cause primary ciliary dyskinesia associated with defective outer and inner dynein arms. *Am. J. Hum. Genet.* **2013**, *93*, 711–720. [CrossRef] [PubMed]
198. Spangler, S.A.; Schmitz, S.K.; Kevenaar, J.T.; de Graaff, E.; de Wit, H.; Demmers, J.; Toonen, R.F.; Hoogenraad, C.C. Liprin-alpha2 promotes the presynaptic recruitment and turnover of RIM1/CASK to facilitate synaptic transmission. *J. Cell Biol.* **2013**, *201*, 915–928. [CrossRef] [PubMed]
199. Saeki, M.; Irie, Y.; Ni, L.; Yoshida, M.; Itsuki, Y.; Kamisaki, Y. Monad, a WD40 repeat protein, promotes apoptosis induced by TNF-alpha. *Biochem. Biophys. Res. Commun.* **2006**, *342*, 568–572. [CrossRef]
200. Liu, G.; Wang, L.; Pan, J. Chlamydomonas WDR92 in association with R2TP-like complex and multiple DNAAFs to regulate ciliary dynein preassembly. *J. Mol. Cell Biol.* **2019**, *11*, 770–780. [CrossRef] [PubMed]
201. Patel-King, R.S.; Sakato-Antoku, M.; Yankova, M.; King, S.M. WDR92 is required for axonemal dynein heavy chain stability in cytoplasm. *Mol. Biol. Cell* **2019**, *30*, 1834–1845. [CrossRef]
202. Itsuki, Y.; Saeki, M.; Nakahara, H.; Egusa, H.; Irie, Y.; Terao, Y.; Kawabata, S.; Yatani, H.; Kamisaki, Y. Molecular cloning of novel Monad binding protein containing tetratricopeptide repeat domains. *FEBS Lett.* **2008**, *582*, 2365–2370. [CrossRef]
203. zur Lage, P.; Stefanopoulou, P.; Styczynska-Soczka, K.; Quinn, N.; Mali, G.; von Kriegsheim, A.; Mill, P.; Jarman, A.P. Ciliary dynein motor preassembly is regulated by Wdr92 in association with HSP90 co-chaperone, R2TP. *J. Cell Biol.* **2018**, *217*, 2583–2598. [CrossRef] [PubMed]
204. Avidor-Reiss, T.; Ha, A.; Basiri, M.L. Transition Zone Migration: A Mechanism for Cytoplasmic Ciliogenesis and Postaxonemal Centriole Elongation. *Cold Spring Harb. Perspect. Biol.* **2017**, *9*, a028142. [CrossRef] [PubMed]
205. Fingerhut, J.M.; Yamashita, Y.M. mRNA localization mediates maturation of cytoplasmic cilia in *Drosophila* spermatogenesis. *J. Cell Biol.* **2020**, *219*, e202003084. [CrossRef] [PubMed]

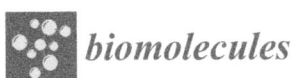

Review

UCS Chaperone Folding of the Myosin Head: A Function That Evolved before Animals and Fungi Diverged from a Common Ancestor More than a Billion Years Ago

Peter William Piper [1,*], Julia Elizabeth Scott [2] and Stefan Heber Millson [2,*]

1. Department of Molecular Biology and Biotechnology, University of Sheffield, Sheffield S10 2TN, UK
2. School of Life Sciences, University of Lincoln, Lincoln LN6 7DL, UK; 16662138@students.lincoln.ac.uk
* Correspondence: peter.piper@sheffield.ac.uk (P.W.P.); smillson@lincoln.ac.uk (S.H.M.)

Abstract: The folding of the myosin head often requires a UCS (Unc45, Cro1, She4) domain-containing chaperone. Worms, flies, and fungi have just a single UCS protein. Vertebrates have two; one (Unc45A) which functions primarily in non-muscle cells and another (Unc45B) that is essential for establishing and maintaining the contractile apparatus of cardiac and skeletal muscles. The domain structure of these proteins suggests that the UCS function evolved before animals and fungi diverged from a common ancestor more than a billion years ago. UCS proteins of metazoans and apicomplexan parasites possess a tetratricopeptide repeat (TPR), a domain for direct binding of the Hsp70/Hsp90 chaperones. This, however, is absent in the UCS proteins of fungi and largely nonessential for the UCS protein function in *Caenorhabditis elegans* and zebrafish. The latter part of this review focusses on the TPR-deficient UCS proteins of fungi. While these are reasonably well studied in yeasts, there is little precise information as to how they might engage in interactions with the Hsp70/Hsp90 chaperones or might assist in myosin operations during the hyphal growth of filamentous fungi.

Keywords: UCS proteins; She4; Hsp90; temperature stress; yeast; filamentous fungi

1. The UCS Protein Function

Myosin molecules need to be subject to a very precise temporal and spatial chaperoning so that they acquire their affinity for actin in the proper context. This is directed, in part, by a chaperone dedicated to the folding of the myosin head, a protein with the characteristic UCS (UNC45, Cro1, She4) domain. This UCS chaperone function was initially identified through the study of *Caenorhabditis elegans Unc-45* ("UNCoordinated") mutants, mutants that display defects in both motility [1,2] and cytokinesis during embryogenesis [3]. This led to the identification of a protein—UNC45—that associates with both Hsp90 and partially folded myosin [4]. The *C. elegans* UNC45 facilitates not just the folding of myosin, but also a regulation of myosin levels by targeting excess or damaged myosin to the proteasome for degradation [5]. It forms linear multimers, a filament assembly scaffold for a precise spatial organisation of the building blocks of myofilament formation and the organisation of sarcomeric repeats [6]. *Drosophila* studies have also highlighted the importance of the UCS protein function, both during late embryogenesis when the initial differentiation of cells into muscle tissue occurs, and at later stages of *Drosophila* development [7–10].

Except in fungi, UNC45 proteins have a 3-domain architecture [6,11] (Figure 1A). At their N-terminus is a tetratricopeptide repeat (TPR), a site for direct binding of the Hsp70 and Hsp90 molecular chaperones. This TPR is dispensable for UNC45 function in C. *elegans* [12] and zebrafish [13] and totally absent in the UCS proteins of fungi (Figure 1A). At the C-terminus, an elongated UCS domain mediates myosin folding, while a central domain aligns the TPR and UCS units to each other (Figure 1A). Direct biochemical proof that it is the UCS domain which mediates myosin folding came from demonstrations that the folding of muscle MHC-B myosin could be efficiently reconstituted in insect cells by the *C. elegans* UNC45, studies that revealed how the binding of the myosin substrate was compromised by the UCS domain mutations of temperature-sensitive *unc-45* mutants of *C. elegans* [14]. The central domain has been associated with a reversible inhibition of the myosin power stroke [15,16].

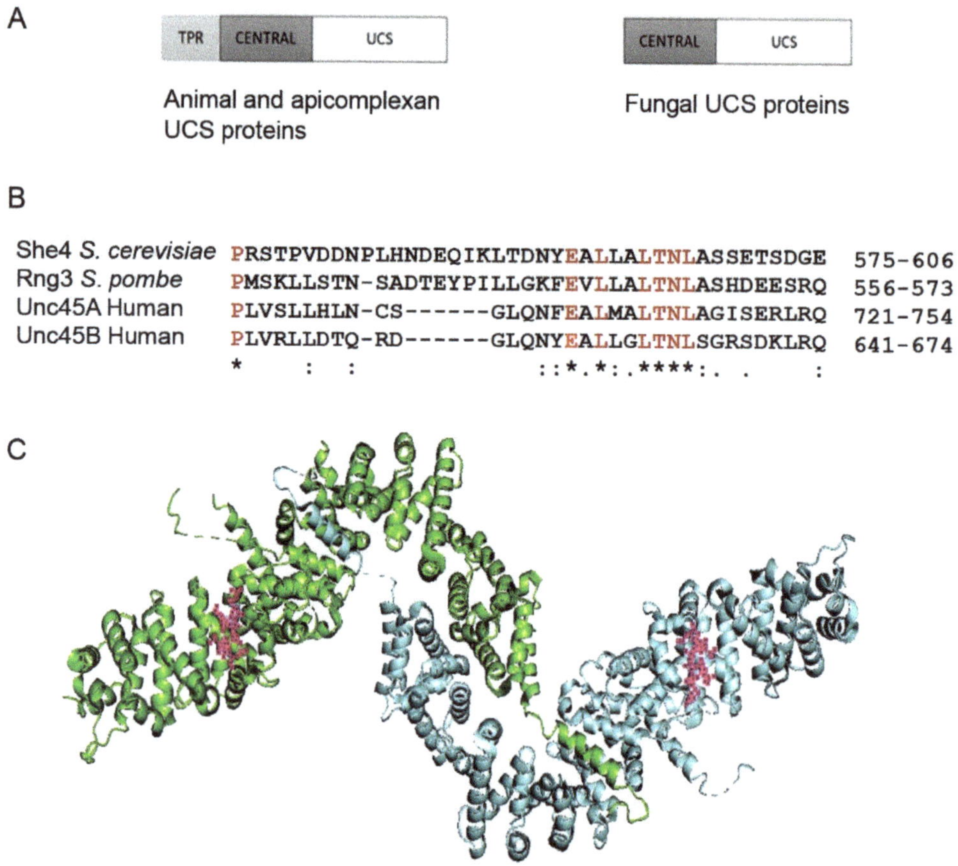

A

| TPR | CENTRAL | UCS |

Animal and apicomplexan UCS proteins

| CENTRAL | UCS |

Fungal UCS proteins

B

```
She4 S. cerevisiae  PRSTPVDDNPLHNDEQIKLTDNYEALLALTNLASSETSDGE   575-606
Rng3 S. pombe       PMSKLLSTN-SADTEYPILLGKFEVLLALTNLASHDEESRQ   556-573
Unc45A Human        PLVSLLHLN-CS------GLQNFEALMALTNLAGISERLRQ   721-754
Unc45B Human        PLVRLLDTQ-RD------GLQNYEALLGLTNLSGRSDKLRQ   641-674
                    *      : :            ::*.*:.****:.     :
```

C

Figure 1. (**A**) Schematic diagram showing the domain structure of UCS proteins in animals and apicomplexan parasites (**left**) and fungi (**right**). (**B**) A small UCS sequence conserved from yeast to man. (**C**) The location (in red) of this **EALLALTNL** sequence in the two molecules within the unit cell of the X-ray crystal structure of She4, the UCS protein of the yeast *Saccharomyces cerevisiae* [17].

The UCS domain consists of repeats of an armadillo/beta-catenin-like motif, an approximately 40 amino acid-long sequence that was first identified in the *Drosophila* segment polarity gene armadillo and the mammalian armadillo homolog beta-catenin. The X-ray crystal structure of the *Drosophila* UNC45 reveals an L-shaped monomer in which a contiguous series of these armadillo repeats are stacked one upon another [7]. Self-association of these stacks causes UNC45 to exist as oligomers in vitro and in vivo [6,11], linear chains of UNC45 units that effectively form an assembly line for the licensing of the folding of myosin heads with a defined periodicity on myofilaments. How the conserved sequences of the flexible UCS interact with myosin is discussed in detail elsewhere [9,14,18].

2. Vertebrate Unc45A (UNC45-GC) and Unc45B (UNC45-SM)

While fungi, flies and worms have just a single UCS protein, vertebrates possess two, the latter denoted as Unc45A (or UNC45-GC) and Unc45B (or UNC45-SM) (reviewed in [9]). Unc45A is expressed in most somatic cells, where it acts upon non-muscle myosin II. Unc45B is expressed primarily in heart and skeletal muscle, where it facilitates the assembly and maintenance of the contractile apparatus [19,20]. Although largely not elaborated here, much attention is now being given to how an altered functioning of Unc45A and Unc45B might be associated with human genetic disorders [21–25].

Studies in zebrafish (*Danio rerio*) have revealed that Unc45A and Unc45B are not functionally redundant [26]. During *D. rerio* development, Unc45B is initially found in the myosin-containing A-band of the sarcomere. Later, in adult *D. rerio*, it is sequestered by the Z-lines in the mature sarcomere, though it is still able to shuttle back to the A-band of the muscle sarcomere in response to either eccentric exercise or damage induced by heat or chemical stress [7,27]. Both in zebrafish [13,26] and in the amphibian *Xenopus tropicalis* [28], the lack of a functional Unc45B results in paralysis, this being associated with loss of the thick and thin filament organisation of skeletal and cardiac muscle. Unc45B is also involved in eye development [29]. It appears essential that the levels of Unc45B should be precisely regulated, since a Unc45B overexpression in the skeletal muscles of zebrafish embryos causes defective myofibril organisation [13]; while in man a defective turnover of Unc45B is associated with hereditary inclusion-body myopathy, the affected individuals having severely disorganised myofibrils [25].

Unc45A is often elevated in tumour cells where it is thought to contribute to their proliferation and metastasis. In ovarian cancer, this elevated Unc45A is correlated with increases in cell motility and trafficked with its target myosin to the leading edges of the migrating cells [30]. Furthermore, Unc45A was recently found to break microtubules (MTs) independently of its effects on non-muscle myosin II and to destabilize MTs independently of its C-terminal UCS domain [31].

3. The UCS Function Evolved before Animals and Fungi Diverged from a Common Ancestor

The UCS chaperone function is generally considered vital for eukaryotic organisms though, as described below, this may not be the case for the yeast *S. cerevisiae*. Despite this, UCS proteins do not display the strong sequence conservation of many other molecular chaperones, such as those of the Hsp70/Hsp90 families. As shown in Figure 1B, a signature sequence central in the UCS domain has been remarkably conserved between the human Unc45A/B and the UCS proteins of fission yeast (*Schizosaccharomyces pombe*) and budding yeast (*S. cerevisiae*). The latter two yeast species diverged from each other more than 350 million years ago [32]. Furthermore, an expression of the human Unc45B—though not the human Unc45A—can provide partial rescue of the loss of UCS protein function in the yeast *S. cerevisiae* [33]. It is difficult to conduct meaningful phylogenetic analysis, such as has been done for myosins [34], on the basis of this short sequence alone in view of the considerable uncertainty as to whether any potential "hits" are functional UCS proteins.

4. Genetic Studies on the UCS Proteins of Ascomycete Fungi; UCS Function in the Absence of the TPR

Rng3, the sole UCS protein of fission yeast (*S. pombe*), has been shown to exist partly in association with polysomes [35]. This reveals that it binds co-translationally to the myosin heavy-chain polypeptides as the latter are synthesised de novo, prior to these myosin molecules acquiring their capacity for actin filament gliding. Compromised Rng3 action, as in certain conditional *RNG3* mutants of *S. pombe*, is associated with dramatically decreased levels of myosin and cortical actin patches, as well as a block to cytokinesis [36–39]. In *S. pombe* Rng3 is essential, as it is needed for the stabilisation of myosin II at the cytokinetic contractile ring [40].

While *S. pombe* has two myosin II species (Myo2 and Myp2), budding yeast (*S cerevisiae*) has just one (Myo1). Furthermore, cytokinesis in *S. pombe* requires both the catalytic and tail domains of this myosin II, while in *S. cerevisiae* just the tail of the sole myosin II (Myo1) can support cytokinesis [41]. This may explain why the UCS protein of *S. cerevisiae* (She4) is nonessential under many conditions of growth, unlike Rng3 of *S. pombe*. The *she4Δ S. cerevisiae* gene deletant is normally moderately temperature-sensitive, but its defective growth at high temperatures is substantially rescued by the osmotic stabilisation of the medium (Figure 2). Thus, while the UCS chaperone is widely considered to provide a critical function in eukaryotic organisms, this appears not to be the case for osmotically stabilised budding yeast.

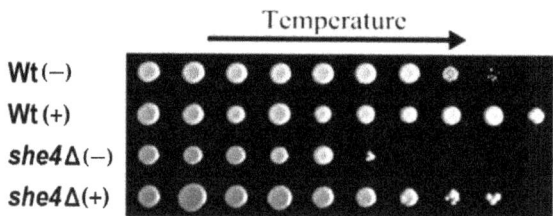

Figure 2. Wild type (Wt) and *she4Δ S. cerevisiae* cells pinned on 2% (w/v) peptone, 1% yeast extract, 2% glucose (YPD), 1.5% agar, and grown 2 days at 30 °C immediately following a prior 48 h growth on liquid YPD either without (−) or with (+) 1.2M sorbitol as osmotic stabiliser, this 48h growth having been conducted under 1.25 °C increases in temperature (left to right 30, 31.25, 32.5, 33.75, 35, 36.25, 37.5, 38.75. 40 and 41.25 °C).

In *S. cerevisiae* She4 acts on the two myosin-I forms (Myo3 and Myo5) and one of two myosin-V isoforms (Myo4) so as to enhance their folding and to reduce their turnover [39,42]. Its function is evidently more important as temperature is increased, since the phenotypes of the *S. cerevisiae she4Δ* mutant are most marked at higher temperatures. At 37–39 °C, *she4Δ* mutant cells exhibit severe defects in the organisation of the actin cytoskeleton (a functional Myo5-green fluorescent protein (GFP) fusion becoming dispersed through the cytosol and displaying an almost total loss of patch-like localisation to actin cortical patches), as well as defective endocytosis (apparent from a relatively weak FM4-64 staining of the vacuole) [42–46]. At slightly higher temperatures (45 °C), these *she4Δ* cells lyse [46]. It is still unclear why the loss of She4 should lead to a defect in cell wall integrity at high temperature (Figure 2). Cells of the *she4Δ* mutant are also defective in mating-type switching during haploid cell divisions, a reflection of the requirement for She4 in the formation of the functional cytoskeleton that can allow the asymmetric localisation of *ASH1* mRNA to daughter cells [47].

The filamentous ascomycete *Podospora anserina* is yet a third fungus in which the UCS protein function has been studied [48]. In this species, it is essential for sexual reproduction, the defective UCS function of the *cro1-1* mutant causing fruiting bodies to contain few asci and giant plurinucleate cells instead of dikaryotic cells after fertilisation. Karyogamy is not impaired, but the resultant polyploid nuclei generally undergo abortive meiosis, the *cro1-1* mutant being compromised in its inability to form septa between the daughter nuclei after each mitosis [48].

5. Myosins in Fungal Growth

In the budding yeast *S. cerevisiae*, a short period of polarised apical growth is followed by an extended isotrophic growth. The latter allows for the delivery of cell wall material over the entire bud surface, thereby leading to an almost spherical daughter cell. In contrast, filamentous fungi generally form hyphae that consist of chains of elongated cells that expand at the apex of the tip cell. During hyphal tip growth, cytoplasmic expansion forces are thought to push the cytoplasm against the flexible apical wall to power the expansion of the plastic apex. Hyphal extension involves the long-distance, polar delivery of Golgi-derived exocytic transport vesicles to this hyphal tip by MT-based kinesin motors (kinesins are not present in *S. cerevisiae*). At the hyphal apex, the fibres of the cell wall, such as chitin or glucan chains, are also synthesised, but as they are not yet cross-linked, the wall is still flexible at this point. Then, as the tip expands, the subapical chitin crystallises and becomes covalently bound to β-1,3-glucans, thereby solidifying the cell wall in the older parts of the growing hyphae.

At the hyphal apex, a forward-moving structure termed the Spitzenkörper determines the direction and rate of hyphal growth. Besides being the destination of exocytic transport vesicles, it also plays a role in endocytosis and membrane recycling (reviewed in [49]). Hyphal tip growth requires not just Spitzenkörper-directed polarised exocytosis at the expanding cell tip, but also the F-actin- and myosin-based transport of secretory vesicles along microfilaments. Actin-binding formin proteins anchor actin filaments to the growing tip and support actin assembly at the plus ends (barbed end) of these actin filaments.

Studies in *S. cerevisiae* [50–52] and *S. pombe* [53–55] have revealed that it is myosin-V motors that move exocytic vesicles towards the F-actin plus ends at plasma membrane regions of growth, whereas myosin-I motors support endocytosis [56]. A similar situation appears to apply in filamentous fungi. In *Aspergillus nidulans*, myosin-V interacts with vesicle transport proteins [57], while in the plant pathogen *Ustilago maydis*, a functional myosin-V-GFP fusion localises to the apical dome of hyphae [58]. In both *A. nidulans* [59–61] and *Candida albicans* [62], myosin-I is essential for hyphal growth and the endocytotic uptake of the endocytic marker dye FM4-64 into the vacuole [61,62]. Interestingly, a mutant form of the *A. nidulans* myosin-I that is almost devoid of ATPase activity can still support hyphal growth, indicating that myosin-I does not "walk" along actin filaments to mediate endocytosis [63]. One can surmise that UCS proteins are probably critical for these myosin-I and myosin-V operations in fungal hyphae, but in the absence of hard data this is still conjecture.

6. Hsp90 in UCS Protein Function

Pioneering in vitro studies on the folding of the myosin motor domain first revealed that mouse Unc45A and Unc45B can both dramatically enhance the Hsp90-dependent folding of a smooth muscle myosin motor domain-GFP fusion, Unc45A being more effective than Unc45B in this regard [64]. Striated muscle Unc45B was also shown to form a stable complex with Hsp90, a complex that selectively bound the partially folded conformation of the myosin motor domain synthesised in a reticulocyte lysate [65].

Unc45A and Unc45B differ in their associations with Hsp90α and Hsp90β, the two forms of cytosolic Hsp90 in vertebrate cells [66]. In many tissues, it is Hsp90β that is expressed constitutively at a high level, whereas Hsp90α is induced primarily in response to stress [66]. These two isoforms of Hsp90 have some distinct functional roles. In mice, Hsp90β [67] is essential for embryonic development [68,69], while a total loss of Hsp90α is fully compatible with viability but causes a block to spermatogenesis [70]. Zebrafish Hsp90α is highly expressed in striated muscle [67], its selective association with Unc45B being essential for the skeletal muscle organisation of embryos [68]. In contrast, it is Hsp90β and Unc45A that predominate in the other tissues of zebrafish [69]. These apparent preferences of Hsp90α for Unc45B and of Hsp90β for Unc45A are an indication of an evolutionary divergence of the respective Hsp90/UCS systems for the folding of non-muscle myosins versus cardiac and skeletal muscle myosins.

Except in fungi, UCS proteins have a TPR domain for direct interaction with the Hsp70/Hsp90 chaperones. Hsp90/Hsp70 binding by *C. elegans* UNC45 is abolished with the loss of this TPR [14]. Nevertheless, an expression of the UCS of this UNC45 alone can rescue *unc-45* null mutants of *C. elegans* arrested in embryonic muscle development, revealing the TPR to be dispensable for UNC45 function in vivo [12]. Tantalisingly, it is thought that the TPR/Hsp90 interaction may be actually inhibitory for the action of UNC45 since titration experiments show that, on a per molecule basis, the UCS alone has a greater activity in vivo in *C. elegans* muscle than the full-length UNC45 protein [12]. Also in zebrafish, loss of the TPR domain of Unc45B has no disruptive effect on myosin thick filament organisation [13]. This Unc45B of zebrafish undergoes an Hsp90-independent interaction with a protein-Apo2 that is required for the integrity of the myosepta and myofiber attachment [71].

Despite the absence of a TPR domain in the UCS proteins of fungi, there is evidence that the latter still associate with Hsp90 although the precise molecular details of these interactions remain unresolved. The *S. pombe* Rng3 binds Hsp90, loss of this interaction being suggested as the reason that a temperature-sensitive mutant of fission yeast Hsp90 (swo1-w1) is defective in actomyosin ring assembly at the restrictive temperature [38]. Certain temperature-sensitive Hsp90 mutants of *S. cerevisiae* also display a defective Myo5-GFP localisation (S.H.M., unpublished). The interactions of the *S. cerevisiae* She4 in the yeast two-hybrid system reveal that in vivo the Hsp90-She4 interaction strengthens dramatically as temperature is raised [46,72,73]. This may be correlated with She4 having a much more prominent role in *S. cerevisiae* at higher temperatures, as mentioned above. Elevated temperature acting to reinforce the Hsp90-She4 interaction might be a consequence of the UCS domain undergoing dramatic topology changes as temperature is increased, as previously observed for the UCS domain of Unc45B [74]. It may also reflect Hsp90/UCS interaction being required, not just for the assembly of a cytoskeleton, but also for the actions of Hsp90 and UFD-2 (ubiquitin fusion degradation 2) in repair of the myofibrillar disorganisation of stress [75].

7. Conclusions

Computational phylogenetics has revealed that fungi are more closely related to animals than plants, with animals and fungi diverging from a common ancestor more than a billion years ago [76]. The conservation of UCS domain structure—animals to fungi—(Figure 1A) suggests that the UCS function evolved prior to this divergence, possibly at the same time as a primordial myosin. The TPR may have been lost subsequently in fungi, as it is still present in the UCS proteins of the apicomplexan parasites *Toxoplasma gondii* and *Plasmodium falciparum* [77]. Apicomplexans are—based on small subunit ribosomal RNA sequencing—older than the three multicellular kingdoms of animals, plants, and fungi.

In this article we highlight the paucity of knowledge as to UCS protein function in fungi, apart from yeasts. The earliest fungi were unicellular marine, flagellated organisms [78]. Animals and fungi both possess uniflagellated reproductive stages (the sperm of animals and the zoospores of chytrid fungi). Flagellar movement is MT-based rather than myosin-dependent, but it is noteworthy that Unc45A was recently found to destabilise MTs in human and rat cells [31], indicating that UCS proteins may influence the functioning of MTs in other species as well. Some unicellular organisms can switch between a flagellar motility and an amoeboid motility [79]. While amoeboid motility is generally considered an animal cell property, it would appear not to have been totally lost in fungi, as it is apparent in a mutant *Neurospora crassa* which is defective in the synthesis of the (1,3)-β-d-glucan needed for cell wall assembly and which cannot form hyphae [80].

Multiple activities contribute to the expression, folding, assembly and interplay of actin and myosin, as well as in maintaining the functionality of actomyosin filaments during situations of stress. While UCS proteins are key in this regard, their interplay with many of the other chaperones and activities for protein turnover is still poorly understood. Screens have identified a number of other chaperones required for muscle integrity in *C. elegans*, including CeHop, CeAha1 and Cep23 [81]. Enabling Hsp70/Hsp90, their accessory components and the systems for protein turnover to establish and maintain the intricate myosin-actin interplay clearly presents a major challenge for the cellular chaperone machinery.

Author Contributions: Writing—original draft preparation, P.W.P.; writing—review and editing, J.E.S. & S.H.M.; supervision, S.H.M. All authors have read and agreed to the published version of the manuscript.

Funding: This research received no external funding.

Institutional Review Board Statement: Not applicable.

Informed Consent Statement: Not applicable.

Data Availability Statement: N/A, review article.

Conflicts of Interest: Authors declare no conflict of interest.

References

1. Barral, J.M.; Bauer, C.C.; Ortiz, I.; Epstein, H.F. Unc-45 mutations in Caenorhabditis elegans implicate a CRO1/She4p-like domain in myosin assembly. *J. Cell Biol.* **1998**, *143*, 1215–1225. [CrossRef] [PubMed]
2. Ao, W.; Pilgrim, D. Caenorhabditis elegans UNC-45 is a component of muscle thick filaments and colocalizes with myosin heavy chain B, but not myosin heavy chain A. *J. Cell Biol.* **2000**, *148*, 375–384. [CrossRef] [PubMed]
3. Kachur, T.; Ao, W.; Berger, J.; Pilgrim, D. Maternal UNC-45 is involved in cytokinesis and colocalizes with non-muscle myosin in the early Caenorhabditis elegans embryo. *J. Cell Sci.* **2004**, *117*, 5313–5321. [CrossRef] [PubMed]
4. Barral, J.M.; Hutagalung, A.H.; Brinker, A.; Hartl, F.U.; Epstein, H.F. Role of the myosin assembly protein UNC-45 as a molecular chaperone for myosin. *Science* **2002**, *295*, 669–671. [CrossRef] [PubMed]
5. Landsverk, M.L.; Li, S.; Hutagalung, A.H.; Najafov, A.; Hoppe, T.; Barral, J.M.; Epstein, H.F. The UNC-45 chaperone mediates sarcomere assembly through myosin degradation in Caenorhabditis elegans. *J. Cell Biol.* **2007**, *177*, 205–210. [CrossRef] [PubMed]
6. Gazda, L.; Pokrzywa, W.; Hellerschmied, D.; Lowe, T.; Forne, I.; Mueller-Planitz, F.; Hoppe, T.; Clausen, T. The myosin chaperone UNC-45 is organized in tandem modules to support myofilament formation in C. elegans. *Cell* **2013**, *152*, 183–195. [CrossRef]
7. Lee, C.F.; Melkani, G.C.; Yu, Q.; Suggs, J.A.; Kronert, W.A.; Suzuki, Y.; Hipolito, L.; Price, M.G.; Epstein, H.F.; Bernstein, S.I. Drosophila UNC-45 accumulates in embryonic blastoderm and in muscles, and is essential for muscle myosin stability. *J. Cell Sci.* **2011**, *124*, 699–705. [CrossRef]
8. Melkani, G.C.; Bodmer, R.; Ocorr, K.; Bernstein, S.I. The UNC-45 chaperone is critical for establishing myosin-based myofibrillar organization and cardiac contractility in the Drosophila heart model. *PLoS ONE* **2011**, *6*, e22579. [CrossRef]
9. Lee, C.F.; Melkani, G.C.; Bernstein, S.I. The UNC-45 myosin chaperone: From worms to flies to vertebrates. *Int. Rev. Cell Mol. Biol.* **2014**, *313*, 103–144.
10. Karunendiran, A.; Nguyen, C.T.; Barzda, V.; Stewart, B.A. Disruption of Drosophila larval muscle structure and function by UNC45 knockdown. *BMC Mol. Cell Biol.* **2021**, *22*, 38. [CrossRef]
11. Lee, C.F.; Hauenstein, A.V.; Gasper, W.C.; Sankaran, B.; Bernstein, S.I.; Huxford, T. Crystal Structure of Drosophila Unc-45, a Putative Myosin Chaperone. *Biophys. J.* **2010**, *98*, 34. [CrossRef]
12. Ni, W.; Hutagalung, A.H.; Li, S.; Epstein, H.F. The myosin-binding UCS domain but not the Hsp90-binding TPR domain of the UNC-45 chaperone is essential for function in Caenorhabditis elegans. *J. Cell Sci.* **2011**, *124*, 3164–3173. [CrossRef]
13. Bernick, E.P.; Zhang, P.J.; Du, S. Knockdown and overexpression of Unc-45b result in defective myofibril organization in skeletal muscles of zebrafish embryos. *BMC Cell Biol.* **2010**, *11*, 70. [CrossRef] [PubMed]
14. Hellerschmied, D.; Lehner, A.; Franicevic, N.; Arnese, R.; Johnson, C.; Vogel, A.; Meinhart, A.; Kurzbauer, R.; Deszcz, L.; Gazda, L.; et al. Molecular features of the UNC-45 chaperone critical for binding and folding muscle myosin. *Nat. Commun.* **2019**, *10*, 4781. [CrossRef] [PubMed]
15. Nicholls, P.; Bujalowski, P.J.; Epstein, H.F.; Boehning, D.F.; Barral, J.M.; Oberhauser, A.F. Chaperone-mediated reversible inhibition of the sarcomeric myosin power stroke. *FEBS Lett.* **2014**, *588*, 3977–3981. [CrossRef]
16. Bujalowski, P.J.; Nicholls, P.; Garza, E.; Oberhauser, A.F. The central domain of UNC-45 chaperone inhibits the myosin power stroke. *FEBS Open Bio.* **2018**, *8*, 41–48. [CrossRef]
17. Shi, H.; Blobel, G. UNC-45/CRO1/She4p (UCS) protein forms elongated dimer and joins two myosin heads near their actin binding region. *Proc. Natl. Acad. Sci. USA* **2010**, *107*, 21382–21387. [CrossRef]
18. Moncrief, T.; Matheny, C.J.; Gaziova, I.; Miller, J.M.; Qadota, H.; Benian, G.M.; Oberhauser, A.F. Mutations in conserved residues of the myosin chaperone UNC-45 result in both reduced stability and chaperoning activity. *Protein Sci.* **2021**, *30*, 2221–2232. [CrossRef]
19. Hutagalung, A.H.; Landsverk, M.L.; Price, M.G.; Epstein, H.F. The UCS family of myosin chaperones. *J. Cell Sci.* **2002**, *115*, 3983–3990. [CrossRef]
20. Price, M.G.; Landsverk, M.L.; Barral, J.M.; Epstein, H.F. Two mammalian UNC-45 isoforms are related to distinct cytoskeletal and muscle-specific functions. *J. Cell Sci.* **2002**, *115*, 4013–4023. [CrossRef]
21. Esteve, C.; Francescatto, L.; Tan, P.L.; Bourchany, A.; de Leusse, C.; Marinier, E.; Blanchard, A.; Bourgeois, P.; Brochier-Armanet, C.; Bruel, A.L.; et al. Loss-of-Function Mutations in UNC45A Cause a Syndrome Associating Cholestasis, Diarrhea, Impaired Hearing, and Bone Fragility. *Am. J. Hum. Genet.* **2018**, *102*, 364–374. [CrossRef] [PubMed]

22. Faivre, L.; Esteve, C.; Francescatto, L.; Tan, P.L.; Bourchany, A.; Delafoulhouze, C.; Marinier, E.; Bourgeois, P.; Brochier-Armanet, C.; Bruel, A.; et al. Description Osteo-Oto-Hepato-Enteric (O2HE) syndrome, a new recessive autosomal syndrome secondary to loss of function mutations in the UNC45A gene. *Eur. J. Hum. Genet. EJHG* **2019**, *27*, 795–796.
23. Donkervoort, S.; Kutzner, C.E.; Hu, Y.; Lornage, X.; Rendu, J.; Stojkovic, T.; Baets, J.; Neuhaus, S.B.; Tanboon, J.; Maroofian, R.; et al. Pathogenic Variants in the Myosin Chaperone UNC-45B Cause Progressive Myopathy with Eccentric Cores. *Am. J. Hum. Genet.* **2020**, *107*, 1078–1095. [CrossRef] [PubMed]
24. Anderson, M.J.; Pham, V.N.; Vogel, A.M.; Weinstein, B.M.; Roman, B.L. Loss of unc45a precipitates arteriovenous shunting in the aortic arches. *Dev. Biol.* **2008**, *318*, 258–267. [CrossRef] [PubMed]
25. Janiesch, P.C.; Kim, J.; Mouysset, J.; Barikbin, R.; Lochmuller, H.; Cassata, G.; Krause, S.; Hoppe, T. The ubiquitin-selective chaperone CDC-48/p97 links myosin assembly to human myopathy. *Nat. Cell Biol.* **2007**, *9*, 379–390. [CrossRef] [PubMed]
26. Comyn, S.A.; Pilgrim, D. Lack of developmental redundancy between Unc45 proteins in zebrafish muscle development. *PLoS ONE* **2012**, *7*, e48861. [CrossRef]
27. Etard, C.; Roostalu, U.; Strahle, U. Shuttling of the chaperones Unc45b and Hsp90a between the A band and the Z line of the myofibril. *J. Cell Biol.* **2008**, *180*, 1163–1175. [CrossRef]
28. Geach, T.J.; Zimmerman, L.B. Paralysis and delayed Z-disc formation in the Xenopus tropicalis unc45b mutant dicky ticker. *BMC Dev. Biol.* **2010**, *1*, 75. [CrossRef]
29. Hansen, L.; Comyn, S.; Mang, Y.; Lind-Thomsen, A.; Myhre, L.; Jean, F.; Eiberg, H.; Tommerup, N.; Rosenberg, T.; Pilgrim, D. The myosin chaperone UNC45B is involved in lens development and autosomal dominant juvenile cataract. *Eur. J. Hum. Genet.* **2014**, *22*, 1290–1297. [CrossRef]
30. Bazzaro, M.; Santillan, A.; Lin, Z.; Tang, T.; Lee, M.K.; Bristow, R.E.; Ie, M.S.; Roden, R.B. Myosin II co-chaperone general cell UNC-45 overexpression is associated with ovarian cancer, rapid proliferation, and motility. *Am. J. Pathol.* **2007**, *171*, 1640–1649. [CrossRef]
31. Habicht, J.; Mooneyham, A.; Hoshino, A.; Shetty, M.; Zhang, X.; Emmings, E.; Yang, Q.; Coombes, C.; Gardner, M.K.; Bazzaro, M. UNC-45A breaks the microtubule lattice independently of its effects on non-muscle myosin II. *J. Cell Sci.* **2021**, *134*, jcs248815. [PubMed]
32. Hoffman, C.S.; Wood, V.; Fantes, P.A. An Ancient Yeast for Young Geneticists: A Primer on the Schizosaccharomyces pombe Model System. *Genetics* **2015**, *201*, 403–423. [CrossRef] [PubMed]
33. Escalante, S.G.; Brightmore, J.A.; Piper, P.W.; Millson, S.H. UCS protein function is partially restored in the Saccharomyces cerevisiae she4 mutant with expression of the human UNC45-GC, but not UNC45-SM. *Cell Stress Chaperones* **2018**, *23*, 609–615. [CrossRef]
34. Hartman, M.A.; Spudich, J.A. The myosin superfamily at a glance. *J. Cell Sci.* **2012**, *125*, 1627–1632. [CrossRef]
35. Amorim, M.J.; Mata, J. Rng3, a member of the UCS family of myosin co-chaperones, associates with myosin heavy chains cotranslationally. *EMBO Rep.* **2009**, *10*, 186–191. [CrossRef] [PubMed]
36. Wong, K.C.Y.; Naqvi, N.I.; Iino, Y.; Yamamoto, M.; Balasubramanian, M.K. Fission yeast Rng3p: An UCS-domain protein that mediates myosin II assembly during cytokinesis. *J. Cell Sci.* **2000**, *113*, 2421–2432. [CrossRef]
37. Lord, M.; Pollard, T.D. UCS protein Rng3p activates actin filament gliding by fission yeast myosin-II. *J. Cell Biol.* **2004**, *167*, 315–325. [CrossRef]
38. Mishra, M.; D'souza, V.M.; Chang, K.C.; Huang, Y.; Balasubramanian, M.K. Hsp90 protein in fission yeast Swo1p and UCS protein Rng3p facilitate myosin II assembly and function. *Eukaryot. Cell* **2005**, *4*, 567–576. [CrossRef]
39. Lord, M.; Sladewski, T.E.; Pollard, T.D. Yeast UCS proteins promote actomyosin interactions and limit myosin turnover in cells. *Proc. Natl. Acad. Sci. USA* **2008**, *105*, 8014–8019. [CrossRef]
40. Stark, B.C.; James, M.L.; Pollard, L.W.; Sirotkin, V.; Lord, M. UCS protein Rng3p is essential for myosin-II motor activity during cytokinesis in fission yeast. *PLoS ONE* **2013**, *8*, e79593.
41. Lord, M.; Laves, E.; Pollard, T.D. Cytokinesis depends on the motor domains of myosin-II in fission yeast but not in budding yeast. *Mol. Biol. Cell* **2005**, *16*, 5346–5355. [CrossRef] [PubMed]
42. Wesche, S.; Arnold, M.; Jansen, R.-P. The UCS Domain Protein She4p Binds to Myosin Motor Domains and Is Essential for Class I and Class V Myosin Function. *Curr. Biol.* **2003**, *13*, 715–724. [CrossRef]
43. Wendland, B.; McCaffery, J.M.; Xiao, Q.; Emr, S.D. A novel fluorescence-activated cell sorter-based screen for yeast endocytosis mutants identifies a yeast homologue of mammalian eps15. *J. Cell Biol.* **1996**, *135*, 1485–1500. [CrossRef]
44. Goodson, H.V.; Anderson, B.L.; Warrick, H.M.; Pon, L.A.; Spudich, J.A. Synthetic lethality screen identifies a novel yeast myosin I gene (MYO5): Myosin I proteins are required for polarization of the actin cytoskeleton. *J. Cell Biol.* **1996**, *133*, 1277–1291. [CrossRef]
45. Toi, H.; Fujimura-Kamada, K.; Irie, K.; Takai, Y.; Todo, S.; Tanaka, K. She4p/Dim1p interacts with the motor domain of unconventional myosins in the budding yeast, Saccharomyces cerevisiae. *Mol. Biol. Cell* **2003**, *14*, 2237–2249. [CrossRef] [PubMed]
46. Gomez-Escalante, S.; Piper, P.W.; Millson, S.H. Mutation of the Ser18 phosphorylation site on the sole Saccharomyces cerevisiae UCS protein, She4, can compromise high-temperature survival. *Cell Stress Chaperones* **2017**, *22*, 135–141. [CrossRef]
47. Long, R.M.; Singer, R.H.; Meng, X.; Gonzalez, I.; Nasmyth, K.; Jansen, R.P. Mating type switching in yeast controlled by asymmetric localization of ASH1 mRNA. *Science* **1997**, *277*, 383–387. [CrossRef]

48. Berteaux-Lecellier, V.; Zickler, D.; Debuchy, R.; Panvier-Adoutte, A.; Thompson-Coffe, C.; Picard, M. A homologue of the yeast SHE4 gene is essential for the transition between the syncytial and cellular stages during sexual reproduction of the fungus Podospora anserina. *EMBO J.* **1998**, *17*, 1248–1258. [CrossRef]
49. Steinberg, G. On the move: Endosomes in fungal growth and pathogenicity. *Nat. Rev. Microbiol.* **2007**, *5*, 309–316. [CrossRef]
50. Govindan, B.; Bowser, R.; Novick, P. The role of Myo2, a yeast class V myosin, in vesicular transport. *J. Cell Biol.* **1995**, *128*, 1055–1068. [CrossRef]
51. Johnston, G.C.; Prendergast, J.A.; Singer, R.A. The Saccharomyces cerevisiae MYO2 gene encodes an essential myosin for vectorial transport of vesicles. *J. Cell Biol.* **1991**, *113*, 539–551. [CrossRef] [PubMed]
52. Schott, D.H.; Collins, R.N.; Bretscher, A. Secretory vesicle transport velocity in living cells depends on the myosin-V lever arm length. *J. Cell Biol.* **2002**, *156*, 35–39. [CrossRef] [PubMed]
53. Motegi, F.; Arai, R.; Mabuchi, I. Identification of two type V myosins in fission yeast, one of which functions in polarized cell growth and moves rapidly in the cell. *Mol. Biol. Cell* **2001**, *12*, 1367–1380. [CrossRef] [PubMed]
54. Mulvihill, D.P.; Edwards, S.R.; Hyams, J.S. A critical role for the type V myosin, Myo52, in septum deposition and cell fission during cytokinesis in Schizosaccharomyces pombe. *Cell Motil. Cytoskelet.* **2006**, *63*, 149–161. [CrossRef]
55. Win, T.Z.; Gachet, Y.; Mulvihill, D.P.; May, K.M.; Hyams, J.S. Two type V myosins with non-overlapping functions in the fission yeast Schizosaccharomyces pombe: Myo52 is concerned with growth polarity and cytokinesis, Myo51 is a component of the cytokinetic actin ring. *J. Cell Sci.* **2001**, *114*, 69–79. [CrossRef]
56. Geli, M.I.; Riezman, H. Role of type I myosins in receptor-mediated endocytosis in yeast. *Science* **1996**, *272*, 533–535. [CrossRef]
57. Renshaw, H.; Juvvadi, P.R.; Cole, D.C.; Steinbach, W.J. The class V myosin interactome of the human pathogen Aspergillus fumigatus reveals novel interactions with COPII vesicle transport proteins. *Biochem. Biophys. Res. Commun.* **2020**, *527*, 232–237. [CrossRef]
58. Weber, I.; Gruber, C.; Steinberg, G. A class-V myosin required for mating, hyphal growth, and pathogenicity in the dimorphic plant pathogen Ustilago maydis. *Plant. Cell* **2003**, *15*, 2826–2842. [CrossRef]
59. McGoldrick, C.A.; Gruver, C.; May, G.S. myoA of Aspergillus nidulans encodes an essential myosin I required for secretion and polarized growth. *J. Cell Biol.* **1995**, *128*, 577–587. [CrossRef]
60. Osherov, N.; Yamashita, R.A.; Chung, Y.S.; May, G.S. Structural requirements for in vivo myosin I function in Aspergillus nidulans. *J. Biol. Chem.* **1998**, *273*, 27017–27025. [CrossRef]
61. Yamashita, R.A.; May, G.S. Constitutive activation of endocytosis by mutation of myoA, the myosin I gene of Aspergillus nidulans. *J. Biol. Chem.* **1998**, *273*, 14644–14648. [CrossRef] [PubMed]
62. Oberholzer, U.; TIouk, L.; Thomas, D.Y.; Whiteway, M. Functional characterization of myosin I tail regions in Candida albicans. *Eukaryot. Cell* **2004**, *3*, 1272–1286. [CrossRef] [PubMed]
63. Liu, X.; Osherov, N.; Yamashita, R.; Brzeska, H.; Korn, E.D.; May, G.S. Myosin I mutants with only 1% of wild-type actin-activated MgATPase activity retain essential in vivo function(s). *Proc. Natl. Acad. Sci. USA* **2001**, *98*, 9122–9127. [CrossRef]
64. Liu, L.; Srikakulam, R.; Winkelmann, D.A. Unc45 activates Hsp90-dependent folding of the myosin motor domain. *J. Biol. Chem.* **2008**, *283*, 13185–13193. [CrossRef] [PubMed]
65. Srikakulam, R.; Liu, L.; Winkelmann, D.A. Unc45b forms a cytosolic complex with Hsp90 and targets the unfolded myosin motor domain. *PLoS ONE* **2008**, *3*, e2137. [CrossRef]
66. Subbarao Sreedhar, A.; Kalmár, É.; Csermely, P.; Shen, Y.-F. Hsp90 isoforms: Functions, expression and clinical importance. *FEBS Lett.* **2004**, *562*, 11–15. [CrossRef]
67. Etard, C.; Behra, M.; Fischer, N.; Hutcheson, D.; Geisler, R.; Strahle, U. The UCS factor Steif/Unc-45b interacts with the heat shock protein Hsp90a during myofibrillogenesis. *Dev. Biol.* **2007**, *308*, 133–143. [CrossRef] [PubMed]
68. Du, S.J.; Li, H.; Bian, Y.; Zhong, Y. Heat-shock protein 90alpha1 is required for organized myofibril assembly in skeletal muscles of zebrafish embryos. *Proc. Natl. Acad. Sci. USA* **2008**, *105*, 554–559. [CrossRef]
69. Krone, P.H.; Evans, T.G.; Blechinger, S.R. Heat shock gene expression and function during zebrafish embryogenesis. *Semin. Cell Dev. Biol.* **2003**, *14*, 267–274. [CrossRef]
70. Grad, I.; Cederroth, C.R.; Walicki, J.; Grey, C.; Barluenga, S.; Winssinger, N.; de Massy, B.; Nef, S.; Picard, D. The molecular chaperone Hsp90α is required for meiotic progression of spermatocytes beyond pachytene in the mouse. *PLoS ONE* **2010**, *5*, e15770. [CrossRef]
71. Etard, C.; Roostalu, U.; Strähle, U. Lack of Apobec2-related proteins causes a dystrophic muscle phenotype in zebrafish embryos. *J. Cell Biol.* **2010**, *189*, 527–539. [CrossRef] [PubMed]
72. Millson, S.H.; Truman, A.W.; Wolfram, F.; King, V.; Panaretou, B.; Prodromou, C.; Pearl, L.H.; Piper, P.W. Investigating the protein-protein interactions of the yeast Hsp90 chaperone system by two-hybrid analysis: Potential uses and limitations of this approach. *Cell Stress Chaperones* **2004**, *9*, 359–368. [CrossRef] [PubMed]
73. Millson, S.H.; Truman, A.W.; King, V.; Prodromou, C.; Pearl, L.H.; Piper, P.W. A two-hybrid screen of the yeast proteome for Hsp90 interactors uncovers a novel Hsp90 chaperone requirement in the activity of a stress-activated mitogen-activated protein kinase, Slt2p (Mpk1p). *Eukaryot. Cell* **2005**, *4*, 849–860. [CrossRef] [PubMed]
74. Bujalowski, P.J.; Nicholls, P.; Barral, J.M.; Oberhauser, A.F. Thermally-induced structural changes in an armadillo repeat protein suggest a novel thermosensor mechanism in a molecular chaperone. *FEBS Lett.* **2015**, *589*, 123–130. [CrossRef] [PubMed]

75. Hellerschmied, D.; Roessler, M.; Lehner, A.; Gazda, L.; Stejskal, K.; Imre, R.; Mechtler, K.; Dammermann, A.; Clausen, T. UFD-2 is an adaptor-assisted E3 ligase targeting unfolded proteins. *Nat. Commun.* **2018**, *9*, 484. [CrossRef]
76. Wang, D.Y.; Kumar, S.; Hedges, S.B. Divergence time estimates for the early history of animal phyla and the origin of plants, animals and fungi. *Proc. Biol. Sci.* **1999**, *266*, 163–171. [CrossRef]
77. Bookwalter, C.S.; Tay, C.L.; McCrorie, R.; Previs, M.J.; Lu, H.; Krementsova, E.B.; Fagnant, P.M.; Baum, J.; Trybus, K.M. Reconstitution of the core of the malaria parasite glideosome with recombinant Plasmodium class XIV myosin A and Plasmodium actin. *J. Biol. Chem.* **2017**, *292*, 19290–19303. [CrossRef]
78. Berbee, M.L.; James, T.Y.; Strullu-Derrien, C. Early diverging fungi: Diversity and impact at the dawn of terrestrial life. *Annu. Rev. Microbiol.* **2017**, *71*, 41–60. [CrossRef]
79. Brunet, T.; Albert, M.; Roman, W.; Coyle, M.C.; Spitzer, D.C.; King, N. A flagellate-to-amoeboid switch in the closest living relatives of animals. *eLife* **2021**, *10*, e61037. [CrossRef]
80. Patel, P.K.; Free, S.J. The Genetics and Biochemistry of Cell Wall Structure and Synthesis in Neurospora crassa, a Model Filamentous Fungus. *Front. Microbiol.* **2019**, *10*, 2294. [CrossRef]
81. Frumkin, A.; Dror, S.; Pokrzywa, W.; Bar-Lavan, Y.; Karady, I.; Hoppe, T.; Ben-Zvi, A. Challenging muscle homeostasis uncovers novel chaperone interactions in Caenorhabditis elegans. *Front. Mol. Biosci.* **2017**, *1*, 21. [CrossRef] [PubMed]

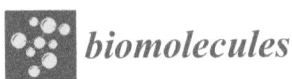

Article

The APE2 Exonuclease Is a Client of the Hsp70–Hsp90 Axis in Yeast and Mammalian Cells

Siddhi Omkar *, Tasaduq H. Wani †, Bo Zheng †, Megan M. Mitchem and Andrew W. Truman *

Department of Biological Sciences, The University of North Carolina at Charlotte, Charlotte, NC 28223, USA; twani@uncc.edu (T.H.W.); bzheng1@uncc.edu (B.Z.); mmitch92@uncc.edu (M.M.M.)
* Correspondence: sparanj2@uncc.edu (S.O.); atruman1@uncc.edu (A.W.T.)
† These authors contributed equally to this work.

Abstract: Molecular chaperones such as Hsp70 and Hsp90 help fold and activate proteins in important signal transduction pathways that include DNA damage response (DDR). Previous studies have suggested that the levels of the mammalian APE2 exonuclease, a protein critical for DNA repair, may be dependent on chaperone activity. In this study, we demonstrate that the budding yeast Apn2 exonuclease interacts with molecular chaperones Ssa1 and Hsp82 and the co-chaperone Ydj1. Although Apn2 does not display a binding preference for any specific cytosolic Hsp70 or Hsp90 paralog, Ssa1 is unable to support Apn2 stability when present as the sole Ssa in the cell. Demonstrating conservation of this mechanism, the exonuclease APE2 also binds to Hsp70 and Hsp90 in mammalian cells. Inhibition of chaperone function via specific small molecule inhibitors results in a rapid loss of APE2 in a range of cancer cell lines. Taken together, these data identify APE2 and Apn2 as clients of the chaperone system in yeast and mammalian cells and suggest that chaperone inhibition may form the basis of novel anticancer therapies that target APE2-mediated processes.

Keywords: Hsp70; Hsp90; APE2; Apn2; cancer; chaperone inhibition

Citation: Omkar, S.; Wani, T.H.; Zheng, B.; Mitchem, M.M.; Truman, A.W. The APE2 Exonuclease Is a Client of the Hsp70–Hsp90 Axis in Yeast and Mammalian Cells. *Biomolecules* **2022**, *12*, 864. https://doi.org/10.3390/biom12070864

Academic Editor: Chrisostomos Prodromou

Received: 2 June 2022
Accepted: 18 June 2022
Published: 21 June 2022

Publisher's Note: MDPI stays neutral with regard to jurisdictional claims in published maps and institutional affiliations.

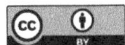

Copyright: © 2022 by the authors. Licensee MDPI, Basel, Switzerland. This article is an open access article distributed under the terms and conditions of the Creative Commons Attribution (CC BY) license (https://creativecommons.org/licenses/by/4.0/).

1. Introduction

The well-conserved Hsp70 and Hsp90 molecular chaperones are critical for the folding, maturation and activity of a large number of "client" proteins [1]. Client proteins are found in diverse cellular pathways, and consequently, chaperones support the maintenance of apoptotic signaling, angiogenesis, autophagy, senescence [1–3]. Although prokaryotes possess a single prototypical Hsp70 and Hsp90 (DnaK and HtpG, respectively), eukaryotes possess several paralogs that differ in their subcellular localization and expression profile [4–6]. In budding yeast, the main cytosolic forms of Hsp70 are Ssa1–4, which arose from multiple gene duplication events. Ssa1 and 2 are constitutively expressed at high levels, whereas Ssa3 and 4 are highly heat inducible [7–9]. The Ssa paralogs are semi-redundant, evidenced by the fact that yeast remain viable as long as they have one paralog expressed at constitutively high levels [7–9]. Despite their relatedness, recent studies suggest that the Ssa paralogs have slightly different client binding profiles [4]. Similarly, humans encode 13 isoforms of Hsp70s from a multigene family with major cytosolic paralogs being HspA8 (constitutive) and HspA1A/HspA1L (inducible) [10–12]. Hsp90 also exists in various forms in cells. In mammalian cells, the inducible Hsp90a and constitutively expressed Hsp90b are the major species in the cytosol, equivalent to yeast Hsp82 and Hsc82, respectively [5,13]. A major stress that cells must deal with to survive are challenges to genome integrity in the form of DNA damage [14]. The sensing of DNA damage and its repair are mediated by an array of proteins that together form the DNA damage response (DDR) pathway [15]. While chaperones support many key signal transduction pathways in the cell, evidence is building to support a particularly critical role for chaperones in the detection and repair of DNA damage. Hsp70 and Hsp90 support DDR by activating and stabilizing a huge number of DDR proteins including p53, CHK1, FANCA, FANCD2,

BRCA1/2, MRN and RNR complexes [16–18]. A common type of DNA damage is the loss of a base from genomic DNA, known as apurinic/apyrimidinic (AP) sites. The repair of such sites involves the recruitment of the related APE1 and APE2 exonucleases (Apn1 and Apn2 in yeast) [19–24]. Although APE1 and APE2 display functional overlap, APE2 possesses an extra C-terminal domain that is absent in APE1 and lacks any redox activity [22]. A recent study examined global protein abundance and epigenetic changes in response to Hsp90 inhibition. Several DDR proteins were among those found to decrease upon ganetespib and AUY922 treatment, including XRCC1, XPC and APE2 [25]. While APE1 becomes associated with Hsp70 during DNA repair to augment endonuclease activity, no such mechanistic connection between chaperones and APE2 has been identified [26]. In this study, we demonstrate a novel interaction between APE2/Apn2 and the Hsp70–Hsp90 system in yeast and mammalian cells. Although there appears to be no preference for which Hsp90 or Hsp70 paralog APE2/Apn2 bind, yeast Apn2 is destabilized in yeast lacking Ssa2, 3 and 4. Inhibition of Hsp90 via ganetespib or Hsp70 via JG-98 triggered a surprisingly rapid reduction of APE2 in a range of cancer cell lines. Understanding the intricacies of chaperone–endonuclease interactions could lead to more targeted and less toxic cancer therapeutics that exploit the genomic instability often seen in tumor cells.

2. Materials and Methods

2.1. Yeast Strains and Growth Conditions

Yeast cultures were grown in either YPD (1% yeast extract) US Biological Life Sciences, Swampscott, MA, USA, 2% glucose (VWR, Radnor, PA, USA), 2% peptone (Thermo Fisher Scientific, Waltham, MA, USA) or in SD (0.67% yeast nitrogen base without amino acids and carbohydrates (US Biological Life Sciences), 2% glucose), supplemented with the appropriate nutrients to select for plasmids and tagged genes. *Escherichia coli* DH5α was used to propagate all plasmids. *E. coli* cells were cultured in Luria broth medium (1% Bacto tryptone, 0.5% Bacto yeast extract, 1% NaCl) and transformed to ampicillin resistance by standard methods. Hsp70 isoform plasmids were transformed into yeast strain *ssa1-4Δ* [27] using PEG/lithium acetate. After restreaking onto media lacking leucine, transformants were streaked again onto media lacking leucine and containing 5-fluoro-orotic acid (5-FOA) (US Biological Life Sciences), resulting in yeast that expressed Hsp70 paralogs as the sole cytoplasmic Hsp70 in the cell. For a full description of yeast strains see Table 1 and for plasmids see Table 2.

2.2. Purification of HA-Tagged Apn2 from Yeast

The protocol followed for HA-IP was taken from [28] with slight modifications. Cells transformed with control pRS316 plasmid or the plasmid-expressing HA-tagged Apn2 [26] were grown overnight in SD-URA media and then re-inoculated into a larger culture of selectable media and grown to an OD_{600} of 0.800. Cells were harvested, and HA-tagged proteins were isolated as follows. Protein was extracted via bead beating in 500 μL protein extraction buffer (50 mM Na-phosphate pH 8.0, 300 mM NaCl, 0.01% Tween-20). Then, 1000 μg of protein extract was incubated with 25 μL anti-HA magnetic beads (Thermo Fisher Scientific) at 30 °C for 30 min. Anti-HA beads were collected by magnet and then washed 3 times with TBS-T and 2 times with protein extraction buffer. After the final wash, the buffer was aspirated, and beads were incubated with 75 μL protein extraction buffer, and 25 μL 5× SDS-PAGE sample buffer sample was denatured for 5 min at 95 °C and boiled for 10–15 min. Next, the beads were collected via magnet, and the supernatant-containing purified HA-Apn2 was transferred to a fresh tube. Then, 20 μL of each sample was analyzed on SDS-PAGE.

2.3. Mammalian Cell Culture and Drug Treatment

The protocol used for transfection and drug treatment was taken from [22] with slight modifications. HEK293T cells were cultured in Dulbecco's modified Eagle's minimal essential medium (DMEM; Invitrogen, Carlsbad, CA, USA) supplemented with 10% fetal bovine serum (FBS; Invitrogen), 100 U/mL penicillin (Invitrogen) and 100 µg/mL streptomycin (Invitrogen). L-GlutaMAX nutrient mixture (Gibco, Waltham, MA, USA, Cat#31765-035) (10% FBS, 100 units of penicillin and 100 units of streptomycin) was used to culture PC3, RPMI 1640 based medium (10% FBS, 100 units of penicillin and 100 units of streptomycin, 1% L-GlutaMAX-I) for LNCaP and DMEM-based medium (10% FBS, 100 units of penicillin and 100 units of streptomycin, 1% L-GlutaMAX-I) for MCF7. All cell lines were incubated at 37 °C in a 5% CO_2 containing atmosphere. Cells were seeded in 6-well plates at $1 \times 10^6/2$ mL per well one day prior to transfection. Cells were transfected by APE2 expression plasmid pcDNA-APE2-HA-BCP [29] with Lipofectamine3000 transfection kit (Invitrogen, Cat#L3000-015), and 2.5 µg of DNA and 7.5 µL of Lipofectamine3000 were used for each well. Briefly, diluted Lipofectamine3000 and DNA plus P3000 with Opti-MEM I (Gibco, Cat#31985-070) were mixed and incubated at room temperature for 15 min and then added to cell culture dropwise. The cells were treated for 0, 2, 4, 8 and 16 h post 48 h transfection with 10 µM JG-98, which is a Hsp70 inhibitor or 10 µM ganetespib (STA-9090, Selleckchem, Houston, TX, USA, Cat#S1159) for Hsp90 inhibition.

2.4. Transfections and Co-Immunoprecipitation in Mammalian Cells

The protocol used for transfection and drug treatment was adapted from [28] with slight modifications. HEK293T cells or specific cancer cells such as PC3, LNCaP and MCF7 were either untransfected (mock) or transfected with plasmids for expression of HA-tagged and/or V5-tagged proteins for constitutive HSPA8 and inducible HSPA1L and HSPA1A using Lipofectamine 3000 (Thermo Fisher Scientific). After 48 h, the cells were washed with 1X PBS, and total cell extract was prepared from the cells using M-PER (Thermo Fisher Scientific) containing EDTA-free protease and phosphatase inhibitor cocktail (Thermo Fisher Scientific) according to the manufacturer's recommended protocol. Protein was quantitated using the Bradford Assay. HA-tagged proteins were purified as follows. First, 200 µg of protein extract was incubated with 25 µL anti-HA magnetic beads (Thermo Fisher Scientific) at 30 °C for 30 min. Anti-HA beads were collected by magnet and then washed 3 times with TBS-T and 2 times with protein extraction buffer. After the final wash, the buffer was aspirated, and beads were incubated with 75 µL protein extraction buffer, and 25 µL 5× SDS-PAGE sample buffer sample was denatured for 5 min at 95 °C and boiled for 10–15 min. Next, the beads were collected via magnet, and the supernatant-containing purified HA-APE2 was transferred to a fresh tube. Finally, 20 µL of each sample was analyzed on SDS-PAGE.

2.5. Western Blotting

First, 20 µg of protein was separated by 4–12% NuPAGE SDS-PAGE (Thermo Fisher Scientific). Proteins were detected using the following antibodies; anti-HA tag (Thermo Fisher Scientific), Anti-FLAG tag (Sigma-Aldrich, St. Louis, MO, USA, USA #F1365), anti-PGK (Thermo Fisher Scientific, #MA5-15738), anti-Ydj1 (Stressmarq Biosciences Inc., Victoria, BC, Canada, #SMC-166D), anti-HDJ2 (Thermo Fisher Scientific, #MA512748). Blots were imaged on a ChemiDoc MP imaging system (Bio-Rad, Hercules, CA, USA). After treatment with Super Signal West Pico Chemiluminescent Substrate (GE Healthcare, Piscataway, NJ, USA). Blots were stripped and reprobed with the relevant antibodies using Restore Western Blot Stripping Buffer (Thermo Fisher Scientific).

3. Results

3.1. Apn2 Interacts with Ydj1, Hsp82 and Ssa1 in Yeast

Previous studies suggested that inhibition of Hsp90 may lead to loss of APE2 in bladder cancer [25]. To determine whether there was a connection between yeast APE2 (Apn2) and chaperones, we purified HA-tagged Apn2 from yeast and probed the complex with anti-HA, anti-Hsp82, anti-Ssa1, and anti-Ydj1 antibodies. We observed a clear association with Ssa1, Hsp82 and Ydj1 (Figure 1A). There are four cytosolic Hsp70s in yeast, Ssa1, 2, 3 and 4, which are highly similar to the amino acid sequence that arose from multiple yeast gene duplication events [4]. While these paralogs have clear functional overlap, they also display differential client preferences [4]. To determine whether all Ssa paralogs can interact with Apn2, we performed co-immunoprecipitation experiments in WT BY4742 yeast cells (Table 1) expressing plasmids-HA-Apn2 and exogenous Flag-Ssa1, 2, 3 or 4 (Figure 1B). In this context, Apn2 bound equally to all Ssa paralogs (Figure 1B). To query whether all four Ssa paralogs could support Apn2 stability, we examined the levels of constitutively expressed HA-Apn2 in $ssa1$–4Δ yeast, expressing only one of the four Ssa proteins (Table 1). The levels of Apn2 were significantly decreased in yeast-expressing Ssa1 as the sole Ssa paralog in the cell (Figure 1C,D). Co-chaperones of Hsp70 play an important role in regulating chaperone activity and specificity [30]. We wondered whether Ydj1, a major co-chaperone of Ssa1–4, may support Apn2 levels in a similar way to its chaperoning of the ribonucleotide complex [28]. To test this possibility, we compared the abundance of Apn2 in WT yeast and those lacking Ydj1 (Table 1). In contrast to the regulation of RNR, the lack of Ydj1 had minimal impact on Ape2 levels (Figure 1E,F).

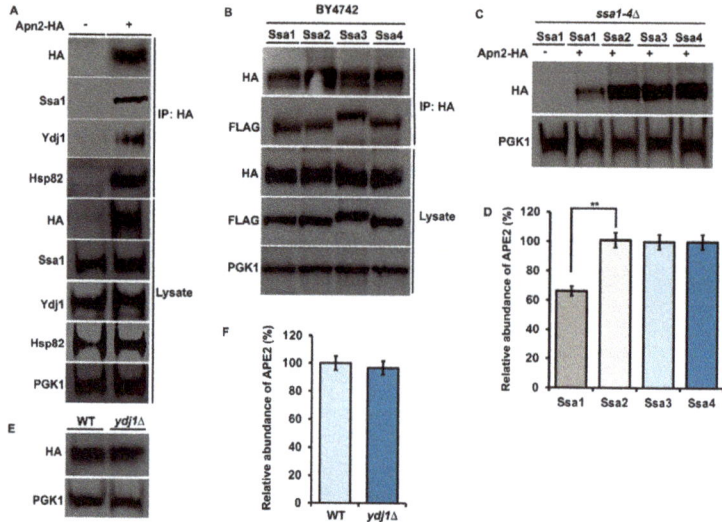

Figure 1. Apn2 interacts with Hsp82, Hsp70 and Ydj1 in yeast. (**A**) Yeast cells expressing Apn-HA were grown to mid-log phase at 30 °C. Lysate from these cells were analyzed by Western blotting with an anti-HA, anti-Ssa1, anti-Ydj1 and anti-Hsp82 antibody. Pgk1 was used as a loading control. Immunoprecipitation was performed using anti-HA magnetic beads, and the interaction was studied. (**B**) WT cells were co-transformed with Apn2-HA and individual Ssa isoforms. Yeast cells were grown to mid-log phase at 30 °C. Lysates were analyzed by Western blotting with HA and FLAG specific antibody. Immunoprecipitation was performed using anti-HA magnetic beads, and interaction between FLAG-Ssa and Apn2-HA was checked using anti-HA and anti-FLAG antibodies on Western blot. (**C**) Yeast expressing the indicated FLAG-Ssa (on a constitutive promoter) in a $ssa1$–4Δ background transformed with Apn2-HA were grown to mid-log phase at 30 °C. Lysates were analyzed by Western blotting with HA- and FLAG-specific antibodies. (**D**) Relative abundance of Apn2-HA was quantitated by taking the ratio of Apn2-HA/PGK1. Data are the mean and SD of three replicate experiments and compared to Ssa2 (** $p < 0.001$) (**E**) WT BY4742 and Ydj1Δ cells, were transformed with HA-Apn2 plasmid. Transformants were grown to mid-log phase at 30 °C. Lysate from these cells was analyzed by Western blotting with an anti-HA and anti-Ydj1 antibody. (**F**) Relative abundance of Apn2-HA was quantitated by taking the ratio of Apn2-HA/PGK1. Data are the mean and SD of three replicate experiments and compared to WT.

3.2. Apn2 Interacts with Both Hsp82 and Is a Client of Hsp90 in Yeast

Our previous results suggested that Apn2 may also be a direct client of Hsp90. To test this hypothesis, we examined Apn2 in yeast expressing a well-characterized temperature sensitive point mutation in Hsp90 [31]. Cells expressing HA-Apn2 in either Hsp82^{G170D} (Table 1) or WT (Table 1) were grown at 25 °C until early mid-log phase and were split into two flasks, one of which was shifted to 39 °C. Cells were lysed after 90 min, and HA-Apn2 levels were examined by Western blot. Incubation at 39 °C caused a significant decrease in HA-Apn2 levels in Hsp82^{G170D} cells, while HA-Apn2 levels remained unchanged in WT cells, confirming Apn2 as a client of Hsp90 (Figure 2A). There are two Hsp90 paralogs in yeast, the heat-inducible Hsp82 and constitutive Hsc82 (Table 1). To assess Apn2 binding preferences for the two Hsp90s, we purified Apn2 from yeast expressing tagged versions of Hsp82 or Hsc82 using anti-HA magnetic beads. Consistent with our results in Figure 1B (above), the binding of Apn2 was equal to both heat-inducible Hsp82 and constitutive Hsc82 (Figure 2C).

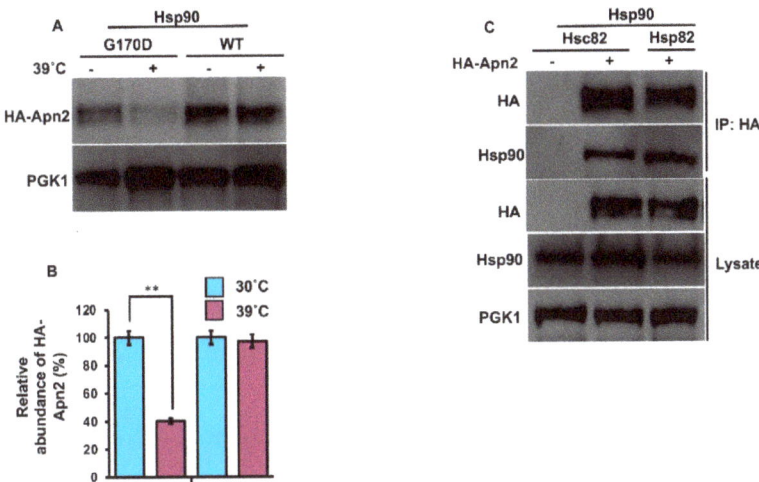

Figure 2. Apn2 interacts with Hsc82 and Hsp82. (**A**) Yeast G170D and P82a cells expressing Apn2-HA were grown to mid-log phase at 30 °C. Cells were stressed at 39 °C, and lysates from unstressed and heat shocked cells were analyzed for Apn2 levels using Western blot with anti-HA antibodies. Pgk1 was used as a loading control. (**B**) Relative abundance of Apn2-HA was quantitated by taking the ratio of Apn2-HA/PGK. Data are the mean and SD of three replicate experiments, and further, unstressed cells were compared to heat shocked cells (** $p < 0.001$). (**C**) Hsc82-Glu and Hsp82-His yeast cells were transformed with Apn2-HA. Cells were grown to mid-log phase at 30 °C. Lysate from these cells was analyzed by SDS-PAGE and Western blotting using anti-HA and yeast anti-Hsc82-specific antibodies. Pgk1 was used as a loading control. Immunoprecipitation was performed using anti-HA magnetic beads, and the interaction was studied.

3.3. Mammalian APE2 Interacts with the Hsp90–Hsp70 Chaperone System

Mammalian APE2 plays a variety of roles in key cellular processes involving the response to a multitude of stressors, including DNA single- and double-strand breaks, base excision repair, and oxidative stress, leading to the activation of DDR complexes and pathways, including ATR and Chk1 [16,18]. The abundance of several DDR proteins, including APE2, decreased in bladder cancer cells treated with Hsp90 inhibitors [25]. To determine if there was a physical interaction between chaperones and APE2, we took a similar approach to that of Figure 1. HEK293 cells were grown to mid-confluence and were transfected with a construct expressing HA-APE2 (Table 2). After 48 h, cells were lysed, and APE2 complexes were purified using anti-HA magnetic beads. SDS-PAGE analysis and Western blotting of APE2 complexes revealed the presence of Hsp70 and Hsp90, which were not observed in the immunoprecipitation from cells lacking HA-APE2 (Figure 3A). Despite the robust interaction of APE2 with the chaperones, the major DNAJA1 co-chaperone was not observed in the APE2 complex (Figure 3A).

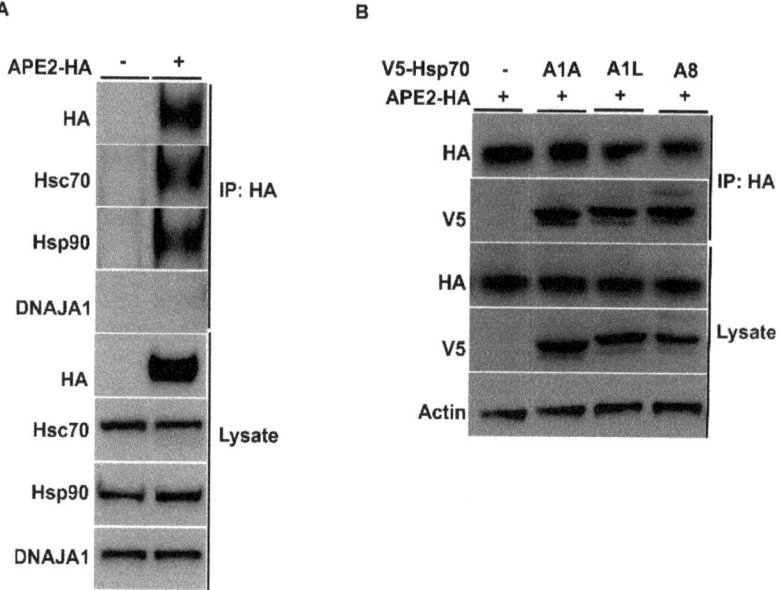

Figure 3. Mammalian APE2 interacts with the Hsp90–Hsp70 chaperone system. (**A**) HEK293 cells were grown to mid-confluence and were transfected with a construct expressing HA-APE2 from a constitutive CMV promoter. After 48 h, cells were lysed, and APE2 complexes were purified using anti-HA-magnetic beads. Lysates from these cells were analyzed by SDS-PAGE and Western blotting using anti-HA, anti-Hsp70, anti-DNAJA1 and anti-Hsp90 specific antibodies. Beta-actin was used as a loading control. Immunoprecipitation was performed using HA beads, and the interaction was studied. (**B**) HEK293 cells were co-transfected with V5-tagged Hsp70 and APE2-HA. Immunoprecipitation was performed using anti-HA-magnetic beads, and the interaction was studied using anti-V5 and anti-HA antibody.

There are a variety of Hsp70 family members expressed in mammalian cells. Although they are highly conserved, they vary in their client selectivity, cellular localization and expression pattern in tissues [11,12,32]. Our previous results suggested that APE2 interacts with HSPA8, the major constitutively expressed isoform of Hsp70 in cells. To determine whether APE2 might be able to bind other HSPA family members, we co-transfected HEK293 cells with plasmids (Table 2) expressing HA-APE2 and V5-tagged HSPA family members that included inducible HSPA1A, HSPA1L and non-inducible HSPA8. After 48 h, we purified HA-APE2 from these cells and subjected the complex to analysis by SDS-PAGE/Western blotting (Figure 3B). Consistent with our results in yeast, APE2 binding was observed between both the constitutive and heat-inducible expressed HSPs in mammalian cells (Figure 3B).

The stability of APE2 in epithelial cells is dependent on Hsp70 and Hsp90 function. Molecular chaperones regulate the folding, maturation and stability of their client proteins [33]. Our previous results implied that APE2 may be a bona fide client of the Hsp90–Hsp70 system. To examine this possibility, we assessed the impact of chaperone inhibition on APE2 abundance. HEK293 cells expressing HA-APE2 were treated with either an inhibitor of Hsp90 (ganetespib) or Hsp70 (JG-98). Cells were harvested at the indicated time points, and APE2 abundance was determined by Western blotting. HEK293 cells treated with ganetespib showed a decrease in APE2 abundance after only 8 h of treatment (Figure 4A). Even more impressive was the rapid decrease in APE2 levels after only 2 h of treatment of JG-98 (Figure 4B). We queried whether this dependence extended to other cancer cell lines including breast cancer (MCF-7) as well as androgen-dependent and androgen-independent prostate cancer (LNCaP and PC-3, respectively). As with our previous experiments, these cell lines were treated with ganetespib, and APE2 levels were assessed through Western blotting at 2 h intervals. In the case of PC-3, MCF7 and LNCaP, the APE2 levels significantly decreased after 2 h of treatment of JG-98 (Figure 5A–F). To similarly understand whether Hsp70 contributed toward APE2 stability, we treated MCF-7, LNCaP and PC-3 cells with the Hsp90 inhibitor and measured APE2 abundance via Western blotting. APE2 levels started to decline significantly after 2 h of treatment with maximum inhibition seen at 16 h (Figure 6A–F).

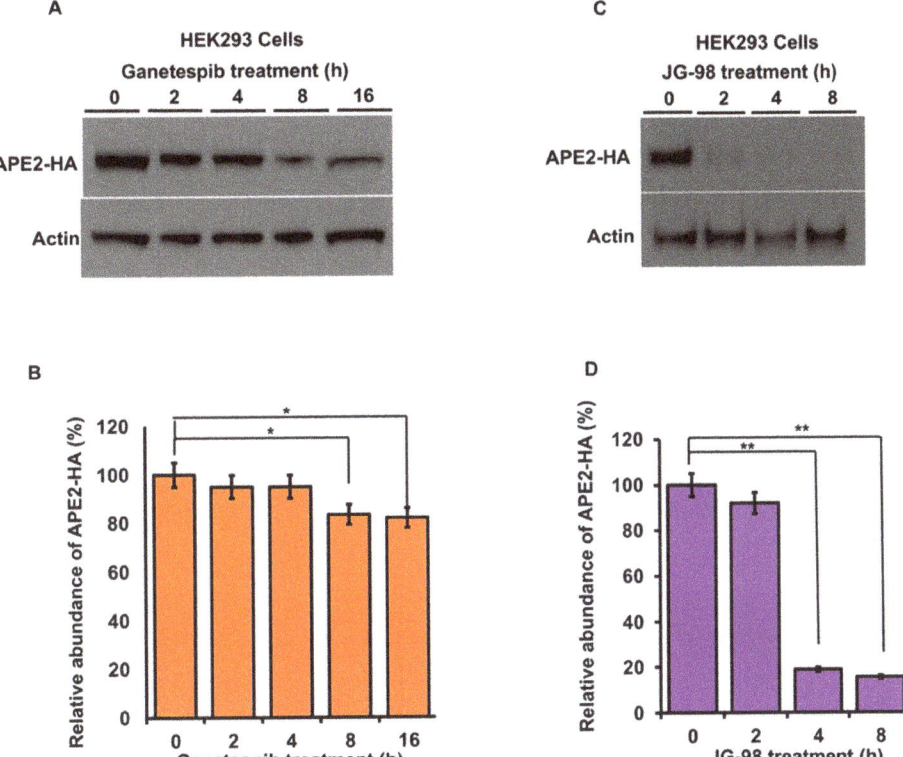

Figure 4. Inhibition of Hsp90 or Hsp70 promote a rapid reduction in APE2 levels. (A) HEK293 cells expressing HA-APE2 were treated with either an inhibitor of Hsp90 (ganetespib) or (C) Hsp70 (JG-98). Cells were harvested at the indicated time points, and APE2 abundance was determined by SDS-PAGE and Western blotting using anti-HA antibody. Beta-actin was used as a loading control. (B,D) The relative abundance of APE2-HA was quantitated by taking the ratio of Apn2-HA/Beta-actin from 3 replicate experiments and compared to untreated HEK293 cells. Data are the mean and SD of three replicate experiments and are compared to untreated. Statistical significance is indicated as (** $p < 0.001$) (* $p < 0.05$).

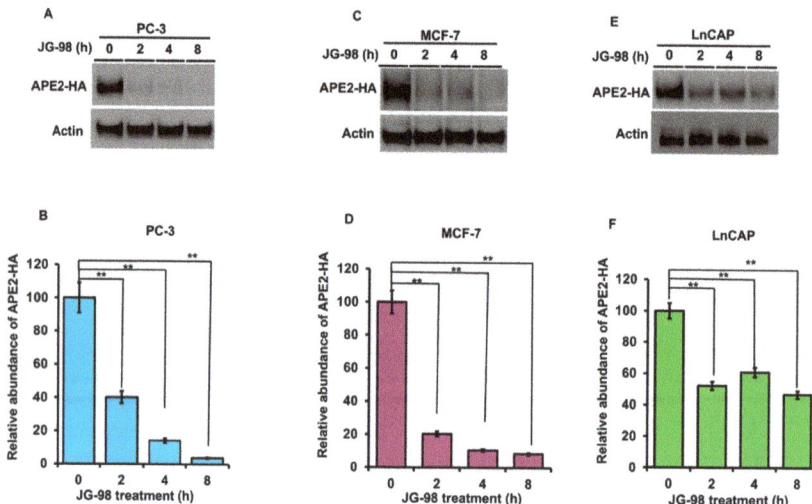

Figure 5. Stability of APE2 in a range of cancer cell lines is dependent on Hsp90 and Hsp70 function. (**A**) PC3 (**C**) MCF7 and (**E**) LnCAP cells expressing HA-APE2 were treated with an inhibitor of Hsp70 (JG-98). Cells were harvested at the indicated time points, and APE2 abundance was determined by SDS-PAGE and Western blotting using anti-HA antibody. Beta-actin was used as a loading control. (**B,D,F**) The relative abundance of APE2-HA was quantitated by taking the ratio of APE2-HA/Beta-actin. Data are the mean and SD of three replicate experiments and are compared to untreated (** $p < 0.001$).

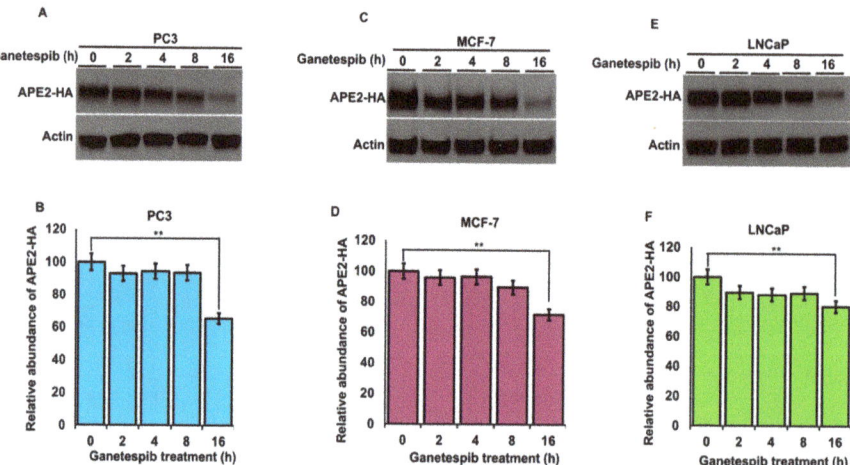

Figure 6. Stability of APE2 in a range of cancer cell lines is dependent on Hsp90 function. (**A**) PC3 (**C**) MCF7 and (**E**) LnCAP cells expressing HA-APE2 were treated with an inhibitor of Hsp90 (ganetespib). Cells were harvested at the indicated time points, and APE2 abundance was determined by SDS-PAGE and Western blotting. Beta-actin was used as a loading control. (**B,D,F**) The relative abundance of APE2-HA was quantitated by taking the ratio of APE2-HA/Beta-actin. Data are the mean and SD of three replicate experiments and are compared to untreated (** $p < 0.001$).

4. Discussion

The ability of cells to repair and maintain their genome is critical for their survival. The response to DNA damage is highly complex and relies on several different signaling cascades comprising multiple proteins [14,15]. The Hsp70–Hsp90 chaperone system binds and regulates several important proteins in this process, including APE1 and P53. Recent efforts in understanding the role of chaperones in DDR have included large-scale proteomics analysis, such as that of Li et al., which examined the abundance of proteins in 5637 bladder cancer cells after treatment with the Hsp90 inhibitors ganetespib (STA9090), or luminespib (AUY-922) [25]. In that study, over 800 proteins were downregulated, including XRCC1, XPC, RAD50, 53BP1 and notably, APE2 [25]. In this study, we have identified a role for the Hsp70 and Hsp90 chaperones in regulating the activity of the APN2/Ape2 exonuclease in yeast and mammalian cells.

4.1. APE2 and Apn2 Display Binding Preferences for Chaperone and Co-Chaperone Paralogs

An unresolved question in chaperone biology is why cells express many highly similar chaperone proteins. In yeast, the four Ssa proteins are highly conserved with over 80% similarity in amino acids sequence [4]. Ssa1 and Ssa2 represent the major cytosolic Hsp70s present under basal conditions, while Ssa3 and Ssa4 are highly heat induced. Several studies have suggested that these chaperone paralogs have overlapping but unique interactomes [34]. Recently, work using the model substrate ribonucleotide reductase (RNR) showed a clear preference for this client in binding Ssa1 and Ssa2 [35]. Although Apn2 binds cytosolic Hsp70 and Hsp90 paralogs equally, cells expressing Ssa1 as their sole cytosolic Ssa1 are unable to support WT levels of Ape2 as depicted by compromised stability in Figure 1B,C. The difference in Apn2 abundance in Ssa2 vs. Ssa1-expressing yeast is particularly interesting considering how similar the two proteins are. However, previous studies have shown that even a single divergent amino acid between Ssa1 and Ssa2 can produce differences in their ability to modulate prion propagation and protein degradation [36]. A recent study observed a parallel defect in septin levels in Ssa1-expressing yeast [37]. Future research, possibly involving a comparative interactome study of Ssa proteins, may shed light on this issue [34].

Cells express a variety of co-chaperones that are critical for stimulation of chaperone ATPase activity and for loading clients onto chaperones for folding [3,30,38]. We show here that Apn2 co-purifies with Ydj1, a major Hsp70 co-chaperone (Figure 1A). In contrast to ribonucleotide reductase whose stability depends on Ydj1 function, loss of Ydj1 does not impact Apn2 stability [28]. It is possible that Apn2 stability in yeast is additionally regulated by other semi-redundant co-chaperones such as Sis1, which has similar yet distinct roles in the cell as Ydj1 [39–42]. This may also explain why in our studies, DNAJA1 the mammalian homologue of Ydj1 does not appear to interact with APE2 (Figure 3A). Going forward, it would be interesting to identify and understand the major co-chaperones responsible for regulating APE2 and Apn2 function in mammalian and yeast cells, respectively.

4.2. Novel Anticancer Strategies Based on Fine-Tuning Chaperone Function

Molecular chaperones are required for the stability and activity of many proteins, including oncoproteins that are critical for cancer progression [43–46]. Recently, APE2 has been revealed to be an important player in regulating genome integrity and cancer progression [20,22,23,29,47,48]. Our study suggests that targeting APE2 activity through inhibition of chaperone function may be a viable anticancer therapy. While in vitro studies such as those presented here clearly show the value of manipulating chaperone function, studies in vivo suggest that complete abolishment of Hsp70 or Hsp90 results in severe toxicity for patients [25,49]. Several alternative approaches to bypass the toxicity issue are currently being pursued [49–51]. The first has been to identify key co-chaperones that regulate oncogenic clients and to develop drugs that inhibit them, such as 116-9e and C-86 [52–54]. While DNAJA1 is not observed in complex with APE2, it is possible that drugs such as 116-9e and C-86 may have a broad enough specificity to be target regulatory co-chaperones of APE2 in cancer. An alternative method for fine-tuning of chaperones may be to manipulate their post-translational modifications (PTMs) [55–57]. Future studies examining the Hsp70/Hsp90-APE2 structure may allow for specific targeting of this interaction via small molecules that bind the interaction interface or alter critical PTMs required for chaperone–exonuclease interaction.

Table 1. Yeast strains used in this study.

Strain	Genotype	Reference/Source
yAT 685	Hsc82 (PP30-HSC82-GLU (MAT a, trp1-289, leu2-3112, his3-200, ura3-52, ade2-101, lys2-801, hsc82::KANMX4, hsp82::KANMX4 LEU2-GPD-HSC82-GLU)	[51]
yAT 686	Hsp82 PP30-HSP82-HIS (MAT a, trp1-289, leu2-3112, his3-200, ura3-52, ade2-101, lys2-801, hsc82::KANMX4, hsp82::KANMX4 LEU2-GPD-HSP82-HIS)	[51]
yAT01	P82a W303–1a hsc82::LEU2 hsp82::LEU2 HIS3-GPD-HSP82a	[31]
yAT05	G170D W303–1a hsc82::LEU2 hsp82::LEU2 HIS3-GPD-hsp82(G170D)a	[31]
yAT38	MATα S288c (BY4742) his3Δ1 leu2Δ0 lys2Δ0 ura3Δ0	Euroscarf
yAT414	MATa (MH272) ssa1Δ::trp1 ssa2::HisG ssa3::HisG ssa4::HisG (ssa1–4) [YCPlac33 SSA1]	[27]
yAT28	MATα S288c (BY4742) ydj1Δ::KanMX4	Euroscarf

Table 2. Plasmids used in this study.

Plasmids	Description	Reference
pNK229	GPD2-Apn2-HA	[18]
pAT778	pRS315PSsa2-Flag-SSA1 (LEU2)	Vector Builder
pAT779	pRS315PSsa2-Flag-SSA2 (LEU2)	Vector Builder
pAT780	pRS315PSsa2-Flag-SSA3 (LEU2)	Vector Builder
pAT781	pRS315PSsa2-Flag-SSA4 (LEU2)	Vector Builder
	APE2-HA	[23]
pAT758	HSPA1A-V5 pcDNA5/FRT/TO	Harm Kampinga
pAT759	HSPA1L-V5 pcDNA5/FRT/TO	Harm Kampinga
pAT763	HSPA8-V5 pcDNA5/FRT/TO	Harm Kampinga

Overall, this work identifies a new client of the Hsp70–Hsp90 axis, the Apn2/APE2 exonuclease. The rapid loss of APE2 in cancer cells upon inhibition of either Hsp90 or Hsp70 provides a path forward for novel therapies that jointly target chaperones and the DNA damage response.

Author Contributions: Conceptualization, A.W.T. and S.O.; methodology, A.W.T.; formal analysis, S.O., B.Z. and T.H.W.; investigation, S.O., B.Z. and T.H.W.; resources, A.W.T.; data curation, S.O.; writing—original draft preparation, S.O. and M.M.M.; writing—review and editing, A.W.T., S.O., T.H.W. and M.M.M.; funding acquisition, A.W.T. All authors have read and agreed to the published version of the manuscript.

Funding: This research was funded by the National Institutes of Health, grant numbers R01GM139885 and R15GM139059.

Institutional Review Board Statement: Not applicable.

Informed Consent Statement: Not applicable.

Data Availability Statement: All data from this study can be found in the main manuscript.

Acknowledgments: We would like to thank Mehdi Mollapour, Daniel Durocher, and Nayun Kim for kindly providing materials for this study.

Conflicts of Interest: The authors declare no competing interests.

References

1. Hartl, F.U.; Bracher, A.; Hayer-Hartl, M. Molecular chaperones in protein folding and proteostasis. *Nature* **2011**, *475*, 324–332. [CrossRef] [PubMed]
2. Balchin, D.; Hayer-Hartl, M.; Hartl, F.U. In vivo aspects of protein folding and quality control. *Science* **2016**, *353*, aac4354. [CrossRef] [PubMed]
3. Rosenzweig, R.; Nillegoda, N.B.; Mayer, M.P.; Bukau, B. The Hsp70 chaperone network. *Nat. Rev. Mol. Cell Biol.* **2019**, *20*, 665–680. [CrossRef]
4. Lotz, S.K.; Knighton, L.E.; Nitika; Jones, G.W.; Truman, A.W. Not quite the SSAme: Unique roles for the yeast cytosolic Hsp70s. *Curr. Genet.* **2019**, *65*, 1127–1134. [CrossRef] [PubMed]
5. Girstmair, H.; Tippel, F.; Lopez, A.; Tych, K.; Stein, F.; Haberkant, P.; Schmid, P.W.N.; Helm, D.; Rief, M.; Sattler, M.; et al. The Hsp90 isoforms from S. cerevisiae differ in structure, function and client range. *Nat. Commun.* **2019**, *10*, 3626. [CrossRef]
6. Kabani, M.; Martineau, C.N. Multiple hsp70 isoforms in the eukaryotic cytosol: Mere redundancy or functional specificity? *Curr. Genom.* **2008**, *9*, 338–348. [CrossRef]
7. Werner-Washburne, M.; Stone, D.E.; Craig, E.A. Complex interactions among members of an essential subfamily of hsp70 genes in Saccharomyces cerevisiae. *Mol. Cell Biol.* **1987**, *7*, 2568–2577. [CrossRef] [PubMed]
8. Werner-Washburne, M.; Becker, J.; Kosic-Smithers, J.; Craig, E.A. Yeast Hsp70 RNA levels vary in response to the physiological status of the cell. *J. Bacteriol.* **1989**, *171*, 2680–2688. [CrossRef]
9. Werner-Washburne, M.; Craig, E.A. Expression of members of the Saccharomyces cerevisiae hsp70 multigene family. *Genome* **1989**, *31*, 684–689. [CrossRef]
10. Hageman, J.; Kampinga, H.H. Computational analysis of the human HSPH/HSPA/DNAJ family and cloning of a human HSPH/HSPA/DNAJ expression library. *Cell Stress Chaperones* **2009**, *14*, 1–21. [CrossRef]
11. Daugaard, M.; Rohde, M.; Jaattela, M. The heat shock protein 70 family: Highly homologous proteins with overlapping and distinct functions. *FEBS Lett.* **2007**, *581*, 3702–3710. [CrossRef] [PubMed]
12. Serlidaki, D.; van Waarde, M.; Rohland, L.; Wentink, A.S.; Dekker, S.L.; Kamphuis, M.J.; Boertien, J.M.; Brunsting, J.F.; Nillegoda, N.B.; Bukau, B.; et al. Functional diversity between HSP70 paralogs caused by variable interactions with specific co-chaperones. *J. Biol. Chem.* **2020**, *295*, 7301–7316. [CrossRef]
13. Sreedhar, A.S.; Kalmar, E.; Csermely, P.; Shen, Y.F. Hsp90 isoforms: Functions, expression and clinical importance. *FEBS Lett.* **2004**, *562*, 11–15. [CrossRef]
14. Lindahl, T. Instability and decay of the primary structure of DNA. *Nature* **1993**, *362*, 709–715. [CrossRef] [PubMed]
15. Ciccia, A.; Elledge, S.J. The DNA damage response: Making it safe to play with knives. *Mol. Cell* **2010**, *40*, 179–204. [CrossRef] [PubMed]
16. Pennisi, R.; Ascenzi, P.; di Masi, A. Hsp90: A New Player in DNA Repair? *Biomolecules* **2015**, *5*, 2589–2618. [CrossRef] [PubMed]
17. Knighton, L.E.; Delgado, L.E.; Truman, A.W. Novel insights into molecular chaperone regulation of ribonucleotide reductase. *Curr. Genet.* **2019**, *65*, 477–482. [CrossRef]
18. Knighton, L.E.; Truman, A.W. Role of the Molecular Chaperones Hsp70 and Hsp90 in the DNA Damage Response. In *Heat Shock Proteins in Signaling Pathways*; Springer: Cham, Switzerland, 2019; Volume 17, pp. 345–358.
19. Whitaker, A.M.; Freudenthal, B.D. APE1: A skilled nucleic acid surgeon. *DNA Repair* **2018**, *71*, 93–100. [CrossRef] [PubMed]
20. Willis, J.; Patel, Y.; Lentz, B.L.; Yan, S. APE2 is required for ATR-Chk1 checkpoint activation in response to oxidative stress. *Proc. Natl. Acad. Sci. USA* **2013**, *110*, 10592–10597. [CrossRef]
21. McNeill, D.R.; Whitaker, A.M.; Stark, W.J.; Illuzzi, J.L.; McKinnon, P.J.; Freudenthal, B.D.; Wilson, D.M., 3rd. Functions of the major abasic endonuclease (APE1) in cell viability and genotoxin resistance. *Mutagenesis* **2020**, *35*, 27–38. [CrossRef]
22. Lin, Y.; McMahon, A.; Driscoll, G.; Bullock, S.; Zhao, J.; Yan, S. Function and molecular mechanisms of APE2 in genome and epigenome integrity. *Mutat. Res. Rev. Mutat. Res.* **2021**, *787*, 108347. [CrossRef] [PubMed]
23. Hossain, M.A.; Lin, Y.; Yan, S. Single-Strand Break End Resection in Genome Integrity: Mechanism and Regulation by APE2. *Int. J. Mol. Sci.* **2018**, *19*, 2389. [CrossRef] [PubMed]
24. Boiteux, S.; Guillet, M. Abasic sites in DNA: Repair and biological consequences in Saccharomyces cerevisiae. *DNA Repair* **2004**, *3*, 1–12. [CrossRef] [PubMed]
25. Li, Q.Q.; Hao, J.J.; Zhang, Z.; Krane, L.S.; Hammerich, K.H.; Sanford, T.; Trepel, J.B.; Neckers, L.; Agarwal, P.K. Proteomic analysis of proteome and histone post-translational modifications in heat shock protein 90 inhibition-mediated bladder cancer therapeutics. *Sci. Rep.* **2017**, *7*, 201. [CrossRef]
26. Mendez, F.; Sandigursky, M.; Kureekattil, R.P.; Kenny, M.K.; Franklin, W.A.; Bases, R. Specific stimulation of human apurinic/apyrimidinic endonuclease by heat shock protein 70. *DNA Repair* **2003**, *2*, 259–271. [CrossRef]
27. Jaiswal, H.; Conz, C.; Otto, H.; Wolfle, T.; Fitzke, E.; Mayer, M.P.; Rospert, S. The chaperone network connected to human ribosome-associated complex. *Mol. Cell Biol.* **2011**, *31*, 1160–1173. [CrossRef]
28. Sluder, I.T.; Nitika; Knighton, L.E.; Truman, A.W. The Hsp70 co-chaperone Ydj1/HDJ2 regulates ribonucleotide reductase activity. *PLoS Genet.* **2018**, *14*, e1007462. [CrossRef] [PubMed]
29. Alvarez-Quilon, A.; Wojtaszek, J.L.; Mathieu, M.C.; Patel, T.; Appel, C.D.; Hustedt, N.; Rossi, S.E.; Wallace, B.D.; Setiaputra, D.; Adam, S.; et al. Endogenous DNA 3′ Blocks Are Vulnerabilities for BRCA1 and BRCA2 Deficiency and Are Reversed by the APE2 Nuclease. *Mol. Cell* **2020**, *78*, 1152–1165 e1158. [CrossRef]

30. Kampinga, H.H.; Craig, E.A. The HSP70 chaperone machinery: J proteins as drivers of functional specificity. *Nat. Rev. Mol. Cell Biol.* **2010**, *11*, 579–592. [CrossRef]
31. Nathan, D.F.; Lindquist, S. Mutational analysis of Hsp90 function: Interactions with a steroid receptor and a protein kinase. *Mol. Cell Biol.* **1995**, *15*, 3917–3925. [CrossRef]
32. Boorstein, W.R.; Ziegelhoffer, T.; Craig, E.A. Molecular evolution of the HSP70 multigene family. *J. Mol. Evol.* **1994**, *38*, 1–17. [CrossRef] [PubMed]
33. Kim, Y.E.; Hipp, M.S.; Bracher, A.; Hayer-Hartl, M.; Hartl, F.U. Molecular chaperone functions in protein folding and proteostasis. *Annu. Rev. Biochem.* **2013**, *82*, 323–355. [CrossRef] [PubMed]
34. Knighton, L.E.; Nitika; Waller, S.J.; Strom, O.; Wolfgeher, D.; Reitzel, A.M.; Truman, A.W. Dynamic remodeling of the interactomes of Nematostella vectensis Hsp70 isoforms under heat shock. *J. Proteom.* **2019**, *206*, 103416. [CrossRef]
35. Knighton, L.E.; Nitika; Omkar, S.; Truman, A.W. The C-terminal domain of Hsp70 is responsible for paralog-specific regulation of ribonucleotide reductase. *PLoS Genet.* **2022**, *18*, e1010079. [CrossRef]
36. Sharma, D.; Masison, D.C. Single methyl group determines prion propagation and protein degradation activities of yeast heat shock protein (Hsp)-70 chaperones Ssa1p and Ssa2p. *Proc. Natl. Acad. Sci. USA* **2011**, *108*, 13665–13670. [CrossRef]
37. Denney, A.S.; Weems, A.D.; McMurray, M.A. Selective functional inhibition of a tumor-derived p53 mutant by cytosolic chaperones identified using split-YFP in budding yeast. *G3* **2021**, *11*, jkab230. [CrossRef]
38. Craig, E.A.; Marszalek, J. How Do J-Proteins Get Hsp70 to Do So Many Different Things? *Trends Biochem. Sci.* **2017**, *42*, 355–368. [CrossRef]
39. Truman, A.W.; Kristjansdottir, K.; Wolfgeher, D.; Hasin, N.; Polier, S.; Zhang, H.; Perrett, S.; Prodromou, C.; Jones, G.W.; Kron, S.J. CDK-dependent Hsp70 Phosphorylation controls G1 cyclin abundance and cell-cycle progression. *Cell* **2012**, *151*, 1308–1318. [CrossRef]
40. Tutar, L.; Tutar, Y. Ydj1 but not Sis1 stabilizes Hsp70 protein under prolonged stress in vitro. *Biopolymers* **2008**, *89*, 171–174. [CrossRef]
41. Walters, R.W.; Muhlrad, D.; Garcia, J.; Parker, R. Differential effects of Ydj1 and Sis1 on Hsp70-mediated clearance of stress granules in Saccharomyces cerevisiae. *RNA* **2015**, *21*, 1660–1671. [CrossRef]
42. Wyszkowski, H.; Janta, A.; Sztangierska, W.; Obuchowski, I.; Chamera, T.; Klosowska, A.; Liberek, K. Class-specific interactions between Sis1 J-domain protein and Hsp70 chaperone potentiate disaggregation of misfolded proteins. *Proc. Natl. Acad. Sci. USA* **2021**, *118*, e2108163118. [CrossRef] [PubMed]
43. Workman, P. Reflections and Outlook on Targeting HSP90, HSP70 and HSF1 in Cancer: A Personal Perspective. *Adv. Exp. Med. Biol.* **2020**, *1243*, 163–179. [CrossRef]
44. Mosser, D.D.; Caron, A.W.; Bourget, L.; Meriin, A.B.; Sherman, M.Y.; Morimoto, R.I.; Massie, B. The chaperone function of hsp70 is required for protection against stress-induced apoptosis. *Mol. Cell Biol.* **2000**, *20*, 7146–7159. [CrossRef] [PubMed]
45. Li, X.; Colvin, T.; Rauch, J.N.; Acosta-Alvear, D.; Kampmann, M.; Dunyak, B.; Hann, B.; Aftab, B.T.; Murnane, M.; Cho, M.; et al. Validation of the Hsp70-Bag3 protein-protein interaction as a potential therapeutic target in cancer. *Mol. Cancer Ther.* **2015**, *14*, 642–648. [CrossRef] [PubMed]
46. Murphy, M.E. The HSP70 family and cancer. *Carcinogenesis* **2013**, *34*, 1181–1188. [CrossRef] [PubMed]
47. Lin, Y.; Bai, L.; Cupello, S.; Hossain, M.A.; Deem, B.; McLeod, M.; Raj, J.; Yan, S. APE2 promotes DNA damage response pathway from a single-strand break. *Nucleic Acids Res.* **2018**, *46*, 2479–2494. [CrossRef] [PubMed]
48. Wallace, B.D.; Berman, Z.; Mueller, G.A.; Lin, Y.; Chang, T.; Andres, S.N.; Wojtaszek, J.L.; DeRose, E.F.; Appel, C.D.; London, R.E.; et al. APE2 Zf-GRF facilitates 3′-5′ resection of DNA damage following oxidative stress. *Proc. Natl. Acad. Sci. USA* **2017**, *114*, 304–309. [CrossRef]
49. Shevtsov, M.; Huile, G.; Multhoff, G. Membrane heat shock protein 70: A theranostic target for cancer therapy. *Philos. Trans. R. Soc. Lond. Ser. B Biol. Sci.* **2018**, *373*, 20160526. [CrossRef]
50. Erlichman, C. Tanespimycin: The opportunities and challenges of targeting heat shock protein 90. *Expert Opin. Investig. Drugs* **2009**, *18*, 861–868. [CrossRef]
51. Piper, P.W.; Millson, S.H.; Mollapour, M.; Panaretou, B.; Siligardi, G.; Pearl, L.H.; Prodromou, C. Sensitivity to Hsp90-targeting drugs can arise with mutation to the Hsp90 chaperone, cochaperones and plasma membrane ATP binding cassette transporters of yeast. *Eur. J. Biochem.* **2003**, *270*, 4689–4695. [CrossRef]
52. Nitika; Blackman, J.S.; Knighton, L.E.; Takakuwa, J.E.; Calderwood, S.K.; Truman, A.W. Chemogenomic screening identifies the Hsp70 co-chaperone DNAJA1 as a hub for anticancer drug resistance. *Sci. Rep.* **2020**, *10*, 13831. [CrossRef] [PubMed]
53. Moses, M.A.; Kim, Y.S.; Rivera-Marquez, G.M.; Oshima, N.; Watson, M.J.; Beebe, K.E.; Wells, C.; Lee, S.; Zuehlke, A.D.; Shao, H.; et al. Targeting the Hsp40/Hsp70 Chaperone Axis as a Novel Strategy to Treat Castration-Resistant Prostate Cancer. *Cancer Res.* **2018**, *78*, 4022–4035. [CrossRef]
54. Wisen, S.; Bertelsen, E.B.; Thompson, A.D.; Patury, S.; Ung, P.; Chang, L.; Evans, C.G.; Walter, G.M.; Wipf, P.; Carlson, H.A.; et al. Binding of a small molecule at a protein-protein interface regulates the chaperone activity of hsp70-hsp40. *ACS Chem. Biol.* **2010**, *5*, 611–622. [CrossRef] [PubMed]
55. Nitika; Porter, C.M.; Truman, A.W.; Truttmann, M.C. Post-translational modifications of Hsp70 family proteins: Expanding the chaperone code. *J. Biol. Chem.* **2020**, *295*, 10689–10708. [CrossRef] [PubMed]

56. Backe, S.J.; Sager, R.A.; Woodford, M.R.; Makedon, A.M.; Mollapour, M. Post-translational modifications of Hsp90 and translating the chaperone code. *J. Biol. Chem.* **2020**, *295*, 11099–11117. [CrossRef] [PubMed]
57. Truman, A.W.; Bourboulia, D.; Mollapour, M. Decrypting the chaperone code. *J. Biol. Chem.* **2021**, *296*, 100293. [CrossRef]

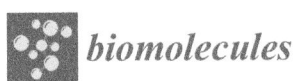

Review

The Role of Hsp90 in Retinal Proteostasis and Disease

Kalliopi Ziaka and Jacqueline van der Spuy *

UCL Institute of Ophthalmology, 11-43 Bath Street, London EC1V 9EL, UK; kalliopi.ziaka.16@ucl.ac.uk
* Correspondence: j.spuy@ucl.ac.uk

Abstract: Photoreceptors are sensitive neuronal cells with great metabolic demands, as they are responsible for carrying out visual phototransduction, a complex and multistep process that requires the exquisite coordination of a large number of signalling protein components. Therefore, the viability of photoreceptors relies on mechanisms that ensure a well-balanced and functional proteome that maintains the protein homeostasis, or proteostasis, of the cell. This review explores how the different isoforms of Hsp90, including the cytosolic Hsp90α/β, the mitochondrial TRAP1, and the ER-specific GRP94, are involved in the different proteostatic mechanisms of photoreceptors, and elaborates on Hsp90 function when retinal homeostasis is disturbed. In addition, several studies have shown that chemical manipulation of Hsp90 has significant consequences, both in healthy and degenerating retinae, and this can be partially attributed to the fact that Hsp90 interacts with important photoreceptor-associated client proteins. Here, the interaction of Hsp90 with the retina-specific client proteins PDE6 and GRK1 will be further discussed, providing additional insights for the role of Hsp90 in retinal disease.

Keywords: chaperone; co-chaperone; heat shock protein; Hsp90; inherited retinal disease; photoreceptor; phototransduction; proteostasis

---

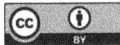

1. Phototransduction and Protein Folding in Photoreceptors (PR)

Photoreceptor cells are highly specialized sensory neurons in the retina, and are essential for converting light into a neural signal, a fundamental process which initiates vision. In the mammalian retina, there are two types of photoreceptor cells, the rods and the cones. Both rods and cones are adjacent to the retinal pigment epithelium (RPE), a monolayer of pigmented cells which is vital for the normal function and survival of photoreceptors [1]. Morphologically, photoreceptors consist of a synaptic terminal, a nuclear region, and an inner segment (IS) and outer segment (OS) which are connected by a connecting cilium (CC). The OS of both cell types consists of closely spaced membranous discs containing photopigment molecules, called opsins, which are coupled to a light-absorbing chromophore (retinal, an aldehyde of vitamin A). Opsins are responsible for tuning the absorption of light to a specific wavelength of the light spectrum. The rod OS contains the rod-specific photopigment rhodopsin, whereas the cone OS contains one of the three cone-opsins, S-opsin, M-opsin, or L-opsin. Rhodopsin, with a peak absorption (λ_{max}) of ~500 nm, functions during dim light conditions allowing scotopic vision, whereas cone opsins are responsible for processing wavelengths ranging from ~350 to 560 nm, thus allowing colour vision [2]. Rods and cones share the same cellular mechanism of light detection, a process known as phototransduction.

Phototransduction is a complex mechanism in which light is converted into an electrical signal through the sequential activation of signalling proteins. In rods, phototransduction is activated by the photoisomerization of the rhodopsin-bound chromophore 11-*cis*-retinal to all-*trans* retinal, inducing a conformational change in rhodopsin to its activated form metarhodopsin II. Metarhodopsin II stimulates the trimeric G-protein transducin by catalysing the exchange of GDP for GTP on the α-subunit. The GTP-associated α-subunit of transducin dissociates from the β and γ subunits and activates PDE6, a phosphodiesterase that hydrolyses cGMP. The decreased concentration of cGMP in the OS results in the closure of cGMP-gated channels in the plasma membrane, and the cessation of sodium and calcium influx, which, in turn, leads to the hyperpolarisation of the rod cell and the inhibition of glutamate release at the synaptic terminal [3]. A series of biochemical reactions is required for photoreceptors to return to their inactive state. This involves another network of proteins which restore the various activated components to their inactive state. G-protein-coupled receptor kinase 1 (GRK1) phosphorylates metarhodopsin II, inducing a conformational change that enables the binding of arrestin, leading to its inactivation. PDE6 is inactivated upon GTP hydrolysis of the transducin α-subunit, a process that is facilitated by the GTPase-activating protein (GAP) complex, consisting of RGS9 (regulator of G-protein-signalling isoform 9) and G-protein β-subunit or G-protein β-subunit-like protein [4]. As a result, free cGMP concentration returns to normal levels (depolarised state) due to the activation of guanylyl cyclase activating proteins (GCAP) and the cGMP-synthesizing enzyme guanylate cyclase (GC). The phototransduction cascade in cone photoreceptors is similar to that in rods and is mediated by homologous phototransduction proteins [5,6]. However, while rods generate a detectable single photon response for maximal sensitivity in dim light conditions, cones are less sensitive than rods and require the simultaneous activation of tens to hundreds of opsin molecules in bright light conditions to generate a detectable response. The high spatial and temporal resolution of cone-mediated vision is made possible by the rapid kinetics of activation and inactivation, the trade-off of which is low amplification and sensitivity. In contrast, the trade-off of the high amplification gain of rods in dim light is their slow kinetics [5,6]. The adaption of rods and cones that shift their dynamic range towards dim and bright light detection respectively places a great metabolic demand on photoreceptors, as the visual cycle requires high amounts of energy for the phototransduction components to coordinate and function together. Moreover, constant triggering of phototransduction causes photooxidative stress to the OS components which need to be constantly replaced to avoid permanent damage. This is achieved by synthesis of new OS disks at the base of the OS and shedding of the OS tips which are phagocytosed by the RPE [7]. Interestingly, RPE cells have the highest phagocytic activity in the body, highlighting the intense metabolic demands of OS renewal [8,9]. To maintain this ability while performing their normal biological function, photoreceptors rely on high levels of protein synthesis, and the correct folding, assembly, trafficking, and degradation of various protein components. High levels of protein synthesis of the phototransduction components occur in the IS which must be continuously translocated through the connecting cilium to their site of action in the OS. The balance of these processes in the photoreceptor cell is called protein homeostasis or "proteostasis".

2. The Importance of Hsp90 Isoforms in Retinal Proteostasis

Proteostasis is maintained and controlled by an extensive network of molecular chaperones, proteolytic systems, and their regulators, termed the proteostasis network (PN). To ensure the correct folding and degradation of misfolded proteins, the PN includes sophisticated protein quality control (PQC) mechanisms, of which the chaperone Hsp90 is a vital component. Hsp90 is an ATP-dependent protein that is universally found in various cellular compartments, such as the cytosol, the ER, and the mitochondria. There are five Hsp90 members, which according to published guidelines for HSP nomenclature are categorised under the HSPC family and include the cytosolic HSPC1 (HSP90AA1), HSPC2 (HSP90AA2), HSPC3 (HSP90AB1), the endoplasmic reticulum (ER) HSPC4 (GRP94), and the mitochondrial HSPC5 (TRAP1) isoforms [10]. These isoforms participate in different PQC systems in the various compartments of the cell with a common aim to support the folding or refolding and stability of client proteins. Hsp90 functions as a dimer, with each protomer within the Hsp90 dimer comprising an N-terminal ATP-binding domain, a middle domain, and a constitutively dimerised C-terminal domain. Hsp90 chaperone activity is coupled with ATP hydrolysis, wherein ATP binds to an open conformation of Hsp90, which induces the transient dimerisation of the N-terminal domains and ATP hydrolysis with subsequent release of the client protein (reviewed by [11,12]). The Hsp90 cycle facilitates the folding, maturation, or assembly of near-native client proteins, of which there are several hundred (https://www.picard.ch/downloads/Hsp90interactors.pdf accessed on 3 July 2022). Hsp90 co-chaperones interact non-covalently with Hsp90 to modulate the Hsp90 cycle or specifically target client proteins to Hsp90 (reviewed by [11,12]).

2.1. Cytosolic Hsp90

The cytosolic isoforms of Hsp90 participate in protein folding as a part of the heat shock response (HSR) and the Hsp90/Hsp70 protein folding machinery (Figure 1). The HSR is an orchestrated process that leads to the rapid transcription of selective genes encoding cytosolic molecular chaperones, also known as heat shock proteins (HSPs). The transcriptional activation of HSPs is regulated by transcription factors known as heat shock factors (HSFs) [13]. HSF1 is the key regulator of the HSR leading to HSP induction in response to stress. In the absence of stress, monomeric HSF1 is maintained in an inactive state by interaction with molecular chaperones in the cytosol, including Hsp90 [14]. In the presence of stress, HSF1 is converted from an inactive monomer to an active DNA-binding trimer, and this trimerization process involves the dissociation of Hsp90 and co-chaperones from its regulatory domain [15]. The trimerized HSF1 translocates to the nucleus and binds to heat shock elements (HSE) in the promoters of target genes that promote the transcription of Hsp90 and other HSPs [16].

In addition to its role in the HSR, cytosolic Hsp90 also functions as part of the Hsp90/Hsp70 protein folding machinery, in which Hsp90 targets client proteins, early folding intermediates in a near native state, and in concert with Hsp70, facilitates the thermodynamically favourable maturation of these clients [17]. In mammalian cells, including photoreceptors, there are two major cytosolic Hsp90 isoforms, the stress-inducible Hsp90α (HSPC1) and the constitutively expressed Hsp90β (HSPC3), which share 85% sequence identity [18] (Figure 1). The less abundant Hsp90α A2 (HSPC2) isoform is identical to Hsp90α with the exception of an N-terminal extension in Hsp90α. A recent study showed that Hsp90α deficiency in mice can cause rhodopsin retention in the IS and eventually lead to retinal degeneration. Further investigation revealed that microtubule-associated protein 1B (MAP1B), which is important for microtubule stabilization, was associated with Hsp90α and significantly reduced in Hsp90-deficient mice by proteasomal degradation. The authors suggested that Golgi organisation and vesicle transportation, which both rely on stable microtubules, are disrupted and this could be the underlying cause of photoreceptor degeneration [19].

2.2. ER-Associated GRP94

The ER has its own network of molecular chaperones which ensure that correctly folded proteins are produced and exit from the organelle for further processing. The glucose-regulated protein 94 (GRP94) (HSPC4) is a key regulator of the ER quality control mechanism and its residence in the ER is facilitated by its distinct C-terminal sequence KDEL, which serves as an ER retrieval signal for the KDEL receptor [20] (Figure 1). GRP94, together with BiP (GRP78), are two of the most abundant proteins in the ER [21] and play a significant role in regulating the ER unfolded protein response (UPR). The UPR involves the activation of a well synchronised set of signalling pathways directed by ER-resident transmembrane proteins that include inositol-requiring protein-1 (IRE1), the protein kinase RNA (PKR)-like ER kinase (PERK), and the activating transcription factor 6 (ATF6) [22] (Figure 1). During stress overload, the UPR branches respond by stimulating the expression of UPR-targeted genes which encode proteins, such as molecular chaperones, folding catalysts, subunits of the translocation machinery (Sec61 complex), ER-associated degradation (ERAD) molecules, and antioxidants. This activation leads to the upregulation of the protein folding and degradation capacity and the inhibition of protein synthesis in order to alleviate the stress and restore the equilibrium in the ER. Specifically in photoreceptors, GRP94 has been shown to be involved in opsin quality control as it forms a complex with mutant opsins and other chaperones (BiP) [23]. Apart from protein folding, ER quality control involves ERAD, a mechanism to detect misfolded proteins and tag them for proteasomal degradation (Figure 1). Evidence from Christianson et al. (2008) [24] showed that GRP94 actively participates in ERAD, when α1-antitrypsin, an ERAD substrate, failed to degrade in GRP94-depleted cells. Misfolded rhodopsin is also subjected to ERAD [25,26], and it has been suggested that GRP94 and BiP might be involved in the recognition of the non-glycosylated ER-retained misfolded opsins [26]. Another important feature of GRP94 is its ability to bind calcium and maintain calcium homeostasis in the ER. The ER quality control machinery is coupled to the storage and utilization of calcium [27]. Most calcium in the ER is stored bound to proteins and GRP94 is one of the most important calcium-binding proteins [20]. A reduction in total calcium levels can strongly affect protein folding and change the molecular chaperone selection in the ER [28–30].

2.3. Mitochondrial TRAP1

The tumour necrosis factor receptor associated protein 1 (TRAP1) is the mitochondria-specific Hsp90 isoform (HSPC5) and has distinct structural and functional properties (Figure 1). Structurally, TRAP1 is similar to the cytosolic Hsp90 isoforms, with the exception of a cleavable N-terminal mitochondrial localization signal and an N-terminal extension or 'strap' that provides stability in its 'closed' conformation [31]. Functionally, TRAP1 participates in the maintenance of mitochondrial integrity, protein folding and response to proteotoxic stress in mitochondria, and protection from oxidative stress damage [31,32]. Similarly to the ER, mitochondria are particularly vulnerable to the disturbance of proteostasis due to their high intrinsic protein folding demands. Hence, they have developed their own protective mechanism to overcome proteotoxic stress, known as the mitochondrial unfolded protein response (UPR^{mt}) [33]. Similar to the HSR and ER-specific UPR, UPR^{mt} is a transient transcriptional change in response to proteotoxic stress that is regulated by mitochondria. It was first described by Martinus et al. (1996) [34] as the transcriptional activation of mitochondria-specific chaperones and depends on mitochondrial-nuclear communication. The activation of UPR^{mt} promotes protein folding, limits protein import, and reduces the translation of mitochondrial proteins. The UPR^{mt} has been most extensively studied in *C. elegans* and there is only a small number of studies that have attempted to characterise it in mammalian cells [34–36]. Similarly to the ER-specific UPR, studies have shown that UPR^{mt} elicits a multi-axis response that is regulated by several proteins and leads to distinct molecular outcomes (reviewed by [37]). However, the exact molecular mechanisms and regulators of the different UPR^{mt} pathways remain largely unexplored, especially in disease. A study in *Drosophila* showed that modulation of TRAP1 expression led to the nuclear translocation of the transcription factor Dve which induced the expression of the mitochondrial chaperonin Hsp60, mitochondrial Hsp70, and a putative protease, CG5045, suggesting that TRAP1 is able to activate the UPR^{mt}. The same study found that TRAP1 modulation could significantly improve health span, potentially by activation of the UPR^{mt} [38]. In recent years, a functional interaction between ER and mitochondria during stress has been the focus of scientific interest. TRAP1 has been shown to have an important role in this ER–mitochondria interaction since it can potentially regulate the ER-associated UPR [39]. In photoreceptors, the elongated mitochondria extend almost the entire length of the IS, and are critical in meeting the high energy demands of photoreceptors for protein synthesis and phototransduction in the OS as well as serving as a calcium store. The photoreceptor TRAP1 is therefore likely to play a critical role in the maintenance of photoreceptor homeostasis and the UPR^{mt} (Figure 1).

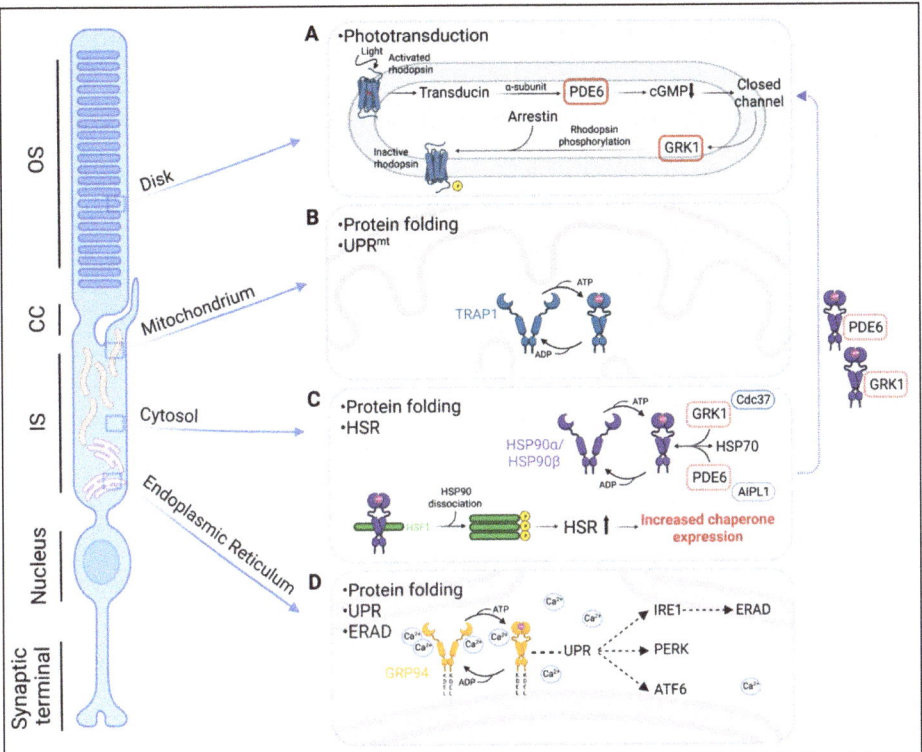

Figure 1. The roles of Hsp90 in photoreceptor proteostasis. (**A**) PDE6 and GRK1 are important components of phototransduction activation and deactivation, respectively. PDE6 and GRK1 are synthesised in the photoreceptor inner segment and translocated to the outer segment via the connecting cilium. Both PDE6 and GRK1 are Hsp90 client proteins. (**B**) The mitochondrial isoform TRAP1 is involved in protein folding and the mitochondrial unfolded protein response (UPR^{mt}). (**C**) The cytosolic isoforms Hsp90α/Hsp90β participate in protein folding in association with the Hsp70 folding machinery, and as a part of the heat-shock response (HSR) by regulating the activation of heat-shock transcription factor 1 (HSF1). During stress, Hsp90 together with other chaperones dissociate from HSF1, which then trimerizes and is activated via phosphorylation. Activated HSF1 translocates to the nucleus and stimulates the expression of molecular chaperones. (**D**) ER-associated GRP94 is important in protein folding and ER protein quality control mechanisms, the UPR, and ER-associated degradation (ERAD). The UPR involves three signalling pathways mediated via ER transmembrane protein folding sensors, the inositol-requiring protein-1 (IRE1), the protein kinase RNA (PKR)-like ER kinase (PERK), and the activating transcription factor 6 (ATF6). Activation of the UPR branches leads to the increased expression of proteins, such as molecular chaperones, folding catalysts, subunits of the translocation machinery (Sec61 complex), ERAD molecules, and antioxidants. Created with BioRender.com.

3. The Role of Hsp90 in Retinal Disease

3.1. Hsp90 and the Stress Response in Retinal Disease

Evidently, Hsp90 is of high importance in the retina because of the many vital roles it has in the different PQC mechanisms of proteostasis. Its importance in retinal homeostasis can be further highlighted by exploring its role in retinal disease paradigms. Currently, 280 genes (316 genes and loci) are associated with inherited retinal degeneration (IRD) (https://sph.uth.edu/retnet/home.htm, accessed on 3 July 2022). The inheritance of IRDs can be autosomal recessive, autosomal dominant, or X-linked, and IRDs can furthermore be progressive or stationary, as well as non-syndromic or part of a wider syndrome. Non-syndromic retinal dystrophies are further classified as macular dystrophies, cone and cone–rod dystrophies, rod–cone dystrophies, or chorioretinopathies [40]. Retinitis pigmentosa (RP) describes a group of retinal degenerative rod–cone dystrophies that are primarily characterized by the loss of rod photoreceptors, as well as the subsequent degeneration of cones. Mutations in rhodopsin are the most common cause of autosomal dominant retinitis pigmentosa (adRP) [2]. The photoreceptor stress machinery has been found to be induced in various models of rhodopsin misfolding. For example, the upregulation of the UPR and of the HSR, including increased levels of Hsp90 and Hsp70, has been observed in the P23H-1 transgenic rat, in which mutant rhodopsin Pro23His (P23H) is misfolded and retained in the ER [41]. Upon treatment with arimoclomol, an HSR co-inducer, Hsp90 and Hsp70 levels were further elevated, and this was associated with decreased rhodopsin aggregation, photoreceptor rescue, and improved visual responses [41]. The role of Hsp90 in the upregulation of the UPR and HSR is likely to be important in other retinal diseases caused by protein misfolding, in which the maintenance and regulation of the vast array of structural and functional proteins is critical for normal photoreceptor homeostasis.

3.2. Hsp90 Inhibition in Retinal Disease

Additional evidence of the significance of Hsp90 in retinal dystrophies, including RP, arise from the consequences of its pharmacological inhibition. Hsp90 inhibition can elicit a dual effect, leading to the proteasome-mediated degradation of its client proteins or the disruption of the chaperone complex with HSF1 and the activation of the HSR, leading to the upregulation of molecular chaperones. Therefore, the potential of Hsp90 inhibitors to manipulate the photoreceptor stress machinery has been explored in various studies. A list of Hsp90 inhibitors that have been used in models of retinal disease is summarized in Table 1. The Hsp90 inhibitor 17-*N*-allylamino-17-demethoxygeldanamycin (17-AAG), also known as tanepsimycin, has been shown to protect against rhodopsin aggregation and toxicity in a cell model of P23H rhodopsin [42]. Two other Hsp90 inhibitors, geldanamycin (GA) and radicicol, also showed a similar effect on alleviating the toxic gain-of-function mechanisms of P23H rhodopsin in vitro, although this effect was less potent compared to 17-AAG [42]. The amelioration of P23H rhodopsin aggregation was not observed in mouse embryonic fibroblasts from HSF-1 knock-out mice, suggesting that the protection depends on HSF1 and the activation of the HSR [43]. In accordance with these findings, the systemic administration of 2-amino-7,8-dihydro-6H-pyrido[4,3-D]pyrimidin-5-one NVPHSP990 (HSP990), a blood brain barrier permeable Hsp90 inhibitor, activated HSF-1 and induced the upregulation of molecular chaperones in the retina of P23H transgenic rats [43]. This HSP990-mediated stimulation of the stress machinery was associated with reduced rhodopsin aggregation and mislocalisation, improved visual function, and photoreceptor survival several weeks after a single drug dose [43]. Hsp90 inhibition has also been reported to be protective in another form of adRP, RP10, which is caused by mutations in the inosine 5′-monophosphate dehydrogenase type 1 (IMPDH1) gene [44]. Systemic delivery of 17-AAG, facilitated by the RNA interference-mediated modulation of the inner blood–retina barrier, protected against photoreceptor degeneration in the Arg224Pro (R224P) mutant IMPDH mouse model, by promoting the expression of HSPs, including Hsp90, which, in turn, reduced the formation of IMPDH aggregates [45]. These studies highlight the potential neuroprotective effects of Hsp90 inhibition in retinal protein misfolding disorders via upregulation of the HSR.

It has also been shown, however, that prolonged inhibition of Hsp90 in the retina may also play a detrimental role in photoreceptor proteostasis as a consequence of the degradation of key Hsp90 client proteins. The rhodopsin mutant Arg135Leu (R135L) is hyperphosphorylated and constitutively bound to arrestin, thereby disrupting vesicular traffic in photoreceptors. 17-AAG enhanced the vectorial transport of R135L rhodopsin to the OS by suppressing the endocytosis defect that characterises this mutation, thereby restoring R135L rhodopsin localization to the WT phenotype in rat retinae [43]. In an in vitro cell model of R135L rhodopsin, Hsp90 inhibition by 17-AAG similarly blocked the recruitment of arrestin to R135L rhodopsin and led to a reduction in the aberrant endocytosis of R135L rhodopsin [43]. Interestingly, this effect was HSF1-independent as 17-AAG rescued the intracellular accumulation of R135L rhodopsin and restored the cytosolic localization of arrestin in HSF-1 knock-out mouse embryonic fibroblasts [43]. It was hypothesized that Hsp90 inhibition may instead mediate its effect on R135L rhodopsin by client-mediated degradation. Indeed, prolonged Hsp90 inhibition with HSP990 in vivo led to a post-translational reduction in GRK1 and PDE6 protein levels, identifying them as Hsp90 clients. Hsp90 inhibition in cells led to the rapid proteasomal degradation of newly synthesised GRK1 confirming a requirement for Hsp90 for GRK1 maturation and function. The effect of Hsp90 inhibition on R135L rhodopsin was therefore attributed to the fact that GRK1 was identified as an Hsp90 client protein, and Hsp90 inhibition decreased GRK1 levels resulting in reduced R135L phosphorylation and subsequently, reduced arrestin binding.

Table 1. List of Hsp90 inhibitors used in models of retinal degeneration.

Compound	Study Outcome	Reference
Geldanamycin	Reduced P23H aggregation and cell death in vitro	Mendes & Cheetham, 2008 [42]
Tanepsimycin 17-AAG	Reduced P23H aggregation and cell death in vitro	Mendes & Cheetham, 2008 [42]
	Reduced protein accumulation in R135L rats	Aguilà et al., 2014 [43]
Radicicol	Reduced P23H aggregation and cell death in vitro	Mendes & Cheetham, 2008 [42]
Alvespimycin 17-DMAG	Prolonged treatment causes photoreceptor cell death in rats	Zhou et al., 2013 [46]
	Induced photoreceptor apoptosis and rhodopsin retention in the IS in wild-type mice	Wu et al., 2020 [19]
HSP990	Reduces P23H aggregation, improves visual function and delays photoreceptor cell death in P23H-1 rats	Aguilà et al., 2014 [43]
	Protects photoreceptors from degeneration caused by aggregating mutant IMPDH1 protein	Tam et al., 2010 [45]

3.3. Ocular Toxicities in Clinical Trials of Hsp90 Inhibition

These findings have important implications for the pharmacological manipulation of molecular chaperones as a therapeutic approach for retinal disease. Despite the plethora of evidence that Hsp90 inhibition can provide protection in the diseased retina as described above, reports from clinical trials in oncology highlight ocular toxicities that have emerged as an important clinical concern (Table 2). Hsp90 N-terminal inhibitors, including ansamycin derivatives (17-dimethylaminoethylamino-17-demethoxygeldanamycin (17-DMAG)), resorcinol derivatives (AT13387, AUY922), and benzamide derivatives (SNX-5422 (PF-04929113)), have been associated with visual disturbances, such as blurred vision, photopsia, night blindness, photophobia, and retinopathy [47–57]. In addition, some preclinical studies have reported that severe retinal degeneration occurred in rats and beagle dogs after treatment with Hsp90 inhibitors [46,58,59]. The oral administration of the Hsp90 scaffold N-terminal inhibitor CH5164840 led to a loss of pupillary light reflex, abnormal electroretinographic (ERG) responses, and histological changes in the photoreceptor outer nuclear layer, including photoreceptor degeneration, in beagle dogs [58]. Similarly, intravenous administration of 17-DMAG or AUY922 promoted photoreceptor cell death in Sprague Dawley (SD) rats in addition to the upregulation of the HSR [46], and AUY92-induced abnormal ERG responses, and photoreceptor OS disorganization in Brown Norway and Wistar rats [59]. However, while ocular effects have been widely reported in preclinical and clinical studies of certain Hsp90 inhibitors, visual disturbances have not been reported for all Hsp90 inhibitors, including 17-AAG and the resorcinol derivative ganetespid. Preclinical studies comparing the ocular toxicity of 17-DMAG, 17-AAG, AUY922, and ganetespid suggest that the extent of ocular toxicity correlates with the retinal biocompatibility and clearance rate of the compound, with high levels of accumulation and prolonged inhibition of Hsp90 in the retina, leading to photoreceptor cell death [46]. Therefore, the inhibition of Hsp90 as a therapeutic approach in the retina is clearly a double-edged sword, whereby Hsp90 inhibition can both induce a neuroprotective response but also lead to ocular toxicity upon prolonged retinal accumulation. The mechanism of retinal toxicity as a consequence of Hsp90 inhibition is poorly understood; however, a possible explanation is that the ocular toxicity observed upon prolonged Hsp90 inhibition might be mediated by the disruption caused to important Hsp90 client proteins in the retina. As described previously, GRK1 biosynthesis requires Hsp90, and prolonged Hsp90 inhibition via systemic administration of HSP990 reduced GRK1 and PDE6 levels post-translationally, suggesting that the Hsp90 client list includes important components of the phototransduction cascade. More recently, Transient Receptor Potential cation channel subfamily M member 1 (TRPM1) has been identified as another potential Hsp90 client protein in the retina [57]. TRPM1 is a constitutively open calcium entry channel primarily expressed in skin melanocytes and retinal ON-bipolar cells in the inner nuclear layer. The treatment of mice with AUY922 resulted in increased apoptosis in the photoreceptor outer nuclear layer, disorganization of the photoreceptor outer segments, disruption of RPE cells, and a dose-dependent decrease in TRPM1 via disruption of the interaction with Hsp90 [57].

Table 2. List of Hsp90 inhibitors used in clinical trials in oncology and their ocular effects. * The observed ocular effects were transient or resolved after treatment discontinuation.

HSP90 Inhibitor Drug	Trial	ClinicalTrials.gov Identifier	Ocular Effect	Reference
Alvespimycin 17-dimethylaminoethylamino-17-demethoxygeldanamycin (17-DMAG)	Phase I trial of 17-DMAG in patients with advanced malignancies	NCT00088868	• blurred vision *	Kummar et al., 2010 [47]
	Phase I trial of 17-DMAG in patients with advanced solid tumors	NCT00248521	• blurred vision • dry eye • keratitis • conjunctivitis or ocular surface disease	Pacey et al., 2011 [50]
Onalespid AT13387	Phase I trial of AT13387 in patients with refractory solid tumors.	NCT00878423	• blurred vision * • flashes * • delayed light dark/accommodation *	Shapiro et al., 2010 [49]
	Phase I study of onalespib in combination with AT7519, a pan-CDK inhibitor, in patients with advanced solid tumors	NCT02503709	• blurry vision and "floaters" *	Do et al., 2020 [56]

Table 2. Cont.

HSP90 Inhibitor Drug	Trial	ClinicalTrials.gov Identifier	Ocular Effect	Reference
Luminespid AUY922 NVP-AUY922	Phase I trial of AUY922 in combination with capecitabine in patients with advanced solid tumors	NCT01226732	• vision darkening * • night blindness *	Bendell et al., 2015 [52]
	Phase I-IB/II trial of NVP-AUY922 as monotherapy or in combination with bortezomib in patients with relapsed or refractory multiple myeloma	NCT00708292	• night blindness • photopsia • visual impairment • retinopathy • blurred vision • cataract • reduced visual acuity	Seggewiss-Bernhardt et al., 2015 [53]
	Phase II trial of AUY922 in patients with refractory gastrointestinal stromal tumors	NCT01404650	• blurred vision * • flashing lights * • delayed light/dark adaptation * • night blindness * • floaters *	Bendell et al., 2016 [54]
	Phase II trial of AUY922 in patients with metastatic gastrointestinal stromal tumor	NCT01389583	• night blindness • blurred vision • flashing light	Chiang et al., 2016 [55] Shen et al., 2021 [57]
SNX-5422 PF-04929113	Phase I study of SNX-5422 in patients with refractory solid tumor malignancies and lymphomas	NCT00644072	• blurred vision • bilateral cataracts	Rajan et al., 2011 [51]

4. Hsp90 Client Proteins in the Retina

Whilst PDE6, GRK1, and TRPM1 have been identified as Hsp90 client proteins in the retina, only PDE6 and GRK1 are specifically expressed in photoreceptor cells and are important components of the phototransduction cascade. An in-depth understanding of the mechanisms underlying the specific recruitment of PDE6 and GRK1 to Hsp90 is crucial to understand the biogenesis of these important phototransduction proteins, not only in the healthy retina but also in retinal diseases associated with these Hsp90 clients, and the review will henceforth focus on mechanistic and structural insights into PDE6 and GRK1 as Hsp90 client proteins. Whilst the Hsp90-PDE6 chaperone complex has been investigated in depth, less is known regarding GRK1 as a specific client for Hsp90 and the role of this association in disease.

4.1. The Hsp90-PDE6 Chaperone Complex

PDE6, a member of the class I family of phosphodiesterases [60], is a heterotetrametric complex, which in rod photoreceptors, comprises the catalytic PDE6α and PDE6β subunits together with two inhibitory PDE6γ subunits. Cone PDE6 comprises two catalytic PDE6α' subunits and two inhibitory PDE6γ' subunits. In the phototransduction cascade, activated transducin relieves the inhibition of the PDE6 catalytic subunits imposed by the inhibitory subunits, leading to cGMP hydrolysis. Mutations in rod PDE6α, PDE6β, and PDE6γ cause autosomal recessive RP and mutations in PDE6β can also cause autosomal dominant congenital stationary night blindness (https://sph.uth.edu/retnet/, accessed on 3 July 2022). In contrast, mutations in cone PDE6α' and PDE6γ' are associated with autosomal recessive cone or cone–rod dystrophy, or achromatopsia (https://sph.uth.edu/retnet/, accessed on 3 July 2022). Interestingly, whilst mutations in the PDE6 subunits cause relatively milder forms of inherited retinal degeneration, mutations in the reported co-chaperone for PDE6, the photoreceptor-specific aryl hydrocarbon receptor interacting protein-like 1 (AIPL1), cause Leber congenital amaurosis (LCA), a severe early onset and rapidly progressive disease leading to photoreceptor degeneration and the loss of vision within the first few years of life [61]. An early observation in *Aipl1* knockout and knockdown mice was the post-transcriptional loss of all three subunits of rod PDE6 prior to the onset of retinal degeneration [62,63]. Cone PDE6 levels were also substantially reduced in cone photoreceptors lacking AIPL1 [64]. In the absence of AIPL1, the rod PDE6 subunits were stably synthesized but subsequently misassembled and targeted for rapid proteasomal degradation [65]. Similarly, whilst the loss of AIPL1 had no effect on the synthesis of the cone PDE6 subunits, the translated subunits were unstable and could not assemble into the holoenzyme [66]. These studies confirmed that AIPL1 is important for the post-translational stability and assembly of both rod and cone PDE6.

4.1.1. AIPL1 Structure

AIPL1 was first identified as a possible Hsp90 co-chaperone due to its homology to the Hsp90 tetratricopeptide repeat (TPR) domain co-chaperone aryl hydrocarbon receptor interacting protein (AIP), with which it shares 49% identity and 69% similarity [61]. AIPL1 and AIP comprise a C-terminal TPR domain and a N-terminal FK506 binding protein (FKBP)-like domain, similar to larger members of the FKBP family of immunophilins, including the Hsp90 TPR domain co-chaperones FKBP51 and FKBP52. The AIPL1 TPR domain consists of three consecutive TPR motifs, and the crystal structure of the human AIPL1 TPR domain revealed that, similar to other Hsp90 TPR domain co-chaperones, the AIPL1 TPR domain adopts a typical TPR fold [67] (Figure 2). Each TPR motif consists of a pair of anti-parallel α-helices such that the consecutive TPR motifs form a series of six anti-parallel α-helices connected by short loops followed by a seventh α-helix, which all together forms a right-handed amphipathic groove. The AIPL1 FKBP-like domain shares the typical FKBP fold comprising a five stranded β sheet forming a half β-barrel surrounding a short α helix and creating a hydrophobic cavity (Figure 2). However, unlike other members of the FKBP family, the FKBP-like domain of AIP and AIPL1 lack peptidyl prolyl isomerase activity and cannot bind immunosuppressant drugs [68,69]. Moreover, the FKBP-like domain of both AIP and AIPL1 uniquely include an extensive insert region linking the last two β strands in the FKBP-like domain [69–71]. In AIP, the insert regions consist of a 19 residue long helical segment followed by a mostly random coil structure and an α-helix [69]. In contrast, the crystal structure of the human AIPL1 FKBP-like domain revealed that the insert region in AIPL1 (residues 90–146) is well structured and comprises three consecutive α-helices (α2, α3 and α4) connected by short loops [71] (Figure 2). Additional differences between the AIP and AIPL1 FKBP-like domains include the absence of an N-terminal α-helix in AIPL1 that is thought to structurally stabilize the AIP FKBP-like fold; and a loop between β4 and α1 that adopts a 'looped-out' conformation in AIPL1 but a 'looped-in' conformation in AIP, wherein a critical hinge residue Trp72 is either flipped in or out, respectively, thus modulating access to a hydrophobic cavity [71] (Figure 2). Finally, the AIPL1 TPR domain is followed by a C-terminal 56 amino acid proline rich domain (PRD), an unstructured random coil that is imperfectly conserved in primates and absent in non-primates [61,72,73] (Figure 2).

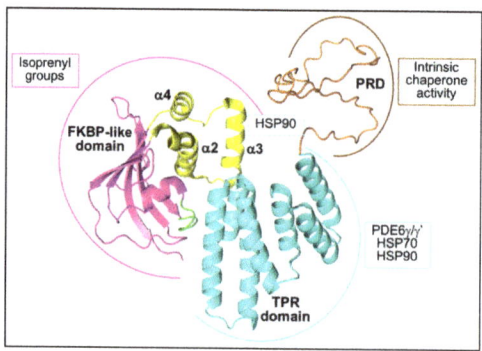

Figure 2. Model of AIPL1. The TPR domain (PDB 6PX0, cyan) and the FKBP-like domain (PDB 5U9A, magenta, yellow, and green) of AIPL1 were superimposed onto FKBP51 (1KT0). The PRD (brown) of

AIPL1 was modelled using the I-TASSER server [74,75]. Helices 2, 3, and 4 of the unique insert region of the AIPL1 FKBP51-like domain (yellow) and the loop between β4 and α1 that adopts a 'looped-out' conformation in AIPL1 (green) are shown. The PRD is required for the intrinsic chaperone activity of AIPL1. The TPR domain mediates the interaction with Hsp90/Hsp70 and the PDE6 inhibitory subunits, whilst Hsp90 may also make contact with the α3 helix in the unique insert region. The FKBP-like domain constitutes a ligand-binding site for isoprenyl groups. Figure courtesy of C. Prodromou, Genome Damage and Stability Centre, University of Sussex.

4.1.2. The Interaction of AIPL1 with Hsp90

Hidalgo-de-Quintana et al. (2008) first provided experimental evidence for the TPR-mediated interaction of full length human AIPL1 with both Hsp90 and Hsp70, with preferential binding to Hsp90 [76]. The TPR consensus residues required for the packing of adjacent α-helices in the TPR motifs and residues involved in tight electrostatic interactions with the C-terminal EEVD TPR acceptor sites of Hsp90 and Hsp70 are conserved in AIPL1. The deletion of the Hsp90 MEEVD pentapeptide or the Hsp70 TIEEVD heptapeptide significantly reduced the interaction of AIPL1 with Hsp90 and Hsp70, respectively, and the MEEVD peptide competitively reduced the interaction of AIPL1 with Hsp90 in quantitative binding assays [76,77]. Moreover, the mutation of lysine 265 to alanine (K265A), a carboxylate clamp residue critical for the tight electrostatic interaction of TPR domain co-chaperones with the C-terminal EEVD motif, significantly reduced the interaction of AIPL1 with Hsp90 and Hsp70 [76,78]. The AIPL1 TPR domain alone can interact with Hsp90 in the absence of the FKBP-like domain, and the disruption of the TPR domain by LCA-associated missense mutations, deletions, insertions, duplications, or C-terminal truncations significantly reduced or abolished the interaction with Hsp90 [77,79]. Therefore, the TPR domain is critical for the interaction of AIPL1 with Hsp90 and features directing the prototypical core TPR domain co-chaperone–chaperone interaction are conserved in AIPL1. Accordingly, Sacristan-Reviriego et al. (2017) showed that human AIPL1 preferentially interacts with Hsp90 in the nucleotide-bound closed conformation and that this interaction is reduced by both apyrase treatment or HSP990 inhibition, indicating that productive Hsp90 ATPase cycles are required for efficient AIPL1 interaction [77]. Moreover, AIPL1 stabilized rod PDE6α to proteasomal degradation in the cytosol and this function was significantly reduced by Hsp90 inhibition with HSP990, GA, or 17-AAG [77]. Similarly, biolayer interferometry (BLI) binding assays recently reported the preferential binding of mouse AIPL1 to adenylyl-imidodiphosphate (AMP-PNP)-bound Hsp90 in a 1:2 stoichiometry [78]. In this study, DMAG treatment significantly impacted the ability of AIPL1 to chaperone cone PDE6α' activity. Altogether, the data point to the preferential interaction of AIPL1 with Hsp90 in the closed conformation and the importance of a functional AIPL1-Hsp90 interaction for PDE6 stability and activity.

In addition to the role of the core TPR domain contacts in mediating the interaction of AIPL1 with the chaperone TPR acceptor site, additional requirements for this interaction have been investigated. In the case of FKBP51 and FKBP52, a region C-terminal to the TPR domain comprising a seventh α-helical extension (α-helix 7) mediates differential binding to Hsp90 and the truncation of FKBP51 and FKBP52 within this α-helical extension at Asn404 and Asn406, respectively, largely abrogated Hsp90 interaction [80]. Interestingly, the removal of the α-helical extension C-terminal to the core TPR domain of human AIPL1 by truncation at the topologically equivalent residue, Glu317 (AIPL1 1-317), reduced but did not abolish the interaction of AIPL1 with Hsp90 and Hsp70 [76]. Similarly, the truncation of the 12 C-terminal residues of mouse AIPL1 (AIPL1 1-316) did not abrogate the binding of AIPL1 to Hsp90 but moderately reduced the affinity for Hsp90 in BLI assays [78]. Notably, this region was however critical for the ability of AIPL1 to chaperone PDE6 in an in vitro heterologous assay for cone PDE6α' function. This suggests that in addition to the core TPR domain contacts, residues within the TPR α-helical extension may be important for functional chaperone complex assembly, although several residues thought to mediate contact of the α-helical extension of FKBP51 with Hsp90 are missing or not conserved in mouse or human AIPL1.

Other regions implicated in the interaction of AIPL1 with Hsp90 include the primate-specific PRD and the α3 helix in the unique insert region of the FKBP-like domain. The deletion of the PRD, whilst having no effect on the structure or thermostability of AIPL1 [68,73], was reported to modestly increase the interaction of AIPL1 with Hsp90 in surface plasmon resonance (SPR) spectroscopy assays. On the other hand, the interaction of AIPL1 with Hsp90 following deletion of the PRD was reported to be comparable to that of full length AIPL1, although a significantly increased interaction was observed with the TPR domain alone in the absence of the PRD [79]. Finally, disease-associated mutations in the AIPL1 PRD had no effect on the interaction with Hsp90 [79]. Whilst the PRD may therefore not play a significant role in the interaction with Hsp90, it does appear to play a critical role in the intrinsic chaperone activity of AIPL1 [68]. AIPL1 was first shown to efficiently suppress the formation of intracellular inclusions comprising misfolded fragments of the AIPL1 interacting partner, NUB1, in a concentration-dependent manner [81]. AIPL1 also suppressed the thermal aggregation of citrate synthase (CS) and protected CS from thermal inactivation, and this effect was lost upon the deletion of the PRD [68]. The AIPL1 suppression of aggregation of the NUB1 fragments was not dependent on Hsp90, as GA had no effect in this assay, but was additive with Hsp70 dependent on AIPL1 C-terminal sequences [76]. Overall, the data suggest that the PRD is critical for AIPL1 intrinsic chaperone activity in association with Hsp70.

A number of studies have also investigated the contribution of the AIPL1 FKBP-like domain to Hsp90 interaction. The AIPL1 FKBP-like domain and TPR domain expressed alone can each fold stably to acquire the native conformation [67,70,71,82]. It has been reported that the AIPL1 FKBP-like domain alone, however, cannot interact with Hsp90 in the absence of the TPR domain [77]. Indeed, the LCA-associated patient mutation, Glu163Stop, which leads to the loss of the entire TPR domain and PRD, completely abolished the interaction of AIPL1 with Hsp90, confirming the critical role of the TPR domain in Hsp90 interaction [77]. However, patient-associated mutations in the FKBP-like domain, including missense mutations and in-frame deletions, diminished the interaction of AIPL1 with Hsp90 and impacted rod PDE6 activity in an indirect assay of cGMP hydrolysis [77,79], suggesting that whilst the FKBP-like domain alone cannot bind Hsp90, it is important for stable ternary chaperone complex formation with full length AIPL1. Interestingly, a very weak but transient interaction of Hsp90 with the N-terminal FKBP-like domain of AIP has been reported, and this interaction was reduced by the deletion of the FKBP-like domain unique insert region [69]. Similarly, the replacement of the α3 helix in the AIPL1 FKBP-like unique insert region with five glycine residues modestly affected the interaction with Hsp90, but critically impacted the activity of cone PDE6α' [78]. A model of the Hsp90-AIPL1 complex based on the cryo-EM structure of the Hsp90-FKBP51 complex placed the α3 helix of the insert region in close proximity to Hsp90, suggesting a moderate contribution of the insert region to the AIPL1–Hsp90 interface [78]. As the TPR acceptor site of Hsp90 can competitively bind a multitude of TPR domain co-chaperones, it has been suggested that contacts with the α3 helix may contribute to the specificity of the interaction of AIPL1 with Hsp90.

4.1.3. The AIPL1-Mediated Targeting of PDE6 to Hsp90

The binding interface between the PDE6 client and Hsp90 has not been investigated. However, several mechanisms have been proposed wherein AIPL1 could specifically target PDE6 to Hsp90. Ramamurthy et al. (2003) first reported that AIPL1 could interact with and facilitate the processing of farnesylated proteins [83]. Notably, the PDE6 catalytic subunits are isoprenylated at the cysteine residue of their C-terminal CAAX box, with the identity of the CAAX box C-terminal residue suggesting that rod PDE6α is farnesylated whilst rod PDE6β and cone PDE6α' are geranylgeranylated. A general role for AIPL1 in protein farnesylation was suggested, since several interactors in a Y2H screen were farnesylated, and mutation of the CAAX box cysteine to induce the loss of farnesylation or promote geranylgeranylation led to the loss of these interactions [83]. Accordingly, AIPL1 was found to interact with rod PDE6α in the mouse retina, and the AIPL1 interaction with PDE6β was reported to be dependent on that with PDE6α [65]. FRET assays with an AMCA conjugated farnesylated cysteine probe, S-farnesyl-L-cysteine methyl ester, revealed a high affinity interaction with the purified FKBP-like but not the TPR domain [70]. Mutation of Cys89 or Leu147 flanking the unique FBKP insert region or the deletion of the insert region (residues 96-143) abolished the interaction with the probe. Similarly, FRET assays confirmed a potent interaction of AIPL1 with an AMCA-conjugated peptide mimic of the PDE6α C-terminus with the cysteine residue modified by S-farnesylation and carboxymethylation [73]. Interestingly, competition assays with an excess of N-acetyl-S-geranylgeranyl-L-cysteine suggested for the first time that AIPL1 may also bind geranylgeranyl. Indeed, the crystal structure of the AIPL1 FKBP-like domain (residues 2-161) in the apo state and in the presence of either S-farnesyl-L-cysteine methyl ester or geranylgeranyl pyrophosphate confirmed the interaction of AIPL1 with these isoprenoid moieties that bind deep within the hydrophobic cavity [71]. There were no significant differences between the apo and isoprenoid-bound structures, with isoprenoid binding inducing only minor conformational changes in the ligand binding domain. Molecular dynamics simulations supported a model wherein the β4-α1 loop adopts a 'looped-in' conformation in the apo structure with the critical Trp72 residue thus occluding the hydrophobic ligand-binding pocket, which then rotates to the 'flipped-out' conformation upon isoprenoid binding [71]. The α2 side chains of the insert region were found to contribute significantly to isoprenoid binding [71], explaining the previous observation that the deletion of the insert region abrogated interaction with a farnesyl probe [70]. Moreover, the mutation of residues in the β4-α1 loop also markedly attenuated isoprenoid binding [71]. These studies thus confirmed the direct interaction of the AIPL1 FKBP-like domain with either farnesyl or geranylgeranyl, suggesting that AIPL1 might specifically target PDE6 to Hsp90 through these interactions. Notably, the mutation of the PDE6α' CAAX-box cysteine to favour either farnesylation or geranylgeranylation had no impact on the ability of AIPL1 to chaperone functional cone PDE6 in in vitro heterologous activity assays, suggesting that the role of AIPL1 is indiscriminate with respect to the identity of the isoprenoid moiety [84]. More recently, a PDE6α Cys857Ser knockin mouse model has been generated that abrogates the farnesylation of rod PDE6α [78]. Interestingly, the levels and targeting of PDE6α and PDE6β to the photoreceptor OS, as well as both the basal and maximal PDE6 activity, were comparable to control mice, in addition to which there was no change in either ERG or optical coherence tomography (OCT) measurements. Moreover, the deletion of the C-terminal 28 residues of cone PDE6α', including the CAAX motif or the loss of isoprenylation by Cys855Ser mutation, had no effect in in vitro assays of AIPL1 chaperoned PDE6 activity. Finally, steric occlusion of the AIPL1 prenyl binding site in an Ile61Phe/Ile151Phe double mutant had no effect on the ability of AIPL1 to chaperone PDE6α' or the Cys855Ser mutant in the heterologous assay. Hence, overall, whilst it is clear that the interaction of the AIPL1 FKBP-like domain with the PDE6 isoprenoid moieties contributes to the formation of the ternary chaperone complex, the exact role of this interaction in PDE6 biogenesis remains unclear. It is noteworthy that whilst the FKBP-like domain of AIPL1 appears to bind either farnesyl or geranylgeranyl groups indiscriminately, only PDE6 is affected in the *Aipl1* knockout and knockdown mouse models (in addition to soluble retinal guanylate cyclase in *Aipl1* knockout cones), despite the wide range of phototransduction components that are isoprenylated, thus suggesting that features other than the interaction of AIPL1 with the PDE6 isoprenoid groups must facilitate the specific recruitment of PDE6 to Hsp90 by AIPL1.

One such possibility is the interaction of AIPL1 with the inhibitory subunits of rod and cone PDE6. The rod PDE6γ subunit was reported to interact with AIPL1 using FRET assays [73]. Subsequently, a conserved C-terminal peptide of rod PDE6γ and cone PDE6γ' was shown to bind the AIPL1 TPR domain but not the AIPL1 FKBP-like domain with association and dissociation kinetics consistent with a 1:1 binding model [67]. Moreover, molecular modelling suggested that the C-terminal 25 residues of the rod and cone inhibitory subunits encompass most, if not all, of the contact with the TPR domain overlapping with the Hsp90 binding site, such that the inhibitory subunits and Hsp90 bind in a mutually exclusive manner [67]. This suggests a model in which the interaction of the PDE6γ/PDE6γ' subunits with the AIPL1 TPR domain impart specificity toward the PDE6 client, as the AIPL1 FKBP-like domain can bind isoprenyl moieties indiscriminately and the Hsp90 TPR acceptor site is bound competitively by TPR domain co-chaperones. This has important implications for modelling the role of AIPL1 and Hsp90 in PDE6 biogenesis in retinal photoreceptors, though it is noteworthy that AIPL1 failed to interact with either rod PDE6γ or cone PDE6γ' in co-immunoprecipitation assays of AIPL1 from mouse retinal explants [65,66].

Overall, these studies highlight the structural and mechanistic basis of PDE6 recruitment to Hsp90 via the PDE6-specific Hsp90 co-chaperone AIPL1. Misfolded PDE6 subunits that cause autosomal recessive retinal disease likely undergo unproductive folding cycles with Hsp90, leading to their post-translational degradation and loss of function.

4.2. The Hsp90-GRK1 Chaperone Complex

In comparison to the Hsp90-PDE6 chaperone complex, the interaction and maturation of GRK1 with Hsp90 as a client protein in retinal photoreceptors is poorly characterised. Mutations in GRK1 are associated with the Oguchi subtype of recessive congenital stationary night blindness (https://sph.uth.edu/retnet/, accessed on 3 July 2022). In the retina, GRK1 is expressed in rod photoreceptors whilst GRK7 is expressed in cone photoreceptors. Both GRK1 and GRK7 are members of the G protein-coupled receptor kinase (GRK) family, serine/threonine-specific protein kinases that mediate the agonist-dependent phosphorylation of G protein-coupled receptors.

GRK1 and GRK7 specifically target the activated state of the G protein-coupled receptors rhodopsin and cone opsin, respectively, and play a key role in the deactivation of the phototransduction cascade and photorecovery after light onset. GRK1 and GRK7 are tethered to the photoreceptor OS phospholipid membranes in close proximity to their substrate by C-terminal isoprenylation. In the dark, GRK1 and GRK7 are bound to and inhibited by recoverin. The activation of the phototransduction cascade leads to the release of calcium from recoverin, which induces a conformational change involving the rotation of a 'myristoyl switch' that results in the calcium-dependent dissociation of recoverin from the membrane and release from GRK, thus enabling GRK to phosphorylate rod and cone opsin [85]. The GRK-mediated phosphorylation of the opsins induces a conformational change in the receptor that in turn allows the binding of arrestin and receptor deactivation through sterically blocking the binding of transducin, effectively switching off the cascade [85].

The GRK family, in addition to the visual kinase subfamily (GRK1, GRK7), includes the β-adrenergic receptor (β-AR) kinase subfamily (GRK2, GRK3) and the GRK4 subfamily (GRK4, GRK5, GRK6). All GRK family members are composed of a short highly conserved ~16 residue N-terminal element unique to this family of kinases [86]. This is followed by a regulator of G protein signalling homology domain (RH) that is interrupted by a highly conserved serine/threonine kinase domain. The catalytic domain of the GRK family, including that of GRK1 and GRK7, has a highly conserved architecture comprising a small N-terminal lobe and a large C-terminal lobe connected by a flexible hinge region that forms a deep nucleotide binding cleft between them, followed by a C-terminal extension (C-tail). The N-terminal lobe comprises a five-stranded β-sheet with a conserved αC helix, whereas the C-terminal lobe comprises six α-helices. A loop within the C-tail forms an active site tether that contributes to the ATP binding site. The substrate mainly interacts with the surface of the C-terminal lobe. The RH domain folds into a bi-lobed helical bundle that bridges the small and large kinase domains [86]. Kinase activation involves a conformational change in which the N-terminal lobe moves towards C-terminal lobe to form a closed state, with the αC-β4 loop thought to act as a hinge point for inter-lobe movement, enabling the rotation between open and closed conformations [87].

Hsp90 has been shown to play a role in the maturation and stabilization of the GRK family members GRK1, GRK2, GRK3, GRK5, and GRK6, with the inhibition of Hsp90 by GA or 17-AAG, leading to rapid proteasomal degradation of the newly synthesized GRKs [43,88]. Similar to GRK1, cone GRK7 is also likely to be an Hsp90 client protein. Hsp90 is known to bind directly to the kinase catalytic domain with Hsp90 binding determinants widely distributed in both lobes. The kinase catalytic domain is one of the most abundant structures in the human proteome, present in more than 500 protein kinases, and has a highly conserved architecture common to serine/threonine and tyrosine kinases. The kinase domain is thus regarded as a universal acceptor site mediating kinase interaction with Hsp90, and it is highly likely, therefore, that the kinase domain of GRK1 and GRK7 similarly directs the interaction with Hsp90. Considerable effort has been invested in identifying the specific features that mediate the recognition of client kinases by Hsp90 [89–94]. Interestingly, no global sequence determinants have been identified for the interaction of kinases with Hsp90, despite the high level of conservation in the kinase domain. Instead, a consensus has emerged in which the intrinsic stability of the kinase domain is an important determinant for Hsp90 interaction. Hsp90 kinase clients were reported to be more thermodynamically unstable than non-clients, with the small-molecule stabilization of the kinase domain reducing the client interaction and mutation of the kinase domain, leading to stronger Hsp90 client binding [89,90,93,94].

Finally, it is well known that cell division cycle 37 (Cdc37) is a ubiquitous kinase-dedicated co-chaperone that is universally employed to direct kinase clients to Hsp90, thereby providing selective recognition of the kinase family [93,94]. Cdc37 has been shown to directly bind the kinase catalytic site, overlapping with the Hsp90 binding. Cdc37 binds to kinase clients in the absence of Hsp90, whereas Hsp90 interacts only weakly without Cdc37. Therefore, Hsp90 and Cdc37 are thought to act in concert in chaperoning client kinases with Hsp90-mediated maturation of kinases strictly dependent on the Cdc37-dependent recruitment of the kinase to Hsp90 [93,94]. Whilst not experimentally tested, it is highly likely that the co-chaperone for GRK1 and GRK7 is Cdc37. Experimental investigation of GRK1 and GRK7 interaction with Hsp90 and Cdc73 will provide further insights and evidence that the features directing client kinase assembly with Cdc73 and Hsp90 are conserved amongst the visual GRKs.

5. Conclusions

In summary, retinal photoreceptors are amongst the most metabolically active cells in the human body. Consequently, high levels of reactive oxygen species accumulate in the photoreceptors, leading to membrane and protein damage. Approximately 10% of the photoreceptor outer segments are turned over daily to replace damaged membranes and proteins. There is therefore an extremely high demand on protein synthesis and turnover in retinal photoreceptor cells requiring high levels of proteostasis. There are currently 280 genes associated with inherited retinal disease, many of which code for proteins of the visual cycle and phototransduction cascade that require high levels of protein synthesis in the photoreceptor inner segment and translocation to the outer segment. Protein quality control is therefore of vital importance in photoreceptor cells and many inherited retinal diseases are protein misfolding disorders. Hsp90 is centrally important to protein folding and quality control in the retinal photoreceptors, including in the cytosol, ER, and in the mitochondria. Indeed, the induction of the HSR via short-term Hsp90 inhibition has been shown to be neuroprotective in in vitro and in vivo models of inherited retinal disease. However, longer term inhibition of Hsp90 in the retina may in fact be detrimental due to the resultant degradation of specific Hsp90 client proteins in the photoreceptors, including PDE6 and GRK1. Mutations in these Hsp90 client proteins themselves lead to retinal disease. Whilst the precise role of Hsp90 in the folding, maturation, or assembly of these retina-specific client proteins is not fully elucidated, this raises the possibility that small molecule manipulation of the Hsp90 cycle to promote the favourable maturation of these client proteins may be a potential therapeutic approach for diseases associated with these clients. In addition, the induction of the HSR in the absence of Hsp90 inhibition might be another favourable avenue for treating protein misfolding disorders in the retina.

Author Contributions: Conceptualization, K.Z. and J.v.d.S.; writing—original draft preparation, K.Z. and J.v.d.S.; writing—review and editing, K.Z. and J.v.d.S.; funding acquisition, J.v.d.S. All authors have read and agreed to the published version of the manuscript.

Funding: This research was funded by the Medical Research Council, UK; grant number [MR/P02582X/1].

Institutional Review Board Statement: Not applicable.

Informed Consent Statement: Not applicable.

Data Availability Statement: Not applicable.

Conflicts of Interest: The authors declare no conflict of interest.

Abbreviations

17-DMAG, 17-Dimethylaminoethylamino-17-demethoxygeldanamycin; 17-AAG, 17-N-allylamino-17-demethoxygeldanamycin; ATF6, activating transcription factor 6; AMP-PNP, adenylyl-imidodiphosphate; AIP, aryl hydrocarbon receptor interacting protein; AIPL1, aryl hydrocarbon receptor interacting protein-like 1; adRP, autosomal dominant retinitis pigmentosa; Cdc37, cell division cycle 37; CS, citrate synthase; CC, connecting cilium; ER, Endoplasmic reticulum; ERAD, ER-associated degradation; FKBP, FK506 binding protein; GRK1, G-protein-coupled receptor kinase 1; GA, geldanamycin; GRP94, glucose-regulated protein 94; GC, guanylate cyclase; GCAP, guanylyl cyclase activating proteins; HSE, heat shock element; HSF, heat shock factor; HSP, heat shock protein; HSR, heat shock response; HSP990, 2-amino-7,8-dihydro-6H-pyrido[4,3-D]pyrimidin-5-one NVPHSP990; IS, inner segment; IMPDH1, inosine 5′-monophosphate dehydrogenase type 1; IRE1, inositol-requiring protein-1; LCA, Leber congenital amaurosis; MAP1B, microtubule-associated protein 1B; UPR^{mt}, mitochondrial unfolded protein response; OCT, optical coherence tomography; OS, outer segment; PRD, proline rich domain; PERK, protein kinase RNA (PKR)-like ER kinase; PQC, protein quality control; PDE6, retinal phosphodiesterase; RPE, retinal pigment epithelium; RP, Retinitis pigmentosa; RGS9, regulator of G-protein-signalling isoform 9; SPR, surface plasmon resonance; TPR, tetratricopeptide repeat; TRAP1, tumor necrosis factor receptor associated protein 1; UPR, unfolded protein response.

References

1. Strauss, O. The Retinal Pigment Epithelium in Visual Function. *Physiol. Rev.* **2005**, *85*, 845–881. [CrossRef]
2. Athanasiou, D.; Aguila, M.; Bellingham, J.; Li, W.; McCulley, C.; Reeves, P.J.; Cheetham, M.E. The molecular and cellular basis of rhodopsin retinitis pigmentosa reveals potential strategies for therapy. *Prog. Retin. Eye Res.* **2018**, *62*, 1–23. [CrossRef] [PubMed]
3. Arshavsky, V.Y.; Lamb, T.D.; Pugh, E.N. G Proteins and Phototransduction. *Annu. Rev. Physiol.* **2003**, *64*, 153–187. [CrossRef] [PubMed]
4. Arshavsky, V.Y.; Wensel, T.G. Timing Is Everything: GTPase Regulation in Phototransduction. *Investig. Opthalmology Vis. Sci.* **2013**, *54*, 7725–7733. [CrossRef] [PubMed]
5. Kefalov, V. Phototransduction: Phototransduction in Cones. *Encycl. Eye* **2010**, 389–396. [CrossRef]
6. Ingram, N.T.; Sampath, A.P.; Fain, G.L. Why are rods more sensitive than cones? *J. Physiol.* **2016**, *594*, 5415–5426. [CrossRef]
7. Spencer, W.J.; Lewis, T.; Pearring, J.N.; Arshavsky, V.Y. Photoreceptor Discs: Built Like Ectosomes. *Trends Cell Biol.* **2020**, *30*, 904–915. [CrossRef]
8. Léveillard, T.; Sahel, J.-A. Metabolic and redox signaling in the retina. In *Cellular and Molecular Life Sciences*; Birkhauser Verlag AG: Basel, Switzerland, 2017; Volume 74, Issue 20; pp. 3649–3665. [CrossRef]
9. Narayan, D.S.; Chidlow, G.; Wood, J.P.M.; Casson, R.J. Glucose metabolism in mammalian photoreceptor inner and outer segments. *Clin. Exp. Ophthalmol.* **2017**, *45*, 730–741. [CrossRef]
10. Kampinga, H.H.; Hageman, J.; Vos, M.J.; Kubota, H.; Tanguay, R.M.; Bruford, E.A.; Cheetham, M.E.; Chen, B.; Hightower, L.E. Guidelines for the nomenclature of the human heat shock proteins. *Cell Stress Chaperones* **2009**, *14*, 105–111. [CrossRef]
11. Biebl, M.M.; Buchner, J. Structure, Function, and Regulation of the Hsp90 Machinery. *Cold Spring Harb. Perspect. Biol.* **2019**, *11*, a034017. [CrossRef]

12. Prodromou, C.; Bjorklund, D.M. Advances towards Understanding the Mechanism of Action of the Hsp90 Complex. *Biomolecules* **2022**, *12*, 600. [CrossRef] [PubMed]
13. Åkerfelt, M.; Morimoto, R.I.; Sistonen, L. Heat shock factors: Integrators of cell stress, development and lifespan. *Nat. Rev. Mol. Cell Biol.* **2010**, *11*, 545–555. [CrossRef]
14. Voellmy, R. On mechanisms that control heat shock transcription factor activity in metazoan cells. *Cell Stress Chaperon.* **2004**, *9*, 122–133. [CrossRef] [PubMed]
15. Gomez-Pastor, R.; Burchfiel, E.T.; Thiele, D.J. Regulation of heat shock transcription factors and their roles in physiology and disease. *Nat. Rev. Mol. Cell Biol.* **2017**, *19*, 4–19. [CrossRef] [PubMed]
16. Prodromou, C. Mechanisms of Hsp90 regulation. *Biochem. J.* **2016**, *473*, 2439–2452. [CrossRef]
17. Luengo, T.M.; Kityk, R.; Mayer, M.P.; Rüdiger, S.G. Hsp90 Breaks the Deadlock of the Hsp70 Chaperone System. *Mol. Cell* **2018**, *70*, 545–552.e9. [CrossRef]
18. Hoter, A.; El-Sabban, M.E.; Naim, H.Y. The HSP90 Family: Structure, Regulation, Function, and Implications in Health and Disease. *Int. J. Mol. Sci.* **2018**, *19*, 2560. [CrossRef]
19. Wu, Y.; Zheng, X.; Ding, Y.; Zhou, M.; Wei, Z.; Liu, T.; Liao, K. The molecular chaperone Hsp90α deficiency causes retinal degeneration by disrupting Golgi organization and vesicle transportation in photoreceptors. *J. Mol. Cell Biol.* **2020**, *12*, 216–229. [CrossRef]
20. Marzec, M.; Eletto, D.; Argon, Y. GRP94: An HSP90-like protein specialized for protein folding and quality control in the endoplasmic reticulum. *Biochim. et Biophys. Acta-Mol. Cell Res.* **2012**, *1823*, 774–787. [CrossRef]
21. Meunier, L.; Usherwood, Y.-K.; Chung, K.T.; Hendershot, L.M. A Subset of Chaperones and Folding Enzymes Form Multiprotein Complexes in Endoplasmic Reticulum to Bind Nascent Proteins. *Mol. Biol. Cell* **2002**, *13*, 4456–4469. [CrossRef]
22. Hetz, C.; Zhang, K.; Kaufman, R.J. Mechanisms, regulation and functions of the unfolded protein response. *Nat. Rev. Mol. Cell Biol.* **2020**, *21*, 421–438. [CrossRef] [PubMed]
23. Anukanth, A.; Khorana, H. Structure and function in rhodopsin. Requirements of a specific structure for the intradiscal domain. *J. Biol. Chem.* **1994**, *269*, 19738–19744. [CrossRef]
24. Christianson, J.C.; Shaler, T.A.; Tyler, R.E.; Kopito, R.R. OS-9 and GRP94 deliver mutant α1-antitrypsin to the Hrd1–SEL1L ubiquitin ligase complex for ERAD. *Nat. Cell Biol.* **2008**, *10*, 272–282. [CrossRef] [PubMed]
25. Kroeger, H.; Messah, C.; Ahern, K.; Gee, J.; Joseph, V.; Matthes, M.T.; Yasumura, D.; Gorbatyuk, M.S.; Chiang, W.-C.; LaVail, M.M.; et al. Induction of Endoplasmic Reticulum Stress Genes, BiP and Chop, in Genetic and Environmental Models of Retinal Degeneration. *Investig. Opthalmology Vis. Sci.* **2012**, *53*, 7590–7599. [CrossRef]
26. Saliba, R.S.; Munro, P.M.G.; Luthert, P.J.; Cheetham, M.E. The cellular fate of mutant rhodopsin: Quality control, degradation and aggresome formation. *J. Cell Sci.* **2002**, *115*, 2907–2918. [CrossRef]
27. Carreras-Sureda, A.; Pihán, P.; Hetz, C. Calcium signaling at the endoplasmic reticulum: Fine-tuning stress responses. *Cell Calcium* **2017**, *70*, 24–31. [CrossRef]
28. Di Jeso, B.; Ulianich, L.; Pacifico, F.; Leonardi, A.; Vito, P.; Consiglio, E.; Formisano, S.; Arvan, P. Folding of thyroglobulin in the calnexin/calreticulin pathway and its alteration by loss of Ca2+ from the endoplasmic reticulum. *Biochem. J.* **2003**, *370*, 449–458. [CrossRef] [PubMed]
29. Mekahli, D.; Bultynck, G.; Parys, J.; De Smedt, H.; Missiaen, L. Endoplasmic-Reticulum Calcium Depletion and Disease. *Cold Spring Harb. Perspect. Biol.* **2011**, *3*, a004317. [CrossRef]
30. Preissler, S.; Rato, C.; Yan, Y.; Perera, L.A.; Czako, A.; Ron, D. Calcium depletion challenges endoplasmic reticulum proteostasis by destabilising BiP-substrate complexes. *eLife* **2020**, *9*, 1–36. [CrossRef]
31. Wengert, L.A.; Backe, S.J.; Bourboulia, D.; Mollapour, M.; Woodford, M.R. TRAP1 Chaperones the Metabolic Switch in Cancer. *Biomolecules* **2022**, *12*, 786. [CrossRef]
32. Felts, S.J.; Owen, B.A.L.; Nguyen, P.; Trepel, J.; Donner, D.B.; Toft, D.O. The hsp90-related Protein TRAP1 Is a Mitochondrial Protein with Distinct Functional Properties. *J. Biol. Chem.* **2000**, *275*, 3305–3312. [CrossRef]
33. Haynes, C.M.; Ron, D. The mitochondrial UPR—Protecting organelle protein homeostasis. *J. Cell Sci.* **2010**, *123*, 3849–3855. [CrossRef]
34. Martinus, R.D.; Garth, G.P.; Webster, T.L.; Cartwright, P.; Naylor, D.J.; Høj, P.B.; Hoogenraad, N.J. Selective Induction of Mitochondrial Chaperones in Response to Loss of the Mitochondrial Genome. *Eur. J. Biochem.* **1996**, *240*, 98–103. [CrossRef] [PubMed]
35. Zhao, Q.; Wang, J.; Levichkin, I.V.; Stasinopoulos, S.; Ryan, M.; Hoogenraad, N.J. A mitochondrial specific stress response in mammalian cells. *EMBO J.* **2002**, *21*, 4411–4419. [CrossRef] [PubMed]
36. Houtkooper, R.; Mouchiroud, L.; Ryu, D.; Moullan, N.; Katsyuba, E.; Knott, G.W.; Williams, R.W.; Auwerx, J. Mitonuclear protein imbalance as a conserved longevity mechanism. *Nature* **2013**, *497*, 451–457. [CrossRef] [PubMed]
37. Münch, C. The different axes of the mammalian mitochondrial unfolded protein response. *BMC Biol.* **2018**, *16*, 81. [CrossRef]
38. Baqri, R.M.; Pietron, A.V.; Gokhale, R.H.; Turner, B.A.; Kaguni, L.S.; Shingleton, A.W.; Kunes, S.; Miller, K.E. Mitochondrial chaperone TRAP1 activates the mitochondrial UPR and extends healthspan in Drosophila. *Mech. Ageing Dev.* **2014**, *141–142*, 35–45. [CrossRef]
39. Takemoto, K.; Miyata, S.; Takamura, H.; Katayama, T.; Tohyama, M. Mitochondrial TRAP1 regulates the unfolded protein response in the endoplasmic reticulum. *Neurochem. Int.* **2011**, *58*, 880–887. [CrossRef]

40. Georgiou, M.; Fujinami, K.; Michaelides, M. Inherited retinal diseases: Therapeutics, clinical trials and end points—A review. *Clin. Exp. Ophthalmol.* **2021**, *49*, 270–288. [CrossRef]
41. Parfitt, D.A.; Aguila, M.; McCulley, C.H.; Bevilacqua, D.; Mendes, H.F.; Athanasiou, D.; Novoselov, S.S.; Kanuga, N.; Munro, P.M.; Coffey, P.J.; et al. The heat-shock response co-inducer arimoclomol protects against retinal degeneration in rhodopsin retinitis pigmentosa. *Cell Death Dis.* **2014**, *5*, e1236. [CrossRef]
42. Mendes, H.F.; Cheetham, M.E. Pharmacological manipulation of gain-of-function and dominant-negative mechanisms in rhodopsin retinitis pigmentosa. *Hum. Mol. Genet.* **2008**, *17*, 3043–3054. [CrossRef] [PubMed]
43. Aguilà, M.; Bevilacqua, D.; McCulley, C.; Schwarz, N.; Athanasiou, D.; Kanuga, N.; Novoselov, S.S.; Lange, C.A.; Ali, R.R.; Bainbridge, J.W.; et al. Hsp90 inhibition protects against inherited retinal degeneration. *Hum. Mol. Genet.* **2014**, *23*, 2164–2175. [CrossRef]
44. Kennan, A.; Aherne, A.; Palfi, A.; Humphries, M.; McKee, A.; Stitt, A.; Simpson, D.A.C.; Demtroder, K.; Orntoft, T.; Ayuso, C.; et al. Identification of an IMPDH1 mutation in autosomal dominant retinitis pigmentosa (RP10) revealed following comparative microarray analysis of transcripts derived from retinas of wild-type and Rho-/- mice. *Hum. Mol. Genet.* **2002**, *11*, 547–558. [CrossRef]
45. Tam, L.C.; Kiang, A.-S.; Campbell, M.; Keaney, J.; Farrar, G.J.; Humphries, M.M.; Kenna, P.F.; Humphries, P. Prevention of autosomal dominant retinitis pigmentosa by systemic drug therapy targeting heat shock protein 90 (Hsp90). *Hum. Mol. Genet.* **2010**, *19*, 4421–4436. [CrossRef] [PubMed]
46. Zhou, D.; Liu, Y.; Ye, J.; Ying, W.; Ogawa, L.S.; Inoue, T.; Tatsuta, N.; Wada, Y.; Koya, K.; Huang, Q.; et al. A rat retinal damage model predicts for potential clinical visual disturbances induced by Hsp90 inhibitors. *Toxicol. Appl. Pharmacol.* **2013**, *273*, 401–409. [CrossRef] [PubMed]
47. Kummar, S.; Gutierrez, M.E.; Gardner, E.R.; Chen, X.; Figg, W.D.; Zajac-Kaye, M.; Chen, M.; Steinberg, S.M.; Muir, C.A.; Yancey, M.A.; et al. Phase I trial of 17-dimethylaminoethylamino-17-demethoxygeldanamycin (17-DMAG), a heat shock protein inhibitor, administered twice weekly in patients with advanced malignancies. *Eur. J. Cancer* **2010**, *46*, 340–347. [CrossRef]
48. Samuel, T.A.; Sessa, C.; Britten, C.; Milligan, K.S.; Mita, M.M.; Banerji, U.; Pluard, T.J.; Stiegler, P.; Quadt, C.; Shapiro, G. AUY922, a novel HSP90 inhibitor: Final results of a first-in-human study in patients with advanced solid malignancies. *J. Clin. Oncol.* **2010**, *28*, 2528. [CrossRef]
49. Shapiro, G.; Kwak, E.L.; Dezube, B.J.; Lawrence, D.P.; Cleary, J.M.; Lewis, S.; Squires, M.; Lock, V.; Lyons, J.F.; Yule, M. Phase I pharmacokinetic and pharmacodynamic study of the heat shock protein 90 inhibitor AT13387 in patients with refractory solid tumors. *J. Clin. Oncol.* **2010**, *28*, 3069. [CrossRef]
50. Pacey, S.; Wilson, R.H.; Walton, M.; Eatock, M.M.; Hardcastle, A.; Zetterlund, A.; Arkenau, H.-T.; Moreno-Farre, J.; Banerji, U.; Roels, B.; et al. A Phase I Study of the Heat Shock Protein 90 Inhibitor Alvespimycin (17-DMAG) Given Intravenously to Patients with Advanced Solid Tumors. *Clin. Cancer Res.* **2011**, *17*, 1561–1570. [CrossRef]
51. Rajan, A.; Kelly, R.J.; Trepel, J.B.; Kim, Y.S.; Alarcon, S.V.; Kummar, S.; Gutierrez, M.; Crandon, S.; Zein, W.M.; Jain, L.; et al. A phase I study of PF-04929113 (SNX-5422), an orally bioavailable heat shock protein 90 inhibitor, in patients with refractory solid tumor malignancies and lymphomas. *Clin. Cancer Res.* **2011**, *17*, 6831–6839. [CrossRef]
52. Bendell, J.C.; Jones, S.F.; Hart, L.; Pant, S.; Moyhuddin, A.; Lane, C.M.; Earwood, C.; Murphy, P.; Patton, J.; Penley, W.C.; et al. A Phase I Study of the Hsp90 Inhibitor AUY922 plus Capecitabine for the Treatment of Patients with Advanced Solid Tumors. *Cancer Investig.* **2015**, *33*, 477–482. [CrossRef] [PubMed]
53. Seggewiss-Bernhardt, R.; Bargou, R.C.; Goh, Y.T.; Stewart, A.K.; Spencer, A.; Alegre, A.; Bladé, J.; Ottmann, O.G.; Fernandez-Ibarra, C.; Lu, H.; et al. Phase 1/1B trial of the heat shock protein 90 inhibitor NVP-AUY922 as monotherapy or in combination with bortezomib in patients with relapsed or refractory multiple myeloma. *Cancer* **2015**, *121*, 2185–2192. [CrossRef] [PubMed]
54. Bendell, J.C.; Bauer, T.M.; Lamar, R.; Joseph, M.; Penley, W.; Thompson, D.S.; Spigel, D.R.; Owera, R.; Lane, C.M.; Earwood, C.; et al. A Phase 2 Study of the Hsp90 Inhibitor AUY922 as Treatment for Patients with Refractory Gastrointestinal Stromal Tumors. *Cancer Investig.* **2016**, *34*, 265–270. [CrossRef] [PubMed]
55. Chiang, N.-J.; Yeh, K.-H.; Chiu, C.-F.; Chen, J.-S.; Yen, C.-C.; Lee, K.-D.; Lin, Y.-L.; Bai, L.-Y.; Chen, M.-H.; Lin, J.-S.; et al. Results of Phase II trial of AUY922, a novel heat shock protein inhibitor in patients with metastatic gastrointestinal stromal tumor (GIST) and imatinib and sunitinib therapy. *J. Clin. Oncol.* **2016**, *34*, 134. [CrossRef]
56. Do, K.T.; Coyne, G.O.; Hays, J.L.; Supko, J.G.; Liu, S.V.; Beebe, K.; Neckers, L.; Trepel, J.B.; Lee, M.-J.; Smyth, T.; et al. Phase 1 study of the HSP90 inhibitor onalespib in combination with AT7519, a pan-CDK inhibitor, in patients with advanced solid tumors HHS Public Access. *Cancer Chemother. Pharmacol.* **2020**, *86*, 815–827. [CrossRef]
57. Shen, C.H.; Hsieh, C.C.; Jiang, K.Y.; Lin, C.Y.; Chiang, N.J.; Li, T.W.; Yen, C.T.; Chen, W.J.; Hwang, D.Y.; Chen, L.T. AUY922 induces retinal toxicity through attenuating TRPM1. *J. Biomed. Sci.* **2021**, *28*, 1–21. [CrossRef]
58. Kanamaru, C.; Yamada, Y.; Hayashi, S.; Matsushita, T.; Suda, A.; Nagayasu, M.; Kimura, K.; Chiba, S. Retinal toxicity induced by small-molecule Hsp90 inhibitors in beagle dogs. *J. Toxicol. Sci.* **2014**, *39*, 59–69. [CrossRef]
59. Roman, D.; VerHoeve, J.; Schadt, H.; Vicart, A.; Walker, U.J.; Turner, O.; Richardson, T.A.; Wolford, S.T.; Miller, P.E.; Zhou, W.; et al. Ocular toxicity of AUY922 in pigmented and albino rats. *Toxicol. Appl. Pharmacol.* **2016**, *309*, 55–62. [CrossRef]
60. Cote, R.H. Photoreceptor phosphodiesterase (PDE6): Activation and inactivation mechanisms during visual transduction in rods and cones. *Pflug. Arch. Eur. J. Physiol.* **2021**, *473*, 1377–1391. [CrossRef]

61. Sohocki, M.M.; Bowne, S.J.; Sullivan, L.S.; Blackshaw, S.; Cepko, C.L.; Payne, A.; Bhattacharya, S.S.; Khaliq, S.; Mehdi, S.Q.; Birch, D.; et al. Mutations in a new photoreceptor-pineal gene on 17p cause Leber congenital amaurosis. *Nat. Genet.* **2000**, *24*, 79–83. [CrossRef]
62. Liu, X.; Bulgakov, O.V.; Wen, X.H.; Woodruff, M.L.; Pawlyk, B.; Yang, J.; Fain, G.L.; Sandberg, M.A.; Makino, C.L.; Li, T. AIPL1, the protein that is defective in Leber congenital amaurosis, is essential for the biosynthesis of retinal rod cGMP phosphodiesterase. *Proc. Natl. Acad. Sci. USA* **2004**, *101*, 13903–13908. [CrossRef] [PubMed]
63. Ramamurthy, V.; Niemi, G.A.; Reh, T.A.; Hurley, J.B. Leber congenital amaurosis linked to AIPL1: A mouse model reveals destabilization of cGMP phosphodiesterase. *Proc. Natl. Acad. Sci. USA* **2004**, *101*, 13897–13902. [CrossRef] [PubMed]
64. Kirschman, L.T.; Kolandaivelu, S.; Frederick, J.M.; Dang, L.; Goldberg, A.F.; Baehr, W.; Ramamurthy, V. The Leber congenital amaurosis protein, AIPL1, is needed for the viability and functioning of cone photoreceptor cells. *Hum. Mol. Genet.* **2009**, *19*, 1076–1087. [CrossRef]
65. Kolandaivelu, S.; Huang, J.; Hurley, J.B.; Ramamurthy, V. AIPL1, a Protein Associated with Childhood Blindness, Interacts with α-Subunit of Rod Phosphodiesterase (PDE6) and Is Essential for Its Proper Assembly. *J. Biol. Chem.* **2009**, *284*, 30853–30861. [CrossRef] [PubMed]
66. Kolandaivelu, S.; Singh, R.K.; Ramamurthy, V. AIPL1, A protein linked to blindness, is essential for the stability of enzymes mediating cGMP metabolism in cone photoreceptor cells. *Hum. Mol. Genet.* **2013**, *23*, 1002–1012. [CrossRef]
67. Yadav, R.P.; Boyd, K.; Yu, L.; Artemyev, N.O. Interaction of the tetratricopeptide repeat domain of aryl hydrocarbon receptor–interacting protein–like 1 with the regulatory Pγ subunit of phosphodiesterase 6. *J. Biol. Chem.* **2019**, *294*, 15795–15807. [CrossRef]
68. Li, J.; Zoldak, G.; Kriehuber, T.; Soroka, J.; Schmid, F.X.; Richter, K.; Buchner, J. Unique Proline-Rich Domain Regulates the Chaperone Function of AIPL1. *Biochemistry* **2013**, *52*, 2089–2096. [CrossRef]
69. Linnert, M.; Lin, Y.-J.; Manns, A.; Haupt, K.; Paschke, A.-K.; Fischer, G.; Weiwad, M.; Lücke, C. The FKBP-Type Domain of the Human Aryl Hydrocarbon Receptor-Interacting Protein Reveals an Unusual Hsp90 Interaction. *Biochemistry* **2013**, *52*, 2097–2107. [CrossRef]
70. Majumder, A.; Gopalakrishna, K.N.; Cheguru, P.; Gakhar, L.; Artemyev, N.O. Interaction of Aryl Hydrocarbon Receptor-interacting Protein-like 1 with the Farnesyl Moiety. *J. Biol. Chem.* **2013**, *288*, 21320–21328. [CrossRef]
71. Yadav, R.P.; Gakhar, L.; Yu, L.; Artemyev, N.O. Unique structural features of the AIPL1–FKBP domain that support prenyl lipid binding and underlie protein malfunction in blindness. *Proc. Natl. Acad. Sci. USA* **2017**, *114*, E6536–E6545. [CrossRef]
72. Sohocki, M.M.; Sullivan, L.S.; Tirpak, D.L.; Daiger, S.P. Comparative analysis of aryl-hydrocarbon receptor interacting protein-like 1 (Aipl1), a gene associated with inherited retinal disease in humans. *Mamm. Genome* **2001**, *12*, 566–568. [CrossRef]
73. Yadav, R.P.; Majumder, A.; Gakhar, L.; Artemyev, N.O. Extended conformation of the proline-rich domain of human aryl hydrocarbon receptor-interacting protein-like 1: Implications for retina disease. *J. Neurochem.* **2015**, *135*, 165–175. [CrossRef] [PubMed]
74. Roy, A.; Kucukural, A.; Zhang, Y. I-TASSER: A unified platform for automated protein structure and function prediction. *Nat. Protoc.* **2010**, *5*, 725–738. [CrossRef] [PubMed]
75. Zhang, Y. I-TASSER server for protein 3D structure prediction. *BMC Bioinform.* **2008**, *9*, 40. [CrossRef] [PubMed]
76. Hidalgo-De-Quintana, J.; Evans, R.J.; Cheetham, M.; Van Der Spuy, J. The Leber Congenital Amaurosis Protein AIPL1 Functions as Part of a Chaperone Heterocomplex. *Investig. Opthalmology Vis. Sci.* **2008**, *49*, 2878–2887. [CrossRef]
77. Sacristan-Reviriego, A.; Bellingham, J.; Prodromou, C.; Boehm, A.N.; Aichem, A.; Kumaran, N.; Bainbridge, J.; Michaelides, M.; Van Der Spuy, J. The integrity and organization of the human AIPL1 functional domains is critical for its role as a HSP90-dependent co-chaperone for rod PDE6. *Hum. Mol. Genet.* **2017**, *26*, 4465–4480. [CrossRef]
78. Yadav, R.P.; Boyd, K.; Artemyev, N.O. Molecular insights into the maturation of phosphodiesterase 6 by the specialized chaperone complex of HSP90 with AIPL1. *J. Biol. Chem.* **2022**, *298*, 101620. [CrossRef]
79. Sacristan-Reviriego, A.; Le, H.M.; Georgiou, M.; Meunier, I.; Bocquet, B.; Roux, A.-F.; Prodromou, C.; Bainbridge, J.; Michaelides, M.; van der Spuy, J. Clinical and functional analyses of AIPL1 variants reveal mechanisms of pathogenicity linked to different forms of retinal degeneration. *Sci. Rep.* **2020**, *10*, 17520. [CrossRef]
80. Cheung-Flynn, J.; Roberts, P.J.; Riggs, D.L.; Smith, D.F. C-terminal Sequences outside the Tetratricopeptide Repeat Domain of FKBP51 and FKBP52 Cause Differential Binding to Hsp90. *J. Biol. Chem.* **2003**, *278*, 17388–17394. [CrossRef]
81. van der Spuy, J.; Cheetham, M. The Leber Congenital Amaurosis Protein AIPL1 Modulates the Nuclear Translocation of NUB1 and Suppresses Inclusion Formation by NUB1 Fragments. *J. Biol. Chem.* **2004**, *279*, 48038–48047. [CrossRef]
82. Yu, L.; Yadav, R.P.; Artemyev, N.O. NMR resonance assignments of the FKBP domain of human aryl hydrocarbon receptor-interacting protein-like 1 (AIPL1) in complex with a farnesyl ligand. *Biomol. NMR Assign.* **2017**, *11*, 111–115. [CrossRef] [PubMed]
83. Ramamurthy, V.; Roberts, M.; Van den Akker, F.; Niemi, G.; Reh, T.A.; Hurley, J.B. AIPL1, a protein implicated in Leber's congenital amaurosis, interacts with and aids in processing of farnesylated proteins. *Proc. Natl. Acad. Sci. USA* **2003**, *100*, 12630–12635. [CrossRef] [PubMed]
84. Gopalakrishna, K.N.; Boyd, K.; Yadav, R.P.; Artemyev, N.O. Aryl Hydrocarbon Receptor-interacting Protein-like 1 Is an Obligate Chaperone of Phosphodiesterase 6 and Is Assisted by the γ-Subunit of Its Client. *J. Biol. Chem.* **2016**, *291*, 16282–16291. [CrossRef] [PubMed]

85. Zang, J.; Neuhauss, S.C.F. The Binding Properties and Physiological Functions of Recoverin. *Front. Mol. Neurosci.* **2018**, *11*, 473. [CrossRef] [PubMed]
86. Chen, Q.; Plasencia, M.; Li, Z.; Mukherjee, S.; Patra, D.; Chen, C.-L.; Klose, T.; Yao, X.-Q.; Kossiakoff, A.A.; Chang, L.; et al. Structures of rhodopsin in complex with G-protein-coupled receptor kinase 1. *Nature* **2021**, *595*, 600–605. [CrossRef]
87. Yeung, W.; Ruan, Z.; Kannan, N. Emerging roles of the αC-β4 loop in protein kinase structure, function, evolution, and disease. *IUBMB Life* **2020**, *72*, 1189–1202. [CrossRef]
88. Luo, J.; Benovic, J.L. G Protein-coupled Receptor Kinase Interaction with Hsp90 Mediates Kinase Maturation. *J. Biol. Chem.* **2003**, *278*, 50908–50914. [CrossRef]
89. Xu, W.; Yuan, X.; Xiang, Z.; Mimnaugh, E.; Marcu, M.; Neckers, L. Surface charge and hydrophobicity determine ErbB2 binding to the Hsp90 chaperone complex. *Nat. Struct. Mol. Biol.* **2005**, *12*, 120–126. [CrossRef]
90. Citri, A.; Harari, D.; Shohat, G.; Ramakrishnan, P.; Gan, J.; Lavi, S.; Eisenstein, M.; Kimchi, A.; Wallach, D.; Pietrokovski, S.; et al. Hsp90 Recognizes a Common Surface on Client Kinases. *J. Biol. Chem.* **2006**, *281*, 14361–14369. [CrossRef]
91. Caplan, A.J.; Mandal, A.K.; Theodoraki, M. Molecular chaperones and protein kinase quality control. *Trends Cell Biol.* **2007**, *17*, 87–92. [CrossRef]
92. Taipale, M.; Jarosz, D.F.; Lindquist, S. HSP90 at the hub of protein homeostasis: Emerging mechanistic insights. *Nat. Rev. Mol. Cell Biol.* **2010**, *11*, 515–528. [CrossRef] [PubMed]
93. Taipale, M.; Krykbaeva, I.; Koeva, M.; Kayatekin, C.; Westover, K.D.; Karras, G.I.; Lindquist, S. Quantitative Analysis of Hsp90-Client Interactions Reveals Principles of Substrate Recognition. *Cell* **2012**, *150*, 987–1001. [CrossRef] [PubMed]
94. Verba, K.A.; Agard, D.A. How Hsp90 and Cdc37 Lubricate Kinase Molecular Switches. *Trends Biochem. Sci.* **2017**, *42*, 799–811. [CrossRef] [PubMed]

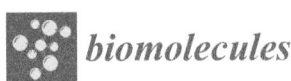

Article

Non-Equilibrium Protein Folding and Activation by ATP-Driven Chaperones

Huafeng Xu

Roivant Sciences, New York, NY 10036, USA; huafeng.xu@roivant.com

Abstract: Recent experimental studies suggest that ATP-driven molecular chaperones can stabilize protein substrates in their native structures out of thermal equilibrium. The mechanism of such non-equilibrium protein folding is an open question. Based on available structural and biochemical evidence, I propose here a unifying principle that underlies the conversion of chemical energy from ATP hydrolysis to the conformational free energy associated with protein folding and activation. I demonstrate that non-equilibrium folding requires the chaperones to break at least one of four symmetry conditions. The Hsp70 and Hsp90 chaperones each break a different subset of these symmetries and thus they use different mechanisms for non-equilibrium protein folding. I derive an upper bound on the non-equilibrium elevation of the native concentration, which implies that non-equilibrium folding only occurs in slow-folding proteins that adopt an unstable intermediate conformation in binding to ATP-driven chaperones. Contrary to the long-held view of Anfinsen's hypothesis that proteins fold to their conformational free energy minima, my results predict that some proteins may fold into thermodynamically unstable native structures with the assistance of ATP-driven chaperones, and that the native structures of some chaperone-dependent proteins may be shaped by their chaperone-mediated folding pathways.

Keywords: chaperones; Hsp70; Hsp90; non-equilibrium; protein folding

Citation: Xu, H. Non-Equilibrium Protein Folding and Activation by ATP-Driven Chaperones. *Biomolecules* **2022**, *12*, 832. https://doi.org/10.3390/biom12060832

Academic Editor: Chrisostomos Prodromou

Received: 24 May 2022
Accepted: 13 June 2022
Published: 15 June 2022

Publisher's Note: MDPI stays neutral with regard to jurisdictional claims in published maps and institutional affiliations.

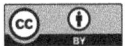

Copyright: © 2022 by the authors. Licensee MDPI, Basel, Switzerland. This article is an open access article distributed under the terms and conditions of the Creative Commons Attribution (CC BY) license (https://creativecommons.org/licenses/by/4.0/).

1. Introduction

A commonly accepted view on protein folding is Anfinsen's thermodynamic hypothesis [1]: the native structure of a protein is uniquely determined by its amino acid sequence, and it is the conformation of the lowest free energy. According to this view, a free energy gap separates the native structure and the denatured conformations, and protein folding is accompanied by a negative free energy change [2]. A protein, left to its own device and given sufficient time, will fold spontaneously to its native structure.

We now know that many proteins depend on the assistance of molecular chaperones for folding into their functional structures inside cells [3–5]. ATP-driven chaperones such as GroEL/GroES [6–8], Hsp70 [9,10], and Hsp90 [11–17] represent an important class of chaperones that consume chemical energy in their functions. Biochemical and structural studies have established that these chaperones undergo a cycle powered by ATP hydrolysis through open and closed conformations [10,18–22]. These chaperones can rescue their protein substrates from misfolded or aggregated structures and accelerate their refolding to their native structures [23–27]. This role of ATP-driven chaperones does not contradict Anfinsen's thermodynamic hypothesis: proteins still fold into the most thermodynamically stable structures, but the chaperones enable them to do so within a physiologically reasonable time [28].

Recent experimental studies suggest that ATP-driven chaperones may play a thermodynamic role besides the kinetic one: they may stabilize proteins in their native structures out of thermal equilibrium, converting the chemical energy of ATP hydrolysis into the conformational free energy of their substrates [26,29]. Coincidental to these experimental studies, theoretical models were published around the same time that predicted such non-equilibrium stabilization [29–31]. In addition to quantitatively recapitulating the experimentally observed acceleration in folding kinetics, these models suggest that ATP-driven chaperones can maintain their protein substrates in their native structures at higher concentrations than thermodynamically permitted in the chaperone-free equilibrium. They explain why ATP hydrolysis is indispensable to the cellular functions of these chaperones, and in the case of Hsp70 [30] and Hsp90 [31], the critical roles of their respective cochaperones.

Here, I define non-equilibrium protein folding to be the phenomenon in which the native fraction of a protein is elevated by an energy-consuming process above its value in thermal equilibrium. Let $f_N = [N]/P_0$ be the steady state fraction of the protein substrate in its native structure in the presence of ATP-driven chaperones, and $f_{N,eq} = [N]_{eq}/P_0$ be the native fraction in the chaperone-free equilibrium, where P_0 is the total protein concentration and $[N]$ is the concentration of the protein in its native structure. Non-equilibrium protein folding occurs if $f_N > f_{N,eq}$, which of course requires energy consumption. I will introduce the gain factor of non-equilibrium folding

$$g \equiv \frac{f_N}{f_{N,eq}} = \frac{[N]}{[N]_{eq}} \qquad (1)$$

which measures the extent of out-of-equilibrium stabilization of the native structure. A protein that primarily occupies the non-native structures in equilibrium (i.e., $f_{N,eq} < 0.5$) but its native structure in the presence of ATP-driven chaperones (i.e., $f_N > 0.5$) would contest Anfinsen's hypothesis.

Note that the native fraction in my definition of non-equilibrium folding includes only the free (i.e., not chaperone-bound) native protein because chaperones primarily bind to proteins that are at least partially unfolded [9,32]. There are, however, examples in which chaperone-bound proteins retain some native activity. For instance, glucocorticoid receptor (GR) can bind to its ligand when it is in complex with Hsp90 [33]. In this case, however, GR may still need to dissociate from Hsp90 to function as an active transcription factor. Thus, in this work, I will only consider non-equilibrium folding to a free, native protein.

Many mechanistic models have been proposed for chaperone-mediated protein folding [27,28,32,34–36]. One prevalent hypothesis regards the chaperones as unfoldases or holdases [37], in that their primary function is to rescue a misfolded or aggregated protein substrate and to hold it in an unfolded state. Upon release from the chaperones, the protein molecule has a certain probability of folding into its native structure [38]. Models based on this hypothesis provide an explanation of how ATP-driven chaperones accelerate the folding of the substrates to their inherently stable native structures, but they do not provide an explicit mechanism for the chaperones to transfer the chemical energy from ATP hydrolysis into the folding free energy of the substrate protein. It has been proposed that the ATP energy is used by the chaperones to achieve ultra-affinity in substrate binding [36].

It is often unclear whether a model will imply non-equilibrium protein folding (i.e., $g > 1$), when microscopic reversibility [31,39] is rigorously enforced. Based on thermodynamic principles, I have previously established one requirement of non-equilibrium protein folding: the substrate protein must undergo a conformational change when it is bound to the chaperone [31]. Supported by biochemical and structural evidence [40–42], this is a key assumption in my models of chaperone-mediated protein folding that couple the conformational dynamics of the protein substrate with the ATP-driven, open-close cycle of the chaperones (Figure 1).

In this work, I introduce an additional requirement that an ATP-driven chaperone must satisfy to perform non-equilibrium protein folding. Specifically, I demonstrate mathematically that an ATP-driven chaperone must break at least one of the four kinetic symmetry conditions (Conditions 1–4 in Section 3.1) to use the energy from ATP hydrolysis for out-of-equilibrium stabilization of substrate proteins in their native structures. As discussed below, Hsp70, Hsp90, and GroEL/GroES each break a different subset of the symmetry conditions, thus they use different mechanisms to perform non-equilibrium folding. Despite the difference in their mechanistic details, I present a unifying principle by which symmetry breaking translates into non-equilibrium folding to the native structures.

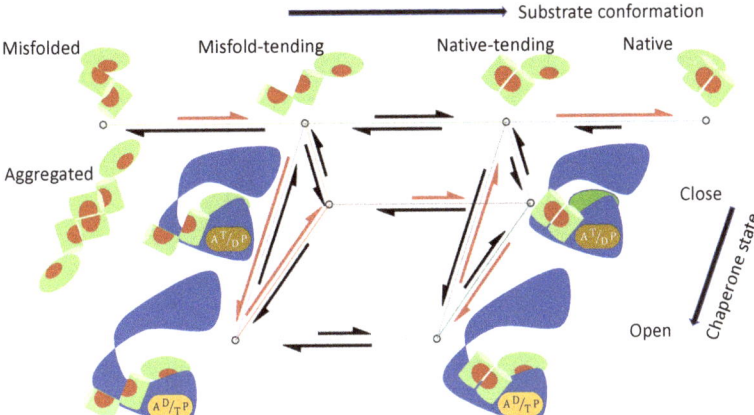

Figure 1. A mechanistic model of chaperone-mediated non-equilibrium protein folding that couples the state cycle of the chaperone and the conformational dynamics of its substrate. The chaperone undergoes a cycle of open and closed conformations, driven by ATP hydrolysis and nucleotide exchange. The protein substrate can transition among four classes of conformations: Misfolded (M), Misfold-tending (U), Native-tending (F), and Native (N). The lengths of the reaction arrows signify the corresponding reaction rates. The red arrows indicate the predominant folding pathway.

In addition, I derive an upper bound on the extent to which an ATP-driven chaperone can elevate the native fraction of a substrate above its chaperone-free equilibrium value (Equation (56)). My results suggest that, for substantial non-equilibrium protein folding (i.e., $g \gg 1$) to occur, the chaperone—with the possible exception of chaperonins such as GroEL/GroES—must bind to an unstable intermediate conformation of the substrate, and the substrate protein must fold slowly on its own.

Whether Anfinsen's hypothesis holds true for an individual protein can be experimentally tested by comparing the protein's activity in the presence and in the absence of functional ATP-driven chaperones; I have previously proposed new experiments that may provide such tests on Hsp70- and Hsp90-mediated folding [30,31]. In this work, I propose a potential proteomics-level experiment that may help identify proteins that depend on ATP-driven chaperones for maintenance of their native structures.

My models of non-equilibrium protein folding imply that the native structures of some proteins may be shaped by the chaperone-mediated folding pathways. They raise the possibility of discovering natural proteins—and engineering novel proteins—that adopt different conformations in the presence and absence of the chaperones.

Assumptions and Notations

To facilitate the exposition, I summarize the assumptions and notations in my model as follows:

- The substrate protein can convert among a set of conformations $\mathbb{S}$, both when it is free in solution and when it is bound to the chaperone. I will use M to denote the misfolded/aggregated conformation and N the native conformation. In addition, I will consider two classes of intermediate conformations: the unfolded and misfold-tending (or aggregation-tending) conformation U, and the non-native but native-tending conformation F. To avoid a proliferation of symbols and to underscore the mechanistic commonality shared by protein folding and activation, in the discussion of kinase activation, I will use M to denote the inactive conformation, N the active conformation, U the inactive-tending conformation, and F the active-tending conformation.

- The chaperone can transition among a set of states $\mathbb{I}$, each state i characterized by its conformational state (e.g., open or closed) and the numbers and the types (ATP vs ADP) of bound nucleotides.

My model includes the following reactions:

- The substrate in conformation S binds to the chaperone in state i with the association rate constant $k_{a,Si}$ and the dissociation rate constant $k_{d,Si}$:

$$S + H_i \underset{k_{d,Si}}{\overset{k_{a,Si}}{\rightleftharpoons}} SH_i \qquad (2)$$

- The free substrate in solution converts between conformation S and conformation S':

$$S \underset{k_{S' \to S}}{\overset{k_{S \to S'}}{\rightleftharpoons}} S' \qquad (3)$$

The corresponding conformational equilibrium constant is

$$K_{SS'} = \frac{k_{S \to S'}}{k_{S' \to S}} \qquad (4)$$

- The substrate bound to the chaperone in state i converts between conformation S and conformation S':

$$SH_i \underset{k_{S' \to S,i}}{\overset{k_{S \to S',i}}{\rightleftharpoons}} S'H_i \qquad (5)$$

- The chaperone transitions between state i and state j when it is bound to a substrate in conformation S:

$$SH_i \underset{k_{S,j \to i}}{\overset{k_{S,i \to j}}{\rightleftharpoons}} SH_j \qquad (6)$$

2. Materials and Methods

2.1. Proof That Symmetry Breaking Is Required for Non-Equilibrium Protein Folding

I will show that, under the symmetry conditions (Conditions 1–4 in Section 3.1), the steady state concentrations of the substrate satisfies, for any pair of conformations S and S',

$$k_{S \to S'}[S] = k_{S' \to S}[S'] \iff \frac{[S']}{[S]} = \frac{k_{S \to S'}}{k_{S' \to S}} = K_{SS'} \qquad (7)$$

where $[S]$ (or $[S']$) is the concentration of the free substrate in conformation S (or S'). Thus, the steady state ratio $[S']/[S]$ is unchanged from that in the chaperone-free equilibrium $[S']_{eq}/[S]_{eq} = K_{SS'}$ for any pair of conformations S and S', including $[N]/[M] = [N]_{eq}/[M]_{eq}$, and the chaperone is unable to increase the native concentration of the substrate above that in the equilibrium.

Letting $[H_i]$ be the concentration of the chaperone in state i and $[SH_i]$ the concentration of the substrate in conformation S bound to the chaperone in state i, the steady state condition for the reactions in Equations (2), (3), (5) and (6) is

$$\begin{aligned}
0 = \frac{d[S]}{dt} &= \sum_i (k_{d,Si}[SH_i] - k_{a,Si}[H_i][S]) + \sum_{S'}(k_{S' \to S}[S'] - k_{S \to S'}[S]) \\
0 = \frac{d[SH_i]}{dt} &= k_{a,Si}[H_i][S] - k_{d,Si}[SH_i] + \sum_{j \neq i}(k_{S,j \to i}[SH_j] - k_{S,i \to j}[SH_i]) \\
&\quad + \sum_{S'}(k_{S' \to S,i}[S'H_i] - k_{S \to S',i}[SH_i])
\end{aligned} \qquad (8)$$

According to Condition 1, the ratio $k_{a,S'i}/k_{a,Si}$ does not depend on i. I denote this ratio as

$$\frac{k_{a,S'i}}{k_{a,Si}} = \gamma_{SS'} K_{SS'}^{-1} \quad (9)$$

where $\gamma_{SS'}$ is a number that does not depend on i.

Consider a hypothetical, restricted system in which the substrate bound to the chaperone cannot change conformations (i.e., setting $k_{S \to S',i} = 0$ for all i and all pairs of S and S' in Equation (8)). Because the reaction $S \rightleftharpoons S'$ is not part of any energy consuming cycle in this restricted system, $[S']/[S] = K_{SS'}$ [31]. Let $\{[S]\} \cup \{[SH_i] | i \in \mathbb{I}\}$ be the steady state concentrations of the substrate in conformation S in this restricted system, I will show that

$$[S'] = K_{SS'}[S] \quad (10)$$
$$[S'H_i] = \gamma_{SS'}[SH_i] \quad (11)$$

are the steady state concentrations of the substrate in conformation S', and that $[SH_i]$ and $[S'H_i]$ satisfy

$$k_{S \to S',i}[SH_i] - k_{S' \to S,i}[S'H_i] = 0 \; \forall i \in \mathbb{I} \quad (12)$$

for the original $k_{S \to S',i} > 0$ and $k_{S' \to S,i} > 0$. Thus, the steady state concentrations of the restricted system are also the solution to the original steady state condition in Equation (8), and Equation (7) holds (it is equivalent to Equation (10)).

To prove Equation (12), consider first an open state i. Thermodynamic cycle closure in the following reaction cycle (which does not consume chemical energy because the chaperone does not change state),

$$\begin{array}{ccc}
S & \underset{k_{S' \to S}}{\overset{k_{S \to S'}}{\rightleftharpoons}} & S' \\
S' + H_i & \underset{k_{d,S'i}}{\overset{k_{a,S'i}}{\rightleftharpoons}} & S'H_i \\
S'H_i & \underset{k_{S \to S',i}}{\overset{k_{S' \to S,i}}{\rightleftharpoons}} & SH_i \\
SH_i & \underset{k_{a,Si}}{\overset{k_{d,Si}}{\rightleftharpoons}} & S + H_i
\end{array} \quad (13)$$

implies that

$$\frac{k_{S' \to S,i}}{k_{S \to S',i}} \frac{k_{a,S'i}}{k_{d,S'i}} \frac{k_{d,Si}}{k_{a,Si}} K_{SS'} = 1 \quad (14)$$

$$\iff k_{S \to S',i} = k_{S' \to S,i} K_{SS'} \frac{k_{a,S'i}}{k_{a,Si}} \frac{k_{d,Si}}{k_{d,S'i}} = k_{S' \to S,i} \gamma_{SS'} \; (\because \text{Equations (9) and (37)})$$

$$\implies k_{S' \to S,i}[S'H_i] - k_{S \to S',i}[SH_i]$$
$$= [SH_i](k_{S' \to S,i} \gamma_{SS'} - k_{S \to S',i}) \; (\because \text{Equation (11)}) \quad (15)$$
$$= 0$$

If i is a closed state such that $k_{a,Si} = k_{a,S'i} = k_{d,Si} = k_{d,S'i} = 0$, Equation (14) no longer holds. According to Condition 4, however, the chaperone can reversibly transition between i and an open state j without the consumption of chemical energy, and, according to Condition 3, the transition rates between i and j do not depend on the conformational state of the bound substrate, i.e.,

$$\frac{k_{S',i \to j}}{k_{S,i \to j}} = \frac{k_{S',j \to i}}{k_{S,j \to i}} = 1 \quad (16)$$

Thus, thermodynamic cycle closure in the following reversible reaction cycle

$$
\begin{aligned}
S &\underset{k_{S'\to S}}{\overset{k_{S\to S'}}{\rightleftharpoons}} S' \\
S' + H_j &\underset{k_{d,S'j}}{\overset{k_{a,S'j}}{\rightleftharpoons}} S'H_j \\
S'H_j &\underset{k_{S',i\to j}}{\overset{k_{S',j\to i}}{\rightleftharpoons}} S'H_i \\
S'H_i &\underset{k_{S\to S',i}}{\overset{k_{S'\to S,i}}{\rightleftharpoons}} SH_i \\
SH_i &\underset{k_{S,j\to i}}{\overset{k_{S,i\to j}}{\rightleftharpoons}} SH_j \\
SH_j &\underset{k_{a,Sj}}{\overset{k_{d,Sj}}{\rightleftharpoons}} S + H_j
\end{aligned}
\qquad (17)
$$

implies

$$\frac{k_{S'\to S,i}}{k_{S\to S',i}} \frac{k_{S,i\to j}}{k_{S,j\to i}} \frac{k_{S',j\to i}}{k_{S',i\to j}} \frac{k_{a,S'j}}{k_{d,S'j}} \frac{k_{d,Sj}}{k_{a,Sj}} K_{SS'} = 1 \qquad (18)$$

$$
\begin{aligned}
&\implies \frac{k_{S'\to S,i}}{k_{S\to S',i}} \frac{k_{a,S'j}}{k_{a,Sj}} \frac{k_{d,Sj}}{k_{d,S'j}} K_{SS'} = 1 \quad (\because \text{Equation (16)}) \\
&\implies \frac{k_{S'\to S,i}}{k_{S\to S',i}} \gamma_{SS'} = 1 \quad (\because \text{Equations (9) and (37)}) \\
&\implies k_{S'\to S,i}[S'H_i] - k_{S\to S',i}[SH_i] \\
&= [SH_i](k_{S'\to S,i}\gamma_{SS'} - k_{S\to S',i}) \quad (\because \text{Equation (11)}) \\
&= 0
\end{aligned}
\qquad (19)
$$

Thus, Equation (12) is true for both open and closed states.

To prove that $\{[S']\} \cup \{[S'H_i] | i \in \mathbb{I}\}$ in Equations (10) and (11) satisfy the steady state condition Equation (8) (swapping S' and S), I only need to show that, for the reactions in Equations (2) and (6), the flux in each reaction involving the substrate in conformation S' is $\gamma_{SS'}$ times the flux of the corresponding reaction involving the substrate in conformation S because $\{[S]\} \cup \{[SH_i] | i \in \mathbb{I}\}$ satisfies Equation (8) and the reactions in Equations (3) and (5) have zero flux (Equations (10) and (12)).

Let $J_{S,ij} = k_{S,i\to j}[SH_i] - k_{S,j\to i}[SH_j]$ be the reactive flux of the state transition for the chaperone bound to a substrate in conformation S (Equation (6)) and $J^a_{Si} = k_{a,Si}[H_i][S] - k_{d,Si}[SH_i]$ be the reactive flux of the substrate in conformation S binding to the chaperone in state i (Equation (2)). The corresponding reactive fluxes for the substrate in conformation S' are

$$
\begin{aligned}
J_{S',ij} &= k_{S',i\to j}[S'H_i] - k_{S',j\to i}[S'H_j] \\
&= \gamma_{SS'}(k_{S,i\to j}[SH_i] - k_{S,j\to i}[SH_j]) \quad (\because \text{Equation (11) and Condition 3}) \\
&= \gamma_{SS'} J_{S,ij}
\end{aligned}
\qquad (20)
$$

and

$$
\begin{aligned}
J^a_{S'i} &= k_{a,S'i}[H_i][S'] - k_{d,S'i}[S'H_i] \\
&= k_{a,S'i}[H_i]K_{SS'}[S] - k_{d,Si}\gamma_{SS'}[SH_i] \quad (\because \text{Equations (10), (11) and (37)}) \\
&= \gamma_{SS'}(k_{a,Si}[H_i][S] - k_{d,Si}[SH_i]) \quad (\because \text{Equation (9)}) \\
&= \gamma_{SS'} J^a_{Si}
\end{aligned}
\qquad (21)
$$

Q.E.D.

2.2. Derivation of the Upper Bound of the Native Concentration at the Steady State of Non-Equilibrium Folding

To derive the upper bound in Equation (51), consider the reactions in Table 1. These are simplifications of the reactions in Equations (2), (3), (5) and (6): only a substrate in intermediate conformations $S = U, F$ can bind to the chaperone (see Section 3.2.1), and only two chaperone states, open (O) and closed (C), are considered. The results hold as long as the substrate binds to all chaperone open states with the same association and dissociation rate constants, i.e.,

$$\begin{aligned} k_{a,Si} &= k_{a,S} \\ k_{d,Si} &= k_{d,S} \end{aligned} \quad \forall \text{ open state } i \tag{22}$$

Table 1. The reactions in chaperone-mediated protein folding. These reactions are depicted in Figure 1. ATP hydrolysis and nucleotide exchange occur and inject chemical energy in the chaperone cycle.

Reaction	Description
$U \underset{k_{M \to U}}{\overset{k_{U \to M}}{\rightleftharpoons}} M$	Misfolding and aggregation; $K_M = k_{U \to M}/k_{M \to U}$
$U \underset{k_{F \to U}}{\overset{k_{U \to F}}{\rightleftharpoons}} F$	Transition between intermediate conformations; $K_F = k_{U \to F}/k_{F \to U}$
$F \underset{k_{N \to F}}{\overset{k_{F \to N}}{\rightleftharpoons}} N$	Folding to native structure; $K_N = k_{F \to N}/k_{N \to F}$
$S + O \underset{k_{d,S}}{\overset{k_{a,S}}{\rightleftharpoons}} SO$	Substrate in $S = U, F$ conformations binding to the open chaperone
$SO \underset{k_{S,C \to O}}{\overset{k_{S,O \to C}}{\rightleftharpoons}} SC$	Transition of chaperone between open and closed states
$UH \underset{k_{F \to U,H}}{\overset{k_{U \to F,H}}{\rightleftharpoons}} FH$	Conversion of protein bound to chaperone in $H = C, O$ states

Let

$$J_{FU} = k_{F \to U}[F] - k_{U \to F}[U] \tag{23}$$

be the reactive flux from F to U. At the steady state, there is no net flux into or out of any molecular species, implying

$$\begin{aligned} J_{FU} &= k_{a,U}[U][O] - k_{d,U}[UO] \\ &= k_{d,F}[FO] - k_{a,F}[F][O] \end{aligned} \tag{24}$$

Because no external chemical energy is consumed in the reaction cycle of

$$U + O \rightleftharpoons UO \rightleftharpoons FO \rightleftharpoons F + O \rightleftharpoons U + O, \tag{25}$$

we have

$$\frac{k_{F \to U,O}}{k_{U \to F,O}} \cdot \frac{k_{a,F}}{k_{d,F}} \cdot \frac{k_{d,U}}{k_{a,U}} \cdot \frac{k_{U \to F}}{k_{F \to U}} = 1 \tag{26}$$

Thus,

$$\begin{aligned} \frac{k_{F \to U,O}[FO]}{k_{U \to F,O}[UO]} &= \frac{k_{F \to U,O}}{k_{U \to F,O}} \cdot \frac{k_{a,F}}{k_{d,F}} \cdot \frac{k_{d,U}}{k_{a,U}} \cdot \frac{k_{U \to F}}{k_{F \to U}} \\ &\quad \cdot \frac{k_{d,F}[FO]}{k_{a,F}[F][O]} \cdot \frac{k_{a,U}[U][O]}{k_{d,U}[UO]} \cdot \frac{k_{F \to U}[F]}{k_{U \to F}[U]} \\ &= \frac{k_{d,F}[FO]}{k_{d,F}[F][O]} \cdot \frac{k_{a,U}[U][O]}{k_{d,U}[UO]} \cdot \frac{k_{F \to U}[F]}{k_{U \to F}[U]} \end{aligned} \tag{27}$$

If J_{FU} in Equations (23) and (24) is positive, all three ratios on the right-hand side of Equation (27) are greater than 1; if $J_{FU} < 0$, they are all smaller than 1. Thus, the reactive flux

$$J_{UF,O} = k_{U \to F,O}[UO] - k_{F \to U,O}[FO] \tag{28}$$

must be of the opposite sign of J_{FU}.

If the chaperone drives the substrate toward the native structure, we have $[F]/[U] > K_F = k_{U \to F}/k_{F \to U}$, implying $J_{FU} > 0$ and $J_{UF,O} < 0$. Because the flux from conformation F to U in free substrates must balance the total flux from conformation U to F in chaperone-bound substrates, the steady state reactive flux of the reaction $UC \rightleftharpoons FC$

$$J_{UF,C} = k_{U \to F,C}[UC] - k_{F \to U,C}[FC] \tag{29}$$

satisfies

$$J_{FU} = J_{UF,C} + J_{UF,O} < J_{UF,C} \tag{30}$$

Thus,

$$k_{F \to U}[F] - k_{U \to F}[U] < k_{U \to F,C}[UC] - k_{F \to U,C}[FC]$$
$$\implies k_{F \to U}[F] < k_{U \to F}\left([U] + \frac{k_{U \to F,C}}{k_{U \to F}}[UC]\right) \equiv k_{U \to F}([U] + \alpha[UC]) \tag{31}$$
$$\implies [F] < K_F \cdot \max(1, \alpha) \cdot ([U] + [UC])$$

We also have, per Equations (23) and (24),

$$J_{FU} = k_{F \to U}[F] - k_{U \to F}[U] = k_{a,U}[O][U] - k_{d,U}[UO] < k_{a,U}[O][U]$$
$$\implies (k_{U \to F} + k_{a,U}[O])[U] > k_{F \to U}[F] \tag{32}$$

At the steady state, there is no net flux in $M \rightleftharpoons U$ or in $F \rightleftharpoons N$, thus

$$\begin{aligned}[M] &= K_M[U] \\ [N] &= K_N[F]\end{aligned} \tag{33}$$

Because

$$[M] + [U] + [UC] + [F] + [N] < P_0 \tag{34}$$

we have

$$\begin{aligned}P_0 &> (K_F^{-1} \max(1,\alpha)^{-1} + 1)[F] + [M] + [N] \quad (\because \text{Equation (31)}) \\ &= (K_F^{-1} \max(1,\alpha)^{-1} + 1)[F] + K_M[U] + K_N[F] \\ &> (K_F^{-1} \max(1,\alpha)^{-1} + 1)[F] + K_M \frac{k_{F \to U}}{k_{U \to F} + k_{a,U}[O]}[F] + k_N[F] \quad (\because \text{Equation (32)})\end{aligned} \tag{35}$$

Thus,

$$[F] < \left(K_M K_F^{-1}\left(1 + \frac{k_{a,U}[O]}{k_{U \to F}}\right)^{-1} + K_F^{-1}\max(1,\alpha)^{-1} + 1 + K_N\right)^{-1} P_0 \tag{36}$$

and plugging in Equation (33) yields the upper bound in Equation (51).

3. Results

3.1. Non-Equilibrium Folding Requires Kinetic Symmetry Breaking

I present a set of four symmetry conditions that, if all satisfied, forbids an ATP-driven chaperone from elevating the native concentration $[N]$ of its substrate above the chaperone-free equilibrium concentration $[N]_{eq}$. A chaperone must break at least one of these symmetry conditions to be able to convert chemical energy into non-equilibrium stabilization of the native structure of the substrate. As I discuss below, different chaperones break different symmetry conditions, corresponding to different mechanisms of non-equilibrium protein folding and activation. The symmetry conditions are as follows:

1. The ratio of association rate constants $k_{a,S'i}/k_{a,Si}$ does not depend on the chaperone state i for all pair of substrate conformations S and S' and for all open state i.
2. The dissociation rate constant $k_{d,Si}$ does not depend on the substrate conformation S, i.e.,
$$k_{d,Si} = k_{d,i} \tag{37}$$
for all open state i and for all conformation S.
3. The transition rates between chaperone states are independent of the conformation of the bound substrate, i.e., $k_{S,i \to j}$ does not depend on S for all pair (i, j).
4. For every closed state i of the chaperone, there is an open state j, such that the chaperone can reversibly transition between states j and i without consuming chemical energy.

In Section 2.1 of Materials and Methods, I prove that, if these four symmetry conditions are all satisfied, the ratio between the concentrations of the free substrate in any two conformations—say, S and S'—at the chaperone-mediated steady state is unchanged from that in the chaperone-free equilibrium, i.e., $[S']/[S] = [S']_{eq}/[S]_{eq}$, which implies $[N]/[M] = [N]_{eq}/[M]_{eq}$. Because chaperone-binding reduces the total concentration of the free substrate, the native concentration of the free substrate will be lower in the presence of chaperones than in the absence of chaperones, i.e., $g < 1$. (As noted in the Introduction, I only consider non-equilibrium folding to a free native protein.)

The above results regarding symmetry conditions hold for an arbitrary number of substrate conformations. For simplicity, I will assume only four representative conformations in the substrate, $\mathbb{S} = \{M \equiv \text{misfolded}, U \equiv \text{misfold-tending}, F \equiv \text{native-tending}, N \equiv \text{native}\}$, in the following discussion.

3.1.1. Requisites for Breaking the Binding and Unbinding Symmetries (Conditions 1 and 2)

The binding symmetry, Condition 1, is trivially satisfied if there is only one open chaperone state to which the substrate binds, or if the substrate binding rate does not depend on the chaperone state, i.e., $k_{a,Si} = k_{a,S}$. Note that the substrate in different conformations S may bind to the chaperone at different rates $k_{a,S}$, e.g., the substrate in an unfolded structure may bind to the chaperone faster than the substrate in a near-native structure, which is a common assumption in models of chaperone-mediated folding [34], but this conformation-selective binding alone does not permit non-equilibrium folding (defined by $g > 1$).

Condition 1 is approximately satisfied if the substrate in different conformations and the chaperone in different states bind using the same interface. In this case, the association rate constant is approximately
$$k_{a,Si} = p_S \times f_i \times k_a \tag{38}$$

where p_S is the probability that the binding surface on the substrate becomes accessible in conformation S, f_i is the probability that the binding surface on the chaperone is accessible in state i, and k_a is the intrinsic binding rate between the two binding surfaces once exposed (Equation (38) assumes that the conformational fluctuations exposing and occluding the binding surfaces are fast compared to the overall binding). The ratio
$$\frac{k_{a,S'i}}{k_{a,Si}} = \frac{p_{S'}}{p_S} \tag{39}$$

thus satisfies Condition 1.

Condition 1 is violated if the substrate binds to different binding surfaces on the chaperone depending on both the substrate conformation and the chaperone (open) state. This requires that the chaperone possesses multiple open states in which different binding surfaces are exposed. There has not been experimental demonstration of any ATP-driven chaperone breaking this symmetry condition.

The unbinding symmetry, Condition 2, is approximately satisfied if the chaperone binds to the substrate in different conformations using the same binding interface. The symmetry is broken if the substrate in different conformations form different protein–protein interactions with the chaperone.

In one limit of such binding interface change, the substrate in the misfold-tending conformation U with a slow dissociation rate $k_{d,U}$ may bind to the open chaperone and, after the chaperone closes, change to the native-tending conformation F in which its chaperone-binding surface is lost, so that, when the chaperone opens again after the ATP-driven cycle, the substrate unbinds rapidly with a fast dissociation rate $k_{d,F} \gg k_{d,U}$. This may happen in chaperones that can retain a substrate without a contact interface while allowing the bound substrate to change conformation from U to F. Hsp90 and GroEL/ES are two such examples: Hsp90 clamps its client kinase between its closed homo dimer with a central hole that may accommodate substantial conformational changes in the client [31,42], and GroEL/ES holds the substrate in its cavity, inside which the substrate may fold [43]. These two chaperones may break Condition 2 by this mechanism and thus perform non-equilibrium protein folding.

Cochaperones that simultaneously bind to the chaperone and to the misfold-tending, but not the native-tending, conformation of the substrate may help break Condition 2. When the substrate in the misfold-tending conformation is bound to the cochaperone, the substrate–cochaperone complex together has an extended chaperone-binding surface with contributions from both the substrate and the cochaperone, which decreases the substrate's dissociation rate from the chaperone. Binding to and unbinding from the cochaperone, a substrate in the misfold-tending conformation has, in effect, a slower dissociation rate than the substrate in the native-tending conformation. One case in point may be that of Cdc37-assisted kinase activation by Hsp90, as discussed in the following.

3.1.2. Cdc37 Enables Hsp90 to Differentiate between the Active-Tending and Inactive-Tending Conformations of a Client Kinase

Cdc37 is a cochaperone that specializes in assisting Hsp90 to activate client kinases [32,44,45]. Experimental evidence suggests that Cdc37 binds to a locally unfolded conformation of the client kinase [46], and that Cdc37 can simultaneously bind to a client kinase and Hsp90 [42,47,48]. Based on the cryo-EM structure of the Hsp90-kinase-Cdc37 complex [42] (Figure 2A), I have previously proposed a simple mechanism for Cdc37 to distinguish between the inactive-tending (U) and active-tending (F) kinase conformations, binding to the former with higher affinity than to the latter: in the inactive-tending conformation, the disordered DFG-loop of the kinase does not interfere with Cdc37 binding, whereas, in the active-tending conformation, the DFG-loop may be ordered into a configuration that results in steric clashes with Cdc37 [31] (Figure 2B,C). Thus, Cdc37 can help Hsp90 retain an inactive-tending client more than an active-tending client, and the effective rate of dissociation from Hsp90 is higher for a client in the active-tending conformation than for a client in the inactive-tending conformation (Figure 2D,E), breaking symmetry Condition 2.

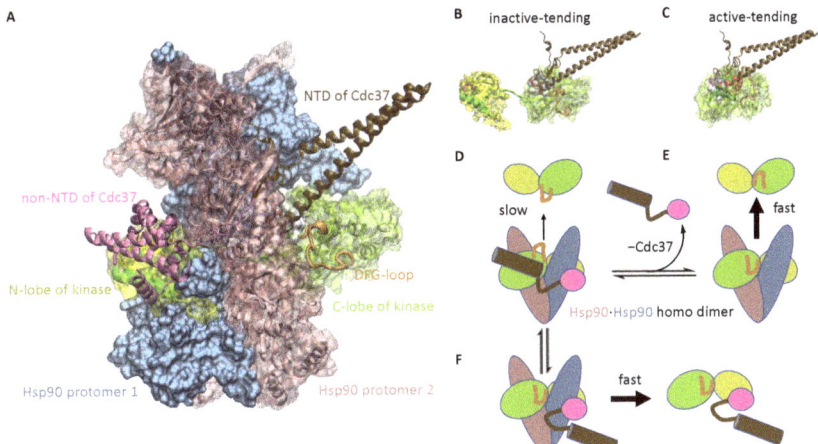

Figure 2. Cochaperone Cdc37 enables a client kinase in different conformations to unbind from Hsp90 at different rates. (**A**) the Hsp90-Cdk4-Cdc37 complex structure (PDB: 5FWM). The closed Hsp90 homo dimer clamps a partially unfolded Cdk4 kinase, and Cdc37 simultaneously binds to Cdk4 and Hsp90; (**B**) Cdc37 can bind to the kinase in the inactive-tending conformation; (**C**) steric clashes prevent Cdc37 from binding to the kinase in the active-tending conformation, due to its DFG-loop configuration and other conformational features; (**D**) Cdc37 helps to retain an inactive-tending kinase molecule inside the open Hsp90, resulting in slow unbinding of the kinase from the Hsp90. The bipartite interaction by NTD and CTD of Cdc37 with the kinase may result in the encirclement of a Hsp90 protomer by the Cdc37-kinase complex, preventing the latter from slipping off Hsp90. (**E**) Without Cdc37, an active-tending kinase molecule unbinds rapidly from the open Hsp90. (**F**) Alternatively, the loss of the interaction between the NTD of Cdc37 and the C-lobe of an active-tending kinase breaks the bipartite interaction between Cdc37 and the kinase, resulting in the release of the Cdc37-kinase complex from Hsp90.

This mechanism implies the following reaction path of Hsp90-mediated kinase activation:

$$U \xrightleftharpoons{+Cdc37} U \cdot Cdc37 \xrightleftharpoons{+Hsp90_{open}} Hsp90_{open} \cdot U \cdot Cdc37 \rightleftharpoons Hsp90_{closed} \cdot U \cdot Cdc37 \xrightleftharpoons{-Cdc37} Hsp90_{closed} \cdot U \rightleftharpoons Hsp90_{closed} \cdot F \xrightarrow{ATP \rightarrow ADP+Pi} Hsp90_{open} \cdot F \xrightleftharpoons{-Hsp90_{open}} F \quad (40)$$

Clearly, this mechanism requires that Cdc37 can dissociate from the Hsp90-kinase complex after Hsp90 closes. This requirement is indeed consistent with the observed structure of the Hsp90-kinase-Cdc37 complex: the closed Hsp90 clamps the client kinase between its N- and C-lobes to prevent the kinase from unbinding, but Cdc37 wraps around the exterior of Hsp90 so that it can disengage from the closed Hsp90 (Figure 2A).

Both the N-terminal domain (NTD) and the C-terminal domain (CTD) of Cdc37 bind to the partially unfolded kinase [49,50]. Individually, NTD and CTD bind to the kinase with low affinities [50] (on the order of 100 μM), but the bipartite interaction between the complete Cdc37 and the kinase results in sub-micromolar affinity. Based on the cryo-EM structure of the Hsp90-kinase-Cdc37 complex, the bipartite interaction may lead to the encirclement of a Hsp90 protomer by the kinase-Cdc37 binary complex, thus preventing the kinase from slipping off Hsp90 (Figure 2D). As discussed above, the NTD of Cdc37 may not bind to the active-tending conformation of the kinase. This not only substantially diminishes the affinity of Cdc37 to the kinase (CTD alone binds with over two-hundred-fold lower affinity), it also breaks the encirclement of the Hsp90 protomer by the Cdc37-kinase binary complex, potentially allowing the latter to dissociate rapidly from Hsp90 (Figure 2F), followed by the conversion of the kinase to the active conformation.

A puzzling observation is that Cdc37 binds to both the inactive B-Raf kinase and the active B-Raf mutant B-Raf^{V600E} (which has the valine at position 600 mutated to a glutamate) with similar affinities [51]: $K_D = 1.0$ µM for the wild-type B-Raf and $K_D = 0.4$ µM for the mutant B-Raf^{V600E} [50]. This can be explained by the above proposal that Cdc37 binds with high affinity to the inactive-tending conformation of the kinase but with comparatively negligible affinity to the other conformations. Consider the conformational equilibrium among the inactive (M), the inactive-tending (U), the active-tending (F), and the active (N) conformations:

$$M \underset{}{\overset{K_M^{-1}}{\rightleftharpoons}} U \underset{}{\overset{K_F}{\rightleftharpoons}} F \underset{}{\overset{K_N}{\rightleftharpoons}} N \tag{41}$$

If Cdc37 binds to the inactive-tending conformation U with a conformation-specific dissociation constant K_D^*, the apparent experimentally measured dissociation constant of Cdc37 binding to the kinase is

$$\begin{aligned} K_D &= \frac{[P][Cdc37]}{[U \cdot Cdc37]} \\ &= \frac{[P]}{[U]} \cdot \frac{[U][Cdc37]}{[U \cdot Cdc37]} \\ &= \frac{K_M K_F^{-1} + K_F^{-1} + 1 + K_N}{K_F^{-1}} \cdot K_D^* \end{aligned} \tag{42}$$

where P represents the kinase in any conformation.

The equilibrium active fraction, on the other hand, is

$$[N]_{eq}/P_0 = \frac{K_N}{K_M K_F^{-1} + K_F^{-1} + 1 + K_N} \tag{43}$$

Thus, it is possible for the wild-type and the mutant kinase to have very different active fractions $[N]_{eq}/P_0$ yet similar K_D's. For example, the hypothetical sets of equilibrium constants in Table 2 would be consistent with the observed Cdc37 affinities of the wild-type B-Raf and the V600E mutant and with the mechanistic hypothesis [52] that the mutation destabilizes the inactive and—less so—the inactive-tending conformation (thus decreasing K_M and increasing K_F).

Table 2. A hypothetical set of equilibrium constants that are consistent with the measured Cdc37 affinities of the wild-type B-raf and the V600E mutant. The dissociation constants are similar between the inactive wild-type and the active mutant.

	K_M	K_F	K_N	K_D^* (µM)	$[N]_{eq}/P_0$	K_D (µM)
wild-type	100	0.1	80	0.0092	0.07	1.0
V600E	10.24	0.4	80	0.0092	0.73	0.4

3.1.3. Cochaperone Hsp40 Enables Differential ATP Hydrolysis by Hsp70 Bound to a Substrate in Different Conformations

Hsp70-mediated protein folding is an example of breaking symmetry Condition 3. The Hsp70 chaperones, such as the bacterial DnaK, adopts an open conformation when its nucleotide binding domain (NBD) is occupied by ATP. Upon ATP hydrolysis, Hsp70 changes to a closed conformation [53,54] (Figure 3A). By itself, Hsp70 has a low basal ATP hydrolysis rate, but the J domain from the Hsp40 cochaperones—also known as J proteins—can stimulate Hsp70 and drastically increase its ATP hydrolysis rate [55,56].

Both Hsp40 and Hsp70 bind to exposed hydrophobic sites on a substrate protein [57,58] (Figure 3A–C). Consequently, a substrate with multiple exposed hydrophobic sites may simultaneously bind to an Hsp70 and an Hsp40. This induces the proximity between the chaperone and the cochaperone, resulting in accelerated ATP hydrolysis in Hsp70 and its transition to the closed state. Because a substrate in the misfold-tending conformation often exposes more hydrophobic sites than a substrate in the native-tending conformation [59], an Hsp70 bound to the former is more likely to be stimulated by a nearby Hsp40 bound to the same substrate molecule than an Hsp70 bound to the latter. By recruiting Hsp40 to accelerate the ATP hydrolysis in Hsp70, a substrate in the misfold-tending conformation induces a higher rate of transition by Hsp70 from the open state to the closed state than a substrate in the native-tending conformation, i.e., $k_{U,\text{open}\to\text{closed}} > k_{F,\text{open}\to\text{closed}}$, breaking symmetry Condition 3 (Figure 3D,E).

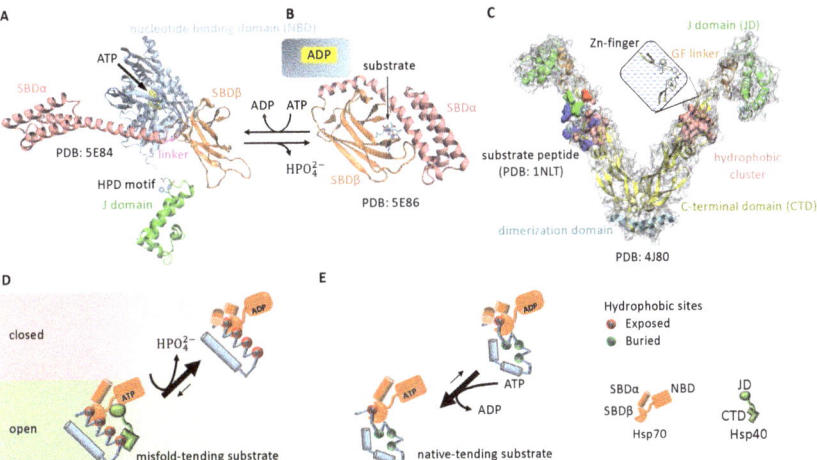

Figure 3. Cochaperone Hsp40 enables Hsp70 to change the balance between its open and closed states in response to the conformation of a bound substrate. (A) the ATP-bound, open state of Hsp70, which allows rapid binding and unbinding of the substrate; (B) the ADP-bound, closed state of Hsp70, with slow binding and unbinding of the substrate. SBD: substrate binding domain. (C) the structure of the Hsp40 cochaperone, including CTD that can bind to exposed hydrophobic sites on a substrate and the J domain that can stimulate the ATP hydrolysis of Hsp70. (D) An Hsp70 bound to a misfold-tending substrate molecule with many exposed hydrophobic sites is likely to be in proximity to an Hsp40 bound to the same substrate molecule, thus the Hsp70 will be stimulated in ATP hydrolysis, which drives the Hsp70 to its ADP-bound, closed state. (E) An Hsp70 bound to a native-tending substrate molecule with few exposed hydrophobic sites is unlikely to have a nearby Hsp40 and thus unlikely to be stimulated in ATP hydrolysis, and nucleotide exchange drives the Hsp70 toward its ATP-bound, open state.

As a result of this symmetry breaking, an Hsp70 bound to a substrate in the misfold-tending conformation is more likely to be closed than one bound to a substrate in the native-tending conformation. Thus, a substrate is on average more quickly released from the Hsp70 if it is in the native-tending conformation than if it is in the misfold-tending conformation. This difference biases the substrate toward the native conformation [30].

3.1.4. Hsp70 and Hsp90 Perform Non-Equilibrium Folding by Preferentially Releasing Substrate Proteins in Native-Tending Conformations

The cochaperone Cdc37 helps break symmetry Condition 2 in Hsp90-mediated kinase activation. The cochaperone Hsp40 helps break symmetry Condition 3 in Hsp70-mediated protein folding. Despite breaking different symmetries, Hsp70 and Hsp90 share the same kinetic consequence: both chaperones release a bound substrate in the native-tending (F) conformation faster than a bound substrate in the misfold-tending (U) conformation.

To see how this kinetic asymmetry promotes the native concentration, consider first a system in which the symmetry conditions are satisfied (Figure 4A). A substrate in the U conformation binds to the chaperone faster than a substrate in the F conformation. As a result, the reactive flux through the ATP-driven cycle of a chaperone bound to a substrate in the U conformation is higher than that through the cycle of a chaperone bound to a substrate in the F conformation. However, kinetic symmetry ensures that, at the steady state, the flux of U binding to the chaperone is the same as the flux of U unbinding from the chaperone; the same holds true for F binding to and unbinding from the chaperone, and there is no net flux between U and F. Under the symmetry conditions, there are two parallel, independent chaperone cycles with respective reactive fluxes:

$$J_{S+\text{Hsp}} = (S \to S \cdot \text{Hsp} \to S \cdot \{\text{states of Hsp} \cdots\} \to S \cdot \text{Hsp} \to S) \text{ for } S = U, F, \quad (44)$$

and

$$J_{U+\text{Hsp}} > J_{F+\text{Hsp}} \quad (45)$$

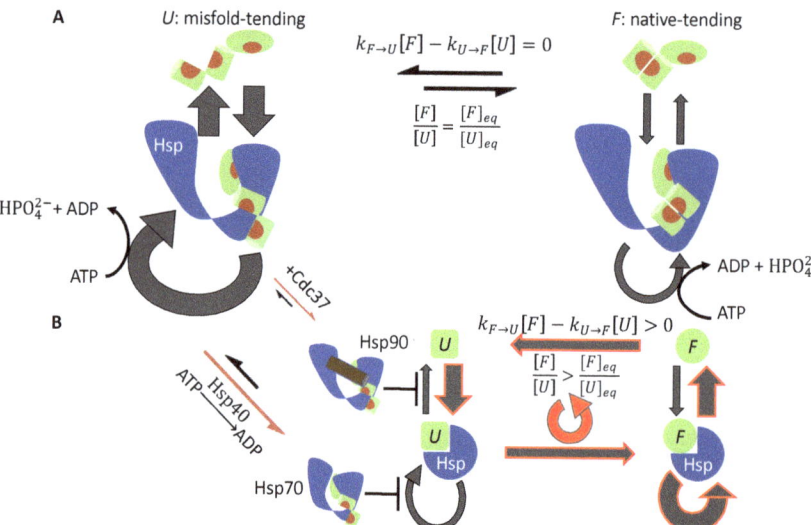

Figure 4. Reactive flux in chaperone-mediated non-equilibrium protein folding. (**A**) Under the symmetry conditions, there are two independent ATP-driven chaperone cycles: one with a higher reactive flux for a substrate in the misfold-tending (U) conformation (left) and one with a lower reactive flux for a substrate in the native-tending (F) conformation (right). There is no net flux between the substrate's two conformations, and the ratio $[F]/[U]$ is the same as its chaperone-free equilibrium value. (**B**) Cochaperones break the kinetic symmetry. The release of a substrate in the U conformation from the chaperone is inhibited: Cdc37 assists Hsp90 with retaining the substrate and Hsp40 stimulates ATP hydrolysis and closure of Hsp70. This restricts the reactive flux to release a substrate in the U conformation, forcing a partial diversion of the flux to the conformation conversion from $U \cdot \text{Hsp}$ to $F \cdot \text{Hsp}$ and resulting in a net reactive flux of $U \to U \cdot \text{Hsp} \to F \cdot \text{Hsp} \to F \to U$ (red cycle), which elevates the ratio $[F]/[U]$ above its chaperone-free equilibrium value.

However, there is no net flux between U and F:

$$J_{UF} = k_{U \to F}[U] - k_{F \to U}[F] = 0 \quad (46)$$

Thus, the ratio between F and U is unchanged from the chaperone-free equilibrium:

$$\frac{[F]}{[U]} = \frac{k_{U\to F}}{k_{F\to U}} = K_{UF} = \frac{[F]_{eq}}{[U]_{eq}} \qquad (47)$$

Symmetry breaking disrupts the independence between this pair of chaperone cycles. The release of a substrate in the U conformation from the chaperone is inhibited: in the case of Hsp90, Cdc37 helps the chaperone retain the bound client kinase; in the case of Hsp70, Hsp40-stimulated ATP hydrolysis and closure in Hsp70 diminish the reactive flux to re-open the chaperone (Figure 4B). This forces part of the reactive flux in $J_{U+\text{HSP}}$ after the binding of the substrate to be diverted into the reactive flux of conformation conversion in the bound substrate:

$$J_{U\cdot\text{Hsp}\to F\cdot\text{Hsp}} > 0 \qquad (48)$$

This in turn leads to a corresponding increase in the reactive flux of the chaperone's release of the substrate in the F conformation, which increases $[F]$ such that

$$\frac{[F]}{[U]} > \frac{[F]_{eq}}{[U]_{eq}} \qquad (49)$$

Thus, symmetry breaking biases the substrate toward the native-tending conformation and elevates the native concentration.

3.1.5. The Potential Role of Sequential Hydrolyses of Multiple ATPs in the Chaperone Cycle

Breaking symmetry Condition 4 permits a net reactive flux along the following path that promotes the native-tending conformation F over the misfold-tending conformation U:

$$U \xrightarrow{+\text{Hsp}_{\text{open}}} U\cdot\text{Hsp}_{\text{open|closed}} \xrightarrow{\text{ATP}\to\text{ADP}+P_i} U\cdot\text{Hsp}_{\text{closed}} \to F\cdot\text{Hsp}_{\text{closed}} \qquad (50)$$
$$\xrightarrow{\text{ATP}\to\text{ADP}+P_i} F\cdot\text{Hsp}_{\text{open}} \xrightarrow{-\text{Hsp}_{\text{open}}} F$$

A non-zero net flux of $U\cdot\text{Hsp}_{\text{closed}} \to F\cdot\text{Hsp}_{\text{closed}}$ does not violate thermodynamic cycle closure in this case because the reaction cycle in Equation (17) is no longer reversible—ATP hydrolysis occurs and chemical energy is consumed in that cycle—and thus Equations (18) and (19) no longer hold.

To break symmetry Condition 4, at least one closed state of the chaperone must be separated from all the open states by ATP hydrolysis. This requires at least two ATP to be hydrolyzed sequentially—not synchronously—per chaperone cycle, and the substrate has to change conformation between two ATP hydrolyses. Examples include Hsp90 that hydrolyzes two ATP molecules sequentially in its cycle [60] and the group II chaperonins in eukaryotes—such as TRiC/CCT—that hydrolyzes up to eight ATPs sequentially [61,62]. The role of such sequential ATP hydrolysis—and the consequent symmetry breaking of Condition 4—in non-equilibrium protein folding is an open question.

3.2. An Upper Bound of Non-Equilibrium Protein Folding and Its Implications

Having established the symmetry breaking requirements for non-equilibrium folding, I now derive an upper bound on the folding capacity of an ATP-driven chaperone. The key result is

$$[N] < \frac{K_N}{K_M K_F^{-1}\left(1 + \frac{k_{a,U}[O]}{k_{U\to F}}\right)^{-1} + K_F^{-1}\max(1,\alpha)^{-1} + 1 + K_N} P_0 \qquad (51)$$

where $[O]$ is the concentration of free chaperone in the open state, the equilibrium constants K_N, K_M, and K_F, the kinetic rate constants $k_{U\to F}$ and $k_{a,U}$, and their corresponding reactions are summarized in Table 1, and

$$\alpha \equiv \frac{k_{U\to F,C}}{k_{U\to F}} \qquad (52)$$

is an acceleration factor to indicate any potential rate change in conformation conversion when the substrate is bound to the closed chaperone. The proof of Equation (51) is given in Section 2.2 of Methods and Materials.

Equation (51) gives a general upper bound applicable to any ATP-driven chaperone. The folding capacity of a specific type of chaperone needs to be calculated by detailed models [30,31], but it cannot exceed that given by Equation (51). This result allows an analysis of the common key factors in non-equilibrium folding without considering the mechanistic details of specific chaperones.

Introducing a combined equilibrium constant for the reaction $U \overset{\tilde{K}_F}{\rightleftharpoons} (F+N)$

$$\tilde{K}_F \equiv \frac{[F]_{eq} + [N]_{eq}}{[U]_{eq}} = (1+K_N)K_F \tag{53}$$

The upper bound in Equation (51) can be written as

$$[N] < \frac{1}{K_M \tilde{K}_F^{-1}\left(1+\frac{k_{a,U}[O]}{k_{U\to F}}\right)^{-1} + \tilde{K}_F^{-1}\max(1,\alpha)^{-1}+1} \cdot \frac{K_N}{1+K_N} P_0 \tag{54}$$

Compare this to the native concentration in the chaperone-free equilibrium

$$\begin{aligned}
[N]_{eq} &= \frac{K_N}{K_M K_F^{-1} + K_F^{-1} + 1 + K_N} P_0 \\
&= \frac{1}{K_M \tilde{K}_F^{-1} + \tilde{K}_F^{-1} + 1} \cdot \frac{K_N}{1+K_N} P_0
\end{aligned} \tag{55}$$

The non-equilibrium gain factor is thus bounded by

$$g = \frac{[N]}{[N]_{eq}} < \frac{K_M \tilde{K}_F^{-1} + \tilde{K}_F^{-1} + 1}{K_M \tilde{K}_F^{-1}\left(1+\frac{k_{a,U}[O]}{k_{U\to F}}\right)^{-1} + \tilde{K}_F^{-1}\max(1,\alpha)^{-1}+1} \tag{56}$$

3.2.1. Chaperones Bind to Unstable Intermediate Conformations of Substrates to Drive Non-Equilibrium Folding

An implication of Equation (56) is that ATP-driven chaperones must bind to an intermediate unfolded conformation (U) of the substrate, not to the misfolded conformation (M) itself, to perform non-equilibrium folding, unless the conformation conversion of a substrate is accelerated when bound to the chaperone (i.e., $k_{U\to F,C} > k_{U\to F}$ hence $\alpha > 1$). This can be demonstrated by contradiction. If the substrate does not have an intermediate misfold-tending conformation and the chaperone directly binds to the misfolded conformation, i.e., M and U are the same, Equation (51) reduces to (by setting $K_M = 0$)

$$[N] < \left(\tilde{K}_F^{-1}\max(1,\alpha)^{-1}+1\right)^{-1} \cdot \frac{K_N}{1+K_N} P_0 \tag{57}$$

and the upper bound of the non-equilibrium gain factor becomes

$$g < \frac{\tilde{K}_F^{-1}+1}{\tilde{K}_F^{-1}\max(1,\alpha)^{-1}+1} \tag{58}$$

In the absence of a mechanism for the substrate to accelerate its conformation conversion when it is bound to the chaperone ($\alpha \leq 1$), $g \leq 1$, the chaperone cannot elevate the native concentration.

To my knowledge, accelerated folding of protein substrates when bound to a chaperone has only been reported for the GroEL/GroES chaperonins [43,63–67]. In general, steric hindrance from the chaperone is more likely to impede rather than to accelerate conformation conversions in a bound substrate; this impedance was observed for the rhodanese protein trapped in GroEL/GroES by a single-molecule experiment [68]. For Hsp90 and Hsp70, there has not been any experimental demonstration that a substrate exhibits faster conformation conversions when bound to the chaperone than when free in the solution. This suggests that chaperones, with the potential exceptions of chaperonins, must bind to intermediate unfolded conformations of the substrate proteins to drive non-equilibrium protein folding.

Assuming $\alpha \leq 1$, the upper bound on the non-equilibrium gain factor becomes

$$g < g_{max} = \frac{K_M(\tilde{K}_F+1)^{-1}+1}{K_M(\tilde{K}_F+1)^{-1}\left(1+\frac{k_{a,U}[O]}{k_{U\to F}}\right)^{-1}+1} \tag{59}$$

For the gain factor to substantially exceed 1, the following must be true:

$$K_M(\tilde{K}_F+1)^{-1} \gg 1 \implies K_M \gg 1 \tag{60}$$

Equation (60) implies that the intermediate conformation U to which the chaperone binds must be intrinsically unstable, and it will predominantly convert to the misfolded conformation M in the absence of the chaperone. This result is intuitive: if the chaperone binds to a dominant conformation of the substrate, it will trap a substantial fraction of the substrate and hinder its folding to the native structure. As a result, the chaperone will be unable to elevate the native concentration. The difficulty to observe the chaperone-binding conformations in biophysical experiments [69] attests to their transiency.

3.2.2. Chaperones Stabilize the Native Structures of Slow-Folding Proteins

Non-equilibrium folding also requires, as implied by Equation (59) and $g \gg 1$,

$$\frac{k_{a,U}[O]}{k_{U\to F}} \gg 1 \iff k_{U\to F} \ll k_{a,U}[O] \tag{61}$$

Taken together, Equations (60) and (61) suggest that chaperones stabilize the native structures of slow-folding proteins. Assuming the binding rate constant to be on the order of $k_{a,U} \sim 10^6$ /M/s, the spontaneous (i.e., without chaperones) refolding rate of the protein, which is approximately $K_M^{-1}k_{U\to F}$, should be much slower than 1 /s to admit effective non-equilibrium folding by chaperones at a concentration of $[O] \sim 1$ µM.

3.2.3. ATP-Driven Chaperones Buffer Destabilizing Mutations

About 18% of protein molecules in the cell harbor at least one missense mutation due to errors in translation [70]. In addition, proteins incur mutations due to germline and somatic gene polymorphism [71]. Given that about 30–40% of random substitutions disrupt protein functions [72,73], most probably by loss-of-folding [74,75], it is likely that many cellular protein molecules have compromised thermal stability and the native structures of some will not be the free energy minima. ATP-driven chaperones may buffer such destabilizing mutations [76,77] and maintain the native concentrations of these proteins by non-equilibrium folding [30].

The missense mutations may alter one or more of the transition rates and the equilibrium constants in protein folding dynamics: e.g., it may decrease the thermal stability of the protein by increasing K_M, decreasing $k_{U\to F}$ or increasing $k_{F\to U}$ (hence decreasing $K_F = k_{U\to F}/k_{F\to U}$), or decreasing K_N. Assuming $\alpha \leq 1$ as discussed above, the maximum native concentration mediated by a chaperone is

$$\begin{aligned}[N]_{max} &= g_{max}[N]_{eq} \\ &= \frac{1}{K_M(\tilde{K}_F+1)^{-1}\left(1+\frac{k_a[O]}{k_{U\to F}}\right)^{-1}+1} \frac{1}{1+\tilde{K}_F^{-1}} \frac{K_N}{1+K_N} P_0\end{aligned} \tag{62}$$

Equation (62) suggests that the capacity of ATP-driven chaperones to buffer a destabilizing mutation depends on both the wild-type substrate's folding kinetics and how the mutation alters the kinetic parameters (Figure 5). For instance, chaperones may be more effective in buffering mutations that slow down the transition from the misfold-tending conformation (U) to the native-tending conformation (F)—i.e., decreasing $k_{U \to F}$ by e.g., stabilizing the U conformation—than mutations that destabilize the native state by decreasing K_N. Such differential buffering may play a role in selecting tolerated genetic variations and shaping their consequences in human disease [78].

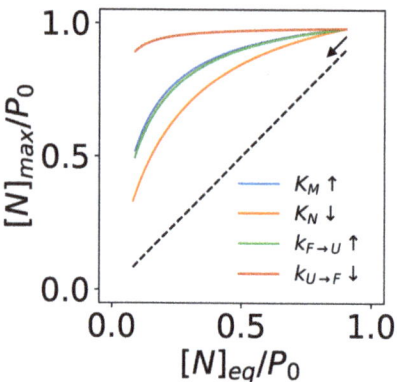

Figure 5. The capacity of ATP-driven chaperones to maintain elevated native fractions in response to destabilizing mutations in a protein substrate. The kinetic parameters of the wild-type protein are $K_M = 10^2$, $K_F = 10$, $K_N = 10^2$, $k_{U \to F} = 0.1\ \text{s}^{-1}$, and $k_a = 10^6\ \text{M}^{-1} \cdot \text{s}^{-1}$; the concentration of the open chaperone is set to $[O] = 1\ \mu\text{M}$.

4. Discussion

Breaking the symmetry Conditions 1–4 is necessary but on its own is insufficient for non-equilibrium folding. $g > 1$ often requires both substantial deviation from the symmetry conditions and other enabling kinetic conditions, as exemplified by Equation (56). Detailed mechanistic models [30,31] are needed to quantitatively predict the extent of non-equilibrium folding. Nonetheless, these symmetry conditions can help assess whether a proposed mechanism of chaperone function will imply non-equilibrium folding.

Unlike equilibrium protein folding, the native yield of non-equilibrium protein folding depends not only on the equilibrium constants but also on the kinetic parameters of the folding reactions and the chaperone cycle. The native concentration of a substrate may change in response to the modulation of the step-wise kinetics of the chaperone cycle [30,31,79] by cochaperones [80], by mutations [81,82] and post-translational modifications [83,84] in the chaperones, and by pharmacological molecules [85]. Such modulations may be used by the cell to regulate proteostasis. They may also offer therapeutic opportunities.

Given both the theoretical models and the experimental evidence suggesting that ATP-driven chaperones can stabilize the native or active structures of substrate proteins out of the thermal equilibrium, Anfinsen's hypothesis does not *need* to be true for protein folding in cells. ATP-driven chaperones may not only kinetically accelerate the folding of proteins to thermodynamically stable native structures, but also actively fold some proteins to native structures that are thermodynamically unstable.

Most proteins have evolved to be marginally stable [86,87]. If ATP-driven chaperones can indeed buffer destabilizing mutations and maintain the native structures and functions of unstable mutants, as discussed in Section 3.2.3, it is then plausible that the native structures of some proteins may have become thermodynamically unstable as a consequence of this chaperone-buffered evolution. They may not stay folded on their own, but depend on the energy-consuming chaperones to maintain their native structures.

How many proteins in a cell take exception to Anfinsen's hypothesis and depend on non-equilibrium folding by a particular ATP-driven chaperone? Emerging proteomics techniques may help answer this question. For example, cell lysates may be subject to proteolytic digestion [88] and the resulting products analyzed by mass spectrometry (MS), identifying proteins with permissible digestion sites, which approximately reflect their state of folding [89]. This proteolysis-MS assay may be repeated for lysates incubated with chaperone inhibitors [90,91] or chaperone agonists [85]. Proteins more susceptible to proteolysis in the presence of chaperone inhibitors—and less susceptible in the presence of chaperone agonists—are candidates that may depend on the chaperone for non-equilibrium folding to their native structures. The lysates should be incubated in the presence of protein synthesis inhibitors so that the analysis can isolate the chaperone's effects on *maintaining* the native structures of its substrates from its effects on the folding of their nascent chains; the former demonstrates non-equilibrium stabilization of thermodynamically unfavorable native structures while the latter may be attributable to kinetic acceleration of protein folding. This analysis may be more applicable to GroEL/GroES and Hsp70 than to Hsp90 because the latter mediates the late-stage folding and activation of its substrates [33,92], which may not be associated with significant changes in the protein disorder detectable by the proteolysis-MS assay.

Implications for Protein Native Structures and Their Folding Pathways

My model of non-equilibrium protein folding and activation suggests the tantalizing possibility that ATP-driven chaperones may play a role in shaping the native structures of some proteins. Consistent with a previous experimental demonstration that chaperones alter the folding pathway of a substrate protein [93], my model implies that an ATP-driven chaperone may bias a substrate protein to fold along pathways that expose few cochaperone binding sites during folding, with consequences for the resulting structures.

Consider two conformations M and N of a substrate protein, where M is the free energy minimum but associated with a folding pathway inhibited by the chaperone, and N has a higher free energy but can be reached through a folding pathway uninhibited by the chaperone (Figure 6). The protein will fold into its free energy minimum conformation M in the absence of the chaperone, but, if the chaperone-induced pathway bias is sufficiently strong, it will fold into the alternative conformation N in the presence of the chaperone. Note that M can be an ensemble of rapidly inter-converting conformations, such as in intrinsically disordered proteins (IDP) or intrinsically disordered protein regions [94–98]. Can ATP-driven chaperones fold some IDPs into well-ordered structures?

It has been proposed that some proteins may fold into native structures that are more kinetically accessible than conformations of the lowest free energy [99]. Indeed, experimental observations have been reported that synonymous codon substitutions result in conformational changes in the translated proteins, due to kinetic changes in the co-translational folding of the nascent chain on the ribosome [100–103]. These results are consistent with the idea that the native structures of some proteins may be determined by kinetics rather than thermodynamics. One implication is that the solution to the structure prediction problem for such proteins in cell may depend on the solution to the protein folding problem, and in-cell protein folding may be an active, energy-dependent process [104]. Predicting the cellular conformation of these proteins—in the presence of ATP-driven chaperones—may require the search for folding pathways that limit the exposures of cochaperone-binding, e.g., hydrophobic, sites.

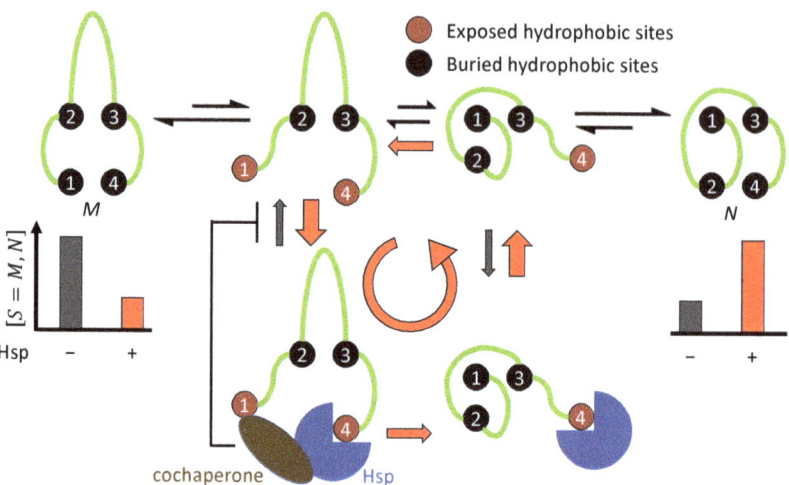

Figure 6. An ATP-driven chaperone (Hsp) may favor the protein folding pathway that exposes few cochaperone binding sites and drive the protein to a different conformation (N) than its most stable conformation (M) in the absence of the chaperone.

5. Conclusions

In this work, I have proposed a theoretical framework to analyze non-equilibrium protein folding by ATP-driven chaperones. The symmetry breaking conditions may help determine whether a chaperone—by a proposed mechanism of action—can convert the energy from ATP hydrolysis to the out-of-equilibrium stabilization of the native structures of its substrate proteins. I have discussed how Hsp70 and Hsp90 may have broken different symmetries and how the symmetry breaking enables them to perform non-equilibrium protein folding and activation. My models predict that some proteins may fold to native structures that do not correspond to the free energy minima, and that their native structures may be shaped by the chaperone-mediated folding pathways. These predictions may be tested by experiments, some of which I have suggested above.

Funding: This research received no external funding.

Data Availability Statement: Not applicable.

Conflicts of Interest: The author declares no conflict of interest.

Abbreviations

The following abbreviations are used in this manuscript:

Hsp40	Heat shock protein 40
Hsp70	Heat shock protein 70
Hsp90	Heat shock protein 90
Cdc37	Cell division cycle 37
cryo-EM	Cryogenic electron microscopy
PDB	Protein data bank

References

1. Anfinsen, C.B. Principles that Govern the Folding of Protein Chains. *Science* **1973**, *181*, 223–230. [CrossRef]
2. Dill, K.A. Dominant forces in protein folding. *Biochemistry* **1990**, *29*, 7133–7155. [CrossRef]
3. Bukau, B.; Weissman, J.; Horwich, A. Molecular Chaperones and Protein Quality Control. *Cell* **2006**, *125*, 443–451. [CrossRef]
4. Hartl, F.U.; Bracher, A.; Hayer-Hartl, M. Molecular chaperones in protein folding and proteostasis. *Nature* **2011**, *475*, 324–332. [CrossRef]

5. Balchin, D.; Hayer-Hartl, M.; Hartl, U.F. In vivo aspects of protein folding and quality control. *Science* **2016**, *353*, aac4354. [CrossRef]
6. Thirumalai, D.; Lorimer, G.H. Chaperonin-Mediated Protein Folding. *Annu. Rev. Biophys. Biomol. Struct.* **2001**, *30*, 245–269. [CrossRef]
7. Lin, Z.; Rye, H.S. GroEL-Mediated Protein Folding: Making the Impossible, Possible. *Crit. Rev. Biochem. Mol. Biol.* **2008**, *41*, 211–239. [CrossRef]
8. Horwich, A.L.; Fenton, W.A. Chaperonin-mediated protein folding: Using a central cavity to kinetically assist polypeptide chain folding. *Q. Rev. Biophys.* **2009**, *42*. [CrossRef]
9. Mayer, M.P. Hsp70 chaperone dynamics and molecular mechanism. *Trends Biochem. Sci.* **2013**, *38*, 507–514. doi: 10.1016/j.tibs.2013.08.001. [CrossRef]
10. Mayer, M.P.; Gierasch, L.M. Recent advances in the structural and mechanistic aspects of Hsp70 molecular chaperones. *J. Biol. Chem.* **2019**, *294*, 2085–2097. [CrossRef]
11. Pearl, L.H.; Prodromou, C. Structure and Mechanism of the Hsp90 Molecular Chaperone Machinery. *Annu. Rev. Biochem.* **2006**, *75*, 271–294. [CrossRef]
12. Pearl, L.H. Review: The HSP90 molecular chaperone—An enigmatic ATPase. *Biopolymers* **2016**, *105*, 594–607. doi: 10.1002/bip.22835. [CrossRef]
13. Radli, M.; Rüdiger, S.G. Dancing with the Diva: Hsp90-Client Interactions. *J. Mol. Biol.* **2018**, *430*, 3029–3040. [CrossRef]
14. Schopf, F.H.; Biebl, M.M.; Buchner, J. The HSP90 chaperone machinery. *Nat. Rev. Mol. Cell Biol.* **2017**, *18*, 345–360. [CrossRef]
15. Chiosis, G.; Dickey, C.A.; Johnson, J.L. A global view of Hsp90 functions. *Nat. Struct. Mol. Biol.* **2013**, *20*, 1–4. [CrossRef]
16. Taipale, M.; Jarosz, D.F.; Lindquist, S. HSP90 at the hub of protein homeostasis: Emerging mechanistic insights. *Nat. Rev. Mol. Cell Biol.* **2010**, *11*, 515–528. [CrossRef]
17. Prodromou, C.; Bjorklund, D.M. Advances towards Understanding the Mechanism of Action of the Hsp90 Complex. *Biomolecules* **2022**, *12*, 600. [CrossRef]
18. Ranson, N.A.; Farr, G.W.; Roseman, A.M.; Gowen, B.; Fenton, W.A.; Horwich, A.L.; Saibil, H.R. ATP-Bound States of GroEL Captured by Cryo-Electron Microscopy. *Cell* **2001**, *107*, 869–879. [CrossRef]
19. Krukenberg, K.A.; Street, T.O.; Lavery, L.A.; Agard, D.A. Conformational dynamics of the molecular chaperone Hsp90. *Q. Rev. Biophys.* **2011**, *44*, 229–255. [CrossRef]
20. Clare, D.K.; Vasishtan, D.; Stagg, S.; Quispe, J.; Farr, G.W.; Topf, M.; Horwich, A.L.; Saibil, H.R. ATP-Triggered Conformational Changes Delineate Substrate-Binding and -Folding Mechanics of the GroEL Chaperonin. *Cell* **2012**, *149*, 113–123. [CrossRef]
21. Kityk, R.; Vogel, M.; Schlecht, R.; Bukau, B.; Mayer, M.P. Pathways of allosteric regulation in Hsp70 chaperones. *Nat. Commun.* **2015**, *6*, 8308. [CrossRef]
22. Alderson, T.; Kim, J.; Markley, J. Dynamical Structures of Hsp70 and Hsp70-Hsp40 Complexes. *Structure* **2016**, *24*, 1014–1030. [CrossRef]
23. Weissman, J.S.; Kashi, Y.; Fenton, W.A.; Horwich, A.L. GroEL-mediated protein folding proceeds by multiple rounds of binding and release of nonnative forms. *Cell* **1994**, *78*, 693–702. [CrossRef]
24. Szabo, A.; Langer, T.; Schröder, H.; Flanagan, J.; Bukau, B.; Hartl, F.U. The ATP hydrolysis-dependent reaction cycle of the Escherichia coli Hsp70 system DnaK, DnaJ, and GrpE. *Proc. Natl. Acad. Sci. USA* **1994**, *91*, 10345–10349. [CrossRef]
25. Doyle, S.M.; Genest, O.; Wickner, S. Protein rescue from aggregates by powerful molecular chaperone machines. *Nat. Rev. Mol. Cell Biol.* **2013**, *14*, 617–629. [CrossRef]
26. Imamoglu, R.; Balchin, D.; Hayer-Hartl, M.; Hartl, F.U. Bacterial Hsp70 resolves misfolded states and accelerates productive folding of a multi-domain protein. *Nat. Commun.* **2020**, *11*. [CrossRef]
27. Rios, P.D.L.; Goloubinoff, P. Hsp70 chaperones use ATP to remodel native protein oligomers and stable aggregates by entropic pulling. *Nat. Struct. Mol. Biol.* **2016**, *23*, 766–769. [CrossRef]
28. Chakrabarti, S.; Hyeon, C.; Ye, X.; Lorimer, G.H.; Thirumalai, D. Molecular chaperones maximize the native state yield on biological times by driving substrates out of equilibrium. *Proc. Natl. Acad. Sci. USA* **2017**, *114*, E10919–E10927. [CrossRef]
29. Goloubinoff, P.; Sassi, A.S.; Fauvet, B.; Barducci, A.; Rios, P. Chaperones convert the energy from ATP into the nonequilibrium stabilization of native proteins. *Nat. Chem. Biol.* **2018**, *14*. [CrossRef]
30. Xu, H. Cochaperones enable Hsp70 to use ATP energy to stabilize native proteins out of the folding equilibrium. *Sci. Rep.* **2018**, *8*, 13213. [CrossRef]
31. Xu, H. ATP-driven Non-equilibrium Activation of Kinase Clients by the Molecular Chaperone Hsp90. *Biophys. J.* **2020**, *119*, 1538–1549. [CrossRef]
32. Verba, K.A.; Agard, D.A. How Hsp90 and Cdc37 Lubricate Kinase Molecular Switches. *Trends Biochem. Sci.* **2017**, *42*, 799–811. [CrossRef]
33. Kirschke, E.; Goswami, D.; Southworth, D.; Griffin, P.; Agard, D. Glucocorticoid Receptor Function Regulated by Coordinated Action of the Hsp90 and Hsp70 Chaperone Cycles. *Cell* **2014**, *157*, 1685–1697. [CrossRef]
34. Todd, M.J.; Lorimer, G.H.; Thirumalai, D. Chaperonin-facilitated protein folding: Optimization of rate and yield by an iterative annealing mechanism. *Proc. Natl. Acad. Sci. USA* **1996**, *93*, 4030–4035. [CrossRef]
35. Hu, B.; Mayer, M.P.; Tomita, M. Modeling Hsp70-Mediated Protein Folding. *Biophys. J.* **2006**, *91*, 496–507. doi: 10.1529/biophysj.106.083394. [CrossRef]

36. Rios, P.D.L.; Barducci, A. Hsp70 chaperones are non-equilibrium machines that achieve ultra-affinity by energy consumption. *eLife* **2014**, *3*, e02218. [CrossRef]
37. Sharma, S.K.; Rios, P.; Christen, P.; Lustig, A.; Goloubinoff, P. The kinetic parameters and energy cost of the Hsp70 chaperone as a polypeptide unfoldase. *Nat. Chem. Biol.* **2010**, *6*, 914–920. [CrossRef]
38. Burston, S.G.; Weissman, J.S.; Farr, G.W.; Fenton, W.A.; Norwich, A.L. Release of both native and non-native proteins from a cis-only GroEL ternary complex. *Nature* **1996**, *383*, 96–99. [CrossRef]
39. Astumian, D.R. Microscopic reversibility as the organizing principle of molecular machines. *Nat. Nanotechnol.* **2012**, *7*, nnano.2012.188. [CrossRef]
40. Sekhar, A.; Velyvis, A.; Zoltsman, G.; Rosenzweig, R.; Bouvignies, G.; Kay, L.E. Conserved conformational selection mechanism of Hsp70 chaperone-substrate interactions. *eLife* **2018**, *7*, e32764. [CrossRef]
41. Park, S.J.; Borin, B.N.; Martinez-Yamout, M.A.; Dyson, H.J. The client protein p53 adopts a molten globule–like state in the presence of Hsp90. *Nat. Struct. Mol. Biol.* **2011**, *18*, 537–541. [CrossRef]
42. Verba, K.A.; Wang, R.Y.R.; Arakawa, A.; Liu, Y.; Shirouzu, M.; Yokoyama, S.; Agard, D.A. Atomic structure of Hsp90-Cdc37-Cdk4 reveals that Hsp90 traps and stabilizes an unfolded kinase. *Science* **2016**, *352*, 1542–1547. [CrossRef] [PubMed]
43. Hayer-Hartl, M.; Bracher, A.; Hartl, F.U. The GroEL–GroES Chaperonin Machine: A Nano-Cage for Protein Folding. *Trends Biochem. Sci.* **2016**, *41*, 62–76. [CrossRef]
44. Siligardi, G.; Panaretou, B.; Meyer, P.; Singh, S.; Woolfson, D.N.; Piper, P.W.; Pearl, L.H.; Prodromou, C. Regulation of Hsp90 ATPase activity by the co-chaperone Cdc37p/p50cdc37. *J. Biol. Chem.* **2002**, *277*, 20151–20159. [CrossRef]
45. Caplan, A.J.; Mandal, A.K.; Theodoraki, M.A. Molecular chaperones and protein kinase quality control. *Trends Cell Biol.* **2007**, *17*, 87–92. [CrossRef]
46. Keramisanou, D.; Aboalroub, A.; Zhang, Z.; Liu, W.; Marshall, D.; Diviney, A.; Larsen, R.; Landgraf, R.; Gelis, I. Molecular Mechanism of Protein Kinase Recognition and Sorting by the Hsp90 Kinome-Specific Cochaperone Cdc37. *Mol. Cell* **2016**, *62*, 260–271. [CrossRef]
47. Sreeramulu, S.; Jonker, H.R.; Langer, T.; Richter, C.; Lancaster, R.C.; Schwalbe, H. The Human Cdc37·Hsp90 Complex Studied by Heteronuclear NMR Spectroscopy. *J. Biol. Chem.* **2009**, *284*, 3885–3896. [CrossRef]
48. Eckl, J.M.; Scherr, M.J.; Freiburger, L.; Daake, M.A.; Sattler, M.; Richter, K. Hsp90·Cdc37 Complexes with Protein Kinases Form Cooperatively with Multiple Distinct Interaction Sites. *J. Biol. Chem.* **2015**, *290*, 30843–30854. [CrossRef]
49. Keramisanou, D.; Kumar, M.V.; Boose, N.; Abzalimov, R.R.; Gelis, I. Assembly mechanism of early Hsp90-Cdc37-kinase complexes. *Sci. Adv.* **2022**, *8*, eabm9294. [CrossRef]
50. Bjorklund, D.M.; Morgan, R.M.L.; Oberoi, J.; Day, K.L.I.M.; Galliou, P.A.; Prodromou, C. Recognition of BRAF by CDC37 and Reevaluation of the Activation mechanism for the Class 2 BRAF-L597R mutant. *bioRxiv* **2022**. [CrossRef]
51. Polier, S.; Samant, R.S.; Clarke, P.A.; Workman, P.; Prodromou, C.; Pearl, L.H. ATP-competitive inhibitors block protein kinase recruitment to the Hsp90-Cdc37 system. *Nat. Chem. Biol.* **2013**, *9*, 307–312. [CrossRef] [PubMed]
52. Kiel, C.; Benisty, H.; Lloréns-Rico, V.; Serrano, L. The yin–yang of kinase activation and unfolding explains the peculiarity of Val600 in the activation segment of BRAF. *eLife* **2016**, *5*, e12814. [CrossRef] [PubMed]
53. Mayer, M.P.; Schröder, H.; Rüdiger, S.; Paal, K.; Laufen, T.; Bukau, B. Multistep mechanism of substrate binding determines chaperone activity of Hsp70. *Nat. Struct. Mol. Biol.* **2000**, *7*, 586–593. [CrossRef]
54. Yang, J.; Nune, M.; Zong, Y.; Zhou, L.; Liu, Q. Close and Allosteric Opening of the Polypeptide-Binding Site in a Human Hsp70 Chaperone BiP. *Structure* **2015**, *23*, 2191–2203. [CrossRef] [PubMed]
55. Laufen, T.; Mayer, M.P.; Beisel, C.; Klostermeier, D.; Mogk, A.; Reinstein, J.; Bukau, B. Mechanism of regulation of Hsp70 chaperones by DnaJ cochaperones. *Proc. Natl. Acad. Sci. USA* **1999**, *96*, 5452–5457. [CrossRef] [PubMed]
56. Wittung-Stafshede, P.; Guidry, J.; Horne, B.E.; Landry, S.J. The J-Domain of Hsp40 Couples ATP Hydrolysis to Substrate Capture in Hsp70. *Biochemistry* **2003**, *42*, 4937–4944. [CrossRef]
57. Rüdiger, S.; Schneider-Mergener, J.; Bukau, B. Its substrate specificity characterizes the DnaJ co-chaperone as a scanning factor for the DnaK chaperone. *EMBO J.* **2001**, *20*, 1042–1050. [CrossRef]
58. Perales-Calvo, J.; Muga, A.; Moro, F. Role of DnaJ G/F-rich Domain in Conformational Recognition and Binding of Protein Substrates. *J. Biol. Chem.* **2010**, *285*, 34231–34239. [CrossRef]
59. Herbst, R.; Schäfer, U.; Seckler, R. Equilibrium Intermediates in the Reversible Unfolding of Firefly (Photinus pyralis) Luciferase. *J. Biol. Chem.* **1997**, *272*, 7099–7105. [CrossRef]
60. Elnatan, D.; Betegon, M.; Liu, Y.; Ramelot, T.; Kennedy, M.A.; Agard, D.A. Symmetry broken and rebroken during the ATP hydrolysis cycle of the mitochondrial Hsp90 TRAP1. *eLife* **2017**, *6*, e25235. [CrossRef]
61. Lopez, T.; Dalton, K.; Frydman, J. The Mechanism and Function of Group II Chaperonins. *J. Mol. Biol.* **2015**, *427*, 2919–2930. [CrossRef] [PubMed]
62. Gestaut, D.; Limatola, A.; Joachimiak, L.; Frydman, J. The ATP-powered gymnastics of TRiC/CCT: An asymmetric protein folding machine with a symmetric origin story. *Curr. Opin. Struct. Biol.* **2019**, *55*, 50–58. [CrossRef] [PubMed]
63. Chakraborty, K.; Chatila, M.; Sinha, J.; Shi, Q.; Poschner, B.C.; Sikor, M.; Jiang, G.; Lamb, D.C.; Hartl, F.U.; Hayer-Hartl, M. Chaperonin-Catalyzed Rescue of Kinetically Trapped States in Protein Folding. *Cell* **2010**, *142*, 112–122. [CrossRef] [PubMed]
64. Tang, Y.C.; Chang, H.C.; Roeben, A.; Wischnewski, D.; Wischnewski, N.; Kerner, M.J.; Hartl, F.U.; Hayer-Hartl, M. Structural Features of the GroEL-GroES Nano-Cage Required for Rapid Folding of Encapsulated Protein. *Cell* **2006**, *125*, 903–914. [CrossRef]

65. Gupta, A.J.; Haldar, S.; Miličić, G.; Hartl, F.U.; Hayer-Hartl, M. Active Cage Mechanism of Chaperonin-Assisted Protein Folding Demonstrated at Single-Molecule Level. *J. Mol. Biol.* **2014**, *426*, 2739–2754. [CrossRef]
66. Baumketner, A.; Jewett, A.; Shea, J. Effects of Confinement in Chaperonin Assisted Protein Folding: Rate Enhancement by Decreasing the Roughness of the Folding Energy Landscape. *J. Mol. Biol.* **2003**, *332*, 701–713. [CrossRef]
67. England, J.L.; Lucent, D.; Pande, V.S. A Role for Confined Water in Chaperonin Function. *J. Am. Chem. Soc.* **2008**, *130*, 11838–11839. [CrossRef]
68. Hofmann, H.; Hillger, F.; Pfeil, S.H.; Hoffmann, A.; Streich, D.; Haenni, D.; Nettels, D.; Lipman, E.A.; Schuler, B. Single-molecule spectroscopy of protein folding in a chaperonin cage. *Proc. Natl. Acad. Sci. USA* **2010**, *107*, 11793–11798. [CrossRef]
69. Rüdiger, S.; Freund, S.M.; Veprintsev, D.B.; Fersht, A.R. CRINEPT-TROSY NMR reveals p53 core domain bound in an unfolded form to the chaperone Hsp90. *Proc. Natl. Acad. Sci. USA* **2002**, *99*, 11085–11090. [CrossRef]
70. Drummond, D.A.; Wilke, C.O. Mistranslation-Induced Protein Misfolding as a Dominant Constraint on Coding-Sequence Evolution. *Cell* **2008**, *134*, 341–352. [CrossRef]
71. Cagan, A.; Baez-Ortega, A.; Brzozowska, N.; Abascal, F.; Coorens, T.H.H.; Sanders, M.A.; Lawson, A.R.J.; Harvey, L.M.R.; Bhosle, S.; Jones, D.; et al. Somatic mutation rates scale with lifespan across mammals. *Nature* **2022**, *604*, 517–524. [CrossRef] [PubMed]
72. Guo, H.H.; Choe, J.; Loeb, L.A. Protein tolerance to random amino acid change. *Proc. Natl. Acad. Sci. USA* **2004**, *101*, 9205–9210.
73. Markiewicz, P.; Kleina, L.; Cruz, C.; Ehret, S.; Miller, J. Genetic Studies of the lac Repressor. XIV. Analysis of 4000 Altered Escherichia coli lac Repressors Reveals Essential and Non-essential Residues, as well as "Spacers" which do not Require a Specific Sequence. *J. Mol. Biol.* **1994**, *240*, 421–433.: 10.1006/jmbi.1994.1458. [CrossRef] [PubMed]
74. Pakula, A.A.; Sauer, R.T. Genetic Analysis of Protein Stability and Function. *Annu. Rev. Genet.* **1989**, *23*, 289–310. [CrossRef] [PubMed]
75. Bloom, J.D.; Labthavikul, S.T.; Otey, C.R.; Arnold, F.H. Protein stability promotes evolvability. *Proc. Natl. Acad. Sci. USA* **2006**, *103*, 5869–5874.
76. Queitsch, C.; Sangster, T.A.; Lindquist, S. Hsp90 as a capacitor of phenotypic variation. *Nature* **2002**, *417*, 618–624. [CrossRef]
77. Aguilar-Rodríguez, J.; Sabater-Muñoz, B.; Montagud-Martínez, R.; Berlanga, V.; Alvarez-Ponce, D.; Wagner, A.; Fares, M.A. The Molecular Chaperone DnaK Is a Source of Mutational Robustness. *Genome Biol. Evol.* **2016**, *8*, 2979–2991.
78. Karras, G.I.; Yi, S.; Sahni, N.; Fischer, M.; Xie, J.; Vidal, M.; D'Andrea, A.D.; Whitesell, L.; Lindquist, S. HSP90 Shapes the Consequences of Human Genetic Variation. *Cell* **2017**, *168*, 856–866.e12. [CrossRef]
79. Zierer, B.K.; Rübbelke, M.; Tippel, F.; Madl, T.; Schopf, F.H.; Rutz, D.A.; Richter, K.; Sattler, M.; Buchner, J. Importance of cycle timing for the function of the molecular chaperone Hsp90. *Nat. Struct. Mol. Biol.* **2016**, *23*, 1020–1028. [CrossRef]
80. Panaretou, B.; Siligardi, G.; Meyer, P.; Maloney, A.; Sullivan, J.K.; Singh, S.; Millson, S.H.; Clarke, P.A.; Naaby-Hansen, S.; Stein, R.; et al. Activation of the ATPase Activity of Hsp90 by the Stress-Regulated Cochaperone Aha1. *Mol. Cell* **2002**, *10*, 1307–1318. [CrossRef]
81. Panaretou, B.; Prodromou, C.; Roe, S.M.; O'Brien, R.; Ladbury, J.E.; Piper, P.W.; Pearl, L.H. ATP binding and hydrolysis are essential to the function of the Hsp90 molecular chaperone in vivo. *EMBO J.* **1998**, *17*, 4829–4836. [CrossRef] [PubMed]
82. Obermann, W.M.; Sondermann, H.; Russo, A.A.; Pavletich, N.P.; Hartl, F.U. In Vivo Function of Hsp90 Is Dependent on ATP Binding and ATP Hydrolysis. *J. Cell Biol.* **1998**, *143*, 901–910. [CrossRef] [PubMed]
83. Backe, S.J.; Sager, R.A.; Woodford, M.R.; Makedon, A.M.; Mollapour, M. Post-translational modifications of Hsp90 and translating the chaperone code. *J. Biol. Chem.* **2020**, *295*, 11099–11117. [CrossRef] [PubMed]
84. Nitika.; Porter, C.M.; Truman, A.W.; Truttmann, M.C. Post-translational modifications of Hsp70 family proteins: Expanding the chaperone code. *J. Biol. Chem.* **2020**, *295*, 10689–10708. [CrossRef] [PubMed]
85. Wisén, S.; Bertelsen, E.B.; Thompson, A.D.; Patury, S.; Ung, P.; Chang, L.; Evans, C.G.; Walter, G.M.; Wipf, P.; Carlson, H.A.; et al. Binding of a Small Molecule at a Protein–Protein Interface Regulates the Chaperone Activity of Hsp70–Hsp40. *ACS Chem. Biol.* **2010**, *5*, 611–622. [CrossRef]
86. Taverna, D.M.; Goldstein, R.A. Why are proteins marginally stable? *Proteins Struct. Funct. Bioinform.* **2002**, *46*, 105–109. [CrossRef]
87. Ghosh, K.; Dill, K. Cellular Proteomes Have Broad Distributions of Protein Stability. *Biophys. J.* **2010**, *99*, 3996–4002. [CrossRef]
88. Park, C.; Marqusee, S. Pulse proteolysis: A simple method for quantitative determination of protein stability and ligand binding. *Nat. Methods* **2005**, *2*, 207–212. [CrossRef]
89. To, P.; Whitehead, B.; Tarbox, H.E.; Fried, S.D. Nonrefoldability is Pervasive Across the E. coli Proteome. *J. Am. Chem. Soc.* **2021**, *143*, 11435–11448. [CrossRef]
90. Leu, J.I.J.; Zhang, P.; Murphy, M.E.; Marmorstein, R.; George, D.L. Structural Basis for the Inhibition of HSP70 and DnaK Chaperones by Small-Molecule Targeting of a C-Terminal Allosteric Pocket. *ACS Chem. Biol.* **2014**, *9*, 2508–2516. [CrossRef]
91. Wen, W.; Liu, W.; Shao, Y.; Chen, L. VER-155008, a small molecule inhibitor of HSP70 with potent anti-cancer activity on lung cancer cell lines. *Exp. Biol. Med.* **2014**, *239*, 638–645. [CrossRef] [PubMed]
92. Jakob, U.; Lilie, H.; Meyer, I.; Buchner, J. Transient Interaction of Hsp90 with Early Unfolding Intermediates of Citrate Synthase Implications for Heat Shock In Vivo. *J. Biol. Chem.* **1995**, *270*, 7288–7294. [CrossRef] [PubMed]
93. Sekhar, A.; Rosenzweig, R.; Bouvignies, G.; Kay, L.E. Hsp70 biases the folding pathways of client proteins. *Proc. Natl. Acad. Sci. USA* **2016**, *113*, E2794–E2801. [CrossRef] [PubMed]
94. Fisher, C.K.; Stultz, C.M. Constructing ensembles for intrinsically disordered proteins. *Curr. Opin. Struct. Biol.* **2011**, *21*, 426–431. [CrossRef]

95. Tompa, P. Unstructural biology coming of age. *Curr. Opin. Struct. Biol.* **2011**, *21*, 419–425. [CrossRef]
96. Oldfield, C.J.; Dunker, A.K. Intrinsically Disordered Proteins and Intrinsically Disordered Protein Regions. *Annu. Rev. Biochem.* **2014**, *83*, 553–584. [CrossRef]
97. Chong, S.H.; Chatterjee, P.; Ham, S. Computer Simulations of Intrinsically Disordered Proteins. *Annu. Rev. Phys. Chem.* **2016**, *68*, 1–18. [CrossRef]
98. Best, R.B. Computational and theoretical advances in studies of intrinsically disordered proteins. *Curr. Opin. Struct. Biol.* **2017**, *42*, 147–154. [CrossRef]
99. Baker, D.; Agard, D.A. Kinetics versus Thermodynamics in Protein Folding. *Biochemistry* **1994**, *33*, 7505–7509. [CrossRef]
100. Kimchi-Sarfaty, C.; Oh, J.M.; Kim, I.W.; Sauna, Z.E.; Calcagno, A.M.; Ambudkar, S.V.; Gottesman, M.M. A "Silent" Polymorphism in the MDR1 Gene Changes Substrate Specificity. *Science* **2007**, *315*, 525–528. [CrossRef]
101. Kim, S.J.; Yoon, J.S.; Shishido, H.; Yang, Z.; Rooney, L.A.; Barral, J.M.; Skach, W.R. Translational tuning optimizes nascent protein folding in cells. *Science* **2015**, *348*, 444–448. [CrossRef]
102. Walsh, I.M.; Bowman, M.A.; Santarriaga, I.F.S.; Rodriguez, A.; Clark, P.L. Synonymous codon substitutions perturb cotranslational protein folding in vivo and impair cell fitness. *Proc. Natl. Acad. Sci. USA* **2020**, *117*, 3528–3534. [CrossRef] [PubMed]
103. Rosenberg, A.A.; Marx, A.; Bronstein, A.M. Codon-specific Ramachandran plots show amino acid backbone conformation depends on identity of the translated codon. *Nat. Commun.* **2022**, *13*, 2815. [CrossRef] [PubMed]
104. Sorokina, I.; Mushegian, A.R.; Koonin, E.V. Is Protein Folding a Thermodynamically Unfavorable, Active, Energy-Dependent Process? *Int. J. Mol. Sci.* **2022**, *23*, 521. [CrossRef] [PubMed]

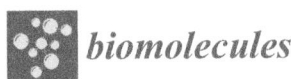

Review

Hsp90 and Associated Co-Chaperones of the Malaria Parasite

Tanima Dutta [1,2,3], Harpreet Singh [4], Adrienne L Edkins [5] and Gregory L Blatch [1,2,5,6,*]

1. The Vice Chancellery, The University of Notre Dame Australia, Fremantle, WA 6160, Australia; tanimadutta85@gmail.com
2. The Institute of Immunology and Infectious Diseases, Murdoch University, Perth, WA 6150, Australia
3. PathWest Nedlands, QEII Medical Centre, Perth, WA 6009, Australia
4. Department of Bioinformatics, Hans Raj Mahila Maha Vidyalaya, Jalandhar 144008, India; harpreetsingh05@gmail.com
5. Biomedical Biotechnology Research Unit, Department of Biochemistry and Microbiology, Rhodes University, Grahamstown 6140, South Africa; a.edkins@ru.ac.za
6. Biomedical Research and Drug Discovery Research Group, Faculty of Health Sciences, Higher Colleges of Technology, Sharjah P.O. Box 7947, United Arab Emirates
* Correspondence: g.blatch@ru.ac.za

Abstract: Heat shock protein 90 (Hsp90) is one of the major guardians of cellular protein homeostasis, through its specialized molecular chaperone properties. While Hsp90 has been extensively studied in many prokaryotic and higher eukaryotic model organisms, its structural, functional, and biological properties in parasitic protozoans are less well defined. Hsp90 collaborates with a wide range of co-chaperones that fine-tune its protein folding pathway. Co-chaperones play many roles in the regulation of Hsp90, including selective targeting of client proteins, and the modulation of its ATPase activity, conformational changes, and post-translational modifications. *Plasmodium falciparum* is responsible for the most lethal form of human malaria. The survival of the malaria parasite inside the host and the vector depends on the action of molecular chaperones. The major cytosolic *P. falciparum* Hsp90 (PfHsp90) is known to play an essential role in the development of the parasite, particularly during the intra-erythrocytic stage in the human host. Although PfHsp90 shares significant sequence and structural similarity with human Hsp90, it has several major structural and functional differences. Furthermore, its co-chaperone network appears to be substantially different to that of the human host, with the potential absence of a key homolog. Indeed, PfHsp90 and its interface with co-chaperones represent potential drug targets for antimalarial drug discovery. In this review, we critically summarize the current understanding of the properties of Hsp90, and the associated co-chaperones of the malaria parasite.

Keywords: *Plasmodium falciparum*; heat shock proteins; cytosolic Hsp90; ATPase; co-chaperones; client proteins

1. Introduction

To combat cellular stress, an elevated expression of chaperones, many of which are heat shock proteins, is observed [1]. In eukaryotes, heat shock protein 90 (Hsp90) and heat shock protein 70 (Hsp70) are the most prominent chaperone families. Together, Hsp90 and Hsp70 collaborate to ensure protein homeostasis by capturing client proteins and facilitating productive folding [2]. Hsp90 has essential functions in cell growth and differentiation, apoptosis, signal transduction, and cell–cell communication [3]. Hsp90 isoforms exist in organisms ranging from bacteria (where it is known as HtpG) to protozoa to higher eukaryotes. Although Hsp90 is not essential for cell survival in the bacterium *Escherichia coli*, it is important for the survival of *Shewanella oneidensis* under heat stress [4]. It is indispensable for viability in the yeast *Saccharomyces cerevisiae* [5], while in higher eukaryotes the Hsp90β, but not the Hsp90α, isoform is essential for survival [6–9]. Hsp90 plays a central role in many cellular networks, along with buffering environmental conditions to promote evolutionary fitness [10].

Plasmodium falciparum is responsible for the most lethal form of human malaria, taking 627,000 lives worldwide in 2020 [11]. Infection begins with a female mosquito injecting sporozoites into human blood. Following the mosquito's 'blood meal', the successful colonization of the liver by sporozoites initiates the parasite life cycle in humans, followed by erythrocyte invasion, which accounts for the pathology of malaria [12,13]. The development of sporozoites takes place within hepatocytes, where they mature into schizonts and then merozoites, which are released and rapidly invade erythrocytes [13,14]. The intra-erythrocytic stage results in alterations of the infected host cells that cause them to adhere to the cell walls of capillaries, thereby preventing them from clearing through the spleen. This structural change poses a risk for the human host, since clusters of infected erythrocytes can create a blockage in blood circulation. After the intra-erythrocytic stage, the gametocyte-infected stage develops, which can infect the mosquito upon blood ingestion [12]. The motile ookinetes penetrates the midgut wall of the mosquito, developing into "oocysts". These cysts then release sporozoites, which migrate to the mosquito's salivary glands and can again infect the human host [12]. During the intra-erythrocytic stage, high temperatures are induced and, therefore, parasite proteins and membranes require cytoprotection for the maintenance of their integrity [15]. Survival of the malaria parasite inside the host and the vector depends on the action of molecular chaperones. The emergence of resistance to the most commonly used antimalarial drugs, coupled with the difficulty in producing an effective vaccine, resulted in an urgent need to develop drugs targeted against novel chemotherapeutic targets [16–18].

There is evidence from saturation-scale mutagenesis screening that all the Hsp90 genes of the malaria parasite are essential [19]. Furthermore, the major cytosolic *P. falciparum* Hsp90 (PfHsp90) is highly expressed during the intra-erythrocytic stage of the parasite life cycle, induced by stress, and plays an essential role in parasite survival and development [7]. Using in vitro cell culture studies, geldanamycin (GA) was found to be highly effective at inhibiting the growth of parasite-infected erythrocytes, and causing an arrest at the ring stage [7,20]. Assuming that PfHsp90 was the primary target of GA, these findings suggest that PfHsp90 plays an important role in malaria parasite growth in erythrocytes [7,20]. In addition, given that transition from early ring to metabolically active trophozoites is regulated by temperature changes, PfHsp90 was also proposed as a major player in the malaria parasite's response to heat shock, and the establishment of infection in erythrocytes [21,22]. Indeed, frequent febrile episodes elevate the level of PfHsp90 expression, and GA inhibition studies suggest that PfHsp90 assists in malaria parasite survival during febrile episodes [23,24]. Interestingly, PfHsp90 is also shown to be essential for liver stage development [25]. Overall, these findings suggest that PfHsp90 is an ideal anti-malaria drug target.

2. Hsp90: Chaperone Activity and Its Conformational Changes

Cytosolic Hsp90 architecture is conserved from bacteria to humans with slight modifications, which are critical for functional differences between Hsp90 paralogs and orthologs [26]. The most common structural feature of all Hsp90 homologs is the presence of an N-terminal nucleotide-binding domain (NTD), along with a C-terminal domain (CTD) and a middle domain (MD) [27] (Figures 1 and 2; Protein Data Bank [PDB] identification [ID] codes: 5FWK and 5FWM). Hsp90 functions as a molecular machine to capture and promote the folding of client proteins through conformational changes regulated by ATPase activity and protein–protein interactions [28]. ATP binds the Hsp90 NTD, and ATP hydrolysis is catalyzed by the NTD and MD. The NTD and MD are joined by a charged linker sequence, which is important for inter-domain communication during chaperone activity [29].

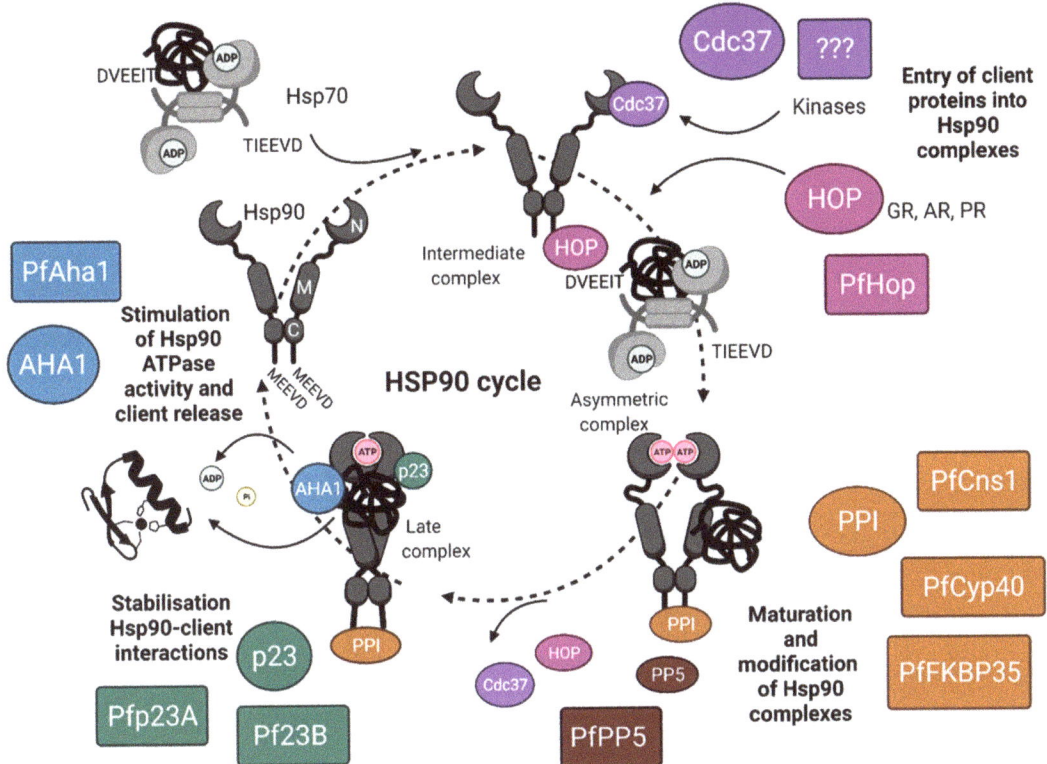

Figure 1. Regulation of the Hsp90 chaperone cycle by co-chaperones. Progression of client proteins through the Hsp90-mediated chaperone folding pathway is regulated by co-chaperones, which act at defined stages in the cycle. Co-chaperones may regulate Hsp90 association with clients, ATPase activity, conformational changes, and post-translational modifications. When inactive, Hsp90 is constitutively dimerized at the C-terminus but not the N-terminus. Entry of client proteins is facilitated by co-chaperones including the Hsp70/Hsp90 organizing protein Hop, which regulates transfer of clients from Hsp70 by binding simultaneously to Hsp70 and Hsp90, to form the intermediate complexes. Hop is conserved in *Plasmodium falciparum* (PfHop, PF3D7_1434300). Kinase clients require the kinase-specific co-chaperone Cdc37; however, a Cdc37-encoding gene has not been identified in the *P. falciparum* genome. On ATP binding, Hsp90 undergoes N-terminal dimerization, and the client protein associates with the middle domain of Hsp90. Bindings of other co-chaperones, including peptidyl-prolyl cis–trans isomerases (PPIase) and protein phosphatase 5 (PP5), associate to form the asymmetric Hsp90 complexes. The *P. falciparum* genome encodes a PP5 isoform (PfPP5, PF3D7_1355500) and multiple PPIase isoforms (PfFKBP35, PF3D7_1247400; PfCns1, PF3D7_1108900; and PfCyp40, PF3D7_1111800). These co-chaperones regulate the post-translational modification and maturation of Hsp90 complexes. Early co-chaperones subsequently dissociate from the complex to be replaced by p23, which stabilizes the late closed Hsp90 complex and the client within the complex, and inhibits ATPase activity. Two homologs of p23 are encoded in the *P. falciparum* genome (Pfp23A, PF3D7_1453700; and Pf23B, PF3D7_0927000). ATP hydrolysis is stimulated by binding of Aha1, resulting in release of the client protein and a return of Hsp90 to the inactive conformation. The *P. falciparum* genome encodes a single Aha1 isoform (PfAha1, PF3D7_0306200). Image created with BioRender.com.

The MD also carries the binding site for Hsp90 clients and co-chaperones. The CTD allows the constitutive dimerization of Hsp90 through two C-terminal helices forming a four-helix bundle [30,31]. One of the most prominent features of Hsp90 chaperone activity is the formation of a V-shape dimer, which helps in the transient N-terminal dimerization that is required for ATP hydrolysis [32] (Figure 1). A C-terminal MEEVD motif is present in all cytosolic Hsp90 paralogs, and is the main site of binding to tetratricopeptide repeat (TPR)-containing co-chaperones [33]. Co-chaperones of eukaryotic Hsp90s typically out-number their respective chaperones, forming complexes with Hsp90 and their client proteins, to promote efficient protein folding and fine-tuning chaperone functions to maintain cellular homeostasis (Figure 1). Consequently, new approaches to inhibit the function of the Hsp90 complex have focused on the disruption of protein–protein interactions with co-chaperones [34].

Hsp90 modulates the stability of several essential cellular proteins, and is a conserved regulator of key protein kinases and nuclear receptors that control the cell cycle and signal transduction events [35–37]. The NTD is rich in β-strands and forms a nucleotide-binding pocket sharing a Bergerat fold with members of the GHKL superfamily (gyrase subunit B [GyrB], histidine kinase, and DNA mismatch repair protein MutL) [38]. This domain can be inhibited competitively by small molecule inhibitors, which target the ATP binding site and, as such, compete with ATP for binding [38–40]. The NTD and MD of Hsp90 undergo key conformational changes, bringing the γ-phosphate of ATP closer to key residues in the MD (e.g., Arg380 in yeast Hsp82), which triggers ATP hydrolysis [41]. Also, Hsp90 has a much higher affinity for ADP than ATP, suggesting that it requires a threshold cellular ATP:ADP ratio for ATPase activity [39,42,43]. In general, all Hsp90s bound to ATP can associate with unfolded/partially folded client proteins. Subsequently, the lid region closes over the ATP binding pocket, and the NTD dimerizes, adopting a closed conformation. The association of the MD in the Hsp90 dimer alters the position of the MD catalytic loop promoting ATP hydrolysis (Figure 1). Upon ATP hydrolysis, the client protein is released to fold spontaneously [2]. The Hsp90 homodimer returns to the unbound open conformation, and is primed for subsequent rounds of ATP hydrolysis and protein folding [38].

3. *P. falciparum* Hsp90s

The *P. falciparum* genome contains four Hsp90 genes, encoding the following PfHsp90 proteins: PfHsp90 (cytosol; PF3D7_0708400), PfTrap1/PfHsp90_M (mitochondrion; PF3D7_1118200), PfGrp94 (endoplasmic reticulum; PF3D7_1222300), and PfHsp90_A (apicoplast; PF3D7_1443900) [44]. Low resolution structural studies suggest that PfHsp90 exists in solution as elongated and flexible dimers [37] (Figure 2). While PfHsp90 shares significant sequence and structural similarity with its eukaryotic homologs, particularly cytosolic human Hsp90β (hHsp90), and contains all the characteristic domains (NTD, charged linker region, MD, CTD, and C-terminal dimerization domain ending in a MEEVD motif), it has several key structural and functional differences [45–47] (Figure 2). In particular, the ATP-binding pocket of PfHsp90 is more hydrophobic, constricted, and basic, relative to hHsp90 [48]. Biochemical studies on PfHsp90 report that, in comparison to hHsp90, it binds ATP with higher affinity (by 30%), is a more active ATPase (with six-fold higher activity), and has significantly higher catalytic efficiency (k_{cat}/K_m of 16.2×10^{-5} min^{-1} μM^{-1}) [49]. While basal ATPase kinetics and, ultimately, the speed of the chaperone cycle are important factors, they are not sufficient for efficient client protein folding by Hsp90 [50,51]. There is evidence that the dwelling time between the open and closed conformations of Hsp90 is critical to ensuring appropriate client protein interaction [50] (Figure 1); and, hence, more detailed biophysical studies are required on PfHsp90. Interestingly, PfHsp90 has a highly (negatively) charged, flexible linker region that is substantially longer than that of hHsp90 [52]. Domain swapping experiments introducing the charged linker from PfHsp90 into yeast or human Hsp90 lead to chimeric proteins, which support viability in yeast but have reduced ATPase activity, and reduced interaction with client proteins and some co-chaperones [52]. It remains to be determined how the intrinsic biochemical properties of PfHsp90 are regulated by different client proteins and their associated co-chaperones. Nevertheless, these initial biochemical findings suggest that the PfHsp90 chaperone cycle may be capable of rapid client protein turnover, which would be highly advantageous to parasite survival under the stressful conditions experienced in the human host. Furthermore, these unique architectural and biochemical features of PfHsp90 suggest that it is a prime drug target for structure-based anti-malarial drug discovery [53].

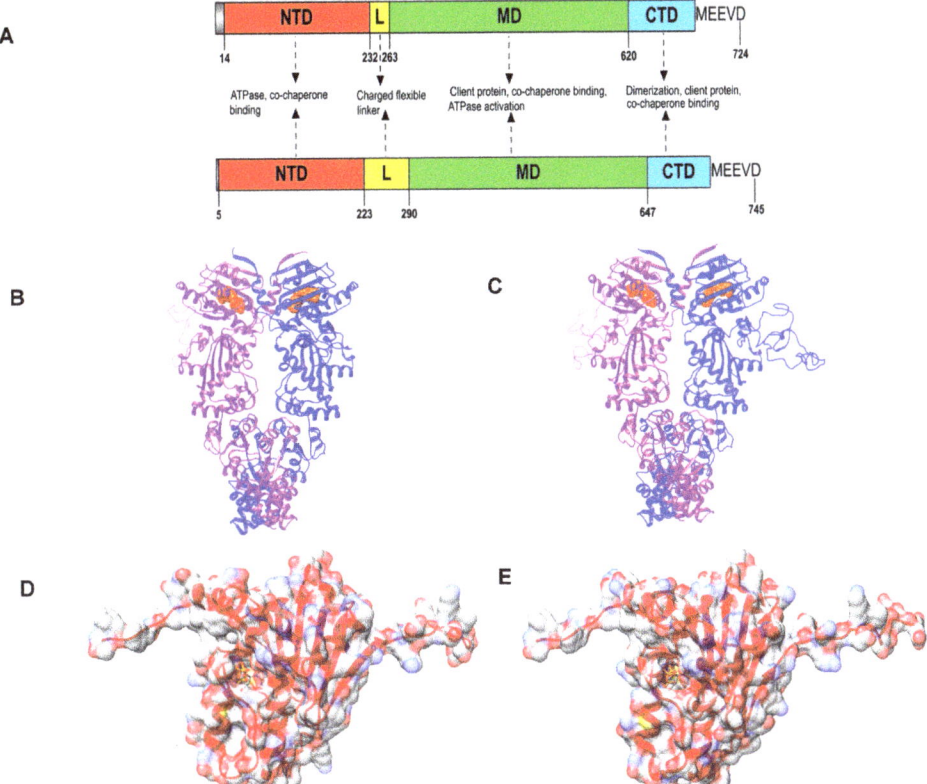

Figure 2. Domain organization and structural view of hHsp90β and PfHsp90. (**A**). Domain organization of hHsp90β (**top**) and PfHsp90 (**bottom**). Structure of full-length dimeric (**B**). hHsp90β and (**C**). PfHsp90 proteins as cartoons. ATP bound to the N-terminal domain (NTD) is shown as red spheres. The two Hsp90 monomers in the models are colored purple and blue. (**D**). hHsp90β and (**E**). PfHsp90 NTD as surface. The surface (with 60% transparency) is colored according to element type and it also depicts the arrangement of secondary structure elements (red color) as cartoons. The bound ATP molecule is represented as sticks, colored according to the element type. Full-length 3D structures of hHsp90β and PfHsp90 were modeled with SWISS-MODEL (SWISS-MODEL: homology modelling of protein structures and complexes. Available online: https://swissmodel.expasy.org/ [accessed on 12 June 2022]) using PDB files 5FWK and 5FWM, respectively, as templates. NTD: N-terminal domain; L: linker region; MD: middle domain; and CTD: C-terminal domain. Element coloring scheme uses red, blue, grey, and yellow for oxygen, nitrogen, carbon, and phosphorous, respectively. Images for 3D structures were rendered using UCSF Chimera 1.10.1 (UCSF Chimera—a visualization system for exploratory research and analysis. Available online: https://www.cgl.ucsf.edu/chimera/ [accessed on 12 June 2022]), while the linear domain layout image was rendered using IBS 1.0 (IBS: an illustrator for the presentation and visualization of biological sequences. Available online: http://ibs.biocuckoo.org/ [accessed on 12 June 2022]).

While co-chaperones of hHsp90 are extensively studied [53], and informed anti-cancer drug discovery [34], there are relatively few studies on PfHsp90 co-chaperones. Increasing our understanding of how PfHsp90 and its co-chaperones interact would greatly assist the development of novel anti-malarial therapies. Table 1 provides a comparison of the known co-chaperones of PfHsp90 to those of hHsp90, and in the following sections these proteins are explored in further detail.

Table 1. Co-chaperones of Hsp90 in *Homo sapiens* and *Plasmodium falciparum*.

Humans	P. falciparum	Known Functions	References
Hop	PfHop (PF3D7_1434300)	Early stage co-chaperone; binds Hsp90 at C-terminus; adaptor for Hsp70 and Hsp90; inhibits ATPase activity	[54,55]
Tah1	PfRPAP3/PfTah1 (PF3D7_0213500)	Component of Rvb1-Rvb2-Tah1-Pih1 (R2TP) complex	[56]
Pih1	PfPih1 (PF3D7_1235000)	Component of Rvb1-Rvb2-Tah1-Pih1 (R2TP) complex	[56]
Cyp40	PfCyp40 (PF3D7_1111800)	Peptidyl prolyl-cis/trans-isomerase	[57]
FKBP38	PfFKBP35 (PF3D7_1247400)	Peptidylprolyl-cis/trans-isomerase	[58,59]
TTC4	PfCns1 (PF3D7_1108900)	TTC4 is known for its interaction with cyclophilin; activated ATPase activity of Hsp70 by binding at TPR domain	[57,60]
p23	Pfp23A (PF3D7_1453700) Pfp23B (PF3D7_0927000)	Late stage co-chaperone, stabilizes closed Hsp90 confirmation; inhibits ATPase activity of Hsp90	[61,62]
Aha1	PfAha1 (PF3D7_0306200)	Potent ATPase activator of Hsp90; promotes client maturation	[57,63]
PP5	PfPP5 (PF3D7_1355500)	Phosphatase activity	[64,65]
Sgt1	PfCBP (PF3D7_0933200)	Kinetochore assembly	[66]
Cdc37	Not found	Early stage co-chaperone; kinase-specific co-chaperone and inhibits ATPase activity of Hsp90	[67]

4. PfHop (Hsp70–Hsp90 Organizing Protein; PF3D7_1434300)

As in other eukaryotes, the PfHsp70 and PfHsp90 protein folding pathways intersect to facilitate the folding of key proteins involved in diverse cellular pathways [22,46]. The interaction between Hsp70 and Hsp90 is regulated by Hop, which has been extensively characterized in the human system [68]. Both Hsp70 and Hsp90 possess C-terminally located EEVD motifs that interact with Hop via its multiple TPR domains [33]. Hop is not required for chaperone-mediated protein folding by Hsp70 and Hsp90 [69], but rather plays an important regulatory role for progression of client proteins through the chaperone cycle [70] (Figure 1). Of the six Hsp70-like proteins encoded by the *P. falciparum* genome, only the cytosol-nuclear localized chaperone PfHsp70-1 possesses the EEVD motif [71], which is crucial for interaction between Hsp70 and Hop. A Hop homologue (PF14_0324) was identified in the *P. falciparum* genome by Acharya and co-workers [44] (Table 1). Overall structural conservation was reported in PfHop, with some variations in the TPR regions [54]. Less conserved segments of Hop outside its TPR domains are shown to influence the overall conformation of the helical turns of the TPR domains, therefore, imparting unique structural features to Hop molecules from different species [72]. Immunofluorescence studies show PfHop to be localized with PfHsp70 and PfHsp90 in the parasite, and PfHsp70-1 complexes contained both PfHsp90 and PfHop by co-immunoprecipitation analysis [54]. PfHop co-localizes with the cytosolic chaperones PfHsp70-1 and PfHsp90 at the blood stages of the malaria parasite, and PfHop is stress-inducible [73,74]. Employing far western, surface plasmon resonance (SPR) and co-immunoprecipitation studies, a direct interaction between PfHop and PfHsp70-1 was identified, which was favored in the presence of ADP rather than ATP [73]. Recent studies on PfHop employing synchrotron radiation circular dichroism (SRCD) and small-angle X-ray scattering reveal that PfHop is a monomeric and elongated protein [55]. PfHop is also found to be unstable at temperatures higher than 40 °C in comparison to its functional partner, PfHsp70-1, which is known to be stable at temperatures as high as 80 °C [55,75].

5. PfTah1 (TPR-Containing Protein Associated with Hsp90; PF3D7_0213500) and PfPih1 (Protein Interacting with Hsp90; PF3D7_1235000)

The R2TP complex is an important multiprotein complex involved in multiple cellular process such as snoRNP biogenesis, PIKK signaling, RNA polymerase II assembly, and apoptosis [56]. Within the R2TP complex, the specialized Pih1 co-chaperone tightly interacts with Rvb1/Rvb2 and with another specialized co-chaperone Tah1 to form the R2TP macromolecular complex. The R2TP complex further interacts with Hsp90 to form the R2TP–Hsp90 complex [56]. A genome-wide screening of *P. falciparum* led to the identification of PfPih1 and PfTah1, which associate with PfHsp90 to form the *Plasmodium* R2TP–Hsp90 complex [47,56] (Table 1). The R2TP complex plays a vital role in both cancer cell proliferation in humans and rapid multiplication of *P. falciparum* [56].

6. Immunophilins: PfCyp40 (Cyclophilin 40/PF3D7_1111800) and PfFKBP35 (FK506-Binding Protein 35/PF3D7_1247400)

Immunophilins are known for their characteristic peptidyl-prolyl cis–trans isomerase (PPI) activity [76]. Cyclophilin 40 (Cyp40) and FK506-binding proteins (FKBPs) were discovered in 1989 as the major receptors of the immunosuppressive drugs Cyclosporine-A and FK506 (tacrolimus), respectively [77,78]. PPIs play an accessory role with the Hsp90 protein folding machinery, and are part of diverse intracellular signaling pathways, ranging from steroid receptors to regulatory tyrosine kinases, critical in cell cycle control [79,80]. In humans, Cyp40, along with FK506-binding proteins FKBP51 and FKBP52, are also components of steroid receptor complexes [81–83]. All three immunophilins (Cyp40, FKBP51, and FKBP52) have conserved N-termini for immunophilin function and a C-terminal domain containing TPR motifs involved in protein–protein interaction [83,84]. They all target Hsp90 through their conserved C-terminal region to form separate steroid receptor complexes containing Hsp90 (Figure 1). Smith and co-workers (1990) [85] explained the dynamic model of steroid receptor assembly, in which the high affinity hormone-binding form of the receptor was regulated through interactions between Hsc70 and Hsp90. The immunophilins are known to regulate the activity of steroid hormone receptors, and their interaction depends on the type of steroid hormone receptor to be activated. FKBP51 preferentially interacts with progesterone and glucocorticoid receptor complexes, while Cyp40 tends to accumulate with estrogen receptor complexes [86]. Mining of the *P. falciparum* 3D7 genome reveals eight putative cyclophilin chaperones with four α-like and four β-like subunits [87]. No *Plasmodium* export element (PEXEL) motifs were found in any of the putative cyclophilins co-chaperones. It was observed that only two have PPIase activity, but all of them prevent aggregation of a model substrate, and are implicated in heat shock resistance in *P. falciparum* [88]. *P. falciparum* Cyp40 (PfCyp40; Table 1) has a predicted C-terminal trans-membrane domain and no export signal [81]. Most of the PfCyps are identified as having no signal peptide and, therefore, would most likely be found in the parasite cytoplasm [89]. Similar to the mammalian counterpart, two PPIase monomers of PfCyp40 are predicted to interact with dimeric PfHsp90 [90].

One of the most highly expressed co-chaperones of hHsp90 across a range of tissues is FKBP38, a membrane-anchored protein distributed predominantly in mitochondria [91,92]. *P. falciparum* FKBP35 (PfFKBP35; Table 1), a putative FKBP38 homologue, is shown to be functional in that it exhibits PPIase activity that is sensitive to inhibition by FK506 and Rap [93]. Pull-down assays reveal that PfFKBP35 interacts with PfHsp90 through its TPR domain, suggesting that PfFKBP35 is a co-chaperone of PfHsp90 [94]. There is limited information on the exact mechanism of inhibitors such as FK506 in the interaction between PfFKBP35 and PfHsp90. PfFKBP35 itself might be responsible for the antimalarial effects of FK506 and Rap. Pharmaco-dynamics analysis suggests that both FK506 and Rap have similar effects on different intra-erythrocytic stages in culture and kinetics of killing or irreversible growth arrest of parasites [95]. Furthermore, X-ray and NMR crystallography experiments show slight differences between PfFKBP35 and another human PPI, FKBP12, which could be critical in the designing of inhibitors that selectively inhibit PfFKBP35 [96]. The structural differences were detected in the $\beta5-\beta6$ segment of the PPIase domain, where PfFKBP35 contains a conserved cysteine and serine residue at amino acid positions 106 and 109, respectively, instead of a histidine (H87) and isoleucine (I90) residue at the corresponding position in human FKBP12, which presents as an architectural FKBP domain. Another study on the design of small molecules, targeting these conserved C106/C105 and S109/S108 residues in PfFKBP35/*Plasmodium vivax* FKBP35 (PvFKBP35) to achieve selectivity, identified a novel ligand D44 (N-(2-Ethylphenyl)-2-(3H-imidazo [4, 5-b] pyridin-2-ylsulfanyl)-acetamide) with potent inhibitory activity against PfFKBP35 [97]. D44 displays approximately 100-fold higher selectivity towards the inhibition of *Plasmodium* FKBPs over human FKBPs (FKBP12 and FKBP52). Structural analysis reveals that the high selectivity towards *Plasmodium* FKBPs is attributed to improved proximity between D44 and the conserved C106/C105 and S109/S108 amino acid residues in PfFKBP35/PvFKBP35. In addition, another study proposed the incorporation of a bulky hydrophobic group at C-11 of FK506, to induce steric clashes with the residues H87 and I90 in FKBP12, as a potential strategy for engineering inhibitors that are selective towards PfFKBP35, while avoiding off-target effects on human FKBP12 [98].

7. Pfp23A (PF3D7_1453700) and Pfp23B (PF3D7_0927000)

The late stage co-chaperone p23 binds to the N-terminal domain of Hsp90, and is important for promoting the closed client-bound conformation of Hsp90 and inhibiting ATPase activity [70] (Figure 1). Pfp23, a 34-kDa phosphoprotein, is highly expressed and phosphorylated in the trophozoite stage of *P. falciparum* intra-erythrocytic development [99]. GST pull-down assays reveal the role of Pfp23 as a co-chaperone of PfHsp90, and this chaperone-co-chaperone interaction is dependent on the presence of ATP [61]. This is similar to the association between Sba1 (p23 yeast homologue) and yeast Hsp90 [100]. More recently, two small acidic co-chaperones, p23 orthologues, were identified in the *P. falciparum* genome [62] (Table 1). It was revealed that Pfp23A and Pfp23B show 13% identity between themselves, and 20% identity with human p23. It was found that Pfp23A has higher thermal stability in comparison to Pfp23B, suggesting structural and functional variability [62]. Both Pfp23A and Pfp23B could inhibit PfHsp90 ATPase activity, although Pfp23A was more effective [62], and although both could prevent aggregation of model substrate proteins (malate dehydrogenase, citrate synthase, and luciferase), the isoforms showed preferences for model client proteins [62]. Site-directed mutagenesis experiments by Chua et al. [61] identified the conserved residues K91, H93, W94, and K96 in Pfp23 as critical for interaction with PfHsp90. Pfp23 was also found to suppress protein aggregation dependent on to its C-terminal tail, showing that it has chaperone activity independent of PfHsp90 [61]. In a separate study to screen cancer inhibitors, the anticancer compound gedunin was identified as a specific inhibitor of p23 [101]. Gedunin binds p23 and abrogates interaction with Hsp90, resulting in cancer cell death. Although gedunin was previously shown to inhibit the chaperone function of Hsp90, the precise inhibitory mechanism is unclear, as gedunin does not bind to the N-terminus or the C-terminus of Hsp90 as most Hsp90-

specific inhibitors do (e.g., ansamycin antibiotics, radicicol, and novobiocin) [102,103]. In addition, gedunin shows antimalarial activity, which may or may not be related to its ability to modulate the interaction of Pfp23 and Hsp90 [104]. The presence of two Pfp23 isoforms with putative functional differences is interesting, and suggests that the mechanism of stabilization of PfHsp90 late stage complexes differs from that of the human Hsp90 complex.

8. PfAha1 (Activator of Hsp90 ATPase/PF3D7_0306200)

The Aha1 co-chaperone binds to the MD and stimulates Hsp90 ATPase activity, promoting client protein activation (Figure 1) [105]. PfAha1 was found using split ubiquitin assays [63] (Table 1). Employing GST pull-down assays, PfAha1 binds PfHsp90 in a manner dependent on $MgCl_2$ and ATP [63]. PfAha1 competes with Pfp23 to interact with PfHsp90 under similar conditions [57]. In contrast to the Pfp23–PfHsp90 interaction, where Pfp23 has an inhibitory effect on the ATPase activity of PfHsp90, PfAha1 stimulates the ATPase activity of PfHsp90 [63], consistent with the function of the human homolog [105]. It was observed by computational modelling that residue N108 in PfAha1 is critical for interaction with PfHsp90, and the mutation of N108 to alanine leads to reduced stimulation of the ATPase activity of PfHsp90 [63]. The PfAha1–PfHsp90 interaction is likely polar in nature, as it is disrupted by high salt concentration. PfAha1 most likely plays a role in the maturation of PfHsp90 client proteins [57]. Furthermore, the presence of PfAha1 suggests that, despite the higher basal ATPase activity of PfHsp90 compared to hHsp90, client release from late stage chaperone complexes is still regulated by ATPase stimulation.

9. PfPP5 (Protein Phosphatase 5/PF3D7_1355500)

PP5 is a TPR-containing co-chaperone that regulates the Hsp90 chaperone cycle through the dephosphorylation of Hsp90 or co-chaperones, such as Cdc37 [106]. Degenerate deoxyoligonucleotide primers were used to identify the protein phosphatase protein in *P. falciparum* for the first time [107] (Table 1). Sequence analysis reveals that PfPP5 has a N-terminal TPR domain followed by a Ser/Thr phosphatase sequence at the C-terminal domain. The PfPP5 Ser/Thr domain is essential for phosphatase activity, and the TPR domain of the protein can act as a negative regulator of phosphatase activity. The N-terminal PfPP5 TPR domain is a potential anti-malaria target for the design of selective inhibitors [107]. This is because PfPP5 possesses an unusually long TPR domain with four TPR motifs, as opposed to the three usually observed in homologs of other species, including human. Using a PfPP5 antibody, both PfPP5 and PfHsp90 were co-immunoprecipitated, which implies that PfPP5 may be part of the Hsp90 chaperone complexes, as observed in mammals [64,65]. PP5 and Aha1 are important in many cellular processes in neurodegenerative diseases in association with Hsp90; therefore, it is important to study this co-chaperone in *P. falciparum* to understand its precise mechanism [108].

In yeast, Ppt1 (PP5 homologue) is demonstrated to specifically dephosphorylate Hsp82 [109]. The deletion of Ppt1 in yeast leads to the hyperphosphorylation of Hsp90 and the reduced efficiency of the Hsp90 chaperone system in activating client proteins (e.g., glucocorticoid receptors, v-Src, and Ste11). In addition, PP5/Ppt1 was also found to dephosphorylate another co-chaperone Cdc37 at the phosphorylated S13 residue, and modulate its activity in recruiting protein kinase clients to Hsp90 [106]. Hence, PP5/Ppt1 was proposed as a positive modulator for the activation of Hsp90 client proteins. In the case of *P. falciparum*, although PfPP5 interacts with PfHsp90 [107], it remains unclear whether PfPP5 exerts its phosphatase activity on PfHsp90. However, the presence of the PfPP5 phosphatase implies that the PfHsp90 complex undergoes phosphorylation by *P. falciparum* kinases.

10. PfCBP (Calcyclin-Binding Protein/PF3D7_0933200) and PfCns1 (Cyclophilin Seven Suppressor 1/PF3D7_1108900)

The calcyclin-binding protein (CBP), suppressor of G2 allele of Skp1 (Sgt1), cyclophilin seven suppressor 1 (Cns1), and tetratricopeptide repeat domain 4 (TTC4) all share significant sequence similarity, contain TPR domains, and are co-chaperones of Hsp90 [110–112]. While related, these co-chaperones each bind differently to Hsp90, and target selective sets of client proteins [57,60,66]. For example, Sgt1 associates with the N-terminus of Hsp90, and specifically recruits leucine-rich-repeat proteins [112]. Bioinformatics analyses applying protein domain homology, identified several putative PfHsp90 co-chaperones related to Sgt1/CBP and TTC4/Cns1, namely, PfCBP and PfCns1, respectively [94] (Table 1). However, further investigation is needed to confirm if these co-chaperones directly interact with PfHsp90 and modulate its chaperone function.

11. Cdc37 (Cell Division Cycle 37) Homolog Potentially Missing in *P. falciparum*

Cdc37 is involved in the recruitment of nascent or unstable kinases to Hsp90 for folding into their active conformation [113,114], and is known to be important for the activation of a diverse group of protein kinases (e.g., Cdk1, Cdk4, Akt, v-Src, Raf, and CK2) [115,116]. Indeed, as many as 65% of the kinases in yeast are reported to require Cdc37 for activation and stabilization [117]. In human cells, 60% of kinases interact with Hsp90, and the recognition of these kinases is mediated by Cdc37 [118]. As many of the kinases have essential signal transduction roles that regulate growth and development, Cdc37 is, thus, recognized as an important component of the Hsp90 chaperone machinery. In addition, Hsp90 chaperone activity itself is integrated with cellular proliferation by phosphorylation. It is, therefore, noteworthy that a Cdc37 homolog has not been found in *P. falciparum* (Table 1). This could mean that other *P. falciparum* co-chaperones are able to functionally compensate for the lack of Cdc37, especially since critical kinases known to associate with Cdc37, such as Cdk1 (PfPK5; MAL13P1·279), Akt (PfPKB; PFL2250c), and CK2 (PfCK2; PF11_0096), are found in *P. falciparum* [94]. The Cdc37 ortholog may be divergent from that of humans and, hence, has not been identified based on sequence identity. Alternatively, *P. falciparum* kinases may have differing chaperone requirements, meaning they can enter the cycle in the absence of Cdc37, or are less reliant on Hsp90 for function.

12. Conclusions

This review suggests that the Hsp90 chaperone, and its associated co-chaperone complexes in *P. falciparum*, are broadly conserved in comparison to other organisms. PfHsp90 displays biochemical differences to hHsp90, which may be targeted for selective inhibition. Importantly, Hsp90 does not function alone, and appropriate proteostasis requires that the chaperone be fine-tuned by co-chaperones. The core co-chaperones regulating client entry, ATPase activity, and Hsp90 conformational regulation at the early, intermediate, and late stages of the chaperone cycle are broadly conserved in *P. falciparum*. However, there are two notable differences that may indicate important areas for future study and evaluation of therapeutic potential.

The first is the presence of two p23 orthologs in *P. falciparum*. While both of these isoforms function similar to p23 in the Hsp90 complex, there are differences in client protein specificity and ATPase inhibition. The requirement of both isoforms for parasite viability, and their individual importance in the PfHsp90 chaperone cycle, have not yet been determined. Since one of the functions of p23 is to inhibit Hsp90 ATPase activity, it may be speculated that the two isoforms arose because of the higher basal ATPase activity of PfHsp90. Given that Pfp23A inhibits the PfHsp90 ATPase activity more than Pfp23B, and that the folding and activation of different clients may require different cycle timing, the two p23 isoforms may have evolved to assist different client protein groups (i.e., the higher ATPase activity of PfHsp90 may allow for more inhibitory steps in the chaperone cycle). A detailed analysis of the co-chaperone functions of these p23 isoforms in vitro and in the parasite would be useful in determining if mechanistic differences do exist, and if they have therapeutic potential.

The second notable difference is the apparent absence of a Cdc37 ortholog in *P. falciparum*. However, since Cdc37 orthologs were identified in other obligate intracellular protozoan parasites (e.g., *Theileria annulata* and *Cryptosporidium parvum*) [119], deeper scrutiny of the *P. falciparum* genome is required. Cdc37 is regarded as one of the most important therapeutic Hsp90 co-chaperones, because of its role in regulating kinase entry into Hsp90 complexes. Kinases are considered important therapeutic targets in both cancer (focusing on human kinases) and malaria, and kinase inhibitors form one of the largest classes of approved drugs. The *P. falciparum* kinome was recently updated, confirming that its kinome is considerably smaller (98 members compared to 497 members in the human kinome) and divergent (38% unique; 46% potentially unique; and 16% human homologs) from that of humans [120]. Therefore, the apparent lack of a Cdc37 ortholog, or the presence of a yet to be identified divergent Cdc37 ortholog or functional equivalent, is likely to reflect differences in the folding requirements of the *P. falciparum* kinome by the Cdc37–PfHsp90 co-chaperone–chaperone machinery. Furthermore, the co-evolution of PfHsp90 and the kinome could have resulted in reduced dependency on a canonical Cdc37 for kinase activation. Indeed, there is evidence that Hsp90 may be able to activate kinases in the absence of Cdc37 [121,122]. Importantly, no study has demonstrated that *P. falciparum* kinases require PfHsp90 in a mechanism analogous to their yeast and human orthologs. Given the importance of kinases to drug discovery, and the fact that many *P. falciparum* kinases are being evaluated as drug targets, it would be interesting to identify a bona fide PfHsp90 kinase client. This could easily be done using available Hsp90 inhibitors in malaria parasite cell lines expressing GFP-tagged kinases. Validation of at least one PfHsp90 kinase client would subsequently support efforts to determine whether or not Cdc37 exists in the malaria parasite. This would be interesting not only from a fundamental perspective, but also in terms of identifying a selective therapeutic target for simultaneous inhibition of multiple kinases.

Taken together, both the conservation and differences in the co-chaperone complexes of PfHsp90 suggest that, as in non-communicable diseases [34], targeting Hsp90–co-chaperone interactions is an exciting new area of research that can both extend our understanding of proteostasis, and identify novel approaches for inhibition.

Author Contributions: Conceptualization, T.D. and G.L.B.; Figure 1, A.L.E.; bioinformatics analyses and Figure 2, H.S.; writing—original draft preparation, T.D.; writing—review and editing, T.D., A.L.E., H.S. and G.L.B. All authors have read and agreed to the published version of the manuscript.

Funding: G.L.B. acknowledges the financial support of Higher Colleges of Technology, UAE (Interdisciplinary Research Grant, IRG), and Rhodes University, South Africa (Rated Researcher Grant). Research activities in the laboratory of A.L.E are supported by a Newton Advanced Fellowship from the Academy of Medical Sciences (UK), and grants from the Resilient Futures Challenge-Led Initiative from the Royal Society (UK) (Grant No CHL\R1\180142), the South African Research Chairs Initiative of the Department of Science and Technology (DST), and the NRF (Grant No 98566), Rhodes University and the Grand Challenges Africa Drug Discovery Programme (which is a partnership between The African Academy of Sciences [AAS], the Bill and Melinda Gates Foundation, Medicines for Malaria Venture [MMV], and the University of Cape Town Drug Discovery and Development Centre [H3D]) (Grant No GCA/DD/rnd3/043).

Conflicts of Interest: The authors declare no conflict of interest.

References

1. Hartl, F.U.; Bracher, A.; Hayer-Hartl, M. Molecular chaperones in protein folding and proteostasis. *Nature* **2011**, *475*, 324–332. [CrossRef] [PubMed]
2. Morán Luengo, T.; Kityk, R.; Mayer, M.P.; Rüdiger, S.G.D. Hsp90 breaks the deadlock of the Hsp70 chaperone system. *Mol. Cell* **2018**, *70*, 545–552.e9. [CrossRef] [PubMed]
3. Pratt, W.B.; Toft, D.O. Regulation of signaling protein function and trafficking by the hsp90/hsp70-based chaperone machinery. *Exp. Biol. Med.* **2003**, *228*, 111–133. [CrossRef] [PubMed]

4. Honoré, F.A.; Méjean, V.; Genest, O. Hsp90 is essential under heat stress in the bacterium *Shewanella oneidensis*. *Cell Rep.* **2017**, *19*, 680–687. [CrossRef]
5. Borkovich, K.A.; Farrelly, F.W.; Finkelstein, D.B.; Taulien, J.; Lindquist, S. Hsp82 is an essential protein that is required in higher concentrations for growth of cells at higher temperatures. *Mol. Cell Biol.* **1989**, *9*, 3919–3930. [CrossRef]
6. Voss, A.K.; Thomas, T.; Gruss, P. Mice lacking HSP90beta fail to develop a placental labyrinth. *Development* **2000**, *127*, 1–11. [CrossRef] [PubMed]
7. Banumathy, G.; Singh, V.; Pavithra, S.R.; Tatu, U. Heat shock protein 90 function is essential for *Plasmodium falciparum* growth in human erythrocytes. *J. Biol. Chem.* **2003**, *278*, 18336–18345. [CrossRef]
8. Rutherford, S.L.; Lindquist, S. Hsp90 as a capacitor for morphological evolution. *Nature* **1998**, *396*, 336–342. [CrossRef]
9. Grad, I.; Cederroth, C.R.; Walicki, J.; Grey, C.; Barluenga, S.; Winssinger, N.; De Massy, B.; Nef, S.; Picard, D. The molecular chaperone Hsp90α is required for meiotic progression of spermatocytes beyond pachytene in the mouse. *PLoS ONE* **2010**, *5*, e15770. [CrossRef]
10. Sangster, T.A.; Salathia, N.; Undurraga, S.; Milo, R.; Schellenberg, K.; Lindquist, S.; Queitsch, C. HSP90 affects the expression of genetic variation and developmental stability in quantitative traits. *Proc. Natl. Acad. Sci. USA* **2008**, *105*, 2963–2968. [CrossRef]
11. WHO. *Guidelines for Malaria*; World Health Organization: Geneva, Switzerland, 2021.
12. Baker, D.A. Malaria gametocytogenesis. *Mol. Biochem. Parasitol.* **2010**, *172*, 57–65. [CrossRef] [PubMed]
13. Vaughan, A.M.; Aly, A.S.; Kappe, S.H. Malaria parasite pre-erythrocytic stage infection: Gliding and hiding. *Cell Host. Microbe.* **2008**, *4*, 209–218. [CrossRef] [PubMed]
14. Venugopal, K.; Hentzschel, F.; Valkiūnas, G.; Marti, M. *Plasmodium* asexual growth and sexual development in the haematopoietic niche of the host. *Nat. Rev. Microbiol.* **2020**, *18*, 177–189. [CrossRef] [PubMed]
15. Barnwell, J.W.; Asch, A.S.; Nachman, R.L.; Yamaya, M.; Aikawa, M.; Ingravallo, P. A human 88-kD membrane glycoprotein (CD36) functions in vitro as a receptor for a cytoadherence ligand on *Plasmodium falciparum*-infected erythrocytes. *J. Clin. Investig.* **1989**, *84*, 765–772. [CrossRef] [PubMed]
16. Daniyan, M.O. Heat shock proteins as targets for novel antimalarial drug discovery. *Adv. Exp. Med. Biol.* **2021**, *1340*, 205–236. [CrossRef] [PubMed]
17. Anokwuru, C.; Makumire, S.; Shonhai, A. Bioprospecting for novel heat shock protein modulators: The new frontier for antimalarial drug discovery? *Adv. Exp. Med. Biol.* **2021**, *1340*, 187–203. [CrossRef]
18. Stokes, B.H.; Dhingra, S.K.; Rubiano, K.; Mok, S.; Straimer, J.; Gnädig, N.F.; Deni, I.; Schindler, K.A.; Bath, J.R.; Ward, K.E.; et al. *Plasmodium falciparum* K13 mutations in Africa and Asia impact artemisinin resistance and parasite fitness. *eLife* **2021**, *10*, e66277. [CrossRef]
19. Zhang, M.; Wang, C.; Otto, T.D.; Oberstaller, J.; Liao, X.; Adapa, S.R.; Udenze, K.; Bronner, I.F.; Casandra, D.; Mayho, M.; et al. Uncovering the essential genes of the human malaria parasite *Plasmodium falciparum* by saturation mutagenesis. *Science* **2018**, *360*, eaap7847. [CrossRef]
20. Kumar, R.; Musiyenko, A.; Barik, S. The heat shock protein 90 of *Plasmodium falciparum* and antimalarial activity of its inhibitor, geldanamycin. *Malar. J.* **2003**, *2*, 30. [CrossRef]
21. Shahinas, D.; Folefoc, A.; Pillai, D.R. Targeting *Plasmodium falciparum* Hsp90: Towards reversing antimalarial resistance. *Pathogens* **2013**, *2*, 33–54. [CrossRef]
22. Shahinas, D.; Pillai, D.R. Role of Hsp90 in *Plasmodium falciparum* malaria. *Adv. Exp. Med. Biol.* **2021**, *1340*, 125–139. [CrossRef] [PubMed]
23. Pavithra, S.R.; Banumathy, G.; Joy, O.; Singh, V.; Tatu, U. Recurrent fever promotes *Plasmodium falciparum* development in human erythrocytes. *J. Biol. Chem.* **2004**, *279*, 46692–46699. [CrossRef] [PubMed]
24. Pallavi, R.; Acharya, P.; Chandran, S.; Daily, J.P.; Tatu, U. Chaperone expression profiles correlate with distinct physiological states of *Plasmodium falciparum* in malaria patients. *Malar. J.* **2010**, *9*, 236. [CrossRef]
25. Posfai, D.; Eubanks, A.L.; Keim, A.I.; Lu, K.Y.; Wang, G.Z.; Hughes, P.F.; Kato, N.; Haystead, T.A.; Derbyshire, E.R. Identification of Hsp90 inhibitors with anti-*Plasmodium* activity. *Antimicrob. Agents Chemother.* **2018**, *62*, e01799-17. [CrossRef]
26. Chen, B.; Zhong, D.; Monteiro, A. Comparative genomics and evolution of the HSP90 family of genes across all kingdoms of organisms. *BMC Genom.* **2006**, *7*, 156. [CrossRef]
27. Verba, K.A.; Wang, R.Y.; Arakawa, A.; Liu, Y.; Shirouzu, M.; Yokoyama, S.; Agard, D.A. Atomic structure of Hsp90-Cdc37-Cdk4 reveals that Hsp90 traps and stabilizes an unfolded kinase. *Science* **2016**, *352*, 1542–1547. [CrossRef] [PubMed]
28. Krukenberg, K.A.; Street, T.O.; Lavery, L.A.; Agard, D.A. Conformational dynamics of the molecular chaperone Hsp90. *Q. Rev. Biophys.* **2011**, *44*, 229–255. [CrossRef]
29. Jahn, M.; Rehn, A.; Pelz, B.; Hellenkamp, B.; Richter, K.; Rief, M.; Buchner, J.; Hugel, T. The charged linker of the molecular chaperone Hsp90 modulates domain contacts and biological function. *Proc. Natl. Acad. Sci. USA* **2014**, *111*, 17881–17886. [CrossRef]
30. Ali, M.M.; Roe, S.M.; Vaughan, C.K.; Meyer, P.; Panaretou, B.; Piper, P.W.; Prodromou, C.; Pearl, L.H. Crystal structure of an Hsp90-nucleotide-p23/Sba1 closed chaperone complex. *Nature* **2006**, *440*, 1013–1017. [CrossRef]
31. Pearl, L.H.; Prodromou, C. Structure and mechanism of the Hsp90 molecular chaperone machinery. *Annu. Rev. Biochem.* **2006**, *75*, 271–294. [CrossRef]

32. Prodromou, C.; Panaretou, B.; Chohan, S.; Siligardi, G.; O'Brien, R.; Ladbury, J.E.; Roe, S.M.; Piper, P.W.; Pearl, L.H. The ATPase cycle of Hsp90 drives a molecular 'clamp' via transient dimerization of the N-terminal domains. *EMBO J.* **2000**, *19*, 4383–4392. [CrossRef] [PubMed]
33. Scheufler, C.; Brinker, A.; Bourenkov, G.; Pegoraro, S.; Moroder, L.; Bartunik, H.; Hartl, F.U.; Moarefi, I. Structure of TPR domain-peptide complexes: Critical elements in the assembly of the Hsp70-Hsp90 multichaperone machine. *Cell* **2000**, *101*, 199–210. [CrossRef]
34. Serwetnyk, M.A.; Blagg, B.S.J. The disruption of protein-protein interactions with co-chaperones and client substrates as a strategy towards Hsp90 inhibition. *Acta Pharm. Sin. B* **2021**, *11*, 1446–1468. [CrossRef] [PubMed]
35. Lindquist, S. Protein folding sculpting evolutionary change. *Cold Spring Harb. Symp. Quant. Biol.* **2009**, *74*, 103–108. [CrossRef]
36. Taipale, M.; Jarosz, D.F.; Lindquist, S. HSP90 at the hub of protein homeostasis: Emerging mechanistic insights. *Nat. Rev. Mol. Cell Biol.* **2010**, *11*, 515–528. [CrossRef]
37. Silva, N.S.M.; Torricillas, M.S.; Minari, K.; Barbosa, L.R.S.; Seraphim, T.V.; Borges, J.C. Solution structure of *Plasmodium falciparum* Hsp90 indicates a highly flexible dimer. *Arch. Biochem. Biophys.* **2020**, *690*, 108468. [CrossRef]
38. Dutta, R.; Inouye, M. GHKL, an emergent ATPase/kinase superfamily. *Trends Biochem. Sci.* **2000**, *25*, 24–28. [CrossRef]
39. Prodromou, C.; Roe, S.M.; O'Brien, R.; Ladbury, J.E.; Piper, P.W.; Pearl, L.H. Identification and structural characterization of the ATP/ADP-binding site in the Hsp90 molecular chaperone. *Cell* **1997**, *90*, 65–75. [CrossRef]
40. Garg, G.; Khandelwal, A.; Blagg, B.S. Anticancer inhibitors of Hsp90 function: Beyond the usual suspects. *Adv. Cancer Res.* **2016**, *129*, 51–88. [CrossRef]
41. Meyer, P.; Prodromou, C.; Hu, B.; Vaughan, C.; Roe, S.M.; Panaretou, B.; Piper, P.W.; Pearl, L.H. Structural and functional analysis of the middle segment of Hsp90: Implications for ATP hydrolysis and client protein and cochaperone interactions. *Mol. Cell* **2003**, *11*, 647–658. [CrossRef]
42. Scheibel, T.; Neuhofen, S.; Weikl, T.; Mayr, C.; Reinstein, J.; Vogel, P.D.; Buchner, J. ATP-binding properties of human Hsp90. *J. Biol. Chem.* **1997**, *272*, 18608–18613. [CrossRef] [PubMed]
43. Young, J.C.; Hartl, F.U. Polypeptide release by Hsp90 involves ATP hydrolysis and is enhanced by the co-chaperone p23. *EMBO J.* **2000**, *19*, 5930–5940. [CrossRef] [PubMed]
44. Acharya, P.; Kumar, R.; Tatu, U. Chaperoning a cellular upheaval in malaria: Heat shock proteins in *Plasmodium falciparum*. *Mol. Biochem. Parasitol.* **2007**, *153*, 85–94. [CrossRef]
45. Edkins, A.L.; Boshoff, A. General structural and functional features of molecular chaperones. *Adv. Exp. Med. Biol.* **2021**, *1340*, 11–73. [CrossRef] [PubMed]
46. Shonhai, A.; Maier, A.G.; Przyborski, J.M.; Blatch, G.L. Intracellular protozoan parasites of humans: The role of molecular chaperones in development and pathogenesis. *Protein. Pept. Lett.* **2011**, *18*, 143–157. [CrossRef]
47. Seraphim, T.V.; Chakafana, G.; Shonhai, A.; Houry, W.A. *Plasmodium falciparum* R2TP complex: Driver of parasite Hsp90 function. *Biophys. Rev.* **2019**, *11*, 1007–1015. [CrossRef]
48. Corbett, K.D.; Berger, J.M. Structure of the ATP-binding domain of *Plasmodium falciparum* Hsp90. *Proteins* **2010**, *78*, 2738–2744. [CrossRef] [PubMed]
49. Pallavi, R.; Roy, N.; Nageshan, R.K.; Talukdar, P.; Pavithra, S.R.; Reddy, R.; Venketesh, S.; Kumar, R.; Gupta, A.K.; Singh, R.K.; et al. Heat shock protein 90 as a drug target against protozoan infections: Biochemical characterization of HSP90 from *Plasmodium falciparum* and *Trypanosoma evansi* and evaluation of its inhibitor as a candidate drug. *J. Biol. Chem.* **2010**, *285*, 37964–37975. [CrossRef]
50. Zierer, B.K.; Rübbelke, M.; Tippel, F.; Madl, T.; Schopf, F.H.; Rutz, D.A.; Richter, K.; Sattler, M.; Buchner, J. Importance of cycle timing for the function of the molecular chaperone Hsp90. *Nat. Struct. Mol. Biol.* **2016**, *23*, 1020–1028. [CrossRef]
51. Xu, H. ATP-driven nonequilibrium activation of kinase clients by the molecular chaperone Hsp90. *Biophys. J.* **2020**, *119*, 1538–1549. [CrossRef]
52. Tsutsumi, S.; Mollapour, M.; Prodromou, C.; Lee, C.T.; Panaretou, B.; Yoshida, S.; Mayer, M.P.; Neckers, L.M. Charged linker sequence modulates eukaryotic heat shock protein 90 (Hsp90) chaperone activity. *Proc. Natl. Acad. Sci. USA* **2012**, *109*, 2937–2942. [CrossRef] [PubMed]
53. Wang, T.; Bisson, W.H.; Mäser, P.; Scapozza, L.; Picard, D. Differences in conformational dynamics between *Plasmodium falciparum* and human Hsp90 orthologues enable the structure-based discovery of pathogen-selective inhibitors. *J. Med. Chem.* **2014**, *57*, 2524–2535. [CrossRef] [PubMed]
54. Gitau, G.W.; Mandal, P.; Blatch, G.L.; Przyborski, J.; Shonhai, A. Characterisation of the *Plasmodium falciparum* Hsp70-Hsp90 organising protein (PfHop). *Cell Stress Chaperones* **2012**, *17*, 191–202. [CrossRef]
55. Makumire, S.; Zininga, T.; Vahokoski, J.; Kursula, I.; Shonhai, A. Biophysical analysis of *Plasmodium falciparum* Hsp70-Hsp90 organising protein (PfHop) reveals a monomer that is characterised by folded segments connected by flexible linkers. *PLoS ONE* **2020**, *15*, e0226657. [CrossRef] [PubMed]
56. Ahmad, M.; Afrin, F.; Tuteja, R. Identification of R2TP complex of *Leishmania donovani* and *Plasmodium falciparum* using genome wide in-silico analysis. *Commun. Integr. Biol.* **2013**, *6*, e26005. [CrossRef]
57. Sahasrabudhe, P.; Rohrberg, J.; Biebl, M.M.; Rutz, D.A.; Buchner, J. The plasticity of the Hsp90 co-chaperone system. *Mol. Cell* **2017**, *67*, 947–961.e5. [CrossRef]

58. Alag, R.; Bharatham, N.; Dong, A.; Hills, T.; Harikishore, A.; Widjaja, A.A.; Shochat, S.G.; Hui, R.; Yoon, H.S. Crystallographic structure of the tetratricopeptide repeat domain of *Plasmodium falciparum* FKBP35 and its molecular interaction with Hsp90 C-terminal pentapeptide. *Protein. Sci.* **2009**, *18*, 2115–2124. [CrossRef]
59. Bianchin, A.; Allemand, F.; Bell, A.; Chubb, A.J.; Guichou, J.F. Two crystal structures of the FK506-binding domain of *Plasmodium falciparum* FKBP35 in complex with rapamycin at high resolution. *Acta Crystallogr. D Biol. Crystallogr.* **2015**, *71*, 1319–1327. [CrossRef]
60. Schopf, F.H.; Huber, E.M.; Dodt, C.; Lopez, A.; Biebl, M.M.; Rutz, D.A.; Mühlhofer, M.; Richter, G.; Madl, T.; Sattler, M.; et al. The co-chaperone Cns1 and the recruiter protein Hgh1 link Hsp90 to translation elongation via chaperoning elongation factor 2. *Mol. Cell* **2019**, *74*, 73–87.e8. [CrossRef]
61. Chua, C.S.; Low, H.; Goo, K.S.; Sim, T.S. Characterization of *Plasmodium falciparum* co-chaperone p23: Its intrinsic chaperone activity and interaction with Hsp90. *Cell Mol. Life Sci.* **2010**, *67*, 1675–1686. [CrossRef]
62. Silva, N.S.M.; Seraphim, T.V.; Minari, K.; Barbosa, L.R.S.; Borges, J.C. Comparative studies of the low-resolution structure of two p23 co-chaperones for Hsp90 identified in *Plasmodium falciparum* genome. *Int. J. Biol. Macromol.* **2018**, *108*, 193–204. [CrossRef] [PubMed]
63. Chua, C.S.; Low, H.; Lehming, N.; Sim, T.S. Molecular analysis of *Plasmodium falciparum* co-chaperone Aha1 supports its interaction with and regulation of Hsp90 in the malaria parasite. *Int. J. Biochem. Cell Biol.* **2012**, *44*, 233–245. [CrossRef] [PubMed]
64. Lindenthal, C.; Klinkert, M.Q. Identification and biochemical characterisation of a protein phosphatase 5 homologue from *Plasmodium falciparum*. *Mol. Biochem. Parasitol.* **2002**, *120*, 257–268. [CrossRef]
65. Zhu, X.; Sun, L.; He, Y.; Wei, H.; Hong, M.; Liu, F.; Liu, Q.; Cao, Y.; Cui, L. *Plasmodium berghei* serine/threonine protein phosphatase PP5 plays a critical role in male gamete fertility. *Int. J. Parasitol.* **2019**, *49*, 685–695. [CrossRef]
66. Johnson, J.L.; Zuehlke, A.D.; Tenge, V.R.; Langworthy, J.C. Mutation of essential Hsp90 co-chaperones SGT1 or CNS1 renders yeast hypersensitive to overexpression of other co-chaperones. *Curr. Genet.* **2014**, *60*, 265–276. [CrossRef]
67. Siligardi, G.; Panaretou, B.; Meyer, P.; Singh, S.; Woolfson, D.N.; Piper, P.W.; Pearl, L.H.; Prodromou, C. Regulation of Hsp90 ATPase activity by the co-chaperone Cdc37p/p50cdc37. *J. Biol. Chem.* **2002**, *277*, 20151–20159. [CrossRef]
68. Bhattacharya, K.; Picard, D. The Hsp70-Hsp90 go-between Hop/Stip1/Sti1 is a proteostatic switch and may be a drug target in cancer and neurodegeneration. *Cell Mol. Life Sci.* **2021**, *78*, 7257–7273. [CrossRef]
69. Bhattacharya, K.; Weidenauer, L.; Luengo, T.M.; Pieters, E.C.; Echeverría, P.C.; Bernasconi, L.; Wider, D.; Sadian, Y.; Koopman, M.B.; Villemin, M.; et al. The Hsp70-Hsp90 co-chaperone Hop/Stip1 shifts the proteostatic balance from folding towards degradation. *Nat. Commun.* **2020**, *11*, 5975. [CrossRef]
70. Dahiya, V.; Rutz, D.A.; Moessmer, P.; Mühlhofer, M.; Lawatscheck, J.; Rief, M.; Buchner, J. The switch from client holding to folding in the Hsp70/Hsp90 chaperone machineries is regulated by a direct interplay between co-chaperones. *Mol. Cell* **2022**, *82*, 1543–1556.e6. [CrossRef]
71. Shonhai, A.; Boshoff, A.; Blatch, G.L. The structural and functional diversity of Hsp70 proteins from *Plasmodium falciparum*. *Protein. Sci.* **2007**, *16*, 1803–1818. [CrossRef]
72. D'Andrea, L.D.; Regan, L. TPR proteins: The versatile helix. *Trends Biochem. Sci.* **2003**, *28*, 655–662. [CrossRef] [PubMed]
73. Zininga, T.; Makumire, S.; Gitau, G.W.; Njunge, J.M.; Pooe, O.J.; Klimek, H.; Scheurr, R.; Raifer, H.; Prinsloo, E.; Przyborski, J.M.; et al. *Plasmodium falciparum* Hop (PfHop) Interacts with the Hsp70 Chaperone in a nucleotide-dependent fashion and exhibits ligand selectivity. *PLoS ONE* **2015**, *10*, e0135326. [CrossRef]
74. Zininga, T.; Pooe, O.J.; Makhado, P.B.; Ramatsui, L.; Prinsloo, E.; Achilonu, I.; Dirr, H.; Shonhai, A. Polymyxin B inhibits the chaperone activity of *Plasmodium falciparum* Hsp70. *Cell Stress Chaperones* **2017**, *22*, 707–715. [CrossRef] [PubMed]
75. Shonhai, A.; Boshoff, A.; Blatch, G.L. *Plasmodium falciparum* heat shock protein 70 is able to suppress the thermosensitivity of an *Escherichia coli* DnaK mutant strain. *Mol. Genet Genom.* **2005**, *274*, 70–78. [CrossRef]
76. Galat, A. Peptidylprolyl cis/trans isomerases (immunophilins): Biological diversity-targets-functions. *Curr. Top. Med. Chem.* **2003**, *3*, 1315–1347. [CrossRef]
77. Siekierka, J.J.; Hung, S.H.; Poe, M.; Lin, C.S.; Sigal, N.H. A cytosolic binding protein for the immunosuppressant FK506 has peptidyl-prolyl isomerase activity but is distinct from cyclophilin. *Nature* **1989**, *341*, 755–757. [CrossRef]
78. Bierer, B.E.; Mattila, P.S.; Standaert, R.F.; Herzenberg, L.A.; Burakoff, S.J.; Crabtree, G.; Schreiber, S.L. Two distinct signal transmission pathways in T lymphocytes are inhibited by complexes formed between an immunophilin and either FK506 or rapamycin. *Proc. Natl. Acad. Sci. USA* **1990**, *87*, 9231–9235. [CrossRef] [PubMed]
79. Duina, A.A.; Marsh, J.A.; Gaber, R.F. Identification of two CyP-40-like cyclophilins in *Saccharomyces cerevisiae*, one of which is required for normal growth. *Yeast* **1996**, *12*, 943–952. [CrossRef]
80. Nair, S.C.; Toran, E.J.; Rimerman, R.A.; Hjermstad, S.; Smithgall, T.E.; Smith, D.F. A pathway of multi-chaperone interactions common to diverse regulatory proteins: Estrogen receptor, Fes tyrosine kinase, heat shock transcription factor Hsf1, and the aryl hydrocarbon receptor. *Cell Stress Chaperones* **1996**, *1*, 237–250. [CrossRef]
81. Lebeau, M.C.; Massol, N.; Herrick, J.; Faber, L.E.; Renoir, J.M.; Radanyi, C.; Baulieu, E.E. P59, an hsp 90-binding protein. Cloning and sequencing of its cDNA and preparation of a peptide-directed polyclonal antibody. *J. Biol. Chem.* **1992**, *267*, 4281–4284. [CrossRef]

82. Peattie, D.A.; Harding, M.W.; Fleming, M.A.; DeCenzo, M.T.; Lippke, J.A.; Livingston, D.J.; Benasutti, M. Expression and characterization of human FKBP52, an immunophilin that associates with the 90-kDa heat shock protein and is a component of steroid receptor complexes. *Proc. Natl. Acad. Sci. USA* **1992**, *89*, 10974–10978. [CrossRef] [PubMed]
83. Ratajczak, T.; Carrello, A.; Mark, P.J.; Warner, B.J.; Simpson, R.J.; Moritz, R.L.; House, A.K. The cyclophilin component of the unactivated estrogen receptor contains a tetratricopeptide repeat domain and shares identity with p59 (FKBP59). *J. Biol. Chem.* **1993**, *268*, 13187–13192. [CrossRef]
84. Goebl, M.; Yanagida, M. The TPR snap helix: A novel protein repeat motif from mitosis to transcription. *Trends Biochem. Sci.* **1991**, *16*, 173–177. [CrossRef]
85. Smith, D.F.; Schowalter, D.B.; Kost, S.L.; Toft, D.O. Reconstitution of progesterone receptor with heat shock proteins. *Mol. Endocrinol.* **1990**, *4*, 1704–1711. [CrossRef]
86. Barent, R.L.; Nair, S.C.; Carr, D.C.; Ruan, Y.; Rimerman, R.A.; Fulton, J.; Zhang, Y.; Smith, D.F. Analysis of FKBP51/FKBP52 chimeras and mutants for Hsp90 binding and association with progesterone receptor complexes. *Mol. Endocrinol.* **1998**, *12*, 342–354. [CrossRef]
87. Mbengue, A.; Bhattacharjee, S.; Pandharkar, T.; Liu, H.; Estiu, G.; Stahelin, R.V.; Rizk, S.S.; Njimoh, D.L.; Ryan, Y.; Chotivanich, K.; et al. A molecular mechanism of artemisinin resistance in *Plasmodium falciparum* malaria. *Nature* **2015**, *520*, 683–687. [CrossRef]
88. Marín-Menéndez, A.; Monaghan, P.; Bell, A. A family of cyclophilin-like molecular chaperones in *Plasmodium falciparum*. *Mol. Biochem. Parasitol.* **2012**, *184*, 44–47. [CrossRef]
89. Florens, L.; Liu, X.; Wang, Y.; Yang, S.; Schwartz, O.; Peglar, M.; Carucci, D.J.; Yates, J.R., 3rd; Wu, Y. Proteomics approach reveals novel proteins on the surface of malaria-infected erythrocytes. *Mol. Biochem. Parasitol.* **2004**, *135*, 1–11. [CrossRef]
90. Pirkl, F.; Buchner, J. Functional analysis of the Hsp90-associated human peptidyl prolyl cis/trans isomerases FKBP51, FKBP52 and Cyp40. *J. Mol. Biol.* **2001**, *308*, 795–806. [CrossRef]
91. Blundell, K.L.; Pal, M.; Roe, S.M.; Pearl, L.H.; Prodromou, C. The structure of FKBP38 in complex with the MEEVD tetratricopeptide binding-motif of Hsp90. *PLoS ONE* **2017**, *12*, e0173543. [CrossRef]
92. Shirane, M.; Nakayama, K.I. Inherent calcineurin inhibitor FKBP38 targets Bcl-2 to mitochondria and inhibits apoptosis. *Nat. Cell Biol.* **2003**, *5*, 28–37. [CrossRef] [PubMed]
93. Kumar, R.; Adams, B.; Musiyenko, A.; Shulyayeva, O.; Barik, S. The FK506-binding protein of the malaria parasite, *Plasmodium falciparum*, is a FK506-sensitive chaperone with FK506-independent calcineurin-inhibitory activity. *Mol. Biochem. Parasitol.* **2005**, *141*, 163–173. [CrossRef] [PubMed]
94. Chua, C.S.; Low, H.; Sim, T.S. Co-chaperones of Hsp90 in *Plasmodium falciparum* and their concerted roles in cellular regulation. *Parasitology* **2014**, *141*, 1177–1191. [CrossRef] [PubMed]
95. Monaghan, P.; Leneghan, D.B.; Shaw, W.; Bell, A. The antimalarial action of FK506 and rapamycin: Evidence for a direct effect on FK506-binding protein PfFKBP35. *Parasitology* **2017**, *144*, 869–876. [CrossRef] [PubMed]
96. Kotaka, M.; Ye, H.; Alag, R.; Hu, G.; Bozdech, Z.; Preiser, P.R.; Yoon, H.S.; Lescar, J. Crystal structure of the FK506 binding domain of *Plasmodium falciparum* FKBP35 in complex with FK506. *Biochemistry* **2008**, *47*, 5951–5961. [CrossRef]
97. Harikishore, A.; Leow, M.L.; Niang, M.; Rajan, S.; Pasunooti, K.K.; Preiser, P.R.; Liu, X.; Yoon, H.S. Adamantyl derivative as a potent inhibitor of *Plasmodium* FK506 binding protein 35. *ACS Med. Chem. Lett.* **2013**, *4*, 1097–1101. [CrossRef]
98. Bharatham, N.; Chang, M.W.; Yoon, H.S. Targeting FK506 binding proteins to fight malarial and bacterial infections: Current advances and future perspectives. *Curr. Med. Chem.* **2011**, *18*, 1874–1889. [CrossRef]
99. Wiser, M.F.; Plitt, B. *Plasmodium berghei*, *P. chabaudi*, and *P. falciparum*: Similarities in phosphoproteins and protein kinase activities and their stage specific expression. *Exp. Parasitol.* **1987**, *64*, 328–335. [CrossRef]
100. Sullivan, W.; Stensgard, B.; Caucutt, G.; Bartha, B.; McMahon, N.; Alnemri, E.S.; Litwack, G.; Toft, D. Nucleotides and two functional states of hsp90. *J. Biol. Chem.* **1997**, *272*, 8007–8012. [CrossRef]
101. Patwardhan, C.A.; Fauq, A.; Peterson, L.B.; Miller, C.; Blagg, B.S.; Chadli, A. Gedunin inactivates the co-chaperone p23 protein causing cancer cell death by apoptosis. *J. Biol. Chem.* **2013**, *288*, 7313–7325. [CrossRef]
102. Hieronymus, H.; Lamb, J.; Ross, K.N.; Peng, X.P.; Clement, C.; Rodina, A.; Nieto, M.; Du, J.; Stegmaier, K.; Raj, S.M.; et al. Gene expression signature-based chemical genomic prediction identifies a novel class of HSP90 pathway modulators. *Cancer Cell* **2006**, *10*, 321–330. [CrossRef] [PubMed]
103. Matts, R.L.; Brandt, G.E.; Lu, Y.; Dixit, A.; Mollapour, M.; Wang, S.; Donnelly, A.C.; Neckers, L.; Verkhivker, G.; Blagg, B.S. A systematic protocol for the characterization of Hsp90 modulators. *Bioorg. Med. Chem.* **2011**, *19*, 684–692. [CrossRef] [PubMed]
104. MacKinnon, S.; Durst, T.; Arnason, J.T.; Angerhofer, C.; Pezzuto, J.; Sanchez-Vindas, P.E.; Poveda, L.J.; Gbeassor, M. Antimalarial activity of tropical *Meliaceae* extracts and gedunin derivatives. *J. Nat. Prod.* **1997**, *60*, 336–341. [CrossRef] [PubMed]
105. Lotz, G.P.; Lin, H.; Harst, A.; Obermann, W.M. Aha1 binds to the middle domain of Hsp90, contributes to client protein activation, and stimulates the ATPase activity of the molecular chaperone. *J. Biol. Chem.* **2003**, *278*, 17228–17235. [CrossRef] [PubMed]
106. Vaughan, C.K.; Mollapour, M.; Smith, J.R.; Truman, A.; Hu, B.; Good, V.M.; Panaretou, B.; Neckers, L.; Clarke, P.A.; Workman, P.; et al. Hsp90-dependent activation of protein kinases is regulated by chaperone-targeted dephosphorylation of Cdc37. *Mol. Cell* **2008**, *31*, 886–895. [CrossRef]
107. Dobson, S.; Kar, B.; Kumar, R.; Adams, B.; Barik, S. A novel tetratricopeptide repeat (TPR) containing PP5 serine/threonine protein phosphatase in the malaria parasite, *Plasmodium falciparum*. *BMC Microbiol.* **2001**, *1*, 31. [CrossRef]

108. Bohush, A.; Bieganowski, P.; Filipek, A. Hsp90 and its co-chaperones in neurodegenerative diseases. *Int. J. Mol. Sci.* **2019**, *20*, 4976. [CrossRef]
109. Wandinger, S.K.; Suhre, M.H.; Wegele, H.; Buchner, J. The phosphatase Ppt1 is a dedicated regulator of the molecular chaperone Hsp90. *EMBO J.* **2006**, *25*, 367–376. [CrossRef]
110. Góral, A.; Bieganowski, P.; Prus, W.; Krzemień-Ojak, Ł.; Kądziołka, B.; Fabczak, H.; Filipek, A. Calcyclin binding protein/siah-1 interacting protein is a Hsp90 binding chaperone. *PLoS ONE* **2016**, *11*, e0156507. [CrossRef]
111. Crevel, G.; Bennett, D.; Cotterill, S. The human TPR protein TTC4 is a putative Hsp90 co-chaperone which interacts with CDC6 and shows alterations in transformed cells. *PLoS ONE* **2008**, *3*, e0001737. [CrossRef]
112. Stuttmann, J.; Parker, J.E.; Noël, L.D. Staying in the fold: The SGT1/chaperone machinery in maintenance and evolution of leucine-rich repeat proteins. *Plant Signal Behav.* **2008**, *3*, 283–285. [CrossRef] [PubMed]
113. Kimura, Y.; Rutherford, S.L.; Miyata, Y.; Yahara, I.; Freeman, B.C.; Yue, L.; Morimoto, R.I.; Lindquist, S. Cdc37 is a molecular chaperone with specific functions in signal transduction. *Genes Dev.* **1997**, *11*, 1775–1785. [CrossRef] [PubMed]
114. Li, T.; Jiang, H.L.; Tong, Y.G.; Lu, J.J. Targeting the Hsp90-Cdc37-client protein interaction to disrupt Hsp90 chaperone machinery. *J. Hematol. Oncol.* **2018**, *11*, 59. [CrossRef] [PubMed]
115. Caplan, A.J.; Mandal, A.K.; Theodoraki, M.A. Molecular chaperones and protein kinase quality control. *Trends Cell Biol.* **2007**, *17*, 87–92. [CrossRef] [PubMed]
116. Lamphere, L.; Fiore, F.; Xu, X.; Brizuela, L.; Keezer, S.; Sardet, C.; Draetta, G.F.; Gyuris, J. Interaction between Cdc37 and Cdk4 in human cells. *Oncogene* **1997**, *14*, 1999–2004. [CrossRef]
117. Bandhakavi, S.; McCann, R.O.; Hanna, D.E.; Glover, C.V. A positive feedback loop between protein kinase CKII and Cdc37 promotes the activity of multiple protein kinases. *J. Biol. Chem.* **2003**, *278*, 2829–2836. [CrossRef]
118. Mandal, A.K.; Lee, P.; Chen, J.A.; Nillegoda, N.; Heller, A.; DiStasio, S.; Oen, H.; Victor, J.; Nair, D.M.; Brodsky, J.L.; et al. Cdc37 has distinct roles in protein kinase quality control that protect nascent chains from degradation and promote posttranslational maturation. *J. Cell Biol.* **2007**, *176*, 319–328. [CrossRef]
119. Johnson, J.L.; Brown, C. Plasticity of the Hsp90 chaperone machine in divergent eukaryotic organisms. *Cell Stress Chaperones* **2009**, *14*, 83–94. [CrossRef]
120. Adderley, J.; Doerig, C. Comparative analysis of the kinomes of *Plasmodium falciparum*, *Plasmodium vivax* and their host *Homo sapiens*. *BMC Genom.* **2022**, *23*, 237. [CrossRef]
121. Boczek, E.E.; Reefschläger, L.G.; Dehling, M.; Struller, T.J.; Häusler, E.; Seidl, A.; Kaila, V.R.; Buchner, J. Conformational processing of oncogenic v-Src kinase by the molecular chaperone Hsp90. *Proc. Natl. Acad. Sci. USA* **2015**, *112*, E3189–E3198. [CrossRef]
122. Xu, H. Non-equilibrium protein folding and activation by ATP-driven chaperones. *Biomolecules* **2022**, *12*, 832. [CrossRef] [PubMed]